Pharmaceutical Biotechnology

Other books of interest

Basic Endocrinology – For Students of Pharmacy and Allied Health Sciences
A. Constanti, A. Bartke and R. Khardori

Immunology – For Pharmacy Students
W.C. Shen and S. Louie

Forthcoming

Drug Delivery and Targeting – For Pharmacists and Pharmaceutical Scientists
A.M. Hillery, A.W. Lloyd and J. Swarbrick

Pharmaceutical Biotechnology
An Introduction for Pharmacists and
Pharmaceutical Scientists

Edited by
Daan J.A. Crommelin *(Department of Pharmaceutics, Utrecht Institute for Pharmaceutical Sciences, Utrecht University, The Netherlands)*
and
Robert D. Sindelar *(Department of Medicinal Chemistry, School of Pharmacy, University of Mississippi, USA)*

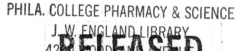 **harwood academic publishers**
Australia • Canada • China • France • Germany • India • Japan • Luxembourg • Malaysia
The Netherlands • Russia • Singapore • Switzerland • Thailand • United Kingdom

British Library Cataloguing in Publication Data

A catalogue record for this book is available from the British Library.

ISBN: 90-5702-249-4 (softcover)

Source acknowledgement for the cover illustration.

The cover illustration shows a ribbon representation of the antigen binding fragment of bactericidal antibody MN12H2 in complex with a synthetic peptide. The peptide is derived from the top of extracellular loop 4 of outer membrane protein PorA of *Neisseria meningitidis* (strain H44/ 76). Heavy and light chain of the antibody are shown in magenta and green and the peptide is shown in yellow. This model is based on an X-ray crystallography study performed by Jean van den Elsen (Antibody Recognition of *Neisseria meningitidis*: a thermodynamic and structural analysis of the interaction between a bactericidal monoclonal antibody and a class 1 outer membrane epitope (1996), thesis, Utrecht University).

Table of Contents

Chapter 2:   **Biophysical and Biochemical Analyses of Recombinant Proteins**

Structure and Analyses of Proteins   *27*

William C. Kenney and Tsutomu Arakawa

Chapter 5:

Pharmacokinetics and Pharmacodynamics of Peptide and Protein Drugs   101

Rene Braeckman

Chapter 6:   **Additional Biotechnology-Related Techniques**   123

Robert D. Sindelar

Chapter 8:

Hematopoietic Growth Factors 185
Jeanne Flynn and Allen W. Rosman

Chapter 9:

Interleukins and Interferons   215

Joseph Tami

Chapter 10: **Insulin**   229
John M. Beals and Paul M. Kovach

Chapter 11: **Growth Hormones**   241
Melinda Marian

Chapter 12:

Vaccines   255

Wim Jiskoot, Gideon F.A. Kersten and E. Coen Beuvery

Chapter 15:   Recombinant Human Deoxyribonuclease   *307*

Melinda Marian and Sharon Baughman

Chapter 16:   Follicle-Stimulating Hormone (FSH)   *315*

Tom Sam and Willem de Boer

Chapter 17:   **Dispensing Biotechnology Products**
Handling, Professional Education and Product Information   321
Gary H. Smith and Peggy Piascik

Chapter 18:   **Biotechnology Products in the Pipeline**   337
Ronald P. Evens and Robert D. Sindelar

Preface

The field of pharmaceutical biotechnology is developing rapidly. For those working in the field of pharmacy and pharmaceutical sciences, completely new techniques and products appear at a rapid pace. This is the result of the interplay between a number of different disciplines, most importantly: molecular biology, molecular genetics, (bio-) engineering, protein, sugar, and nuclear acid chemistry and, last but not least, the pharmaceutical sciences.

The total worldwide sales of biotechnology-produced pharmaceuticals continue to increase significantly. For instance, in 1990 US sales amounted to approximately $2.0 billion. Sales increased to $5.1 billion in 1994 and $7.7 billion in 1995, compared to $85 billion total US pharmaceuticals sales. Growth in the use of biotech compounds surpasses the growth of conventional pharmaceutical products. Estimates predict that sales of biotech pharmaceuticals in the US will approach $16 billion by 2004.

Not only sales figures distinguish biotech compounds. Many of them are indicated for the treatment or prevention of serious life threatening diseases, e.g., cancer, viral infection, or hereditary deficiencies, or for previously untreatable conditions. These compounds often dramatically improve the patients' quality of life.

We believe that there is a strong need for an introductory textbook on pharmaceutical biotechnology that provides detailed coverage of both the basic science and clinical use of biotechnology-produced pharmaceuticals. Therefore, the goal of this book is to provide the readers with an introductory text to familiarize themselves with biotechnology-related issues and terms. There is a strong focus on those issues related to the pharmaceutical profession and the pharmaceutical sciences. One target group is those pharmacists who wish to update their knowledge of biotechnology. A second target group is the present generation of pharmacy students at our universities. Thirdly, pharmaceutical scientists who have not been in contact with modern biotechnology and wish to familiarize themselves with the principles of this fast moving field are targeted. We are hopeful that this book will be used at universities, in life-long learning courses and in the professional environment of the pharmacist and pharmaceutical scientist all over the world.

Chapter topics were discussed at length with a number of academic and industrial experts. It was decided to start with a rather comprehensive introduction to biotechnology with issues relevant to the target groups (Chapter 1). As pharmaceutical biotech products are mainly (glyco)proteins, attention is paid to typically chemical aspects of (glyco) proteins to help the reader to understand the intricacies of the (physico)chemistry of these high molecular weight compounds (Chapter 2).

The advent and development of biotech products has created a number of unique pharmaceutical problems. The production, downstream processing and characterization of biotech products are in many ways very different from the way 'conventional' low molecular weight products are handled. The same applies to the delivery and pharmacokinetic aspects of proteins (Chapters 3 to 5).

Chapter 6 consists of an introduction to a number of additional biotechnology-based methodologies important to pharmacy and the pharmaceutical sciences. These include bioengineered animals, protein engineering, antisense approaches, glycobiology and the immense impact of biotechnology on the drug discovery process.

The exciting field of gene therapy is reviewed in Chapter 7. The reader is led through the fascinating world of gene delivery to somatic cells and introduced to the potentials and limitations of the present generation of gene transfection strategies.

In Chapters 8 to 16 recently registered recombinant proteins are discussed in multiple sections in terms of their chemistry, pharmacology and therapeutic indications.

In Chapter 17 the issue of how to handle pharmaceutical biotech products in the practice setting is discussed and sources for professional and patient information and education are provided.

Finally, in Chapter 18, experts provide the reader with a glimpse at products in the biotech pipeline.

For educational purposes, each chapter is concluded with a number of self-assessment questions and a number of literature references for further reading. The multi-color printing of the art work in this book (which was made possible by an educational grant from Amgen, Inc.) should assist the reader in mastering the subject matter. To help the reader with the many abbreviations and acronyms in the text, a list of abbreviations is added as well.

We encourage the reader to suggest to us how we can improve coming editions of this book both in terms of topics to be discussed or deleted and in terms of errors that undoubtedly were made in spite of our careful checking.

The marketing of recombinant human insulin in the early 1980s and the development of monoclonal antibody-based kits ushered in a new era in pharmacy. Rapidly evolving developments in the techniques and products of biotechnology necessitate a solid understanding by pharmacists, future pharmacists and pharmaceutical scientists. We believe that this text will contribute to this understanding.

Daan J.A. Crommelin and Robert D. Sindelar

Acknowledgment: Harwood Academic Publishers are grateful to Amgen, Inc. (USA) for providing a generous educational grant for this book.

Contributors

• **John R. Adair**
Axis Genetics plc
Babraham, Cambridge, UK

• **Tsutomu Arakawa**
Department of Protein Chemistry
Amgen Inc., Thousand Oaks
California, USA

• **Sharon Baughman**
Department of Pharmacokinetics
and Metabolism, Genentech, Inc.
San Francisco, California, USA

• **John M. Beals**
Biopharmaceutical Product
Development, Lilly Research
Laboratories, Eli Lilly and Company
Indianapolis, Indiana, USA

• **E. Coen Beuvery**
Laboratory for Product and
Process Development, National
Institute of Public Health and
Environmental Protection (RIVM)
Bilthoven, The Netherlands

• **Willem de Boer**
Regulatory Affairs, NV Organon
Oss, The Netherlands

• **Abraham Bout**
IntroGene B.V., Leiden
The Netherlands

• **Rene Braeckman**
Department of Pharmacokinetics
and Pharmacodynamics
Chiron Corp., Emeryville
California, USA

• **Daan J.A. Crommelin**
Department of Pharmaceutics
Utrecht Institute for
Pharmaceutical Sciences (UIPS)
Utrecht University
The Netherlands

• **Ronald P. Evens**
Professional Services, Amgen Inc.
Thousand Oaks, California, USA

• **Jeanne Flynn**
Professional Services, Amgen Inc.
Thousand Oaks, California, USA

• **Norberto A. Guzman**
The R.W. Johnson
Pharmaceutical Research
Institute, Johnson and Johnson
Raritan, New Jersey, USA

• **Wiel P.M. Hoekstra**
Department of Molecular Cell
Biology, Utrecht University
The Netherlands

• **Khurshid Iqbal**
The West Company, Lionville
Pennsylvania, USA

• **Wim Jiskoot**
Laboratory for Product and
Process Development, National
Institute of Public Health and
Environmental Protection (RIVM)
Bilthoven, The Netherlands

• **Robert Jordan**
Centocor BV and Centocor
Malvern, Pennsylvania, USA

• **Farida Kadir**
Department of Pharmaceutics
Utrecht University
The Netherlands

• **William C. Kenney**
Department of Protein Chemistry
Amgen Inc., Thousand Oaks
California, USA

• **Gideon F.A. Kersten**
Laboratory for Product and
Process Development, National
Institute of Public Health and
Environmental Protection (RIVM)
Bilthoven, The Netherlands

• **Paul M. Kovach**
Biopharmaceutical Product
Development, Lilly Research
Laboratories, Eli Lilly and Company
Indianapolis, Indiana, USA

• **Melinda Marian**
Department of Pharmacokinetics
and Metabolism, Genentech, Inc.
San Francisco, California, USA

• **Nishit B. Modi**
Department of Pharmacokinetics
and Metabolism, Genentech, Inc.
San Francisco, California, USA

• **Peggy Piascik**
College of Pharmacy, University
of Kentucky, Lexington, USA

• **Allen W. Rosman**
Professional Services, Amgen Inc.
Thousand Oaks, California, USA

• **Tom Sam**
Regulatory Affairs, NV Organon
Oss, The Netherlands

• **Robert D. Sindelar**
Department of Medicinal
Chemistry, School of Pharmacy
University of Mississippi, USA

• **Sjef C.M. Smeekens**
Department of Molecular Cell
Biology, Utrecht University
The Netherlands

• **Gary H. Smith**
College of Pharmacy, University
of Arizona, Tucson, USA

• **Joseph Tami**
formerly at the Departments of
Medicine/Hematology and
Pharmacology, University of
Texas Health Science Center
San Antonio, USA;
Currently: Drug Development
Isis Pharmaceuticals
California, USA

• **Sven Warnaar**
Centocor CBV and Centocor
Malvern, Pennsylvania, USA

• **David S. Ziska**
School of Pharmacy, University
of Mississippi, Jackson, USA

• **Robert A. Zivin**
The R.W. Johnson
Pharmaceutical Research
Institute, Johnson and Johnson
Raritan, New Jersey, USA

Acknowledgements

The editors gratefully acknowledge the advice and assistance of colleagues, each recognized to possess a considerable range of knowledge in one or more topics covered in this book, who served as chapter/section reviewers.

- **Allison, A.C.**, Ph.D.
DAWA Inc, Belmont, California USA

- **Boulamwini, J.K.**, Ph.D.
Department of Medicinal Chemistry, School of Pharmacy University of Mississippi, USA

- **De Boer, A.**, Ph.D. M.D.
Department of Pharmacoepidemiology and Pharmacotherapy Utrecht University The Netherlands

- **Danhof, M.**, Ph.D.
Department of Pharmacology Leiden/Amsterdam Center for Drug Research, The Netherlands

- **Dingermann, Th.**, Ph.D.
Institut für Pharmazeutische Biologie, Johann Wolfgang Goethe-Universität, Frankfurt Germany

- **Frøkjaer, S.**, Ph.D.
Department of Pharmaceutics The Royal Danish School of Pharmacy, Copenhagen Denmark

- **Groves, M.J.**, Ph.D.
Institute for Tuberculosis Research, College of Pharmacy University of Illinois, USA

- **Hudson, R.A.**, Ph.D.
Department of Medicinal and Biological Chemistry, College of Pharmacy, University of Toledo Ohio, USA

- **Koeller, J.M.**, M.S.
Clinical Pharmacy Programs University of Texas Health Science Center, USA

- **Kung, P.C.**, Ph.D.
T Cell Sciences, Inc. Needham, Massachusetts USA

- **Louie, S.G.**, Pharm.D.
Department of Clinical Pharmacy School of Pharmacy University of Southern California, USA

- **Rimoldi, J.M.**, Ph.D.
Department of Medicinal Chemistry, School of Pharmacy University of Mississippi, USA

- **Speedie, M.**, Ph.D.
College of Pharmacy University of Minnesota Minneapolis, USA

- **Wafelman, A.R.**, Ph.D.
Department of Clinical Pharmacy and Toxicology, Academisch Ziekenhuis Leiden The Netherlands

- **Wagner, E.**, Ph.D.
Bender and Co., Vienna Austria

- **Zuidema, J.**, Ph.D.
Department of Biopharmaceutics Utrecht University The Netherlands

Abbreviations

3-D	three dimensional	CG	chorionic gonadotropin
^{125}I-hGH	iodine labeled human growth hormone	CGD	chronic granulomatous disease
A	(d)ATP(deoxy)adenosine 5'-triphosphate (Chapter 1)	$C_H(1,2,3)$	constant region(s) of heavy chain of IgG
A	adenine	CHO	Chinese hamster ovary
Å	angstroms	C_L	constant region of light chain of IgG (e.g., Chapter 13)
AA	amino acid(s)		
AAV	adeno-associated virus	CL	elimination clearance from central compartment (Chapter 5)
ABO	blood group antigens		
ADA	adenosine deaminase	CL_d	distributional clearance (Chapter 5)
ADCC	antibody dependent cellular cytotoxicity	CL_e	linear clearance for distribution of drug to the effector compartment and elimination from the effector compartment (Chapter 5)
ADME	absorption, distribution, metabolism, excretion		
ADP	adenosine diphosphate		
AG-LCR	asymmetric gap ligation chain reaction	CMI	cell-mediated immunity
AHF	antihemophiliac factor/factor VIII	CML	chronic myelogenous leukemia
AIDS	acquired immune deficiency syndrome	CMV	cytomegalovirus
ALS	amyotrophic lateral sclerosis	CNS	central nervous system
AMI	acute myocardial infarction	Con A	concanavalin A
AML	acute myelogenous leukemia	CRI	chronic renal insufficiency
AP	alkaline phosphatase	CSF(s)	colony stimulating factor(s)
APC	antigen presenting cell	CT	cholera toxin
apoE	apolipoprotein E	CTL	cytotoxic T-lymphocyte
APSAC	acylated plasminogen-streptokinase activator	CTP	cytidine 5'-triphosphate
ARDS	adult respiratory distress syndrome	D_5W	dextrose 5% in water
Asn	asparagine	DAB_{389} CD4	a fusion protein
Asp	aspartic acid	DAB_{389} EGF	a fusion protein
ATP	adenosine 5'-triphosphate	DAB_{389} hGM-CSF	fused peptide sequence of human GM-CSF
AUC	area under the curve	DAB_{389} IL-2	IL-2 fusion protein; also called IL-2 fusion toxin
batching	preparing batches		
BCG	bacille Calmette-Guérin	DAB_{389} IL-4	a fusion protein
BCGFII	B-cell growth factor	DAB_{389} IL-6	a fusion protein
BDNF	brain-derived neurotrophic factor	dATP	deoxyadenosine 5'-triphosphate
BMT	bone marrow transplantation	dCTP	deoxycytidine 5'-triphosphate
BRMs	biological response modifiers	ddNTP	dideoxyribonucleotide triphosphate
BSA	bovine serum albumin	DF	denatured form
C	(d)CTP(deoxy)cytidine 5'-triphosphate (Chapter 1)	DF	diafiltration
C	cytosine	dGTP	deoxyguanosine 5'-triphosphate
C	plasma concentration (Chapter 5)	ΔG_u	free energy
CAM	cell adhesion molecules	di	supplied diluent (Chapter 7)
CCK	cholecystokinin	DNA	deoxyribonucleic acid
CD	circular dichrism (e.g., Chapter 2)	DNase	deoxyribonuclease (I)
CD	cluster designation (term to label surface molecules of lymphocytes) (e.g., Chapter 9)	DNF	do not freeze (Chapter 7)
		dNTP	deoxyribonucleotide triphosphate
CDC	complement dependent cytotoxicity	DSC	differential scanning calorimetry
cDNA	copy DNA/complementary deoxyribonucleic acid	DTP	diphtheria-tetanus-pertussis
CDR	complementarity determining region	dTTP	deoxythymidine 5'-triphosphate
C_E	concentration in effect compartment (Chapter 5)	E	effect (Chapter 5)
CETP	cholesterol (cholesteryl) ester transfer protein	E_o	baseline effect (Chapter 5)
CF	cystic fibrosis	EBV	Epstein-Barr virus
CFTR	cystic fibrosis transmembrane conductance regulator	EC_{50}	concentration that produces 50% of maximum inhibition or stimulation (Chapter 5)
CFU	colony-forming unit	EDF	eosinophil differentiation factor
CFU-GM	granulocyte-macrophage progenitor cells	EDTA	ethylenediaminetetraacetic acid

EGF	epidermal growth factor	hGH	human growth hormone
EI	electrospray ionization	hGH-N	normal hGH gene
ELISA	enzyme-linked immunosorbent assay	hGH-V	variant hGH gene
E_{max}	maximum inhibition or stimulation (Chapter 5)	HIC	hydrophobic interaction chromatography
EPO	erythropoietin (Epoetin alfa)	His	histidine
ERK/MAP	extracellular signal-regulated kinase/mitogen activated protein kinase	HIV	human immunodeficiency virus
		HMWP	high molecular weight protein
ES	pluripotent embryonic stem cells	HPLC	high-performance liquid chromatography
EU	endotoxin unit	HPRT	hypoxanthine phosphoribosyl transferase
ex da	see expiration date on package (Chapter 7)	HRP	horseradish peroxidase
F(ab')$_2$	proteolysis product of IgG (cf. Chapter 13)	HSA	human serum albumin
Fab	proteolysis product of IgG (cf. Chapter 13)	HSCs	hematopoietic stem cells
Fc	constant fragment (of immunoglobulins)	HSV-tk	herpes simplex virus-thymidine kinase
FDA	Food and Drug Administration	HTS	high-throughput screening
FEV_1	mean forced expiratory volume in one second	IA	intra-arterial
FGF	fibroblast growth factor	IC	intracoronary
FH	familial hypercholesterolemia	ICAM-1	intercellular adhesion molecule-1
FPLC	fast protein liquid chromatography	ICSI	intracytoplasmic sperm injection
FSH	follicle-stimulating hormone	IFN	interferon(s)
FTIR	Fourier transform infrared spectroscopy	IFN α	interferon α
F_V	variable domains of light and heavy chains	IFN β	interferon β
FVC	forced vital capacity	IFN γ	interferon γ
G	(d)GTP(deoxy)guanosine 5'-triphosphate (Chapter 1)	Ig	immunoglobulin
G	guanine	IgE	immunoglobulin E
G-CSF	granulocyte colony-stimulating factor	IGF	insulin-like growth factor
G-LCR	gap ligation chain reaction	IGF-I	insulin growth factor-I
Ga-DF	gallium-desferal	IGF-II	insulin growth factor-II
GCV	gancyclovir	IGFBP	IGF binding protein
GEMM	granulocyte, erythrocyte, monocyte and megakaryocyte	IgG	immunoglobulin G
GERD	gastroesophageal reflux disease	IL	interleukin(s)
GF	growth factor	IL	intralesional (Chapter 17)
GH	growth hormone	IL-1	interleukin-1
GHBP	growth hormone binding protein	IL-1 ra	IL-1 receptor antagonist
GHD	growth hormone deficiency	IL-2	interleukin-2
GHRH	growth hormone releasing hormone	IL-2R	interleukin-2 receptor
GIFT	gamete intra-fallopian transfer	IL-3	interleukin-3
GIT/GI tract	gastrointestinal tract	IM	inner membrane (Chapter 1)
GlcNAc	N-acetyl-glucosamine	im	intramuscular
GLP	good laboratory practice	IO	intra-orbital
GM-CSF	granulocyte-macrophage colony-stimulating factor	IP	intraperitoneal
GMP	good manufacturing practice	IPTG	iso-propyl-ß-thiogalactoside
GnRH	gonadotropin releasing hormone	IPV	inactivated polio vaccine
GO	glucose-oxidase	ISS	idiopathic short stature
Gp/GP	glycoprotein	ITP	idiopathic thrombocytopenic purpura
GPIIb-IIIa	integrin $\alpha_{IIb}\beta_3$, the fibronectin receptor	ITR	inverted terminal repeat
GRF	growth hormone releasing factor	iv/IV	intravenous
GTP	guanosine 5'-triphosphate	IVB	intravenous bolus (Chapter 17)
GvHD	graft versus host disease	IVF	*in vitro* fertilization
HACA	human anti-chimeric antibody	IVIF	intravenous infusion (Chapter 17)
HAMA	human anti-mouse antibodies	IVIN	intravenous injection (Chapter 17)
HBsAg	hepatitis B surface antigen	K_{O1} and K_{1O}	rate constants (Chapter 5)
Hct	hematocrit	K_d	rate constant resembling distribution and transduction delays (Chapter 5)
HEPA	high efficiency particulate air filters		
hG-CSF	human granulocyte colony-stimulating factor	kD	kilodalton

K_{out}	first order rate constant for effect disappearance (Chapter 5)	PAI	plasminogen activator inhibitors
LAF	lymphocyte activating factor	PAI-1	plasminogen activator inhibitor type-1
LAK	leucocyte activated killer (cells)	PBPC	peripheral blood progenitor cells
LCR	ligation chain reaction	PCR	polymerase chain reaction
LDL	low-density lipoprotein	PCTA	percutaneous transluminal coronary angioplasty
LDLR	low-density lipoprotein receptor	PD	pharmacodynamics
LH	luteinizing hormone	PDGF	platelet-derived growth factor
LPD	lymphoproliferative disorders	PEG IL-2	PEGylated interleukin-2/polyethylene glycol modified interleukin-2
LPS	lipopolysaccharide	PG	peptidoglycans (Chapter 1)
LRP	(low density) lipoprotein receptor-related protein	pI	iso-electric point, negative logarithm
LTR	long terminal repeat	pit-hGH	pituitary-derived human growth hormone
LYZ	lysozyme	PIXY-321	fusion protein between GM-CSF/IL-3
M cells	microfold cells	PK	pharmacokinetics
M-CSF	macrophage colony-stimulating factor	PNA	peptide nucleic acid
MAb(s)	monoclonal antibody(s)	PP	polypropylene
MALDI	matrix-assisted laser desorption ionization	PT	prothrombin time
MAP	multiple antigen peptide	PTH	parathyroid hormone (recombinant human)
MCB	master cell bank	PTO	United States Patent and Trademark Office
MDR-1	multiple drug resistance	PVC	polyvinyl chloride
Meg	megakaryocyte	PVDF	polyvinylidine difluoride
Met-GH	methionin human growth hormone	pwd	powder (Chapter 17)
met-rhGH	methionyl recombinant human growth hormone, contains N-terminal methionine	rAAT	recombinant α_1-antitrypsin
		RAC	US Recombinant DNA Advisory Committee
mfg	contact manufacturer (Chapter 17)	rAHF	recombinant anti-hemophilia factor
MGDF	megakaryocyte growth and development factor	RB	roller bottle
MHC	major histocompatibility complex	rDNA	recombinant deoxyribonucleic acid/recombinant-DNA
MMR	measles-mumps-rubella	Ref	refrigerator (Chapter 17)
MPS	mononuclear phagocyte system	rG-CSF	recombinant granulocyte colony-stimulating factor (filgrastim)
M_r	relative molecular mass		
mRNA	messenger ribonucleic acid/messenger RNA	RGD	amino acid sequence Arg-Gly-Asp (arginine-glycine-aspartic acid)
MTP-PE	muramyltripeptide-phosphatidylethanolamine		
MuLV	murine leukemia virus	rGM-CSF	recombinant granulocyte-macrophage colony-stimulating factor
mUPA	murine urokinase-type plasminogen activator		
M_w	relative molecular mass	rhDNase	recombinant human deoxyribonuclease I
NA	not available (Chapter 17)	rhGH	recombinant human growth hormone, natural sequence
NF	natural form		
NF-κB	transcription factor in B- and T-cells	rhIL-11	recombinant human interleukin-11
NFs	neurotrophic factors	RIA	radioimmunoassay
NGF	nerve growth factor	rIFN γ	recombinant interferon γ
NIH	National Institutes of Health	R_{in}	zero order appearance rate (Chapter 5)
NK	natural killer	RMS	root mean square
NOESY	2-D nuclear Overhauser effect NMR technique	RNA	ribonucleic acid
NPH	neutral protamine Hagedorn	RNase P	ribonuclease P
NS	normal saline (Chapter 17)	RNase H	ribonuclease H
NSAIDs	nonsteroidal anti-inflammatory drugs	R_{out}	first order disappearance rate (Chapter 5)
NZS	neocarzinostatin	RP-HPLC	reversed-phase high performance liquid chromatography
ODNs	oligodeoxynucleotides	RT	reverse transcriptase
OLA	oligonucleotide ligation assay	RT	room temperature (only Chapter 17)
OM	outer membrane (Chapter 1)	rt-PA	recombinant tissue-type plasminogen activator
OMP	outer membrane protein	RT-PCR	reverse transcription polymerase chain reaction
ori	origin of replication	RTU	ready to use solution (Chapter 17)
PAGE	polyacrylamide gel electrophoresis	SBWFI	sterile bacteriostatic water for injection (Chapter 17)
		SC	suspension culture

sc/SC	subcutaneous	T_g	glass transition temperature
SCF	stem cell factor (also known as c-kit ligand and steel factor)	TGF	tissue growth factor
scF$_V$	single chain antibody ('stabilised' F$_V$)	T_h-cell	T-helper cell
SCN	severe chronic neutropenia	Ti	tumor inducing
scu PA	single chain urokinase plasminogen activator	TIL	tumor infiltrating lymphocytes
SDS-PAGE	(SDS-Page) sodium dodecyl sulfate polyacrylamide-gel electrophoresis	TIMI	thrombolysis in myocardial infarction
		TNF α	tumor necrosis factor α
Ser	serine	TPO	thrombopoietin
sIL2R	soluble interleukin-2 receptor	TR	terminal repeats
SLE	systemic lupus erythematosus	TRAP	thrombin receptor activating peptide
SOD	superoxide dismutase	TRF	T-cell replacement factor
sol	solution (Chapter 17)	TSH	thyroid-stimulating hormone
SQ	subcutaneous injection (Chapter 17)	TSP	thrombospondin
SQI	subcutaneous infusion (Chapter 17)	U	uracil
SSC	large scale suspension culture process	U	UTP/uridine 5'-triphosphate (Chapter 1)
STI	soy bean trypsin inhibitor	UF	ultrafiltration
SWFI	sterile water for injection (Chapter 17)	uPA	urokinase-type plasminogen activator
T/dTTP	deoxythymidine 5'-triphosphate (Chapter 1)	UTP	uridine 5'-triphosphate
T	thymine	UV	ultraviolet
t-PA	tissue plasminogen activator	V_β	volume of distribution of peripheral compartment of two-compartment kinetic model (Chapter 5)
$t_{1/2\alpha}, t_{1/2\beta}$	half lives in α and β phase of two compartment kinetic model (Chapter 5)		
		V_E	apparent volume of distribution in the effect compartment (Chapter 5)
T_3, T_4	thyroid hormones		
TAC	T-cell activating antigen	V_H	variable region of heavy chain of IgG
TAS	transcription-based amplification system	V_L	variable region of light chain of IgG
TCGF	T-cell growth factor	WCB	working cell bank
T_{DTH}	delayed type hypersensitivity T-cells	WHO	World Health Organization
T_e	eutectic temperature	WHO-IUIS	World Health Organization-International Union of Immunologic Societies
TFF	tangential flow filtration		
TFPI	tissue factor pathway inhibitor		

I Molecular Biotechnology

by: Wiel P.M. Hoekstra and Sjef C.M. Smeekens

Introduction

Biotechnology has been defined in many different ways. Specific definitions for pharmaceutical biotechnology can be deduced directly from these definitions. In general biotechnology implies the use of microorganisms, plants and animals or parts thereof for the production of useful compounds. Consequently, pharmaceutical biotechnology should be considered as biotechnological manufacturing of pharmaceutical products.

Various forms of biotechnology existed already in ancient times. The Bible documents this ancient origin of biotechnology, informing us about Noah who apparently knew how to make wine from grapes. Based merely on experience but without understanding of the underlying principles, bioproducts were for many ages homemade in a traditional fashion.

Insight in the nature of the traditional processes was achieved about 1870 when Pasteur made clear that chemical conversions in these processes are performed by living cells and should thus be considered as biochemical conversions. Biotechnology became science! In the decades after Pasteur knowledge increased when the role of enzymes as catalysts for most of the biochemical conversions became apparent. Based on that knowledge, tools became available to control and optimize the traditional processes to a certain extent.

A further and very important breakthrough took place after the development of molecular biology. The notion, brought forward by the pioneers in molecular biology around 1950, that DNA encodes proteins and in this way controls all cellular processes was the impetus for a new period in biotechnology. The fast evolving DNA technologies, after the development of the recombinant DNA technology in the seventies, allowed biotechnologists to control gene expression in the organisms used for biotechnological manufacturing. Moreover, the developed technologies opened ways to introduce foreign DNA into all kinds of organisms. As will be shown later, genetically modified organisms constructed in that way opened up completely new possibilities for biotechnology. The new form of biotechnology, based on profound knowledge of the DNA molecule and the availability of manipulation technologies of DNA, is frequently described as "molecular biotechnology". The possibilities of the molecular approaches for further development of biotechnology were immediately apparent, albeit that the expectations sometimes were overestimated. At the same time biotechnology became the subject of public debate. An important question in the debate deals with potential risks: do genetically modified organisms as used in production facilities pose unknown risks for an ecosystem and for the human race itself? Moreover, a profound ethical question was brought forward: is it right to modify the genetic structure of living organisms?

In this chapter we will focus mainly on the new biotechnology by describing its means and goals. As to the question concerning potential risks of the technology, we will confine ourselves to stating that all sorts of measurements are taken to avoid risks while using genetically modified organisms. The ethical aspects, interesting as they are, are beyond the scope of this chapter.

The Cell

Although biotechnology does not exclusively make use of cells but also of complete organisms or of cell constituents, knowledge of basic cell biology is required to understand biotechnology to its full extent.

Cells from all sorts of organisms are used in biotechnology. Not only prokaryotic cells like simple unicellular bacteria are used, but also eukaryotic cells, like cells of higher microorganisms, plants and animals, are exploited. Those cell types are not dealt with in detail. The unifying concepts in cell biology and the diversification as far as relevant for pharmaceutical biotechnology will be the main topic of discussion in Chapter 1.

The Prokaryotic Cell

The prokaryotes, to which the bacteria belong, represent the simplest cells in nature. A schematic illustration (Figure 1.1) depicts a prokaryotic cell. Such a cell is in fact no more than cytoplasm surrounded by some surface layers, generally described as the cell envelope. In the bacterial world one distinguishes two main types of organisms. They

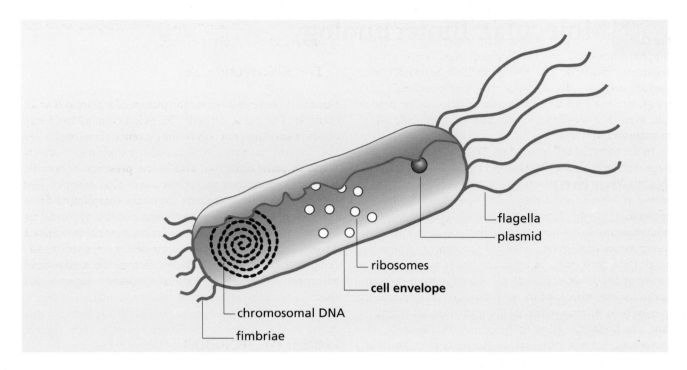

Figure 1.1. Cross-section (artificial) through a bacterial cell. The surface structures (fimbriae and flagella) are not essential structures but allow the cells to adhere and to move.

are called Gram-positive or Gram-negative based on different behavior in a classical cell staining technique. The fundamental differences between these two prokaryotic types are mainly apparent in the structure of the cell envelope.

The bacterial cell envelope consists of a cytoplasmic membrane and of a very characteristic wall structure called the peptidoglycan layer. The cells of Gram-positive organisms are multilayered with peptidoglycan while only one or two such layers are found in cells of Gram-negative organisms. However, the clearest distinction between the two types of bacterial cells is that in Gram-negative organisms the cell is surrounded by a very specific extra membrane layer, called outer membrane (OM) (Figure 1.2). Next to the cytoplasmic membrane, also called the inner membrane (IM), the OM is a permeation barrier for substances that are transported into or out of the cell.

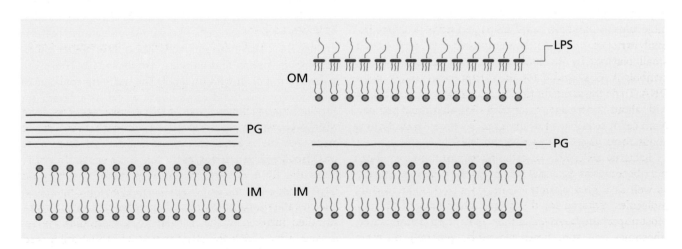

Figure 1.2. Cell envelope G⁺ cell (left) and G⁻ cell (right). G⁺ = Gram-positive; G⁻ = Gram-negative; PG = peptidoglycan; LPS = lipopolysaccharide; OM = outer membrane; IM = inner membrane.

A prominent and very particular chemical constituent of the OM is the compound named lipopolysaccharide (LPS). Biopharmaceutical products gained from Gram-negative organisms must be extensively purified especially when they are used as a pharmaceutical for man or animal (Chapter 4), since LPS set free during the isolation of the product has, even in a very low concentration, severe toxic effects to man and animals.

In the bacterial cell most of the DNA is organized in one large circular molecule. The bacterial DNA is not surrounded by a nuclear membrane and is not as complex in organization as DNA in eukaryotic cells. One generally refers to bacterial DNA as chromosomal DNA, analogous to the nomenclature in eukaryotic cells. Bacteria may, apart from the chromosomal DNA, harbor autonomously replicating small DNA molecules, called plasmids. Functions that are essential for a bacterial cell are usually encoded by the chromosome, whereas functions encoded by plasmids are generally in no way essential. Nevertheless, plasmids endow the bacterial cell with properties that may be very important for the survival of the bacteria. Antibiotic resistances and production of toxic proteins, for example, are well known plasmid encoded traits. As we will see later, plasmids are used in biotechnology as important and basic tools for the recombinant DNA technology.

When we refer to plasmids as small DNA molecules, this is of course in comparison to the size of the chromosomal DNA. Besides, one has to realize that plasmids vary in size. Small plasmids, generally the relevant ones for biotechnology, harbor about 6000 DNA building units, called nucleotides. Chromosomal DNA of a bacterium contains at least 1000 times more nucleotides. The DNA content of an animal or plant cell on the other hand exceeds several hundred times that of a bacterial cell. Moreover, the DNA of the former cells is no longer organized in one molecule, but in several linear chromosomes. A popular way to illustrate this fast growing complexity of DNA molecules in nature is based on pages and books. One can easily write on one page the composition of the DNA of a small plasmid by its nucleotide composition, using the symbols A, C, G and T for the various nucleotides in the DNA. To do the same for the bacterial chromosome, a book with about 1000 pages is needed. For an animal cell or a plant cell it requires a few hundred books, each containing about 1000 pages to describe the DNA.

Bacterial cells, like all cells, harbor in their cytoplasm the ribosomes as essential structures for protein synthesis, as well as a great variety of enzymes and other (macro) molecules required for the proper physiology of the cell. Most important, however, is that, apart from chromosome, ribosomes and sometimes plasmids, generally no other distinct structures are visible in the cytoplasm of the bacterial cell, even when studied with an electron microscope.

Furthermore, there are no compartments present in the cytoplasm of the prokaryotic cell.

The Eukaryotic Cell

Figure 1.3 presents a schematic picture of a plant cell as an example of an eukaryotic cell. The eukaryotic cell has a very complex structure, not only by the presence of cell organelles like the nucleus, mitochondria and chloroplast (exclusively found in plant cells), but also by the presence of specific internal membranes and of vacuoles. This complex and compartmentalized structure implies a complicated functional behavior and is one of the reasons that in the initial phase of modern biotechnology simple bacterial cells, easier to handle and more simple to modify, were prominently used. Nowadays, molecular biotechnologists use all sorts of eukaryotic cells, exploiting the fast growing insights in cell biology.

Gene Expression

Genetic information, chemically determined by the DNA structure, is transferred to daughter cells by DNA replication and is expressed by transcription (conversion of DNA into RNA) followed by translation (conversion of RNA into protein). This set of processes is found in all cells and proceeds generally in similar ways. It is one of the main unifying concepts in cell biology. The pioneers of molecular biology called that series of events the "central dogma" of biology. It was found later that retroviruses, a special class of animal RNA viruses, encode an enzyme that catalyses the conversion of RNA into complementary DNA. This enzyme, called the reverse transcriptase since it directs, so to say, the reverse of the transcription, therefore enables an information flow from RNA into DNA. Reverse transcriptase became, as will be shown later, a very important tool for DNA technology.

The various DNA linked processes are schematically depicted below:

$$\text{DNA} \leftrightarrows \text{RNA} \rightarrow \text{protein}$$

The "central dogma" was based on investigations done with bacteria and viruses. Later it was found that in eukaryotic organisms many genes are expressed differently from what was predicted by the dogma in the strict sense. In some cases the RNA derived by transcription of a eukaryotic DNA segment is subject to a process called splicing before it leaves the nucleus. During this process certain parts, the so-called introns, of the nascent RNA molecules are removed, after which the other parts (the exons) are linked together and form the effective RNA for the protein synthesis (Figure 1.4).

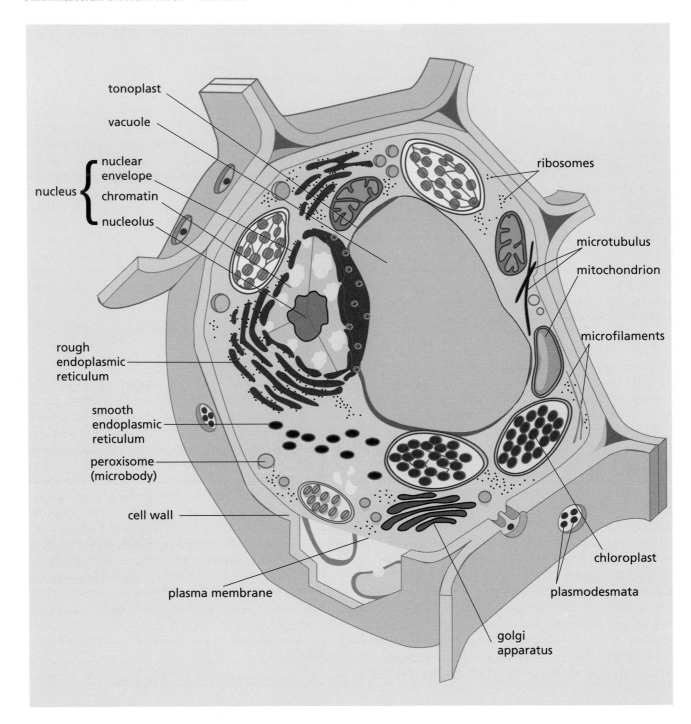

Figure 1.3. Plant Cell, schematic view.

Furthermore, it is important to realize that a nascent protein, the direct result of the translation, is not necessarily identical to the protein functional in the cell as enzyme or structural protein. Most proteins as we find them in the cell are modified by post-translational events. Nascent polypeptides are, for example, trimmed by peptidases; in some cases lipidic groups are linked to the protein, while in eukaryotic cells modification through linking of sugar groups (glycosylation) is a common event. Such post-translational modifications are important features with regard to the specific function of the protein.

Precise knowledge of the information flow in the cell is very important for biotechnology, since it offers possibilities to control cellular processes at the level of gene expres-

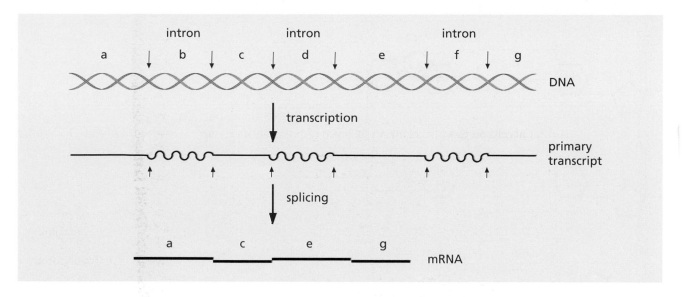

Figure 1.4. RNA splicing.

DNA Replication

sion. Therefore, the essentials of elements and processes involved in the flow of genetic information will be described below.

Although DNA may be differently organized in various organisms one or more double-stranded DNA molecules in a helix conformation are the predominant structures. Strands of DNA are composed of four specific building elements, the deoxyribonucleotides dATP, dCTP, dGTP and dTTP (shortly written as A, C, G and T) linked by phosphodiester bonds. The two strands in the DNA helix are held together through hydrogen bonds between the nucleotides in the various strands. The DNA strands in the helix are complementary in their nucleotide composition: an A in one strand is always facing a T in the other one, while a C is always facing a G (Figure 1.5). Moreover, the strands in double stranded DNA run antiparallel: the 5'-P end of the one strand faces the 3'-OH end of the complementary strand and the other way round.

During cell division the genetic information in a parental cell is transferred to the daughter cells by DNA replication. Essential in the very complex DNA replication process is the action of DNA polymerases. During replication each DNA strand is copied into a complementary strand that runs antiparallel. The topological constraint for replication due to the double helix structure of the DNA is solved by unwinding of the helix, catalysed by the enzyme helicase. In a set of biochemical events deoxyribonucleotide monomers are added one by one to the end of a growing DNA strand in a 5' to 3' direction.

DNA replication starts from specific sites, called origins of replication (*ori*). The bacterial chromosome and many plasmids have only one such site. In the much larger eukaryotic genomes there can be hundreds of *ori's* present. For circular DNA molecules like bacterial chromosomes and plasmids there are two possible ways for the replication. Semi conservative replication (Figure 1.6a) proceeding in the closed circle as such (Figure 1.6b) is one way. The constraint brought forward by the rotation as a consequence of the unwinding (there is no free end!) is resolved by the activity of a special class of enzymes, the topoisomerases. Alternatively, replication proceeds via a rolling circle model. In that case the replication starts by cutting one of the DNA strands in the *ori* region and then proceeds as indicated in Figure 1.6c.

Bacterial plasmids are defined as autonomously replicating DNA molecules. The basis for that statement is the presence of an *ori* site in the plasmids. The qualification autonomous, however, does not imply that a plasmid is independent from host factors for replication and expression. Some plasmids depend on very specific host factors and consequently they can only replicate in specific hosts. Other plasmids are less specific as to their host factor requirements and are able to replicate in a broad set of hosts. As will be demonstrated later, this difference in host range is meaningful when plasmids are exploited in biotechnology.

Transcription

Genetic information is located in the genes formed by discrete segments of the cellular DNA. In a process called

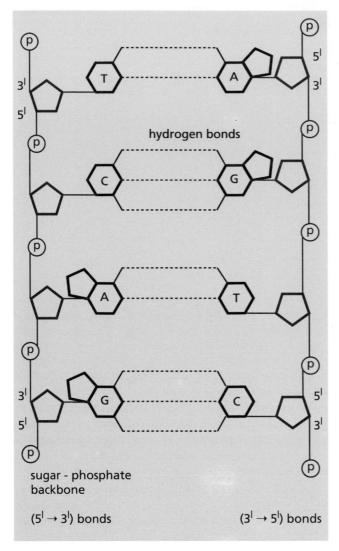

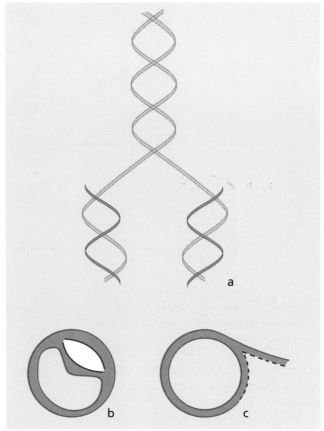

Figure 1.6. a. DNA replication (general picture); b. Closed circle replication; c. Rolling circle model.

Figure 1.5. Schematic DNA structure showing polarity and complementarity.

transcription (presented schematically in Figure 1.7), genes are copied into a complementary length of ribonucleic acid (RNA) by the enzyme RNA polymerase. Most of the RNA molecules, the messenger RNAs (mRNAs), specify the amino acid composition of the cellular proteins. Other RNA molecules derived by transcription, ribosomal RNA (rRNA) and transfer RNA (tRNA), participate as auxiliary molecules for translation.

The discovery of how the specific arrangement of nucleotides in the gene codes the sequence of amino acids in the polypeptide, the unravelling of the genetic code, is one of the milestones of the DNA époque. It was found that triplets of nucleotides in the DNA, and consequently in the mRNA, code for the amino acid composition of a protein. Most important was finding that the genetic code was (almost) universal in nature. A given triplet of nucleotides, a so-called codon, in mRNA codes for the same amino acid in nearly all organisms.

In the mRNA molecules there is more information than merely the triplets required for the encoded protein. The protein encoding information is preceded by a piece of RNA that allows binding to the ribosome, while after the triplet encoding the C-terminal amino acid there is some RNA that functions in the termination of the transcription process. Thus, signals are required to guarantee within this mRNA molecule a proper start and finish for the polypeptide synthesis. Near the 5'-end of the mRNA a specific triplet, coding for the amino acid methionine, dictates the proper start of the polypeptide synthesis and near the 3'-end a specific triplet (a stop codon) dictates a proper finish of the polypeptide synthesis. The genetic code, on the basis of the triplets in the mRNA, is presented in Table 1.1. One can see that there are three different stop codons. Moreover, it is clear from this Table 1.1 that the code is highly redundant: for certain amino acids there are several codons. Whenever there is a choice between various codons for one amino acid, different organisms tend to show different prefer-

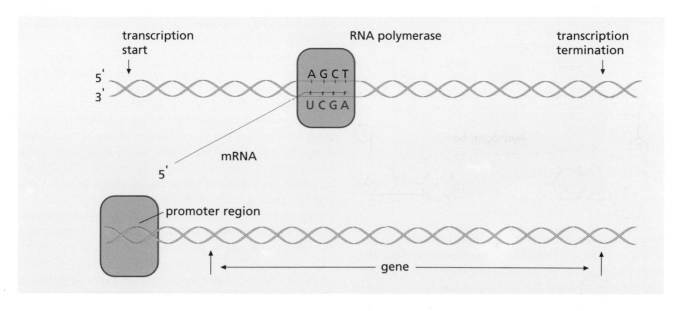

Figure 1.7. Transcription. Upper part shows ongoing transcription. Note that in the RNA, instead of T the nucleotide U acts as the complement of A in the DNA. The lower panel depicts the start, involving specific binding of RNA polymerase to the promoter region.

ences. Later it will become clear that this organism dependent codon preference has consequences for certain biotechnological processes.

Transcription starts with the binding of the enzyme RNA polymerase at a specific site, called promoter, imme-

First position (5'-end)	Second position				Third position (3'-end)
	U	C	A	G	
U	Phe	Ser	Tyr	Cys	U
	Phe	Ser	Tyr	Cys	C
	Leu	Ser	Stop	Stop	A
	Leu	Ser	Stop	Trp	G
C	Leu	Pro	His	Arg	U
	Leu	Pro	His	Arg	C
	Leu	Pro	Gln	Arg	A
	Leu	Pro	Gln	Arg	G
A	Ile	Thr	Asn	Ser	U
	Ile	Thr	Asn	Ser	C
	Ile	Thr	Lys	Arg	A
	Met	Thr	Lys	Arg	G
G	Val	Ala	Asp	Gly	U
	Val	Ala	Asp	Gly	C
	Val	Ala	Glu	Gly	A
	Val	Ala	Glu	Gly	G

Table 1.1. The 'universal' genetic code. Note: the bold codons are used for initiation.

diately upstream from a gene or from a set of genes transcribed as an operational unit (an operon). Promoters vary in their efficiency to bind RNA polymerase. Some promoters, the strong promoters, are highly efficient while others are weak and often require additional factors for effective binding of RNA polymerase. Promoter structures, in prokaryotes as well as in eukaryotes, have been studied in great detail. Based on such studies it is now feasible in biotechnology, as shown later, to fuse very effective promoter structures to any gene that one wishes to be expressed.

After binding of the RNA polymerase, the DNA helix is partially unwound and subsequently the transcription process starts. RNA synthesis then proceeds with the ribonucleotides ATP, GTP, CTP and UTP as building units. One DNA strand in the gene, the so called template strand, serves as the matrix for this RNA synthesis. Like in the DNA synthesis, the RNA synthesis runs antiparallel in the direction 5' to 3' and proceeds in a complementary way. The latter implies that a G in the matrix DNA leads to C in the RNA, a C leads to a G, a T to an A while an A in the DNA shows up as a U in the RNA. The transcription may stop either on the basis of intrinsic structural features of the RNA at the end of the gene or the operon or by the intervention of a specific terminating protein factor at this site.

Transcription can be regulated at various stages in the process. The intrinsic properties of the promoter, next to various kinds of proteins that can either repress or stimulate the binding of RNA polymerase, regulate the transcription start. Transcription termination can also be regulated. Termination may, under the influence of physiological factors, occur at a premature stage. Alternatively, the

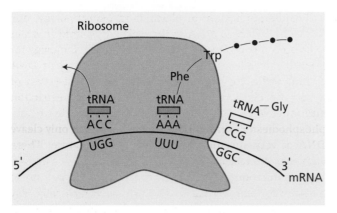

Figure 1.8. Schematic picture of ongoing translation. The amino acid Phe is linked to the growing peptide chain. The tRNA that delivered the previous amino acid Trp is leaving the ribosome complex. The next amino acid to be linked will be Gly, according the mRNA code.

normal termination signal could be ignored (a process called read-through). This may lead to various lengths of transcripts starting from the same promoter. Finally, gene activity can also be regulated at the level of the formed mRNA. All transcripts are subject to degradation, but rates of degradation can vary widely: some transcripts have a short half-life time while others are very stable. Biotechnologists try to influence the expression of a gene encoding a relevant protein at each of these regulation levels in order to achieve optimal production.

Translation

Translation, presented schematically in Figure 1.8, is a complex cellular process where mRNA molecules, ribosomes, tRNA molecules, amino acids, aminoacyl synthetases and a number of translation factors act together in a highly coordinated way. The ribosome, an organelle built from rRNA molecules and proteins, is the cellular structure where the various compounds for the protein synthesis assemble.

The building elements of the proteins, the amino acids, are used in the protein synthesis in a form adapted for a convenient interaction with the mRNA. The adaptation of the amino acid is achieved by coupling it to a specific tRNA molecule through the catalytic action of specific aminoacyl synthetases. The adapted amino acid is linked to the 3'-OH terminus of a specific tRNA molecule. Each tRNA molecule contains in a characteristic loop of the molecule a specific triplet. This triplet is complementary and runs antiparallel to the codon for the linked amino acid and is consequently designated the anticodon. Coupling through base pairing of the anticodon in the tRNA to the codon in

the mRNA is the way amino acids are positioned according to the code in the mRNA.

Translation starts with the formation of a specific initiation complex. In a bacterial cell this consists of a 30S ribosomal subunit, a tRNA carrying the amino acid methionine, GTP and various initiation factors all at the position of the start codon AUG of the mRNA. To form this initiation complex the 5'-end region of the bacterial messenger is important. This region, which itself is not translated, harbors a specific ribosome binding site. To the initiation complex a 50S ribosomal subunit is subsequently bound, creating a functional 70S ribosome. Translation then proceeds, with the help of specific elongation factors, in such a way that the 70S ribosomes are transported along the mRNA molecule stepwise over a distance of one triplet. This stepwise transport guarantees that protein synthesis proceeds in a coordinated way dictated by the (triplet) codons. The amino acids, delivered by the specific tRNA molecules, are linked together, one after the other, by peptide bond formation. Meanwhile the tRNA carriers are set free again.

At the end of an mRNA molecule there are one or more stop codons. These triplets do not accept any tRNA-aminoacyl molecule and are therefore terminating signals for protein synthesis. After termination the protein is released from the 70S ribosome. The ribosomes then fall apart in their 30S and 50S subunits which may be used in a further translation cycle.

Although there is a common general picture for translation in prokaryotes and eukaryotes there are nevertheless various distinct differences, especially in the nature of initiation and elongation factors. A very clear distinction is a direct consequence of the difference in DNA organization between pro- and eukaryotes. In the prokaryotic cell, mRNA is already available for the ribosomes while it is still in the process of transcription. In the eukaryotic cell, on the other hand, the mRNA is only available for translation after it is completely synthesized and after it is transported through the nuclear membrane. Consequently, transcription and translation are coupled processes in the prokaryotic cell, while these processes occur separately in the eukaryotic cell.

Recombinant DNA Technology

After it was established that DNA is the chemical constituent for the hereditary properties of the cell and after the discovery that (bacterial) cells can spontaneously take up DNA, investigators immediately tried to manipulate the genetic properties of all kind of cells. To achieve this, they simply added foreign DNA to microbial cells, plant cells or animal cells. All these attempts failed. There are two reasons for this lack of success. First of all, only a limited number of bacterial species is able to take up DNA spontaneously; most bacteria and certainly animal and plant species are unable to do this. Secondly, foreign DNA, if taken up at all, is in general not maintained in the receptor cell. DNA brought into a cell from outside will only be maintained if it is able to replicate autonomously, or if it is integrated in the recipient genome. In all other cases foreign DNA will not be propagated in the cell culture and will eventually disappear by degradation through the activity of cellular nucleases.

Genetic modification of organisms became feasible later on when recombinant DNA technologies were developed. This enabled the fusion of any DNA fragment to DNA molecules able to maintain themselves by autonomous replication (such molecules are called replicons). The various techniques developed to introduce recombinant DNA molecules into all sorts of biological cells led to successful genetic modification strategies.

Replicons used as carriers for foreign DNA fragments are termed vectors. The vectors exploited in the DNA technology include mainly plasmids from bacteria or yeast, or DNA from bacteriophages, animal viruses or plant viruses. Especially small microbial plasmids are very popular as vectors in biotechnology, since they can easily be isolated as intact circular double stranded molecules. Plasmids with a broad host range, mentioned before, are very attractive since they can be used in various hosts and consequently enable a flexible application of the DNA technology.

For the application of plasmids in biotechnology, one has to fuse foreign DNA to the isolated plasmid in order to create a recombinant DNA molecule. The technology for this, the so-called recombinant DNA technology or DNA cloning technology, became feasible after the discovery of a specific class of nucleases, the so-called restriction endonucleases. Next to nucleases able to cleave any phosphodiester bond in DNA, nucleases which only cleave DNA at very specific sites are present in nature. These enzymes, the restriction enzymes, were discovered around 1970 in microorganisms. Their function is to discriminate between foreign DNA and self DNA. Microbial cells may in real life be confronted with DNA from an unrelated cell via various genetic transfer systems. Although all DNA is built likewise, DNA can be marked specifically at particular sites by a characteristic pattern of methylated or glucosylated nucleotides. This DNA marking, which does not interfere with the coding and replicating functions, is host specific. Restriction enzymes have the remarkable property to recognize DNA on the basis of the specific host marking. When DNA is transferred and the marking does not fit with the recipient cell, such DNA will be recognized and cut at specific sites by the restriction enzyme. Once the DNA is cut it will be further degraded in the cell. As is the case in many biological systems, things are never absolute: some DNA molecules may escape from the action of the restriction enzymes and by getting a proper marking they can be rescued.

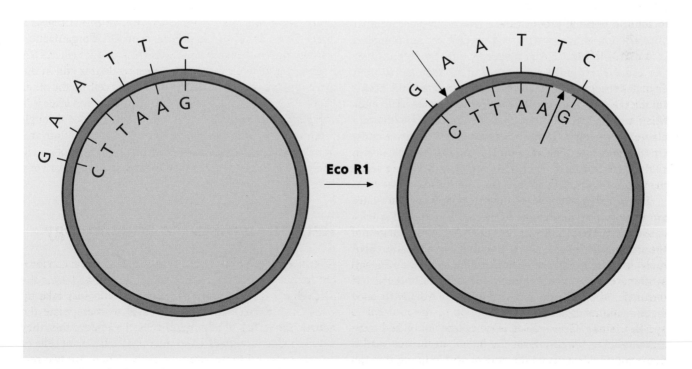

Figure 1.9. Treatment of a plasmid with a unique Eco R1 site. This restriction enzyme will open the plasmid and makes it amenable for manipulation.

The very selective action of the restriction enzymes is the basis for their application in the recombinant DNA technology. Addition of a restriction enzyme to a plasmid without proper marking will convert the closed circular molecule to linear fragments, provided that the plasmid harbors recognition sites for the chosen restriction enzyme. In Figure 1.9 this is depicted for a special, but representative case. A plasmid with only one recognition site for the restriction enzyme *Eco*R1 is treated with this enzyme. The double-stranded DNA is then asymmetrically cut at the recognition site, encompassing 6 bases namely GAATTC, which leads to linear DNA with typical short single-stranded ends. If foreign DNA — isolated either from microbial, plant or animal cells — with recognition sites for the enzyme *Eco*R1 is likewise cut with this enzyme, fragments with single-stranded ends characteristic for *Eco*R1 are formed. When the open vector and the foreign DNA fragments are brought together under appropriate physico-chemical conditions, the various single stranded ends may recombine due to the presence of complementary bases. A possible reaction product could be a plasmid to which a specific foreign DNA fragment, as a passenger, is linked. Although the DNA pieces in such construct are interlinked by base pairing, they do not form a closed circular molecule. The enzyme DNA ligase, present in all sorts of cells and able to catalyse the formation of phosphodiester bonds, is used to create a closed circular recombinant DNA molecule.

According to the technology presented schematically in Figure 1.10, recombinant DNA molecules consisting of vector and passenger DNA can be created. A great number of restriction enzymes with very specific recognition sites is available to cut DNA at a specific site. Some enzymes, like *Eco* R1, recognize a sequence of six base pairs, other enzymes recognize just four bases. Some, again like *Eco*R1, cut the DNA asymmetrically while others create blunt ends when cutting DNA. Although DNA fragments with complementary single stranded ends (so called cohesive ends) are the most favorable ones for linking, DNA ligase is also able to link fragments with blunt ends. In Table 1.2 some representative restriction enzymes are listed.

Recombinant DNA molecules are biologically of no interest as long as they reside in the reaction tube. Transfer of the construct to a living cell, however, may change the situation drastically. If the vector that served for the construct is able to replicate in the host, all daughter cells will inherit a precise copy (a clone) of the recombinant DNA molecule. Therefore the term "cloning" is frequently used for the technology described above.

The cloning technique is very suitable to obtain large amounts of a specific DNA fragment, by fusing such a fragment to an appropriate vector and transferring the construct to a host that can easily be cultivated to high cell

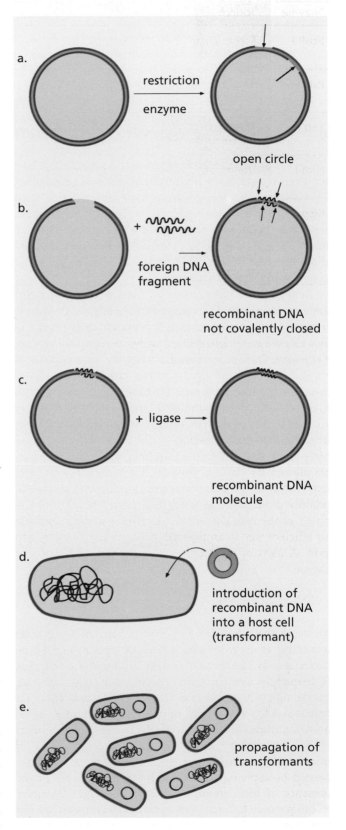

a. restriction enzyme → open circle

b. + foreign DNA fragment → recombinant DNA not covalently closed

c. + ligase → recombinant DNA molecule

d. introduction of recombinant DNA into a host cell (transformant)

e. propagation of transformants

Figure 1.10. Principle of cloning a foreign DNA fragment.

Enzyme	Source	Cutting sequence
EcoR I	*Escherichia coli*	G↓AATT C C TTAA↑G
Pst I	*Providencia stuartii*	C TGCA↓G G↑ACGT C
Taq I	*Thermus aquaticus*	T↓CG A A GC↑T
Hinf I	*Haemophilus influenzae*	G↓AN*T C C TNA↑G
Msp I	*Moraxella species*	C↓CG G G GC↑C
Hae III	*Haemophilus aegyptus*	GG↓CC CC↑GG

Table 1.2. Some restriction enzymes, their origin and their recognition site. Note: open space in the recognition site indicates the endonucleolytic cut by the enzyme.
* N means: no base preference.

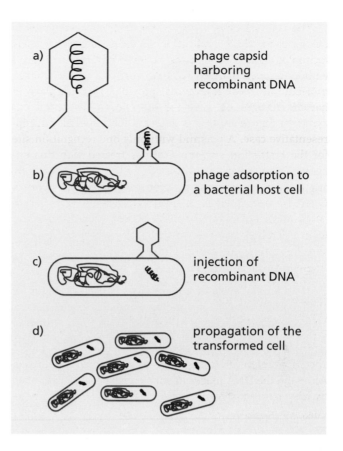

Figure 1.11. Phage as a mediator for transfer of recombinant DNA.

a) phage capsid harboring recombinant DNA

b) phage adsorption to a bacterial host cell

c) injection of recombinant DNA

d) propagation of the transformed cell

densities. The recombinant DNA molecules, which can then be isolated from the cell mass, form an abundant source for the specific DNA fragment. Moreover and most important for pharmaceutical biotechnology, if the cloned piece of foreign DNA harbors an intact gene with appropriate signals for gene expression, the modified host cells may, based on the universal character of gene expression, produce proteins encoded by the foreign DNA. This is the power of the recombinant DNA technology in a nutshell: an efficient way to amplify DNA fragments and a way to gain all sorts of gene products from hosts that one can choose.

DNA Transfer

As stated above transfer of a recombinant DNA molecule to a cell is an essential step in the DNA technology. Some bacterial cells, like those of the species *Bacillus subtilis* that is frequently used in industrial biotechnology, are able to take up DNA under physiological conditions. This process is described as natural transformation. In most cases, however, microbial cells have to be forced by an unusual regimen to take up DNA. For example, in the case of microorganisms such non-physiological conditions are created by applying a heat shock to the host cells in the presence of high amounts of Ca^{2+} ions. An alternative technique used to force DNA uptake is electroporation. For that purpose DNA and cells are brought together in a cuvette which is then subjected to a vigorous electrical

discharge. Under those artificial conditions the cell envelope is forced to open itself, after which DNA may enter through the "holes" that are created. The brute force in these techniques kills a large fraction of the cells, but sufficient cells survive, among which are several that took up DNA. The technique of electroporation is widely applicable and frequently used.

Next to direct transfer of recombinant DNA molecules as such, there is for transfer to bacterial cells the possibility to package DNA in a bacteriophage capsid and then to mimic the normal bacteriophage infection procedure (Figure 1.11). Transfer to bacterial cells can also be achieved by making use of conjugation. Conjugation is a process where DNA transfer takes place by cell-cell mating. For conjugation a special class of plasmids is required, so-called conjugative plasmids. If a cell with such a plasmid — the donor — meets a cell without such plasmid — the recipient — they may form together cell aggregates. In the so called mating aggregate the plasmid from the donor has the ability to transfer itself, as a consequence of a conjugative replication process according to the rolling circle model, to the recipient cell. By manipulating the conjugative plasmids

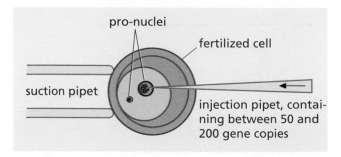

Figure 1.12. Injection of foreign DNA into a fertilized cell.

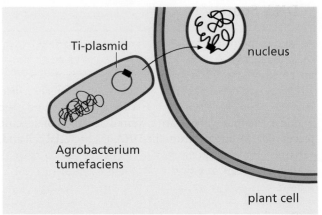

Figure 1.13. Plant cell modification by Ti-plasmid. Part of the Ti-plasmid (marked) is transferred to the plant cell and may be stably integrated in the plant DNA.

one may create donors harboring recombinant DNA molecules which can then rather efficiently be transferred by cell-cell contact.

If an animal virus or a plant virus is used as vector for the recombinant DNA technology, one may exploit natural virus infection processes to transfer DNA to an animal or a plant cell (cf. Chapter 7). As is the case in microorganisms, DNA transfer to animal cells can be forced by a treatment with large amounts of Ca^{2+}-ions or by another chemical treatment. Next to that, it is possible to inject DNA with a syringe into the nucleus of the cell. The latter technique (one could speak of a kind of micro-surgery) is feasible due to the relative large dimensions of the animal cells compared to bacteria and is also applied to plant cells. The technique is illustrated in Figure 1.12. The cell is brought on the tip of a thin glass tube and is fixed to the tube by suction at the other end of the tube. By means of a micromanipulator a small syringe filled with DNA is directed to the nucleus of the fixed cell and then the DNA is injected into the nucleus.

A very successful way to transfer DNA into plant systems is based on a very special type of conjugation. The soil bacterium, *Agrobacterium tumefaciens*, harbors a conjugative plasmid called Ti (acronym for tumor inducing). If such a bacterium infects wounded tissues of certain plants, part of the Ti-plasmid is transferred to a plant cell in a conjugation-like process. This transfer is followed by integration of the transferred DNA into the genome of the plant. The infected plant cells lose normal growth control and develop a tumor (a plant disease called crown gall). By manipulating the Ti-plasmid, such that its tumor inducing properties are lost and foreign DNA fragments are linked to it, any DNA can be transferred in a convenient way from the modified *Agrobacterium* donor to a plant cell. Figure 1.13 illustrates this remarkable process, where, in fact, biological kingdom barriers are crossed in a natural fashion.

Since the wall of the plant cell is the main barrier for uptake of DNA, one has exploited protoplasts of plant cells (i.e. plant cells lacking walls) to introduce DNA. Protoplasts can take up DNA quite easily. It is feasible to regenerate from protoplasts that took up DNA intact, genetically modified plant cells. Finally, a very artificial method to introduce DNA in plant tissue has been developed quite recently. Microprojectiles covered with DNA are shot with a gun into plant cells. In fact, many plant species that can not readily be genetically modified with any of the methods mentioned above can be modified using this rather bizarre gun method.

The various techniques that are used to transfer DNA are generally not very efficient and may cause, as stated before, extensive killing of cells. Moreover, the fate of the transferred DNA is not always predictable. For example, in some cases the introduced DNA is subject to nuclease mediated breakdown, while in animal or plant cells the introduced DNA does not always reach the nucleus, nor is it always integrated in a proper way. All methods to transfer DNA yield, in general, only a few cells that are vital and more or less stably modified. Therefore, selection techniques are highly desirable to find these rare cells. Most selection techniques use a marker on the vector that codes for a selective property. Markers which code for a resistance towards a specific antibiotic substance are frequently used. If the cell that has to be modified is sensitive towards that antibiotic, the few modified cells from the transfer trial can easily be selected by bringing samples of the treated cells (either microbial cells, plant cells or animal cells) in a medium containing the relevant antibiotic. Only the cells that took up DNA and do maintain that DNA in their progeny will proliferate, all other cells are killed or, at least, do not grow. An alternative selection method uses recipient cells with specific growth deficiencies and vectors carrying genes which overcome such deficiencies.

DNA Sources

As stated before, any DNA can be used to construct recombinant DNA molecules. In protein production based on recombinant DNA technology very distinct pieces of DNA are required. Referring to the metaphor described before in this chapter, only a few lines on a specific page in one of the many books are required. Isolation of specific pieces of DNA directly from the DNA of a bacterial cell and, certainly, of a plant or an animal cell implies a very tedious search. How can one find a DNA fragment of interest in a more convenient way? There are several strategies.

Synthetic DNA

It is feasible to use synthetic DNA as a source for the desired recombinant DNA sequence. If one seeks DNA that codes for a specific protein, the amino acid sequence of that protein is sometimes known. With the genetic code as guide one may synthesize the coding DNA by organic synthesis and use that DNA to construct an appropriate recombinant DNA molecule. Although the technique to unravel the amino acid composition of proteins and the possibilities of the organic DNA synthesis have improved over the past years, the organic DNA synthesis approach is only feasible to clone genes coding small proteins. For example, the synthetic approach has been used successfully for large scale production of human insulin, as will be described later.

The synthetic DNA approach allows the choice, whenever there are more triplets available for a certain amino acid, of the triplet that is used most frequently in the host that is selected for the production. In other words this technique allows one to master the codon usage problem, mentioned earlier in this chapter.

cDNA

An alternative for direct isolation of cellular DNA coding for a specific protein is the copy DNA (cDNA) approach. This important development in DNA technology became apparent when the enzyme reverse transcriptase was exploited as a tool.

Genes are not always expressed in the cell, nor are they expressed everywhere in the organism. Some genes are only expressed in a certain stage of cell growth, or under very specific environmental conditions, or expressed only in very specific tissues of an organism. The mRNA molecules in a cell thus represent a minority of all the available genes, namely those that are actually expressed. Knowledge of the cell physiology or knowledge of the specific biological tasks of animal and plant tissues, enables the isolation of a particular and characteristic set of mRNA molecules.

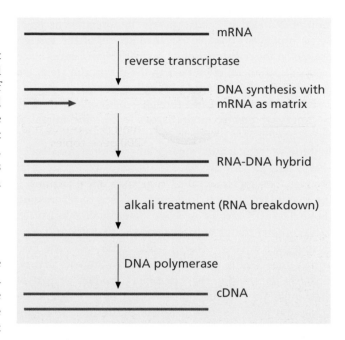

Figure 1.14. Synthesis of cDNA.

Conversion of these mRNA molecules by the enzyme reverse transcriptase into DNA leads to synthesis of the genes that were expressed. These DNA molecules, called c(opy) DNA molecules, to distinguish them from the natural DNA molecules, can be used for gene cloning. Provided that the search starts with the right kind of cell culture conditions or with the appropriate tissues the cDNA strategy can be very efficient. It is illustrated in Figure 1.14.

cDNA cloning has some obvious consequences. In contrast to a gene that is directly isolated from the chromosome, cDNA lacks a promoter region. Furthermore, in the case of genes harboring exons and introns, cDNA is built only from exons. The lack of the authentic promoter requires that in the cloning strategy a promoter should be fused to the cDNA in order to achieve gene expression. Mostly a strong promoter that can be controlled in such a way to be switched on and off, depending on environmental or tissue condition, is fused to cDNA.

Control over foreign gene expression by using a suitable promoter is very essential. Foreign proteins may disturb the physiology of the host cell as a result of uncontrolled gene expression and cause a premature stop of cell development. Therefore, a promoter like the *lac* promoter is frequently used in bacterial cells to direct the synthesis of a foreign protein. This promoter is only switched on when an appropriate inducer like iso-propyl-ß-thiogalactoside (IPTG) is added to the medium. Cultivation of the cells in absence of the inducer allows optimal cell growth since the possible deleterious foreign gene product is not produced. When high cell numbers are present in the culture, the inducer is added and consequently the foreign gene product is produced. Possible negative effects of the foreign protein on the cell are minimal in their consequences since high cell numbers, often near to the maximum yield, are present when the harmful production started.

In an animal or a plant a foreign gene should preferably be expressed only in certain tissues to keep the animal or the plant vital or to be able to isolate the protein efficiently. In those biotechnological applications where mammals like sheep, goat or cow are used as host for pharmaceutical products (an approach called "pharmaceutical farming"), the mammary gland is frequently used as an expression tissue. The cDNA for an objective protein is therefore fused to a promoter that is only expressed in that tissue. Transferring such a DNA construct into embryos of the host animal may lead to genetically modified animals that exclusively deliver the pharmaceutical product as part of their milk. This production route enables an efficient isolation and allows relatively simple purification strategies (cf. Chapter 6).

The lack of introns in the cDNA has the advantage that cDNA may lead to a functional gene product even in organisms where splicing does not occur (like in prokaryotic cells) or where splicing is ambiguous or unreliable.

DNA Libraries

The mRNA approach is not feasible if precise knowledge of gene expression is lacking and does not allow cloning of DNA that is not expressed. A general approach to master very complex DNA molecules for recombinant DNA technology is to create a DNA library. To do so, random DNA fragments from a bacterial, plant or animal cell are fused to a vector and then transferred to an appropriate host. By isolating from a bacterial cell, for example, DNA fragments that on average amount 1% of total DNA and linking these fragments individually to a vector, one may create together a few hundred different recombinant DNA molecules which represent the total bacterial chromosome. Using the "DNA-book" metaphor again: the original bacterial "DNA book" with about 1000 pages is divided in about 150 small booklets of, e.g., 10 pages each. These booklets tell, with some overlap and without an *a priori* ordering, the same story as told in the complete book. The immediate advantage of this approach is that large molecules are split in suitable smaller pieces linked to a replicon.

An individual host with a specific recombinant DNA molecule thus harbors a fragment of the total DNA on a replicating vector. By preselecting from the library the cells carrying gene(s) or DNA of interest, one may obtain a smaller molecule harboring little more than the DNA of interest by trimming the fragment isolated from these cells. By subsequent cloning of such smaller fragments one may

achieve the final goal: a recombinant DNA molecule with a very distinct piece of foreign DNA. It is noteworthy to mention in this respect that DNA libraries are available from many organisms. Likewise cDNA libraries exist from many tissues such as the human brain. By analysis of the various fragments, insight into the genetic structure of all sorts of organisms is rapidly growing. In this respect the present unravelling of the human genome, a project involving scientists all over the world, is worth mentioning.

Production by Recombinant DNA Technology

Only two of the many examples available of the production of biopharmaceuticals by the recombinant DNA technology will be treated here: the production of human insulin and the production of the human growth hormone (hGH). The pharmaceutical aspects of both proteins are discussed in more detail in Chapters 10 and 11, respectively.

The large scale production of human insulin nicely illustrates the synthetic DNA approach. Moreover, this example shows clearly that, besides knowledge of the coding gene, detailed knowledge of the protein to be produced is required.

The structural gene for human insulin is 1430 nucleotides long, while the gene is intervened (introns) by sequences of 179 and 786 nucleotides. The protein encoded by the gene is 110 amino acids in length. However, the mature protein encompasses a total of 51 amino acids. It consists of two separate chains: an A chain of 21 amino acids and a B chain of 30 amino acids. Chains A and B are held together by S bonds between the cysteines on the adjacent chains. The human insulin protein is apparently extensively processed after translation. Processing proceeds in two steps. The primary product, called preproinsulin, is 110 amino acids long in accordance with the prediction from the DNA sequence. During the membrane translocation of the protein the "pre" part of the protein, a stretch of 24 amino acids serving as the leader sequence for membrane translocation, is cleaved off. The remaining protein, 86-amino acids long, is called proinsulin. This protein is further processed in pancreatic cells, while an internal fragment (called the C or connecting chain) of 33 amino acids together with a few assorted amino acids is enzymatically removed. The A and B chains that are left are associated through S-bonds and form the mature and biologically active insulin.

The strategy for the gene cloning according to the detailed knowledge of the mature protein, was to clone and produce the chains A and B separately. The information for the fragment A was synthesized by linking a set of appropriate oligonucleotides. This DNA was then by ligation fused to the end of the gene *lacZ* in the plasmid pBR322, a very well known *E. coli* cloning vector. At the fusion point between *lacZ* and the information for chain A a codon for the amino acid methionine was built in, for reasons that will be explained later on. The information for fragment B was (for strategic reasons) synthesized in two steps. Firstly, the N terminal coding part was synthesized by linking oligonucleotides. This fragment was fused to the plasmid pBR322 and propagated in *E. coli* as such. Secondly, the C-terminal coding part was synthesized and also propagated after ligating it to pBR322. The two DNA fragments were then isolated from the respective recombinant DNA molecules. Both parts were linked together and fused at the end of the *lacZ* gene in the plasmid pBR322. Again the codon for the amino acid methionine was built in at the fusion point.

The linking of the information for A and B to the *lacZ* gene, part of the well known lactose-operon, has two advantages. First of all, both fragments depend for their expression on the regimen of the *lacZ* gene, which allows an effective and controlled expression. Secondly, the peptides A and B are synthesized as products fused to ß-galactosidase. Since especially small foreign peptides in a bacterial cell are very vulnerable to proteolytic breakdown, the fusion strategy is an effective mean to prevent breakdown. Treatment of the isolated fusion proteins with the agent cyanogen bromide allows the isolation of the fragments A and B. This agent has the ability to cleave peptides whenever the amino acid methionine is present and cleaves immediately after this amino acid. Since neither fragment A nor B of insulin contains methionine and the cloning strategy guaranteed the presence of methionine at the fusion point, the isolation of peptides A and B as such is relatively simple. The final step consists of mixing A and B and allowing the S bonds to form spontaneously. Figure 1.15 presents the procedure of insulin production with the help of synthetic DNA.

The strategy to clone and produce hGH shows some other interesting features. First of all, the production was initiated by making cDNA out of a mRNA pool derived from the human pituitary, the tissue where this peptide hormone is synthesized. The cDNA molecule coding for the hGH was isolated and, since it contained information of 24 amino acids that should guarantee transport in the human body, it was reduced with an appropriate restriction enzyme. However, in this procedure the coding information for some of the amino acids essential for the activity of the mature hormone was lost. This missing part of information lost from the original cDNA molecule was chemically synthesized and fused to the fragmented cDNA molecule in order to get the full information for the mature hGH. Next, the construct was linked to a bacterial vector in such a way that it was fused to a strong promoter. In some constructs information coding for a bacterial leader

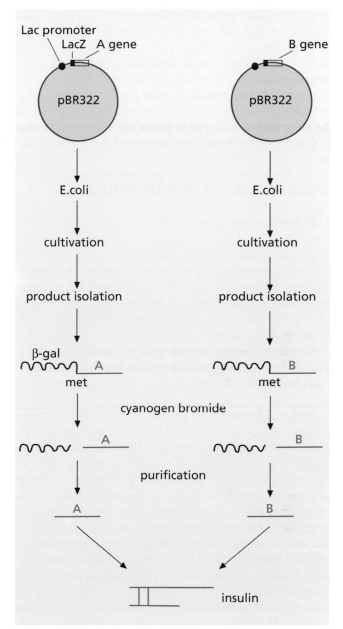

Figure 1.15. Synthesis of insulin by synthetic DNA.

sequence was linked to the hGH gene. A bacterial leader peptide (a N-terminal sequence of about 20 amino acids) is able to induce translocation of the protein over the cytoplasmic membrane. The leader peptide has rather specific physico-chemical properties and enables a protein to cross the cytoplasmic membrane barrier during which the leader peptide is cleaved off. The reason for attaching a leader peptide is that in certain production strategies one wishes to obtain products that are released from the cytoplasm to be able to perform a convenient purification strategy afterwards. If the hGH gene is linked to an appropriate leader peptide and expressed in the host *E. coli*, hGH molecules will show up in the space between the IM and the OM, the so-called periplasmic space. It is possible to damage the OM in such a way that the contents of the periplasm are set free. Then, purification of hGH is rather easy and cheaper than purification of h$\overline{G}$H as a product in the cytoplasm of *E. coli*. Cloning strategies that guarantee membrane translocation are frequently selected in order to release a protein from the cytoplasm.

Specific DNA Techniques

DNA Sequencing

The development of technologies for detailed nucleotide sequence determination of DNA molecules has been of immense importance. This knowledge opens the way for very precise DNA modifications, like changing individual nucleotides in order to change an individual amino acid in a protein (cf. Chapter 6).

In 1977 two different methods were published for DNA sequencing. The Maxam and Gilbert method is based on chemical degradation of DNA, whereas the Sanger method, also called the chain termination method, uses DNA replication enzymology. The Sanger method is the most popular method and is described here. It uses a DNA polymerase enzyme normally involved in DNA replication. DNA polymerases are template dependent, meaning that they need a single stranded DNA molecule which they will copy according to the A-T and G-C base pairing rules, and are primer dependent, meaning that they need a free 3′-hydroxyl group of an oligonucleotide as a starting point for the incorporation of deoxyribonucleotide triphosphates (dATP, dCTP, dTTP and dGTP). The primer is a short, chemically synthesized molecule, about 20 nucleotides in length which is complementary and antiparallel to a segment in the single-stranded DNA molecule to be sequenced. Under the right conditions it will hybridize and thus provide a specific starting point for the elongation reaction by the polymerase.

The method depends in essence on the inclusion in the reaction mixture of a so-called dideoxyribonucleotide triphosphate (ddNTP). These molecules not only lack the 2′ hydroxyl group on the ribose as is normal in DNA, but also the 3′ hydroxyl group; hence the name *di*-deoxy. These ddNTPs can be incorporated into DNA strands by DNA polymerase. However, since the lacking 3′-hydroxyl group is required for DNA elongation, the DNA molecules which have incorporated such a ddNTP are no longer substrate for further chain elongation: the chain terminates with a ddNTP and this principle is used for the sequencing reaction. Per reaction four tubes are set up which contain template, primer and the four dNTPs. To the four tubes

ddNTP is added. To the first tube ddATP is added, to the second tube ddTTP, to the third tube ddCTP and to the fourth tube ddCTP. The ratio of dNTP versus ddNTP in each tube is chosen in such a way that a small number of templates in each tube will incorporate the specific ddNTP and will no longer be substrates for elongation (chain termination). Therefore in each tube a fraction of the strands will terminate with the specific ddNTP present in that particular tube. The length of the terminated strands is determined by the oligonucleotide primer, which sets a fixed starting point, and the ddNTP incorporated. In the first reaction tube, for example, fragment lengths are determined by the position of the various A nucleotides in the template. After the synthesis reaction the contents of the four individual sequencing tubes are applied to a high resolution polyacrylamide gel electrophoresis system which separates individual elongation products based on their length. Tube 1 reveals the positions of A, tube 2 of C, tube 3 of T and tube 4 of G. The reaction products can be visualized either by autoradiography in case a small aliquot of radioactively labeled dNTP has been incorporated in all reactions (usually α-^{32}P-dCTP) or by fluorography in case a fluorescent group has been chemically added to the sequencing primer during its synthesis. Especially, the latter method is very well suited for automation. Currently, sequencing machines are commercially available which, in one run, can sequence over 800 nucleotides. In such machines 20-40 runs can be loaded and analyzed simultaneously which tremendously enhances productivity. Needless to say, sequences are handled, analyzed and stored electronically. Three interlinked computer sequence databases are operational in the world which are freely accessible via Internet.

DNA Hybridization

To gain insight into the DNA composition, sequencing is the final approach. There is, however, a possibility to acquire information about DNA structure by hybridization with the help of so-called DNA probes. In essence the probe is a specific single-stranded DNA fragment. Such a probe will form double-stranded DNA (in other words will hybridize) whenever it encounters a single stranded complementary piece of DNA under appropriate conditions. There are many applications for DNA probes.

If, for example, one wishes to see which recombinant DNA molecule in an extensive DNA library harbors a gene of interest, one might use a DNA probe. DNAs from the library are converted into single stranded DNA and then confronted with a probe that reflects a very characteristic segment of the desired gene. Hybridization will, provided that the probe has the required specificity, only occur with target DNA molecules that harbor the gene of interest.

The use of DNA hybridization probes in diagnostic testing in humans can be illustrated by using cystic fibrosis (CF) as an example. The frequency of this heritable and deadly disease is approximately once in 2000 live births making it the most frequent genetic disorder among Caucasians. The cloning of the gene in 1989 based on its position on the human genetic map was a *tour de force* involving several laboratories. It enabled the molecular analysis of the genetic defect, revealing that approximately 70% of the diseased genes contain an identical mutation: a three base pair deletion in the protein coding gene resulting in the loss of a phenylalanine amino acid at position 508 of the 1480 amino acid-long protein. This mutation was named CFdel508 and the knowledge gained was used to design oligonucleotide probes for rapid screening purposes.

These single-strand DNA probes are complementary to the normal and CFdel508 regions of the CF gene shown below. The symbols L, E, etc. represent various amino acids (see Chapter 2). F, e.g., stands for phenylalanine.

Normal:

5′-AAA GAA AAT ATC ATC TTT GGT GTT-3′
   L   E   N   I   I   F   G   V

Mutant (CFdel508):

5′-AAA GAA AAT ATC AT- --T GGT GTT-3′
   L   E   N   I   I   G   V

DNA isolated from e.g. white blood cells of suspected carriers or amnion fluid is boiled to make it single stranded and then immobilized on filter paper. Next, hybridization with normal and CFdel508 specific probes clarifies whether one has the disease, in which case both the maternal and the paternal genes are affected, whether one is a carrier of the disease, in which one of the two genes is affected (heterozygosy), or whether one is normal at this genomic position.

Variation on this technology allows for the automated and simultaneous screening for many genetic diseases for which the molecular lesions are known. Kits which contain all the reagents necessary for a particular test are commercially available.

PCR Technology

For the detection of DNA or for testing the presence of mutations in DNA the probe method described above is very powerful. Within the current probe techniques, however, a substantial amount of DNA is required to allow the detection of target DNA. The PCR (polymerase chain reaction) technology became very popular in recent years to acquire large amounts of DNA.

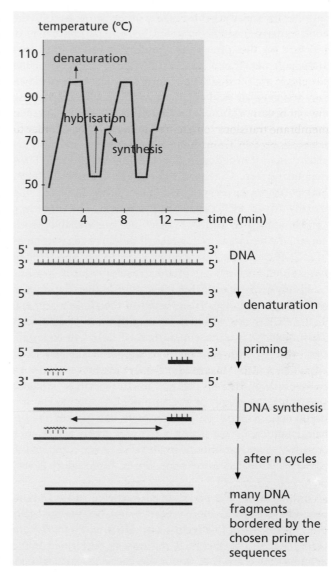

Figure 1.16. PCR-method. Upper panel: sequence of heating, hydridizing, synthesis. Below: synthesis events.

In the PCR technology target DNA is amplified by *in vitro* DNA synthesis, occurring in a number of fast repeating steps. The reaction starts with the conversion of the double-stranded target DNA to single-stranded DNA and uses specific oligonucleotides as primers to allow DNA polymerase to do its job. The choice of the oligonucleotide primers, hybridizing with each of both target strands, will determine the left and right limits of the DNA to be amplified.

Each PCR cycle (illustrated in Figure 1.16) consists of three steps each requiring only 1–3 minutes. In the first step the target DNA must be made single stranded and this is done by heating the sample to 92°C. The second step involves the specific hybridization of the two primers to the complementary single-stranded DNA. The optimal temperature for this process is about 55°C. In the third step DNA polymerase will extend the primer sequence using the single stranded DNA as a template. The optimal extension temperature is about 72°C since the DNA polymerase chosen is derived from a thermophilic bacterium, *Thermus aquaticus*, which normally grows in hot springs at temperatures above 80°C. This DNA polymerase is extremely resistant against heat denaturing and survives the 92°C DNA denaturing step. All reagents (target DNA, primers, dNTPs and polymerase) are put in a tube which is sealed and usually 20–30 PCR cycles are performed. The procedure can be automated and PCR machines are available which control the temperature for each of the three separate steps of a PCR cycle. Such machines can process hundreds of tubes simultaneously and produce results within 2–4 hours.

Ideally each cycle of DNA replication doubles the amount of DNA which is located in between the chosen primers. Thirty PCR cycles will give an amplification of 2^{30} times. This means that minute quantities of DNA can be amplified with specific primers to easily detectable levels. It should be realized that the specificity of the reaction is fully determined by the PCR primers and these primers will also determine the length of the amplified fragment. The tremendous sensitivity of the technique has sparked the development of a great number of applications where such sensitivity is of paramount importance. Also, compared to many other detection methods, the PCR procedure is very fast.

For example, the presence of microbial pathogens in raw and processed food products can be unequivocally determined using this technology. DNA is extracted from this material and the PCR reaction is performed using primers which are specific for the suspected pathogen(s). Detailed knowledge of DNA sequences of all sorts of genes in all sorts of organisms allows the development of such specific primers, the main prerequisite for diagnostic PCR technology. If specific amplified DNA products can be detected, this is proof that the pathogen is present in the material. Also in clinical material (blood, urine, etc.) the technique is used extensively as a rapid and sensitive test for the presence of bacterial and viral pathogens. A third area where PCR has become standard technology is in forensic science. At a crime scene often minute quantities of potentially important evidence is found (single hairs, blood drops, semen stains, etc.) and PCR technology can be used to get enough DNA to show the origin of this material. These are but a few examples of the use of PCR technology. PCR is often an essential step in elaborate diagnostic and detection procedures and novel applications are continuously being developed.

As for the application of the PCR technology for diagnosis of pathogens, one has to realize that for most purposes the intent is to detect viable pathogens. The PCR technology obviously cannot distinguish DNA from vital or dead material and in that respect it is not always an adequate technique. The PCR technique is a very sensitive one since minute amounts of DNA are highly amplified. This high sensitivity may limit the discriminative power of the technique when applied for diagnostic purposes. For example, it may detect minor contaminants in the samples. Moreover, DNA contaminants may be introduced during the performance of the tests. It is therefore a major concern in the application of PCR to avoid DNA contaminations that could cause false positive reactions.

Modified PCR techniques and related methodologies are discussed in Chapter 6.

Cell Cultures

Biotechnology depends heavily on techniques to cultivate pro- and eukaryotic cells, since these cells are sources of bioproducts or of mediators of various bioconversions. The scale of culturing is an important issue in biotechnology. Experience from small scale cultures is not directly transferable to large scale culturing in manufacturing industries. What can be cultivated in small flasks in a research laboratory cannot always be cultivated efficiently on an industrial scale. Simply enlarging the culture devices from small flasks to tanks containing many thousand liters is not enough. Cultivation on an industrial level requires very sophisticated and delicate process technologies (cf. Chapter 3).

Cultivation of Microbes

Some microbial species are very popular in biotechnology since they can be cultivated in an easy and safe way. To microbial species with a long lasting tradition in biotechnology belong bacterial species like *Clostridium acetobutyricum, Corynebacterium sp., Xanthomonas sp., Bacillus sp., Lactobacillus sp.* as well as the fungi *Saccharomyces cerevisiae* (baker's yeast), *Penicillium sp.* and *Aspergillus sp.*.

In general, microbes can be cultivated either in vessels or tanks filled with an appropriate liquid growth medium or on plates containing a growth medium solidified with agar (cf. Chapter 3). Culturing in this way implies that the conditions for the growing cells gradually diminish, since nutrients are depleted by the growing cells and growth inhibiting metabolites gradually accumulate. Consequently, microbial growth under these conditions will stop after a while. However, there are culture devices, the continuous culture apparatus, which allow indefinite growth of the microorganisms. This is achieved by continuously adding fresh medium to the culture, meanwhile removing growing cells and metabolites by an overflow device. Under a

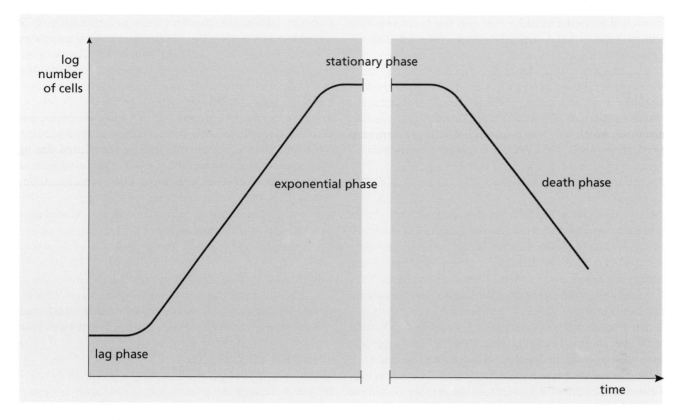

Figure 1.17. Bacterial growth curve.

proper regimen of addition and removal, a "steady state" situation where cells continuously grow is created. The suggestive name for such cultures is "continuous culture". Most industrial biotechnology, however, is based on culturing in tanks without a supply and overflow device. Such culture devices are called "batch cultures".

Figure 1.17 presents a typical picture of bacterial growth in a batch culture. There are several characteristic phases in the so called bacterial growth curve. Bacteria generally do not immediately start multiplying when they are inoculated in a fresh medium. A phase, called the lag phase, where cells do not divide but gradually adapt to the specific growth conditions in the medium precedes the phase where all cells start to divide. This phase, the actual growth phase, is called the logarithmic or exponential phase. The exponential growth phase is for many biotechnological applications very relevant since most of the genes are then optimally expressed. The exponential phase is followed by the stationary phase, where active growth comes to an end due to depletion and spoilage of the medium.

The stage where the exponential growth is about to end is of interest for some biotechnological purposes. At that stage, for reasons that are not completely understood, some microorganisms start the synthesis of so called secondary metabolites. These metabolic products are, according to their name, not essential for the basic cellular metabolism, but may be very relevant as bioproducts. Secondary metabolites relevant for pharmaceutical biotechnology are antibiotics as produced by some microorganisms.

After some time the stationary phase is followed by a phase where the bacteria die off. This stage is clearly not of great interest for biotechnology.

The bacterial growth curve is not directly applicable for microbes that do not reproduce by binary fission. However, a lag phase preceding a phase of active growth and followed by a stationary phase is generally found.

Also in biotechnology time is money and maximum cell yields are therefore required. Thus one tries to keep the lag phase as short as possible and to postpone the onset of the stationary phase. The first goal is achieved by inoculating the tank with cells that, by proper preculturing, are optimally adapted to the medium in the tank. The second goal is achieved in various ways. A successful approach, especially when cells are limited in outgrowth by medium depletion, consists of adding fresh medium near the end of the exponential phase. This technique is called 'fed batch culture'.

To achieve optimal growth of microorganisms it is not only essential to provide a medium with the proper nutrients, but also conditions like pH, oxygen tension and temperature have to be chosen appropriately and should be controlled while cultivating. Last but not least, infection with other microorganisms should be prevented. This requires strict sterility measures and work protocols.

To give an idea about the impressive performance of fast growing microbial cells, such cells may grow with doubling times of about 30 minutes and cultures can easily reach densities of 10^9 cells per mL. If one cultivates bacterial cells on plates, a colony on such plate, appearing after one day or so, might easily harbor millions of cells.

Animal Cell Cultures

Animal cells can be isolated out of a particular tissue after a protease (trypsin) treatment. When such cells are transferred to glass or plastic they will adhere and start growing, if supplied with a suitable liquid growth medium. A cell culture of this type is called a "primary" culture. Such cultures will die after a while and are thus not very useful for biotechnology.

Some animal cell types, however, become exceptional in their growth characteristics when they are cultivated. The main characteristic is that the cell becomes immortal. Such cells are used to prepare "continuous" cell lines. They may survive for months or even years, as long as they are diluted and recultured at frequent intervals. Some cells of malignant origin or originating from normal cells transformed by a virus like the Epstein Barr virus are immortal and grow to high cell densities. For pharmaceutical biotechnology the latter cell lines may be of limited value since they are of malignant nature and may release transforming viruses as a contaminant for the pharmaceutical product. Most useful are non-malignant immortalized cell lines, e.g. 3T3 fibroblasts.

Some cell lines depend on a solid support for their growth, others can be cultivated in suspension which may be advantageous for biotechnology. Successful cultivation of animal cells *in vitro* requires a suitable, in general very complex, growth medium providing not only all nutritional requirements for the cells but also a number of specific growth factors and hormones. The pH must be buffered around 7.0 and proper osmotic conditions isotonic with the cell cytoplasm are required (cf. Chapter 3).

Animal cell cultivation is certainly much more complicated than cultivation of common microorganisms. For pharmaceutical biotechnology there are various safe cell lines available, each with their specific characteristics.

The production of monoclonal antibodies may serve to illustrate an application of animal cell culture within the framework of pharmaceutical biotechnology (cf. Chapter 13). Antibodies are synthesized in the body of man and animals as a consequence of the confrontation with antigens. In an antigen there are in general different parts (so called epitopes), each able to provoke the synthesis of a particular antibody molecule. Consequently, a mixture of antibodies is normally formed in the spleen, the antibody delivering tissue, as a result of the confrontation with an antigenic molecule. However, an individual antibody synthesizing cell, a particular lymphocyte cell, will only produce one very specific type of antibody molecule. If one could propagate such an individual lymphocyte, identical and very specific antibodies, so called monoclonal antibodies, would be obtained. However, lymphocytes can not be cultivated as immortal cell lines. It was a major milestone in science when one succeeded to fuse *in vitro* an antibody synthesizing lymphocyte, isolated from the spleen, with a fast proliferating tumor cell. Such fused cells, called hybridomas, combine the ability of the lymphocyte to produce a specific type of antibody with the ability of the tumor cell to grow as an immortal cell line. Cultivation of hybridomas and concurrent production of monoclonal antibodies is feasible either by injecting such cells in mice or rats or, preferably, as an animal cell culture. In Figure 1.18 the strategy of the hybridoma technology is presented.

Plant Cell Cultures

Plants have always been an important source of pharmacologically active compounds. The complex structure of many of these compounds precludes their chemical synthesis, certainly on a commercial scale. Many active compounds are extracted from intact plants or plant parts. Such compounds usually are present in very low quantities and this has triggered research into the use of alternative production methods.

Cell biologists have tried to produce high levels of active compounds in plant cell cultures but this has not been an easy task. Apart from the problems associated with large scale cell cultures, a major problem with plant cells is that they can not be kept in the differentiated state. When fully differentiated plant tissues are excised to initiate a cell culture this differentiated state is usually lost. Often the compound of interest is made only in specialized tissues in the intact plants. Use of these tissues for cell culture initiation results in a significant decrease in the production of the compound of interest. The addition of plant hormones (e.g. auxins and cytokinins) may alleviate this problem, but up until now efficient production of pharmaceutically interesting compounds in plant cell culture systems is rare. Systems that are available are usually based on procedures involving repeated selection of cell lines with the highest production potential.

Production capacity of cell lines can be further improved by feeding to the culture strategically chosen cheaply available precursors for the compound of interest. The cells then perform the final and chemically most demanding biosynthetic steps. A better understanding of cellular dif-

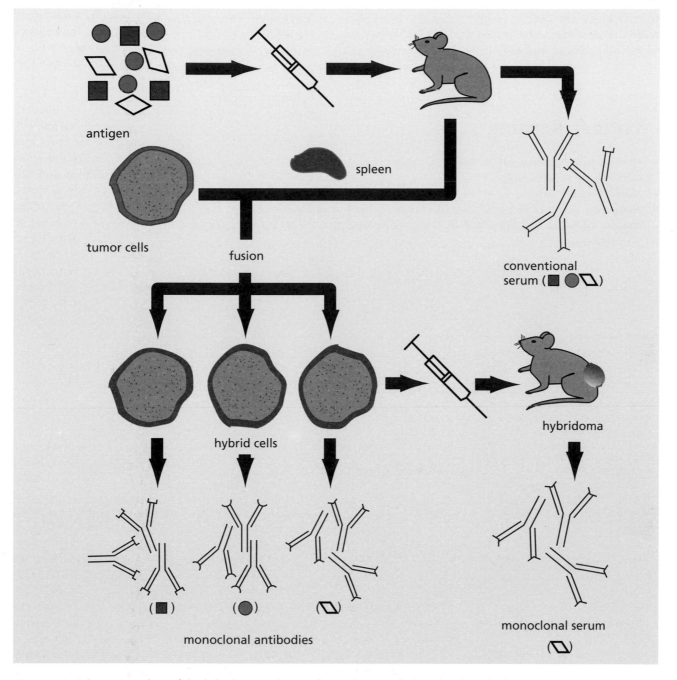

antigen

tumor cells

spleen

fusion

conventional serum (■ ● ◇)

hybrid cells

hybridoma

monoclonal antibodies

(■) (●) (◇)

monoclonal serum

(◇)

Figure 1.18. Schematic outline of the hybridoma technique for production of monoclonal antibodies.

ferentiation processes combined with genetic modification technology of plant cells may help in overcoming these problems and allow for a more efficient use of plant cell cultures in pharmaceutical biotechnology. To circumvent the plant culturing problems one might exploit the recombinant DNA technology, described before. Several of the plant genes which encode enzymes involved in biosynthesis of pharmaceutically active compounds have been cloned. Expression of such genes in heterologous host systems opens an *ex planta* way for enzymatic synthesis of active compounds.

Concluding Remarks

Growing knowledge in the physiology of microbial, animal and plant cells together with detailed insight in gene structure and function has opened new ways for pharmaceutical biotechnology. This chapter is merely an introductory illustration of new approaches based on DNA technology. In order to appreciate and exploit the achievements of cell biology and recombinant DNA technology, further reading is required. The books listed below are just a few out of a large number of excellent books available. ∎

Further Reading

- **Alberts B, Brag D, Lewis J, Raff M, Roberts K, Watson J.** (1994). *Molecular biology of the cell*, 3rd ed., Garland Publ. Inc., New York
- **Brown TA.** (1991). *Gene cloning*, 2nd ed., Chapman and Hall, London
- **Primrose SB.** (1991). *Molecular Biotechnology*, Blackwell Scientific Publications, Oxford
- **Watson J, Gilman M, Wikowski J, Zolle M.** (1992). *Recombinant DNA*, 2nd ed., Freeman and Company, New York

Self-Assessment Questions

Question 1: A bacterial strain carrying a foreign structural gene with its own promoter on an appropriate plasmid does not yield a substantial amount of the encoded gene product.
What factors could explain this failure?

Question 2: What kind of bacterial plasmid is needed in order to function as an optimal vector for DNA cloning in a particular bacterial host?

Question 3: Potential hosts for the biotechnological production by the recombinant-DNA technology of a human protein, lacking functional post-translational modifications, and to be used as a biopharmaceutical are:
a. Escherichia coli K-12
b. Bacillus subtilis
c. Saccharomyces cerevisiae *(a yeast)*
d. Aspergillus nidulans *(a fungus)*
e. plant cells
f. animal cells
Which one(s) would you prefer? Why?

Question 4: Same question as above but now the protein is for its biological activity dependent on specific post-translational modifications.

Question 5: To gain microbial products in biotechnology one may use batch cultures or alternatively continuous cultures. What are the differences between these culture methods and what are the practical consequences of these differences?

Question 6: If one uses a batch culture for production, what kind of measures have to be taken in order to achieve an efficient production yield?

Question 7: If one wants to isolate an animal gene for the purpose of producing the gene product in a bacterial host, what would be the most appropriate isolation procedure?

Question 8: A foreign product, encoded by a recombinant plasmid, appears harmful for the bacterial host which should produce that product. What kind of measures should be taken, in order to gain nevertheless substantial amounts of that product?

Question 9: The PCR technology, using specific primers for Salmonella typhimurium, reveals a clear signal in: 1) a food product, or ii) in a pharmaceutical product produced through biotechnology. What conclusions can be drawn as to the safety of the food product, or of the pharmaceutical product?

Question 10: DNA probes may reveal genetic diseases. Is this feasible with all genetic diseases?

Answers

Answer 1: There are various possible explanations, at each stage of the gene expression something may go wrong or occur with low efficiency. For example:
a) it might be that the authentic promoter of the foreign gene does not (optimally) function in the specific host.
b) it might be that the foreign gene contains introns. Since the bacterial host is not able to cope with introns, a functional gene product is not feasible.
c) the construct may yield a mRNA without appropriate translational signals e.g. a ribosome binding signal. Fusion of the gene towards a leading fragment of a functional bacterial gene might at least overcome the translational start problem. In that case a fused gene product may be produced in substantial amounts.

        d) the mRNA molecule may appear to be very unstable. In that case the gene expression is doomed to be low.

        e) the foreign gene product is produced in the bacterial host, but appears very unstable as it is degraded by one or more of the bacterial proteases. Therefore, one frequently uses bacterial strains with minimal proteolytic activity as production hosts.

Answer   2: The crucial demands are that the plasmid is able to replicate (preferably as a multicopy plasmid) in the specific host and that it is maintained in a stable fashion in the host. Advantages for the optimal application are the presence on the plasmid of selective markers (mostly antibiotic resistance determinants) and a range of restriction sites. A relatively small size of the plasmid will allow rather simple experimental procedures.

Answer   3: The product should be produced in a safe and economic way. Since the product is not depending on post translational modifications, prokaryotic hosts like *E. coli* K-12 or *B. subtilis* are attractive (from the point of safety and economics, based on long lasting biotechnological experience). The fact that *E. coli* is a Gram-negative host causes extra efforts when it comes to purification of the product. A safe biopharmaceutical should be completely free of LPS. Taking this into consideration *B. subtilis* is preferable. The eukaryotic micro-organisms *S. cereviseae* and *A. nidulans* could be options in companies with a lot of experience with these organisms (and most likely with specific patents around the application of such organisms). Plant and animal cells are, *a priori*, not specifically required and are not appropriate, since plant and animal cell cultures are production-wise very demanding.

Answer   4: In this case the prokaryotic organisms can not be used, since they have only a very limited post-translational modification activity. Animal cells could fulfil the post-translational modifications as can the human cells responsible for the protein production. They are therefore, despite high costs, most desirable. However, it is known that *Aspergillus* species are remarkably active in post-translational modification, and it is certainly worthwhile to consider these organisms since they can be cultivated in an economic way.

Answer   5: In the batch culture device the medium is gradually depleted and various (unwanted) metabolites of the growing cells appear, while in the continuous culture device there is a continuous nutrient supply and removal of cells and growth inhibiting metabolites. The practical consequence for cultivation in a batch device is that the production inevitably comes to an end and regular restarts (time and money consuming) of the culture are required. Continuous cultures on the other hand do not need restarts and have the outlook to be more economic. However, the control and handling of a (large scale) continuous culture is complicated.

Answer   6: Prevent an extensive lag phase. This is achieved by using an inoculum for the culture that is optimally adapted to the conditions in the batch device. In addition, one may try to postpone an early onset of the stationary phase, for example by adding extra nutrients after a while.

Answer   7: If the gene encodes a rather small protein with a known amino acid sequence, one may chemically synthesize the gene. If the gene product is a large protein this is not feasible. Since one has to keep in mind that the gene might be endowed with introns, it seems most appropriate to start by isolating mRNA from appropriate sources. mRNA should then be converted into cDNA.

Answer 8: In that case the foreign gene should be controlled by a bacterial promoter that can be switched "on" and "off" at will. Cultivation of the cells under conditions where the promoter is "off", allows cells to grow. When cells are present in large amounts and still metabolically active, the promoter is switched "on" , for example, by addition of a specific promoter activity, inducing agent to the medium.

Answer 9: The signal achieved by PCR reveals specifically the presence of DNA. This DNA might be present as such or set free from *Salmonella* cells, either alive or dead. The safety of a food product depends on the presence of harmful bacterial cells that are alive or, in some instances, on the presence of a toxin produced by the bacterium. Therefore, PCR technology analysis is not conclusive to answer the question whether the food is safe or not. As to the biopharmaceutical, the safety regulations are more stringent as drug safety may be jeopardized by the presence of bacterial constituents (e.g. endo- or exotoxins). Therefore, PCR revealing Salmonella *typhimurium* DNA in a biopharmaceutical is very alarming.

Answer 10: No; only for genetic diseases with a well known and well defined genetic basis, a probe can be developed and used as a detection tool. So far, most genetic diseases are not known at the level of the DNA. Some diseases are known to be the result of rather complex DNA changes and their detection will, therefore, be not amenable for straightforward DNA probing.

2 Biophysical and Biochemical Analyses of Recombinant Proteins

Structure and Analyses of Proteins

by: William C. Kenney and Tsutomu Arakawa

Introduction

For a recombinant protein to become a human therapeutic, its biophysical and biochemical characteristics must be substantially understood. These properties serve as bases for comparison of lot-to-lot reproducibility, for establishing the range of allowable conditions for the protein, and for identifying stability characteristics arising from long-term storage.

A number of tools are available to characterize recombinant proteins. Various spectrophotometric techniques can be utilized to determine the biophysical properties of proteins and a number of analytical techniques are available to examine their biochemical and biological integrity. Where possible, the results of these experiments are compared to those obtained using naturally occurring proteins in order to be confident that the recombinant protein has the desired characteristics of the naturally occurring one.

Protein Structure

Primary Structure

Most proteins which are developed as therapeutic drugs perform specific functions by interacting with other small and large molecules, e.g., cell surface receptors, binding proteins, nucleic acids, carbohydrates and lipids. The functional properties of proteins are derived by their folding into distinct three-dimensional structures. Protein folding occurs based on polypeptide sequence in which twenty different amino acids are connected through peptide bonds in a specific way. This alignment of twenty amino acids, called a primary sequence, has in general all the necessary information for folding into a distinct tertiary structure. Because these twenty amino acids possess different side chains, polypeptides with widely diverse properties are obtained.

All of the twenty amino acids consist of a C_α carbon to which an amino group, a carboxyl group, a hydrogen and a side chain bind in L configuration (Figure 2.1). These amino acids are joined by condensation to yield a peptide bond consisting of a carboxyl group of an amino acid joined

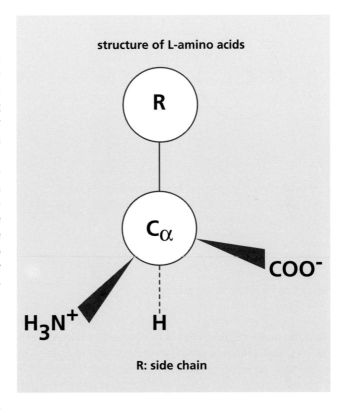

structure of L-amino acids

R

C_α

H_3N^+ H   COO⁻

R: side chain

Figure 2.1. Structure of L-amino acids.

with the amino group of the next amino acid (Figure 2.2). The condensation gives an amide group, NH, at the N-terminal side of C_α and a carbonyl group, C=O, at the C-terminal side. These groups, as well as the amino acyl side chains, play important roles in protein folding. Due to their ability to form hydrogen bonds, they make major energetic contributions to the formation of two important secondary structures, α-helix and β-sheet. The peptide bonds between various amino acids are very much equivalent, however, so that they do not determine which part of a sequence should form α-helix or β-sheet. Sequence-dependent secondary structure formation is determined by the side chains.

The twenty amino acids commonly found in proteins are shown in Figure 2.3. They are described by their full names and three- and one-letter codes. Their side chains

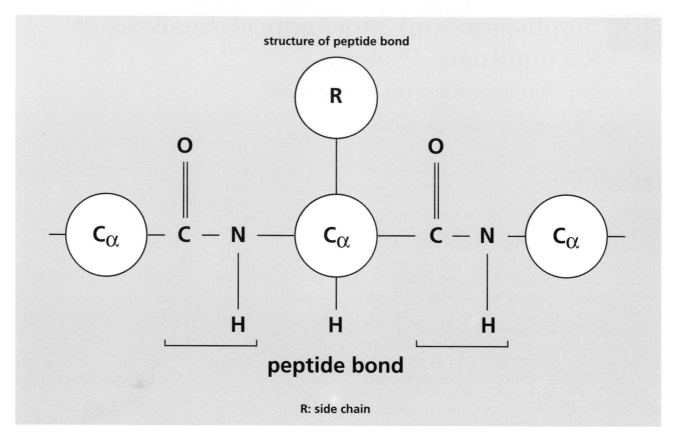

Figure 2.2. Structure of peptide bond.

are structurally different in such a way that at neutral pH, aspartic and glutamic acids are negatively charged and lysine and arginine are positively charged. Histidine is positively charged, the extent of which depends on the pH. At pH 7.0, on average about half of the side chains are positively charged. Tyrosine and cysteine are protonated and uncharged at neutral pH, but become negatively charged above pH 10 and 8, respectively.

Polar amino acids consist of serine, threonine, asparagine, and glutamine as well as cysteine, while non-polar amino acids consist of alanine, valine, phenylalanine, proline, methionine, leucine, and isoleucine. Glycine behaves neutrally while cystine, the oxidized form of cysteine, is characterized as hydrophobic. Although tyrosine and tryptophan often enter into polar interactions, they are better characterized as non-polar, or hydrophobic as described later.

These twenty amino acids are incorporated into an unique sequence based on the genetic code, as the following example in Figure 2.4 shows. This is an amino acid sequence of granulocyte-colony stimulating factor (G-CSF), which selectively regulates proliferation and maturation of neutrophils. Although the exact property of this protein depends on the location of each amino acid, hence each side chain

in the three-dimensional structure, the average property can be estimated simply from its amino acid composition, as shown in Table 2.1; i.e., a list of the total number of each amino acid contained in this protein molecule.

Using the pK_a values of these side chains and one amino and carboxyl terminus, one can calculate total and net charges of a protein as a function of pH, i.e., a titration curve. Since cysteine can be oxidized to form a disulfide bond or can be in a free form, accurate calculation above pH 8 requires knowledge of the status of cysteinyl residues in the protein. The titration curve thus obtained is only an approximation, since some charged residues may be buried and the effective pKa values depend on the location of each residue. Nevertheless, the calculated titration curve gives a clue as to the overall charged state of a protein at a given pH and hence its solution property. The other molecular parameters such as isoelectric point, molecular weight, extinction coefficient, partial specific volume and hydrophobicity can also be estimated from the amino acid composition, as shown in Table 2.1.

The primary structure of a protein, i.e., the sequence of the twenty amino acids, can lead to the three-dimensional structure because the amino acids have diverse physical

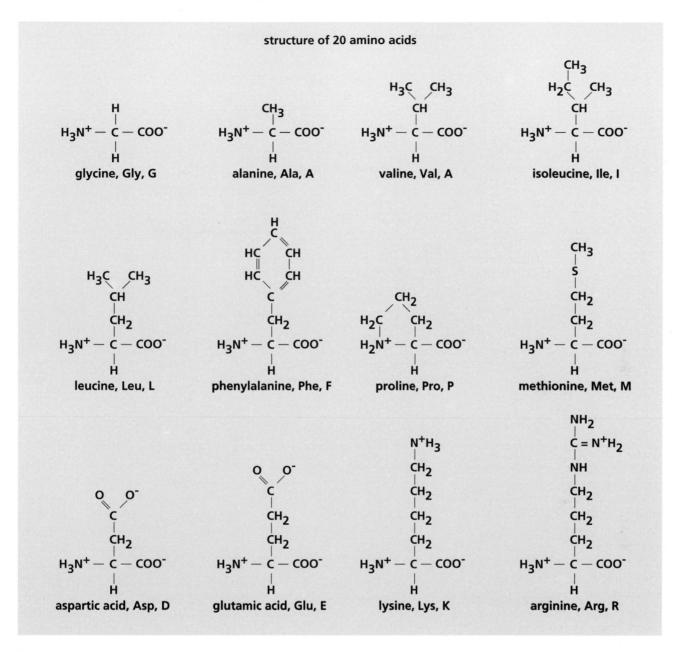

Figure 2.3a. Structure of 20 amino acids.

properties. First, each type of amino acid has the tendency to be more preferentially incorporated into certain secondary structures. The frequencies of each amino acid found in α-helix, β-sheet and β-turn, secondary structures that are discussed later in this chapter, can be calculated from a number of proteins whose three-dimensional structures have been solved. These are listed in Table 2.2. The β-turn has a distinct configuration consisting of four sequential amino acids and there is a strong preference for specific amino acids in these four positions. For example, although

asparagine has an overall high frequency of occurrence in a β-turn, it is most frequently observed in the first and

TPLGPASSLPQSFLLKCLEQVRKIQGDGAALQEKLCATYK	40
LCHPEELVLLGHSLGIPWAPLSSCPSQALQLAGCLSQLHS	80
GLFLYQGLLQALEGISPELGPTLDTLQLDVADFATTIWQQ	120
MEELGMAPALQPTQGAMPAFASAFQRRAGGVLVASHLQSF	160
LEVSYRVLRHLAQP	

Figure 2.4. Amino acid sequence of granulocyte-colony stimulating factor.

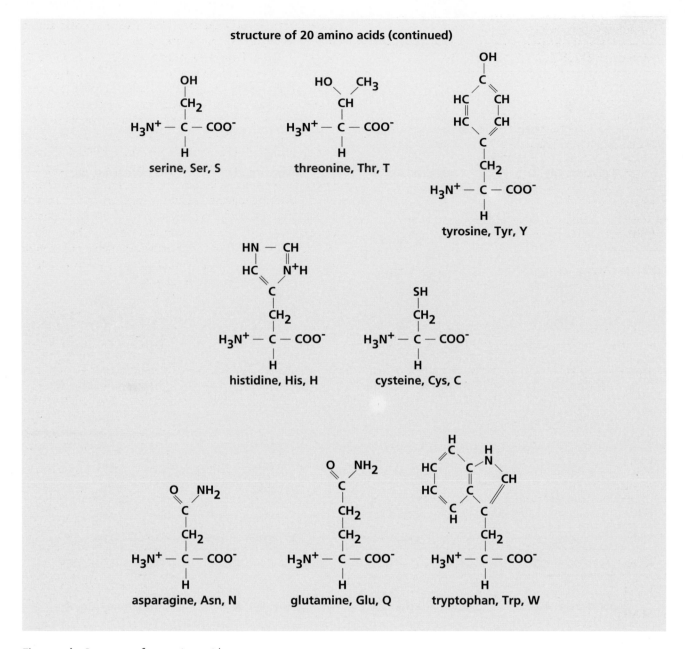

structure of 20 amino acids (continued)

serine, Ser, S

threonine, Thr, T

tyrosine, Tyr, Y

histidine, His, H

cysteine, Cys, C

asparagine, Asn, N

glutamine, Glu, Q

tryptophan, Trp, W

Figure 2.3b. Structure of 20 amino acids.

third position of a β-turn. This characteristic of asparagine is consistent with its side chain as a potential and only site of N-linked glycosylation. Effects of glycosylation on the biological and physicochemical properties of proteins are extremely important; however, their contribution to structure is not readily predictable based on the amino acid composition.

Based on these numbers, one can predict the folding of polypeptide segments as to which type of secondary structure they prefer to form. As shown in Figure 2.5, there are a number of methods developed to predict the secondary structure from the primary sequence of the proteins. Using G-CSF as an example, regions of α-helix, β-sheets, turns, hydrophilicity, and antigen sites can be suggested.

Another property of amino acids, which impacts on protein folding, is the hydrophobicity of their side chains. Although non-polar amino acids are basically hydrophobic, it is important to know how hydrophobic they are. This property has been determined by measuring the partition coefficient or solubility of amino acids in water and organic solvents and normalizing such parameters relative to glycine. Relative to the side chain of glycine, H, such normalization

Parameter	Value
Molecular weight	18673
Total number of amino acids	174
1 microgram	53.5 picomoles
Molar extinction coefficient	15820
1 A(280)	1.18 mg/ml
Isoelectric point	5.86
Charge at pH 7	- 3.39

Table 2.1a. Amino acid composition and structural parameters of granulocyte colony stimulating factor.

shows how strongly the side chains of non-polar amino acids prefer the organic phase to the aqueous phase. A representation of such measurements is shown in Table 2.3. The values indicate the increase in free energies in bringing the side chains from organic solvent to water. Transfer of tryptophan and tyrosine to water causes a loss of substantial energy. Conversely, transfer of those residues from water to organic solvent results in a decrease of energy. Although it is unclear how comparable the hydrophobic property is between an organic solvent and the interior of protein molecules, the hydrophobic side chains favor clustering together, resulting in a core structure with a property similar to an organic solvent. These hydrophobic characteristics of non-polar amino acids and hydrophilic characteristics of polar amino acids generate a partition of amino acyl residues into a hydrophobic core and hydrophilic surface, resulting in overall folding.

Amino acid	Number	% by weight	% by frequency
A Ala	19	7.23	10.92
C Cys	5	2.76	2.87
D Asp	4	2.47	2.30
E Glu	9	6.22	5.17
F Phe	6	4.73	3.45
G Gly	14	4.28	8.05
H His	5	3.67	2.87
I Ile	4	2.42	2.30
K Lys	4	2.75	2.30
L Leu	33	20.00	18.97
M Met	3	2.11	1.72
N Asn	0	0.00	0.00
P Pro	13	6.76	7.47
Q Gln	17	11.66	9.77
R Arg	5	4.18	2.87
S Ser	14	6.53	8.05
T Thr	7	3.79	4.02
V Val	7	3.71	4.02
W Trp	2	1.99	1.15
Y Tyr	3	2.62	1.72

Table 2.1b. Amino acid composition and structural parameters of granulocyte colony stimulating factor.

α-helix		β-sheet		β-turn		β-turn position 1		β-turn position 2		β-turn position 3		β-turn position 4	
Glu	1.51	Val	1.70	Asn	1.56	Asn	0.161	Pro	0.301	Asn	0.191	Trp	0.167
Met	1.45	Ile	1.60	Gly	1.56	Cys	0.149	Ser	0.139	Gly	0-.190	Gly	0.152
Ala	1.42	Tyr	1.47	Pro	1.52	Asp	0.147	Lys	0.115	Asp	0.179	Cys	0.128
Leu	1.21	Phe	1.38	Asp	1.46	His	0.140	Asp	0.110	Ser	0.125	Tyr	0.125
Lys	1.16	Trp	1.37	Ser	1.43	Ser	0.120	Thr	0.108	Cys	0.117	Ser	0.106
Phe	1.13	Leu	1.30	Cys	1.19	Pro	0.102	Arg	0.106	Tyr	0.114	Gln	0.098
Gln	1.11	Cys	1.19	Tyr	1.14	Gly	0.102	Gln	0.098	Arg	0.099	Lys	0.095
Trp	1.08	Thr	1.19	Lys	1.01	Thr	0.086	Gly	0.085	His	0.093	Asn	0.091
Ile	1.08	Gln	1.10	Gln	0.98	Tyr	0.082	Asn	0.083	Glu	0.077	Arg	0.085
Val	1.06	Met	1.05	Thr	0.96	Trp	0.077	Met	0.082	Lys	0.072	Asp	0.081
Asp	1.01	Arg	0.93	Trp	0.96	Gln	0.074	Ala	0.076	Tyr	0.065	Thr	0.079
His	1.00	Asn	0.89	Arg	0.95	Arg	0.070	Tyr	0.065	Phe	0.065	Leu	0.070
Arg	0.98	His	0.87	His	0.95	Met	0.068	Glu	0.060	Trp	0.064	Pro	0.068
Thr	0.83	Ala	0.83	Glu	0.74	Val	0.062	Cys	0.053	Gln	0.037	Phe	0.065
Ser	0.77	Ser	0.75	Ala	0.66	Leu	0.061	Val	0.048	Leu	0.036	Glu	0.064
Cys	0.70	Gly	0.75	Met	0.60	Ala	0.060	His	0.047	Ala	0.035	Ala	0.058
Tyr	0.69	Lys	0.74	Phe	0.60	Phe	0.059	Phe	0.041	Pro	0.034	Ile	0.056
Asn	0.67	Pro	0.55	Leu	0.59	Glu	0.056	Ile	0.034	Val	0.028	Met	0.055
Pro	0.57	Asp	0.54	Val	0.50	Lys	0.055	Leu	0.025	Met	0.014	His	0.054
Gly	0.57	Glu	0.37	Ile	0.47	Ile	0.043	Trp	0.013	Ile	0.013	Val	0.053

Table 2.2. Frequency of occurrence of 20 Amino acids in α-helix, β-sheet and β-turn. Taken and edited from Chou PY and Fasman GD, 1978, Ann. Rev. Biochem. 47, 251–276 with permission from Annual Reviews, Inc.

Secondary Structure

α-HELIX

Immediately evident in the primary structure of protein is that each amino acid is linked by a peptide bond. The amide, NH, is a hydrogen donor and the carbonyl, C=O, is a hydrogen acceptor, and they can form a stable hydrogen bond when they are positioned in an appropriate configu-ration of the polypeptide chain. Such structures of the polypeptide chain are called secondary structure. Two main structures, α-helix and β-sheet, accommodate such stable hydrogen bonds. The main chain forms a right-handed helix, because only the L-form of amino acids are in pro-teins, and makes one turn per 3.6 residues. The overall length of α-helices can vary widely. Figure 2.6 shows an example of a short α-helix. In this case, the C=O group of residue 1 forms a hydrogen bond to the NH group of

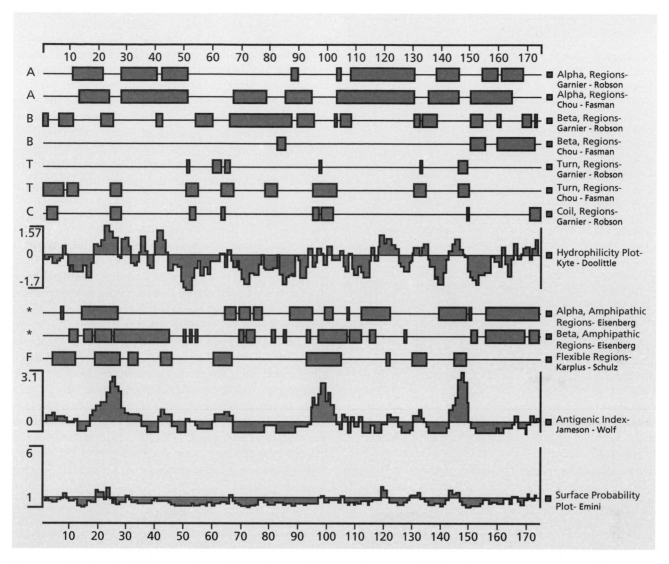

Figure 2.5. Predicted secondary structure of granulocyte-colony stimulating factor. Obtained using a program "DNA Star" (DNASTAR Inc., Madison, WI).

residue 5 and C=O group of residue 2 forms a hydrogen bond with the NH group of residue 6. Thus, at the start of an α-helix, four amide groups are always free and at the end of an α-helix four carboxyl groups are also free. As a result, both ends of an α-helix are highly polar.

Moreover, all the hydrogen bonds are aligned along the helical axis. Since both peptide NH and C=O groups have dipole moments pointing in the same direction, they will add to a substantial dipole moment throughout the entire α-helix, with the negative partial charge at the C-terminal side and the positive partial charge at the N-terminal side.

The side chains project outward from the α-helix. This means that all the side chains surround the outer surface of an α-helix and interact with each other and with side chains of other regions which come in contact with these side chains. These interactions, so-called long-range interactions, can stabilize the α-helical structure and act as a folding unit. Often an α-helix serves as a building block for the three-dimensional structure of globular proteins by bringing hydrophobic side chains to one side of a helix and hydrophilic side chains to the opposite side of the same helix. Distribution of side chains along the α-helical axis can be viewed using the helical wheel. Since one turn in an α-helix is 3.6 residue long, each residue can be plotted every 360/3.6 = 100° around a circle (viewed from the top of α-helix), as shown in Figure 2.7. Such a plot shows the projection of the position of the residues onto a plane perpendicular to the helical axis. One of the helices present in erythropoietin is shown in Figure 2.7, using an open circle for hydrophobic side chains and an open rectangle

Amino acid side chain	cal/mole
Tryptophan	3400
Norleucine	2600
Phenylalanine	2500
Tyrosine	2300
Dihydroxyphenylalanine	1800
Leucine	1800
Valine	1500
Methionine	1300
Histidine	500
Alanine	500
Threonine	400
Serine	- 300

Table 2.3. Hydrophobicity scale: transfer free energies of amino acid side chains from organic solvent to water. Taken from Nozaki Y and Tanford C, 1971, J. Biol. Chem., 246, 2211–2217 with permission from American Society of Biological Chemists.

for hydrophilic side chains. It becomes immediately obvious that one side of the α-helix is highly hydrophobic, suggesting that this side forms an internal core, while the other side is relatively hydrophilic most likely exposed to the surface. Since many biologically important proteins function by interacting with other macromolecules, the information obtained from the helical wheel is extremely useful. For example, mutations of amino acids in the solvent-exposed side may lead to identification of regions responsible for biological activity while mutations in the internal core may lead to altered protein stability.

β-SHEET STRUCTURE

The second major structural element found in proteins is the β-sheet. In contrast to the α-helix, which is built up from a continuous region with a peptide hydrogen bond linking every fourth amino acid, the β-sheet is comprised of peptide hydrogen bonds of different regions of the polypeptide which may be far apart in sequence. β-strands can interact with each other in one of two ways as shown in Figure 2.8, i.e., either parallel or antiparallel. In a parallel β-sheet, each strand is oriented in the same direction with peptide hydrogen bonds formed between the strands, while in antiparallel β-sheets, the polypeptide sequences are oriented in the opposite direction. In both structures, the C=O and NH groups project into opposite sides of the polypeptide chain, and hence a β-strand can interact from either side of that particular chain to form peptide

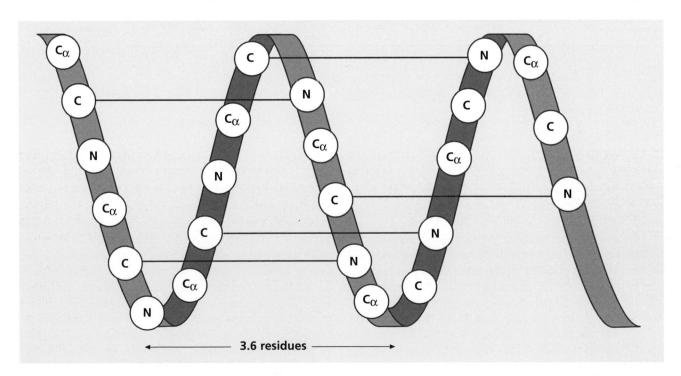

Figure 2.6. Schematic illustration of the structure of α-helix.

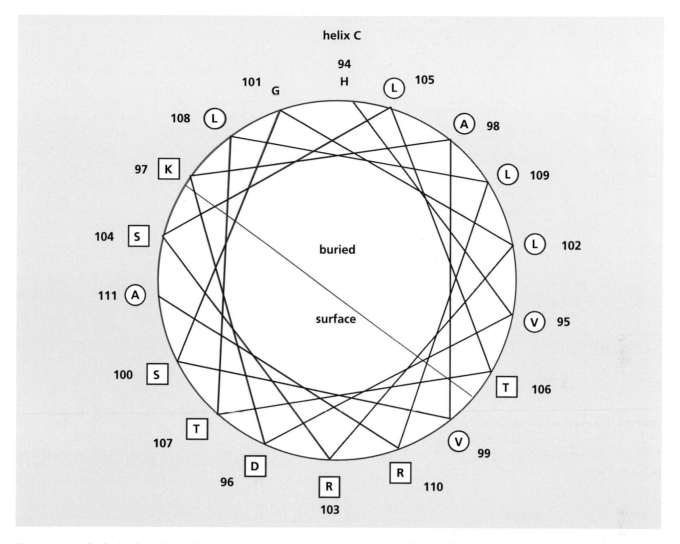

Figure 2.7. Helical wheel analysis of erythropoietin sequence, from His94 to Ala111 (Elliott, S., personal communication).

hydrogen bonds with adjacent strands. Thus, more than two β-strands can contact each other either in a parallel or in an antiparallel manner, or even in combination. Such clustering can result in all the β-strands lining a plane as a sheet. The β-strands which are at the edges of the sheet have unpaired alternating C=O and NH groups.

Side chains project perpendicularly to this plane in opposite directions and can interact with other side chains within the same β-sheet or with other regions of the molecule, or are exposed to the solvent.

In almost all known protein structures, β-strands are right-handed twisted. This way, the β-strands adapt into widely different conformations. Depending on how they are twisted, all the side chains in the same strand or in different strands do not necessarily project into the same direction.

LOOPS AND TURNS

Loops and turns form more or less linear structures, and interact with each other to form a folded three-dimensional structure. They are comprised of an amino acid sequence which is usually hydrophilic and exposed to the solvent. These regions consist of β-turns (reverse turns), short hairpin loops, and long loops. Many hairpin loops are formed to connect two antiparallel β-strands.

As shown in Figure 2.5, the amino acid sequences which form β-turns are relatively easy to predict, since turns must be present periodically to fold a linear sequence into a globular structure. Amino acids found most frequently in the β-turn are usually not found in α-helical or β-sheet structures. Thus, proline and glycine represent the least observed amino acids in these typical secondary structures,

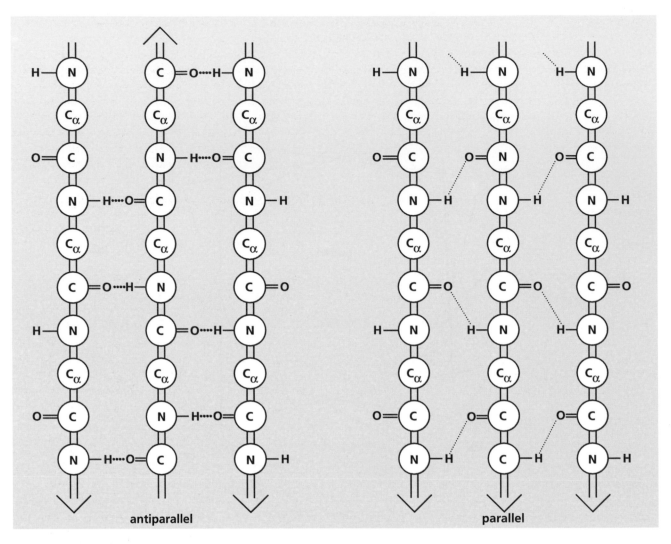

Figure 2.8. Schematic illustration of the structure of antiparallel (left side) and parallel (right side) β-sheet. Arrow indicates the direction of amino acid sequence from the N-terminus to C-terminus.

however, proline has an extremely high frequency of occurrence at the second position in the β-turn while glycine has a high preference at the third and fourth position of a β-turn.

Although loops are not as predictable as β-turns, those amino acids with high frequency for β-turns also can form a long loop. Even though difficult to predict, loops are an important secondary structure, since they form a highly solvent exposed region of the protein molecules and allow the protein to fold onto itself.

Tertiary Structure

Combination of the various secondary structures in a protein results in its three-dimensional structure. Many proteins fold into a fairly compact, globular structure. The way

secondary structures in most globular proteins are packed is rather limited in number.

Folding of a protein molecule into a distinct three-dimensional structure determines its function. Enzyme activity requires exact coordination of catalytically important residues in the three-dimensional space. Binding of antibody to antigen and those of growth factors and cytokines to their receptors all require a distinct, specific surface for high affinity binding. These interactions do not occur if the tertiary structures of antibodies, growth factors and cytokines are altered.

A unique tertiary structure of a protein can often result in assembly of the protein into a distinct quaternary structure consisting of a fixed stoichiometry of protein within the complex. Assembly can occur between the same proteins or between different polypeptide chains. Each molecule in the complex is called a subunit. Actin and tubulin self-associate into F-actin and microtubule, while hemoglobin is a tetramer consisting of two α and two β subunits. Among the cytokines and growth factors, interferon-γ is a homodimer, while platelet-derived growth factor is a homodimer of A or B chain or a heterodimer of A and B chains. The formation of a quaternary structure occurs via non-covalent interaction or through disulfide bonds between the subunits.

Forces

Interactions occur between groups in proteins which are responsible for formation of their secondary, tertiary and quaternary structures. Either repulsive or attractive interactions can occur between different groups. Repulsive interactions consist of steric hindrance, electrostatic effects and increased entropy. Like-charges repel each other and bulky side chains, although they do not repel each other, cannot occupy the same space. Folding is against the nature which moves toward randomness, i.e., increasing entropy. Folding leads to a fixed position of each atom and hence a decrease in entropy. Repulsive interactions are overcome by attractive interactions, i.e., hydrophobic interactions, hydrogen bonds, electrostatic interaction and van der Waals interactions. Hydration of proteins, discussed in the next section, also plays an important role in protein folding.

These interactions are all relatively weak and can be easily broken and formed, hence, folded protein structures arise from a fine balance between these repulsive and attractive interactions. This stability of the folded structure is a fundamental concern in developing protein therapeutics.

HYDROPHOBIC INTERACTIONS

The hydrophobic interaction reflects a summation of the van der Waals attractive forces among non-polar groups in the protein interior, which change the surrounding water structure necessary to accommodate these groups when they become exposed. The transfer of non-polar groups from the interior to the surface comprises a large decrease in the entropy term so that hydrophobic interactions are essentially entropically driven. The resulting large positive free energy change prevents the transfer of nonpolar groups from the largely sheltered interior to the more solvent exposed exterior of the protein molecule. Thus, nonpolar groups preferentially reside in the protein interior while the more polar groups are exposed to the surface and surrounding environment. The partitioning of different amino acyl residues between the inside and outside of a protein correlates well with the hydration energy of their side chains, that is, their relative affinity for water. This illustrates the aspect of solvent effects on hydrophobic interactions (cf. Table 2.3).

HYDROGEN BONDS

The hydrogen bond is ionic in character since it depends strongly on the sharing of a proton between two electronegative atoms (generally oxygen and nitrogen atoms). Hydrogen bonds may form either between a protein atom and a water molecule or exclusively as protein intramolecular hydrogen bonds. Intramolecular interactions can have significantly greater free energies (because of entropic considerations) than intermolecular hydrogen bonds, so the contribution of all hydrogen bonds in the protein molecule to the stability of protein structures can be substantial. In addition, when the hydrogen bonds occur in the interior of protein molecules, the bonds become stronger due to the hydrophobic environment.

ELECTROSTATIC INTERACTIONS

Electrostatic interactions occur between any two charged groups. According to Coulomb's law, if the charges are of the same sign, the interaction is repulsive with an increase in energy, but if they are opposite in sign it is attractive, with a lowering of energy. Electrostatic interactions are strongly dependent upon distance, according to Coulomb's law, and dielectric constant of the medium. The numerous charged groups present on protein molecules can provide overall stability by the electrostatic attraction of opposite charges, for example, between negatively charged carboxyl groups and positively charged amino groups. Thus, the free energy derived from electrostatic interactions is actually a property of the whole structure, not just of any single amino acid residue or cluster. Electrostatic interactions are much stronger in the interior of the protein molecule because of a lower dielectric constant.

VAN DER WAALS INTERACTIONS

Weak van der Waals interactions exist between atoms (except the bare proton), whether they are polar or nonpolar. They arise from net attractive interactions between permanent dipoles and/or induced (temporary and fluctuating) dipoles. However, when two atoms approach each other closely, the repulsion between their electron clouds becomes strong and counterbalances the attractive forces. This repulsive force is highly sensitive to the distance between two atoms.

Hydration

Water molecules are bound to proteins internally and externally. Some water molecules occasionally occupy small internal cavities in the protein structure, and are hydrogen-bonded to peptide bonds and side chains of the protein and often to a prosthetic group, or cofactor, within the protein.

The protein surface is extensive and consists of a mosaic of polar and nonpolar amino acids, and it binds a large amount of water molecules, i.e., it is hydrated, from the surrounding environment. As described in the previous section, water molecules trapped in the interior of protein molecules are bound more tightly to hydrogen-bonding donors and acceptors because of a lower dielectric constant.

Solvent around the protein surface clearly has a general role in hydrating peptide and side chains but might be expected to be rather mobile and non-specific in its interactions. Well-ordered water molecules can make significant contributions to protein stability. One water molecule can hydrogen-bond to two groups distant in the primary structure on a protein molecule, acting as a bridge between these groups. Such a water molecule may be highly restricted in motion, and can contribute to the stability, at least locally, of the protein, since such tight binding may be available only when these groups assume the proper configuration to accommodate a water molecule that is present only in the native state of the protein. Such hydration can also decrease the flexibility of the groups involved.

There is evidence also for solvation of hydrophobic groups on the protein surface. So-called hydrophobic hydration occurs because of the unfavorable nature of the interaction between water molecules and hydrophobic surface, resulting in clustering of water molecules. Since this is energetically unfavorable, such hydrophobic hydration does not contribute to the protein stability. However, this hydrophobic hydration facilitates hydrophobic interaction. This unfavorable hydration is diminished as the various hydrophobic groups come in contact either intramolecularly or intermolecularly, leading to folding of intrachain structures or protein-protein interactions.

Both the loosely and strongly bound water molecules can have an important impact not only on protein stability but also protein function. For example, certain enzymes function in non-aqueous solvent, provided that a small amount of water, just enough to cover the protein surface, is present. Hydrated water can modulate the dynamics of surface groups. Such dynamics may be critical for enzyme function. Dried enzymes are in general inactive and become active after they absorb 0.2 g water per g protein. This amount of water is only sufficient to cover surface polar groups, yet may give flexibility for function.

Evidence that water bound to protein molecules has different properties from bulk water was demonstrated by the presence of non-freezable water. Thus, when a protein solution is cooled below –40°C, a fraction of water, ~0.3 g water/g protein, does not freeze and can be detected by high resolution NMR. Several other techniques also detect a similar amount of bound water. This unfreezable water reflects the unique property of bound water that prevents it from adapting an ice structure.

Protein Folding

Proteins become functional only when they assume a distinct tertiary structure. Many physiologically and therapeutically important proteins present their surface for recognition by the interacting molecules such as substrates, receptors, and cell-surface adhesion macromolecules. When recombinant proteins are produced in *Escherichia coli*, they often form inclusion bodies into which they are deposited as insoluble proteins. Formation of such insoluble states does not naturally occur in cells where they are normally synthesized and transported. Therefore, an *in vitro* process is required to refold insoluble recombinant proteins into the native, physiologically active state. This is usually accomplished by solubilizing the insoluble proteins with detergents or denaturants followed by purification and removal of these reagents concurrent with refolding the proteins (cf. Chapter 3).

Unfolded states of proteins are usually highly stable and soluble when occurring in the presence of denaturing agents. Once the proteins are folded correctly, they are also relatively stable. During the transition from the unfolded form to the native state, the protein must go through a multitude of other transition states in which it is not fully folded and denaturants or solubilizing agents are at low concentrations or even absent.

Refolding of proteins can be achieved in various ways. Dilution of proteins at high denaturant concentration into aqueous buffer will decrease both denaturant and protein concentration simultaneously. Addition of aqueous buffer to denaturant-protein solution also causes a decrease in concentrations of both denaturant and protein. The difference in these procedures is that in the first case both denaturant and protein concentrations are the lowest at the beginning of dilution and gradually increase as the process continues. In the second case, both denaturant and protein concentrations are highest at the beginning of dilution and gradually decrease as the dilution proceeds. Dialysis or diafiltration of proteins in the denaturant against an aqueous buffer resembles the second case, since the denaturant concentration decreases as the procedure continues. In this case, however, the protein concentration remains unchanged. Refolding can also be achieved by first binding the protein in denaturants to a solid phase, i.e., a column matrix, and then equilibrating it with an aqueous buffer. In this case, protein concentrations are not well-defined. Each procedure has advantages and disadvantages and may be applicable for one protein, but not to another.

If proteins in the native state have disulfide bonds, cysteines must be correctly oxidized. Such oxidation may be done in various ways, e.g., air oxidation, glutathione catalyzed disulfide exchange, or adduct formation followed by reduction and oxidation or by disulfide reshuffling.

Protein folding has been a topic of intensive research since Anfinsen's demonstration that ribonuclease can be refolded from the fully reduced and denatured state in *in vitro* experiments. This can be achieved only if the amino acid sequence itself contains all the information necessary for folding into the native structure. This is the case, at least partially, for many proteins. Most proteins, however, do not refold in a simple one-step process, rather they refold via various intermediates which are relatively compact and possess varying degrees of secondary structures, but lack a rigid tertiary structure. Intrachain interactions of these preformed secondary structures eventually lead to the native state, however, the absence of a rigid structure in these preformed secondary structures also can expose a cluster of hydrophobic groups to those of other polypeptide chains, instead of their own polypeptide segments, resulting in intermolecular aggregation. High efficiency in the recovery of native protein depends heavily on how this aggregation of intermediate forms is minimized. Use of chaperones or polyethylene glycol has been found quite effective for this purpose. The former are proteins which aid in the proper folding of other proteins by stabilizing intermediates in the folding process and the latter serves to solvate the protein during folding and diminishes interchain aggregation events.

When recombinant proteins are expressed in eukaryotic cells and secreted into media, the proteins are in general folded into the native conformation. If the proteins have sites for N-linked or O-linked glycosylation, they undergo varying degrees of glycosylation depending on host cells used and level of expression. For many glycoproteins, glycosylation is not essential for folding, since they can be refolded into the native conformation without carbohydrates, nor is glycosylation often necessary for receptor binding and hence biological activity. However, glycosylation can alter the biological and physicochemical properties of proteins such as pharmacokinetics, solubility, and stability.

Techniques for Characterizing Folding

Conventional techniques used to obtain information on the folded structure of proteins are circular dichroism (CD), fluorescence, and Fourier transform infrared spectroscopies (FTIR). CD and FTIR are widely used to estimate the secondary structure of proteins. The α-helical content of a protein can be readily estimated by CD in the far UV region (180–260 nm) and by FTIR. FTIR signals from loop structures, however, occasionally overlap with those arising from an α-helix. The β-sheet gives weak CD signals, which are variable in peak positions and intensities due to twists of interacting β-strands, making far UV CD unreliable for evaluation of these structures. On the other hand, FTIR can reliably estimate the β-structure content as well as distinguish between parallel and antiparallel forms.

CD in the near UV region (250–340 nm) reflects the environment of aromatic amino acids, i.e., tryptophan, tyrosine and phenylalanine and of disulfide structures. Fluorescence spectroscopy yields information on the environment of tyrosine and tryptophan residues. In many cases, CD and fluorescence signals are drastically altered upon refolding and hence can be used to follow formation of the tertiary structure of a protein.

None of these techniques can give the folded structure at the atomic level, i.e., they give no information on the exact location of each amino acid residue in the three-dimensional structure of the protein. This can only be determined by X-ray crystallography or NMR. The above mentioned spectroscopic methods, however, are fast and require lower protein concentrations than either NMR or X-ray crystallography, and are amenable to examine the protein under widely different conditions. When a naturally occurring form of the protein is available, these techniques, in particular near UV CD and fluorescence spectroscopies, can quickly address whether the refolded protein assumes the native folded structure.

Temperature dependence of these spectroscopic properties also gives a clue about protein folding. Since the folded structures of proteins are built upon cooperative interactions of many side chains and peptide bonds in a protein molecule, elimination of one interaction by heat can cause cooperative elimination of other interactions, leading to unfolding of protein molecules, i.e., many proteins undergo a cooperative thermal transition over a narrow temperature range. Conversely, if the proteins are not fully folded, they may undergo non-cooperative thermal transitions as observed by a gradual signal change over a wider range of temperature. Microcalorimetry is a powerful technique for these studies, since cooperative thermal unfolding usually gives a sharp endotherm peak with increasing temperature.

Hydrodynamic properties of proteins change greatly upon folding, going from elongated and expanded structures to compact globular ones. Sedimentation velocity and size exclusion chromatography are two frequently used techniques to evaluate hydrodynamic properties, although the latter is much more accessible. Sedimentation coefficient (how fast a molecule migrates in a centrifugal field) is a function of the molecular weight and hydrodynamic size of the proteins while elution position in size exclusion chromatography (how fast it migrates through pores) depends on only the hydrodynamic size. In both methods, comparison of sedimentation coefficient or elution position with that of a globular protein with an identical molecular weight (or upon appropriate molecular weight normalization) gives information on how compactly the protein is folded.

For oligomeric proteins, determination of the molecular weight of the associated states and establishment of the quaternary structure can be used to assess the folded structure. For strong interactions, specific protein association requires that intersubunit contact surfaces perfectly match each other. Such an associated structure, if obtained by covalent bonding, may be determined simply by sodium dodecylsulfate polyacrylamide gel electrophoresis. If protein association involves non-covalent interactions, sedimentation equilibrium or light scattering experiments can assess this phenomenon. Although these techniques have been used for many decades with some difficulty, emerging technologies in analytical ultracentrifugation and laser light scattering, and appropriate software to analyze the results, have greatly facilitated their general use.

Site specific chemical modification and proteolytic digestion are also powerful techniques for studying the folding of proteins. The extent of chemical modification or proteolytic digestion depends on whether the specific sites are exposed to the solvent or are buried in the interior of the protein molecules and thus inaccessible to these modifications. For example, trypsin cleaves peptide bonds on the C-terminal side of basic residues. Although most proteins contain several basic residues, brief exposure of the

native protein to trypsin usually generates only a few peptides, as cleavage occurs only at the accessible basic residues, whereas the same treatment can generate many more peptides when done on the denatured (unfolded) protein, since all the basic residues are now accessible.

Protein Stability

Although proteins may be folded into a distinct three-dimensional structure, the folded structure does not necessarily mean that it retains this structure in aqueous solution indefinitely. This is because proteins are neither chemically nor physically stable. The protein surface is chemically highly heterogeneous and contains reactive groups. Long term exposure of these groups to environmental stresses causes various chemical alterations. Many proteins including growth factors and cytokines have cysteine residues. If some of them are in a free, or sulfhydryl, form, they may undergo oxidation and disulfide exchange. Oxidation can also occur on methionyl residues. Hydrolysis can occur on peptide bonds and on amides of asparagine

	Physical property effected	Method of analysis

Oxidation
  Cys
    Disulfide
      intrachain
      interchain
  Met, Trp, Tyr
	hydrophobicity
	size
	hydrophobicity
		RP-HPLC, SDS-PAGE
		size exclusion chromatography
		mass spectrometry

Peptide bond Hydrolysis	size	size exclusion chromatography SDS-PAGE
N to O migration Ser, Thr	hydrophobicity chemistry	RP-HPLC inactive in Edman reaction
α-Carboxy to β-Carboxy migration Asp, Asn	hydrophobicity chemistry	RP-HPLC inactive in Edman reaction
Deamidation Asn, Gln	charge	ion exchange chromatography
Acylation α-amino group, ε-amino group	charge	ion exchange chromatography mass spectrometry
Esterification/Carboxylation Glu, Asp, C-terminal	charge	ion exchange chromatography mass spectrometry
Secondary structure changes	hydrophobicity aggregation	RP-HPLC size exclusion chromatography

Table 2.4. Common reactions affecting stability of proteins.

and glutamine residues. Other chemical modifications can occur on peptide bonds, tryptophan, tyrosine, and amino and carboxyl groups. Table 2.4 lists a number of reactions that can occur during purification and storage of proteins and methods that can be used to detect such changes.

Physical stability of a protein is expressed as the difference in free energy, ΔG_u, between the native (N) and denatured (D) states. Thus, protein molecules are in equilibrium between the above two states. As long as this unfolding is reversible and ΔG_u is positive, it does not matter how small the ΔG_u is. In many cases, this reversibility does not hold. This is always seen when ΔG_u is decreased by heating. Most proteins denature upon heating and aggregation results in irreversible denaturation. Thus, unfolding is made irreversible by aggregation:

$$N \;\Leftrightarrow\; D \;\Rightarrow\; \text{Aggregation}$$
$$\Delta G_u \qquad k$$

Therefore, any stresses that decrease ΔG_u and increase k will cause accumulation of irreversibly inactivated forms of the protein. Such stresses may include chemical modifications as described above and physical parameters such as pH, ionic strength, protein concentration, and temperature. Development of suitable formulations that prolong the shelf-life of a recombinant protein is essential when it is to be used as a human therapeutic.

The use of protein stabilizing agents to enhance storage stability of proteins has become customary. These compounds affect protein stability by increasing ΔG_u. However, they may also increase k and hence their net effect on long-term storage of proteins depends on the protein as well as on the storage conditions.

When the irreversible process occurs due to aggregation, minimizing the irreversible step should increase the stability and may be attained by the addition of mild detergents. In this case the effects of detergents on ΔG_u also must be evaluated.

Another approach to enhance storage stability of proteins is to lyophilize, or freeze-dry, the proteins. Lyophilization can minimize the aggregation step during storage, since either chemical modification or aggregation is reduced in the absence of water. The effects of a lyophilization process itself on ΔG_u and k are not fully understood and hence such a process must be optimized for each protein therapeutic (cf. Chapter 4).

Analytical Techniques

Blotting Techniques

Blotting methods have an important niche in biotechnology. They are used to detect very low levels of unique molecules in a milieu of proteins, nucleic acids, and other cellular components. They can detect aggregates or breakdown products occurring during long-term storage and they can be used to detect components from the host cells used in producing recombinant proteins.

Biomolecules are transferred to a membrane, and this membrane is then probed with specific reagents to identify the molecule of interest. Membranes used in protein blots are made of a variety of materials including nitrocellulose, nylon, and polyvinylidine difluoride (PVDF) all of which avidly bind protein.

Liquid samples can be analyzed by methods called dot blots or slot blots. A solution containing the biomolecule of interest is filtered through a membrane which captures the biomolecule. The difference between a dot blot and a slot blot is that the former uses a circular or disk format while the latter is a rectangular configuration. The latter method allows for more precise quantitation of the desired biomolecule by scanning methods and relating the integrated results to that obtained with known amounts of material.

Often the sample is subjected to some type of fractionation such as polyacrylamide gel electrophoresis (see below) prior to the blotting step. An early technique, Southern blotting, named after the discoverer, E.M. Southern, is used to detect DNA fragments. When this procedure was adapted to RNA fragments and to proteins, other compass coordinates were chosen as labels for these procedures, i.e., northern blots for RNA and western blots for proteins. Western blots involve the use of labeled antibodies to detect specific proteins.

TRANSFER OF PROTEINS

Following polyacrylamide gel electrophoresis, transfer of proteins from the gel to the membrane can be accomplished in a number of ways. Originally, blotting was achieved by capillary action. In this commonly used method, the membrane is placed between the gel and absorbent paper. Fluid from the gel diffuses or wicks toward the absorbent paper and the protein is captured by the intervening membrane. A blot, or impression, of the protein within the gel is thus made.

Transfer of proteins to the membrane can occur under the influence of an electric field as well. The electric field is applied perpendicular to the original field used in separation so that the maximum distance the protein needs to migrate is only the thickness of the gel, and hence transfer of proteins can occur very rapidly. This latter method is called electroblotting.

DETECTION SYSTEMS

Once the transfer has occurred, the next step is to identify the presence of the desired protein. In addition to various

1 Transfer protein to membrane by diffusion or electroblotting.

2 Block residual protein binding sites on membrane with extraneous proteins such as milk proteins.

3 Treat membrane with antibody which recognizes the protein of interest. If this antibody is labeled with a detecting group then go to step 5.

4 Incubate membrane with secondary antibody which recognizes primary antibody used in step 3. This antibody is labeled with a detecting group.

5 Treat the membrane with suitable reagents to locate the site of membrane attachment of the labeled antibody in step 4 or step 5.

Table 2.5. Major steps in blotting proteins to membranes.

1 Antibodies are labeled with radioactive markers such as ^{125}I.

2 Antibodies are linked to an enzyme such as horseradish peroxidase (HRP) or alkaline phosphatase (AP). On incubation with substrate an insoluble colored product is formed at the location of the antibody. Alternatively, the location of the antibody can be detected using a substrate which yields a chemiluminescent product, an image of which is made on photographic film.

3 Antibody is labeled with biotin. Streptavidin or avidin is added to strongly bind to the biotin. Each streptavidin molecule has four binding sites. The remaining binding sites can combine with other biotin molecules which are covalently linked to HRP or to AP.

Table 2.6. Detection methods used in blotting techniques.

colorimetric staining methods, the blots can be probed with reagents specific for certain proteins, as for example, antibodies to a protein of interest. This technique is called immunoblotting. In the biotechnology field, immunoblotting is used as an identity test for the product of interest. An antibody that recognizes the desired protein is used in this instance. Secondly, immunoblotting is sometimes used to show the absence of host proteins. In this case, the antibodies are raised against proteins of the organism in which the recombinant protein has been expressed. This latter method can attest to the purity of the desired protein.

Table 2.5 lists major steps needed for the blotting procedure to be successful. Once transfer of proteins is completed, residual protein binding sites on the membrane need to be blocked so that antibodies used for detection react only at the location of the target molecule, or antigen, and not at some non-specific location. After blocking, the specific antibody is incubated with the membrane.

The antibody reacts with a specific protein on the membrane only at the location of that protein because of its specific interaction with its antigen. When immunoblotting techniques are used, methods are still needed to recognize the location of the interaction of the antibody with its specific protein. A number of procedures can be used to detect this complex (see Table 2.6).

The antibody itself can be labeled with a radioactive marker such as ^{125}I and placed in direct contact with X-ray film. After exposure of the membrane to the film for a suitable period, the film is developed and a photographic negative is made of the location of radioactivity on the membrane. Alternatively, the antibody can be linked to an enzyme which upon addition of appropriate reagents catalyzes a color or light reaction at the site of the antibody. These procedures entail purification of the antibody and specifically labeling it. More often, "secondary" antibodies are used. The primary antibody is the one which recognizes the protein of interest. The secondary antibody is then an antibody that specifically recognizes the primary antibody. Quite commonly, the primary antibody is raised in rabbits. The secondary antibody may then be an antibody raised in another animal, such as a goat, which recognizes rabbit antibodies. Since this secondary antibody recognizes rabbit antibodies in general, it can be used as a generic reagent to detect rabbit antibodies to a number of different proteins of interest that have been raised in rabbits. Thus, the primary antibody specifically recognizes and complexes a unique protein, and the secondary antibody, suitably labeled, is used for detection.

The secondary antibody can be labeled with a radioactive or enzymatic marker group and used to detect several different primary antibodies. Thus, rather than purifying a number of different primary antibodies, only one secondary antibody needs to be purified and labeled for recognition of all the primary antibodies. Because of their wide use, many common secondary antibodies are commercially available in kits containing the detection system and follow routine, straightforward procedures.

In addition to antibodies raised against the amino acyl constituents of proteins, specific antibodies can be used which recognize unique post-translational components in proteins as, for example, phosphotyrosyl residues, which are important during signal transduction, and carbohydrate moieties of glycoproteins.

Figure 2.9 illustrates a number of detection methods that can be used on immunoblots. The primary antibody, or if convenient, the secondary antibody, can have an appropriate label for detection. They may be labeled with a

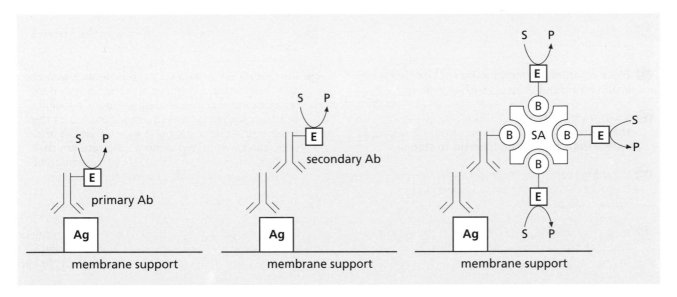

Figure 2.9. Common immunoblotting detection systems used to detect antigens, Ag, on membranes. Abbreviations used: Ab, antibody; E, enzyme, such as horseradish peroxidase or alkaline phosphatase; S, substrate; P, product, either colored and insoluble or chemiluminescent; B, biotin; SA, streptavidin.

radioactive tag as mentioned previously. Secondly, these antibodies can be coupled with an enzyme such as horseradish peroxidase (HRP) or alkaline phosphatase (AP). Substrate is added and is converted to an insoluble, colored product at the site of the protein-primary antibody-secondary antibody-HRP product. An alternative substrate can be used which yields a chemiluminescent product. A chemical reaction leads to the production of light which can expose photographic or X-ray film. The chromogenic and chemiluminescent detection systems have comparable sensitivities to radioactive methods. The former detection methods are displacing the latter method since problems associated with handling radioactive material and radioactive waste solutions are eliminated.

As illustrated in Figure 2.9, streptavidin, or alternatively avidin, and biotin can play an important role in detecting proteins on immunoblots. This is because biotin forms very tight complexes with streptavidin and avidin. Secondly, these proteins are multimeric and contain four binding sites for biotin. When the latter molecule is covalently linked to proteins such as antibodies and enzymes, streptavidin binds to the covalently bound biotin, thus recognizing the site on the membrane where the protein of interest is located.

Immunoassays

ELISA

Enzyme-linked immunosorbent assay (ELISA) provides a means to quantitatively measure extremely small amounts of proteins in biological fluids and serves as a tool for analyzing specific proteins during purification. This procedure takes advantage of the observation that plastic surfaces are able to adsorb low but detectable amounts of proteins. This is a solid phase assay, therefore, in which antibodies to a desired protein are allowed to absorb to the surface of microtitration plates. Each plate can contain up to 96 wells so that multiple samples can be assayed. After incubating the antibodies in the wells of the plate for a specific period of time, excess antibody is removed, and residual protein sites on the plastic are blocked by incubation with an inert protein. Several microtitration plates can be prepared at one time since the antibodies coating the plates retain their binding capacity for an extended period. During the ELISA, sample solution containing the protein of interest is incubated in the wells and is captured by the antibodies coating the well surface. Excess sample is removed and other antibodies which now have an enzyme linked to them are added to react with the bound antigen. The format described above is called a sandwich assay since the antigen of interest is located between the antibody on the titer well surface and the antibody containing the linked enzyme. Figure 2.10 illustrates a number of formats that can be used in an ELISA. A suitable substrate is added and the enzyme linked to the antibody-antigen-antibody-well complex converts this compound to a colored product. The amount of product obtained is proportional to the enzyme adsorbed in the well of the plate. A standard curve can be prepared if known concentrations of antigen are tested in this system, and the amount of antigen in unknown samples can be estimated from this standard

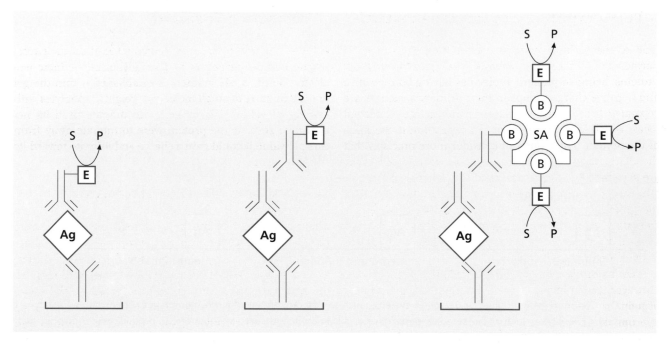

Figure 2.10. Examples of several formats for ELISA in which the specific antibody is adsorbed to the surface of a microtitration plate. See Figure 9 for abbreviations used. The antibody is represented by the Y type structure. The product, P, is colored and the amount generated is measured with a spectrometer or plate reader.

curve. A number of enzymes can be used in ELISAs, however, the most common ones are horseradish peroxidase and alkaline phosphatase. A variety of substrates for each enzyme are available which yield colored products when catalyzed by the linked enzyme. Absorbance of the colored product solutions is measured on plate readers, instruments which rapidly measure the absorbance in all 96 wells of the microtitration plate, and data processing can be automated for rapid throughput of information.

The above ELISA format is only one of many different methods. For example, the microtitration wells may be coated directly with the antigen rather than having a specific antibody attached to the surface. Quantitation is made by comparison with known quantities of antigen used to coat individual wells.

Another approach, this time subsequent to binding of antigen either directly to the surface or to an antibody on the surface, is to use an antibody specific to the immunoglobulin binding the protein antigen, that is, a secondary antibody. This latter antibody contains the linked enzyme used for detection. The advantage to this approach is that such antibodies can be obtained in high purity and with the desired enzyme linked to them from commercial sources. Thus, a single source of enzyme-linked antibody can be used in assays for different protein antigens. Should a sandwich assay be used, then antibodies

from different species need to be used for each side of the sandwich. A possible scenario is that rabbit antibodies are used to coat the microtitration wells; mouse antibodies, possibly a monoclonal antibody, are used to complex with the antigen and then a goat anti-mouse immunoglobulin containing linked HRP or AP is used for detection purposes.

As with immunoblots discussed above, streptavidin, or avidin, can be used in these assays if biotin is covalently linked to the antibodies and enzymes (Figure 2.10).

If a radioactive label is used in place of the enzyme in the above procedure, then the assay is a solid phase radioimmunoassay (RIA). As stated before, assays are moving away from use of radioisotopes because of problems with safety and disposal of radioactive waste and since nonradioactive assays have comparable sensitivities.

Electrophoresis

Analytical methodologies to measure protein properties stem from those used in their purification (cf. Chapter 3). The major difference lies in the fact that systems used for analyses have higher resolving powers than those used in purification. The two major methods for analysis have their bases in chromatographic or electrophoretic techniques.

POLYACRYLAMIDE GEL ELECTROPHORESIS

One of the earliest methods for analysis of proteins is polyacrylamide gel electrophoresis (PAGE). In this method, proteins, being amphoteric molecules having both positive and negative charge groups in their primary structure, are separated based on their net electrical charge. A second factor which is responsible for the separation is the mass of the protein. Thus, one can consider more precisely that the charge to mass ratio of proteins determines how they are separated in an electrical field. The charge of the protein can be controlled by the pH of the solution in which the protein is separated. The farther away the protein is from its pI value, that is, the pH at which it has a net charge of zero, the greater is the net charge and hence the greater is its charge to mass ratio.

The major component of polyacrylamide gels is water. However, they provide a flexible support so that after a protein has been subjected to an electrical field for an appropriate period of time it provides a matrix to hold the proteins in place until they can be detected with suitable reagents. By adjusting the amount of acrylamide that is used in these gels, one can affect the migration of material within the gel. The more acrylamide, the more hindrance for the protein to migrate in an electrical field.

The addition of a detergent, sodium dodecyl sulfate, to the electrophoretic separation system allows for the separation to take place primarily as a function of size of the protein. Sodium dodecyl sulfate complexes with proteins, resulting in unfolding of the proteins, and the amount of detergent that is complexed is proportional to the size of the protein. The larger the protein, the more detergent that is complexed. SDS is a negatively charged molecule, and the net effect when proteins are in a solution of SDS is that the charge of the protein is overwhelmed by that of the SDS complexed with it so that the proteins take on net negative charges proportional to their molecular weight.

Polyacrylamide gel electrophoresis in the presence of sodium dodecyl sulfates is commonly known as SDS-PAGE. All the proteins take on a net negative charge, with larger proteins binding more SDS but with the charge to mass ratio being fairly constant among the proteins.

Since all proteins have essentially the same charge to mass ratio, how can separation occur? This is done by controlling the concentration of acrylamide in the pathway of proteins migrating in an electrical field. The greater the acrylamide concentration the more difficult it is for large protein molecules to migrate relative to smaller protein molecules. This is sometimes thought of as a sieving effect since the greater the acrylamide concentration, the smaller the pore size within the polyacrylamide gel. Indeed, if the acrylamide concentration is sufficiently high, some high molecular weight proteins may not migrate within the gel at all.

ISOELECTRIC FOCUSING

Another method to separate proteins based on their electrophoretic properties is to take advantage of their isoelectric point. A pH gradient is established within the gel using a mixture of small molecular weight ampholytes with varying pI values. The protein will migrate until its net charge is zero. If the protein were to migrate away from this pH value it could gain a charge and migrate toward its pI value again.

2-DIMENSIONAL GEL ELECTROPHORESIS

The above methods can be combined into a procedure called 2-D gel electrophoresis. Proteins are first fractionated by isoelectric focusing based upon their pI values. They are then subjected to SDS-PAGE perpendicular to the first dimension and fractionated based on the molecular weights of proteins. SDS-PAGE cannot be placed before isoelectric focusing since once SDS binds to and denatures the proteins they no longer migrate based on their pI values.

DETECTION OF PROTEINS WITHIN POLYACRYLAMIDE GELS

Although the polyacrylamide gels provide a flexible support for the proteins, with time they will diffuse and spread within the gel. Consequently, it is usual practice to fix the proteins or trap them at the location that they migrated. This is accomplished by placing the gels in a fixing solution in which the proteins become insoluble.

There are many methods to stain proteins in gels, but the two most common and well-studied methods are either staining with Coomassie blue or by a method using silver. The latter method is used if increased sensitivity is required. The principle of Coomassie blue stain is hydrophobic interaction of a dye with the protein, thus the gel takes on a color wherever a protein is located. Using standard amounts of proteins, the amount of protein or contaminant may be estimated.

Quantitation using the silver staining method is less precise, although due to the increased sensitivity of this method, very low levels of contaminants can be detected.

CAPILLARY ELECTROPHORESIS

With recent advances in instrumentation and technology, capillary electrophoresis has gained an increased presence in the analyses of recombinant proteins. Rather than having a matrix as in polyacrylamide gel electrophoresis through which the proteins migrate, they are free in solution in an electric field within the confines of a capillary tube with a diameter of 25–50 micrometers. The capillary tube passes

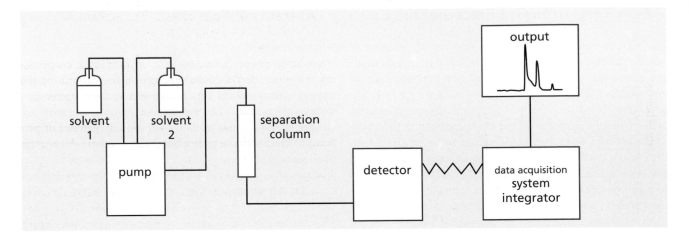

Figure 2.11. Components of a typical chromatography station. The pump combines solvents 1 and 2 in appropriate ratios to generate a pH, salt concentration, or hydrophobic gradient. Proteins that are fractioned on the column pass through a detector which measures their occurrence. Information from the detector is used to generate chromatograms and the relative amount of each component.

through an ultraviolet light or fluorescence detector that measures the presence of proteins migrating in the electric field. The movement of one protein relative to another is a function of the molecular mass and the net charge on the protein. The latter can be influenced by pH and analytes in the solution. This technique has yet to gain acceptance for routine analyses because of difficulties in reproducibility of the capillaries and in validating this system. Nevertheless, it is a powerful analytical tool for the characterization of recombinant proteins during process development and in stability studies.

Chromatography

Chromatography techniques are used extensively in biotechnology not only in protein purification procedures (cf. Chapter 3), but also in assessing the integrity of the product. Routine procedures are highly automated so that comparisons of similar samples can be made. An analytical system consists of an autosampler which will take a known amount (usually a known volume) of material for analysis and automatically place it in the solution stream headed toward a separation column used to fractionate the sample. Another part of this system is a pump module which provides a reproducible flow rate. In addition, the pumping system can provide a gradient which changes properties of the solution such as pH, ionic strength, and hydrophobicity. A detection system is located at the outlet of the column. This measures the relative amount of protein exiting the column. Coupled to the detector is a data acquisition system which takes the signal from the detector and integrates it into a value related to the amount of material (see Figure 2.11). When the protein appears, the signal begins to in-

crease, and as the protein passes through the detector, the signal subsequently decreases. The area under the peak of the signal is proportional to the amount of material which has passed through the detector. By analyzing known amounts of protein, an area versus amount of protein plot can be generated and this may be used to estimate the amount of this protein under other circumstances. Another benefit of this integrated chromatography system is that low levels of components which appear over time can be estimated relative to the major desired protein being analyzed. This is a particularly useful function when the long-term stability of the product is under evaluation.

Proteins have a multitude of properties which can be used to advantage in chromatographic analyses. The following describes how some of these properties can be used.

SIZE EXCLUSION CHROMATOGRAPHY

As the name implies, this procedure separates proteins based on their size or molecular weight or shape. The matrix consists of very fine beads containing cavities and pores accessible to molecules of a certain size or smaller, but inaccessible to larger molecules. The principle of this technique is the distribution of molecules between the volume of solution within the beads versus the volume of solution surrounding the beads. Small molecules have access to a larger volume than do large molecules. As solution flows through the column, molecules can diffuse back and forth, depending upon their size, in and out of pores. Smaller molecules can reside within the pores for a finite period of time whereas larger molecules, unable to enter these spaces, continue along in the fluid stream. Intermediate-sized molecules spend an intermediate amount of

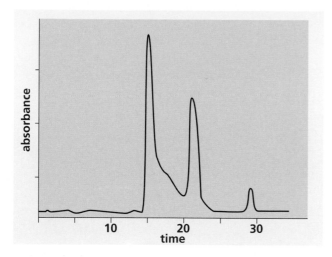

Figure 2.12. Size exclusion chromatography of a recombinant protein which on storage yields aggregates and smaller peptides (see text).

time within the pores and can be fractionated from large molecules which cannot access the matrix space at all and small molecules which have free access to this volume and spend the most time within the beads. Protein molecules can distribute between the volume within these beads and the excluded volume based on the size and shape of the protein. This distribution is based on the relative concentration of the protein in the beads versus the excluded volume.

Over time, proteins can undergo a number of changes which affect their size. A peptide bond within the protein can hydrolyze yielding two smaller polypeptide chains. More commonly, size exclusion chromatography is used to assess aggregated forms of the protein. Figure 2.12 shows an example of this. The peak at 22 minutes represents the native protein. The peak at 15 minutes is aggregated protein and that at 28 minutes depicts degraded protein yielding smaller polypeptide chains. Aggregation can occur when a protein molecule unfolds to a slight extent and exposes surfaces which are attracted to complementary surfaces on adjacent molecules. This interaction can lead to dimerization or doubling of molecular weight or to higher oligomers. From the chromatographic profile, the mechanism of aggregation often can be implicated. If dimers, trimers, tetramers, etc. are observed, then aggregation occurs by stepwise interaction of a monomer with a dimer, trimer, etc. If dimers, tetramers, octamers, etc. are observed, then aggregates can interact with each other. Sometimes, only monomers and high molecular weight aggregates are observed, suggesting that intermediate species are kinetically of short duration and protein molecules susceptible to aggregation combine into very large molecular weight complexes.

REVERSED-PHASE HIGH PERFORMANCE LIQUID CHROMATOGRAPHY

This method takes advantage of the hydrophobic properties of proteins. The functional groups on the column matrix contain from one to up to eighteen carbon atoms in a hydrocarbon chain. The more carbon atoms, the more hydrophobic is the matrix. The hydrophobic patches of proteins interact with the hydrophobic chromatographic matrix. Proteins are then eluted from the matrix by increasing the hydrophobic nature of the solvent passing through the column. Acetonitrile is a common solvent used, although other organic solvents such as ethanol also may be used. The solvent is made acidic by addition of trifluoroacetic acid since proteins have increased solubility at pH values further removed from the pI, or isoelectric point, of the proteins. A gradient with increasing concentration of hydrophobic solvent is passed through the column. Different proteins have different hydrophobicities and are eluted from the column at varied hydrophobic potential of the solvent.

This technique can be very powerful. It may detect the addition of a single oxygen atom to the protein, as when a methionyl residue is oxidized, or when the hydrolysis of an amide moiety on a glutamyl or asparginyl residue occurs. Disulfide bond formation or shuffling also changes the hydrophobic characteristic of the protein. Hence, RP-HPLC can be used not only to assess the homogeneity of the protein but also to follow degradation pathways occurring during long-term storage.

Reversed-phase chromatography of proteolytic digests of recombinant proteins may serve to identify this protein. Enzymatic digestion yields unique peptides which elute at different retention times or at different organic solvent concentration. Moreover, the map, or chromatogram, of peptides arising from enzymatic digestion of one protein is quite different from the map obtained from another protein. Several different proteases such as trypsin, chymotrypsin, and other endoproteinases are used for these identity tests.

HYDROPHOBIC INTERACTION CHROMATOGRAPHY

A companion to RP-HPLC is hydrophobic interaction chromatography (HIC), although in principle this latter method is normal-phase chromatography, i.e., an aqueous solvent system rather than an organic one is used to fractionate proteins. The hydrophobic characteristics of the solution are modulated by inorganic salt concentrations. Ammonium sulfate and sodium chloride are often used since these compounds are highly soluble in water. In the presence of high salt concentrations, proteins are attracted to hydrophobic surfaces on the matrix of resins used in this technique. As the salt concentration decreases, proteins have less affinity for the matrix and eventually elute from the column. This method lacks the resolving power of RP-HPLC but is a more gentle method, since low pH values or organic solvents can be detrimental to some proteins.

ION EXCHANGE CHROMATOGRAPHY

This technique takes advantage of the electronic charge properties of proteins. Some of the amino acyl residues are negatively charged and others are positively charged. The net charge of the protein can be modulated by the pH of its environment relative to the pI value of the protein. At a pH value lower than the pI, the protein has a net positive charge, whereas at a pH value greater than the pI, the protein has a net negative charge. Opposites attract in ion-exchange chromatography. The resins in this procedure can contain functional groups with positive or negative charges. Thus, positively charged proteins bind to negatively charged matrices and negatively charged proteins bind to positively charged matrices. Proteins are displaced from the resin by increasing salt, e.g., sodium chloride, concentrations. Proteins with different net charges can be separated from one another during elution with an increasing salt gradient. The choice of charged resin and elution conditions are dependent upon the protein of interest.

In lieu of changing the ionic strength of the solution, proteins can be eluted by changing the pH of the medium, i.e., with the use of a pH gradient. This method is called chromatofocusing and proteins are separated based on their pI values. When pH reaches the pI value of a specific protein, it has a net neutral charge and is no longer attracted to the charged matrix and is eluted.

OTHER CHROMATOGRAPHIC TECHNIQUES

Other functional groups may be attached to chromatographic matrices to take advantage of unique properties of certain proteins. These affinity methodologies, however, are more often used in the manufacturing process than in analytical techniques. Methods that consider the size, charge, and hydrophobic nature of the protein can define its homogeneity and be used in stability assessment.

Bioassays

Paramount to development of a protein therapeutic is to have an assay that identifies its biological function. Chromatographic and electrophoretic methodologies can address the homogeneity of a biotherapeutic and be useful in

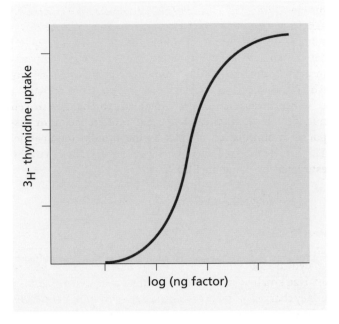

Figure 2.13. An *in vitro* bioassay showing a mitogenic response in which radioactive thymidine is incorporated into DNA in the presence of an increasing amount of a protein factor.

investigating stability parameters; however, it is also necessary to ascertain that the protein has acceptable bioactivity. Bioactivity can be determined either *in vivo*, i.e., administering the protein to an animal and ascertaining some change within the body, or *in vitro*, in which a response of a specific receptor or microbiological or tissue cell line is measured when the therapeutic protein is present. An example of the latter type of bioassay can be an increase in DNA synthesis as measured by incorporation of radioactivity labeled thymidine. The protein factor binds to receptors on the cell surface which triggers secondary messengers to send signals to the cell nucleus to synthesize DNA. The binding of the protein factor to the cell surface is dependent upon the amount of factor present. Figure 2.13 presents a dose response curve of thymidine incorporation as a function of concentration of the factor. At low concentrations, the factor concentration is too low to trigger a response. As the concentration increases, incorporation of thymidine occurs, and at higher concentrations the amount of thymidine incorporation ceases to increase as DNA synthesis is occurring at the maximum rate. Bioassays can be readily quantitated, and a standard curve can be obtained using known quantities of the protein factor. Comparison of other solutions containing unknown amounts of the factor with this standard curve will yield quantitative estimates of the factor concentration. By relating the bioactivity units to the amount of protein used in the measurement the specific activity, or units/mg, can be obtained. Through experience and development of the protein therapeutic, a value is obtained for fully functional protein. Subsequent comparisons to this value can be used to ascertain any loss in activity during stability studies, or changes in activity when amino acyl residues of the protein are modified.

Other *in vitro* bioassays can measure changes in cell number or production of another protein factor in response to stimulation of cells by the protein therapeutic. The amount of the secondary protein produced can be estimated by using an ELISA.

Mass Spectrometry

Recent advances in the measurement of the molecular masses of proteins have made this technique an important analytical tool. While this method was used in the past to analyze small volatile molecules, the molecular weights of highly charged proteins having masses of over 100 kilodaltons (kD) can now be accurately determined.

Because of the precision of this method, post-translational modifications such as acetylation or glycosylation can be predicted. New protein forms that arise during stability studies can suggest the nature of this form. For example, an increase in mass of 16 mu (mass units) suggests that an oxygen atom has been added to the protein as happens when a methionyl residue is oxidized to a methionyl sulfoxide residue. The molecular mass of peptides obtained after proteolytic digestion and separation by HPLC can indicate from which region of the primary structure they are derived. If peptides have molecular masses differing from that expected from the primary sequences, the nature of the modification to that peptide can be implicated. Moreover, molecular mass estimates can be taken on peptides obtained from unfractionated proteolytic digests. Molecular masses that differ from expected values indicate that some peptide has been altered, that glycosylation or other modification has been altered, or that the protein under investigation still contains contaminants.

Another way that mass spectrometry can be used as an analytical tool is in sequencing of peptides. A recurring structure, the peptide bond, in peptides tends to yield fragments of the mature peptide which differ stepwise by an amino acyl residue. The difference in mass between two fragments indicates the amino acid removed from one fragment to generate the other. Except for leucine and isoleucine, each amino acid has a different mass and hence a sequence can be read from the mass spectrograph. Stepwise removal can occur from either the amino terminus or carboxy terminus.

By changing three basic components of the mass spectrometer, the ion source, the analyzer and the detector, different types of measurement may be undertaken. Typical ion sources which volatilize the proteins are electrospray ionization, fast atom bombardment, and liquid secondary ion. Common analyzers include quadrupole, magnetic sector, and time of flight. The function of the analyzer is to separate the ionized biomolecules based on their mass to charge ratio. The detector measures a current whenever impinged upon by charged particles. Electrospray ionization (EI) and matrix-assisted laser desorption (MALDI) are two sources that can generate high molecular weight volatile proteins. In the former method, droplets are generated by spraying or nebulizing the protein solution into the source of the mass spectrometer. As the solvent evaporates, the protein remains behind in the gas phase and passes through the analyzer to the detector. In MALDI, proteins are mixed with a matrix which vaporizes when exposed to laser light, thus carrying the protein into the gas phase.

Since proteins are multi-charge compounds, a number of components are observed representing mass to charge forms, each differing from the next by one charge. By imputing various charges to the mass to charge values, a molecular mass of the protein can be estimated. The latter step is empirical since only the mass to charge ratio is detected and not the net charge for that particular particle.

Concluding Remarks

With the advent of recombinant proteins as human therapeutics, the need for methods to evaluate their structure, function, and homogeneity has become paramount. Various biophysical methods are used to arrive at the primary, secondary, and tertiary structure of the protein. Bioassays establish its activity, and a number of analytical techniques determine the quality, purity and stability of the recombinant product. ■

Further Reading

- **Butler JE.** (1991). *Immunochemistry of Solid-Phase Immunoassay*, CRC Press, Boca Raton, Fla.
- **Crabb JW.** (1995). *Techniques in Protein Chemistry VI*, Academic Press, San Diego, Calif.
- **Coligan J, Dunn B, Ploegh H, Speicher D, Wingfield P.** (1995). *Current Protocols in Protein Science*, J. Wiley & Sons, New York, N.Y.
- **Creighton TE.** (1989). *Protein Structure: A Practical Approach*, IRL Press, Oxford, England.
- **Crowther JR.** (1995). *ELISA, Theory and Practice*, Humana Press, Totowa, N.J.
- **Dunbar BS.** (1994). *Protein Blotting: A Practical Approach*, Oxford University Press, New York, N.Y.
- **Gregory RB.** (1994). *Protein-Solvent Interactions*, Marcel Dekker, New York, N.Y.
- **Hames BD, Rickwood D.** (1990). *Gel Electrophoresis of Proteins: A Practical Approach*, 2nd ed., IRL Press, New York, N.Y.
- **Landus JP.** (1994). *Handbook of Capillary Electrophoresis*, CRC Press, Boca Raton, Fla.
- **McEwen CN, Larsen BS.** (1990). *Mass Spectrometry of Biological Materials*, Dekker, New York, N.Y.
- **Price C, Newman DJ.** (1991). *Principles and Practice of Immunoassay*, Stockton Press, New York, N.Y.
- **Schulz GE, Schirmer RH.** (1979). *Principles of Protein Structure*, Springer-Verlag, New York, N.Y.
- **Shirley BA.** (1995). *Protein Stability and Folding*, Humana Press, Totowa, N.J.

Self-Assessment Questions

Question 1: *What is the net charge of granulocyte-colony stimulating factor at pH 2.0, assuming that all the carboxyl groups are protonated?*

Question 2: *Based on the above calculation, do you expect the protein to unfold at pH 2.0?*

Question 3: *Design an experiment using blotting techniques to ascertain the presence of a ligand to a particular receptor.*

Question 4: *What is the transfer of proteins to a membrane such as nitrocellulose or PDVF called?*

Question 5: *What is the assay in which the antibody is adsorbed to a plastic microtitration plate and then is used to quantitate the amount of a protein using a secondary antibody conjugated with horseradish peroxidase named?*

Question 6: *In 2-dimensional electrophoresis, what is the first method of separation?*

Question 7: *What is the method for separating proteins in solution based on molecular size called?*

Answers

Answer 1: Based on the assumption that glutamyl and aspartyl residues are uncharged at this pH, all the charges come from protonated histidyl, lysyl, arginyl residues, and the amino terminus, i.e., 5 His + 4 Lys + 5 Arg + N-terminal = 15.

Answer 2: Whether a protein unfolds or remains folded depends on the balance between the stabilizing and destabilizing forces. At pH 2.0, extensive positive charges destabilize the protein, but whether such destabilization is sufficient or insufficient to unfold the protein depends on how stable the protein is in the native state. The charged state alone cannot predict whether a protein will unfold.

Answer 3: A solution containing the putative ligand is subjected to SDS-PAGE. After blotting the proteins in the gel to a membrane, it is probed with a solution containing the receptor. The receptor, which binds the ligand, may be labeled with agents suitable for detection or, alternatively, the complex can subsequently be probed with an antibody to the receptor and developed as for an immunoblot. Note that the reciprocal of this can be done as well, in which the receptor is subjected to SDS-PAGE and the blot is probed with the ligand.

Answer 4: This method is called blotting. If an electric current is used then the method is called electroblotting.

Answer 5: This assay is called an ELISA, enzyme-linked immunosorbent assay.

Answer 6: Either isoelectric focusing or native polyacrylamide electrophoresis. The second dimension is performed in the presence of the detergent sodium dodecyl sulfate.

Answer 7: Size exclusion chromatography.

3 Production of Biotech Compounds
Cultivation and Downstream Processing

by: Farida Kadir

Introduction

The growing therapeutic use of proteins in the pharmaceutical industry has created an increasing need for practical and economical processing techniques. As a result biotechnological production methods have advanced tremendously in recent years. When producing proteins for therapeutic use, a number of issues must be considered related to manufacture, purification and characterization of the products. Biotechnological products for therapeutic use have to meet strict specifications, especially when used via the parenteral route (Walter and Werner, 1993).

In this chapter aspects of cultivation and purification during production will be dealt with briefly. For further details the reader is referred to the literature mentioned.

Cultivation

Expression Systems

Expression systems for proteins of therapeutic interest include pro- and eucaryotic cells (bacterial, yeast and animal cells). The choice of a particular system will be determined to a large extent by the nature of the desired protein product.

In principle, any protein can be produced using genetically engineered organisms, but not every type of protein can be produced by any cell type. For example, proteolytic cleavage in bacterial expression systems may lead to a degraded product. Moreover, bacteria are not capable of producing glycoproteins because they lack the capacity to glycosylate. A solution to these problems is to use mammalian cells as a production vehicle. These cells possess a machinery to produce a wide range of biologically active macromolecules which are comparable to those in human cells. Features of proteins of different biological origin are listed in Table 3.1 (Walter *et al.* 1992).

Cultivation Systems

In general cells can be cultivated either in vessels containing an appropriate liquid growth medium in which the cells are either attached to microspheres, or free in suspen-

Protein feature	Procaryotic Bacteria	Eucaryotic Yeast	Eucaryotic Mammalian cells
Concentration	high	high	low
Molecular weight	low	high	high
S-S bridges	limitation	no limitation	no limitation
Secretion	no	yes/no	yes
Aggregation state	inclusion body	singular, native	singular, native
Folding	misfolding	correct folding	correct folding
Glycosylation	no	possible	possible
Retrovirus	no	no	possible
Pyrogen	possible	no	no

Table 3.1. Features of proteins of different biological origin.

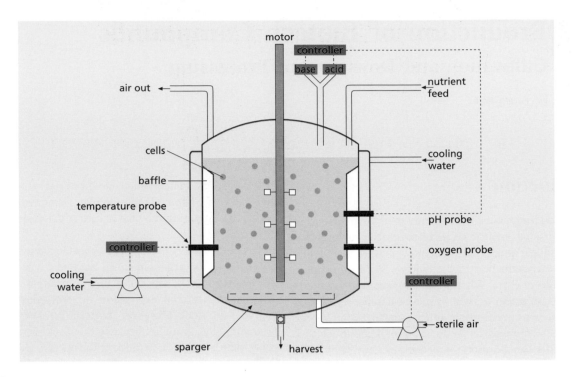

Figure 3.1a. Schematic representation of a stirred-tank bioreactor (adapted from Klegerman and Groves, 1992).

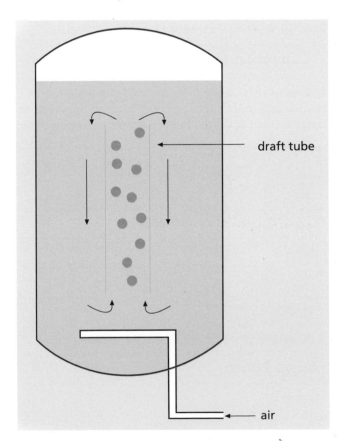

Figure 3.1b. Schematic representation of an airlift bioreactor (adapted from Klegerman and Groves, 1992).

sion or in an immobilized state as monolayers, or entrapped in matrices (usually solidified with agar). The culture method will determine the scale of the separation and purification methods. Production-scale cultivation is commonly performed in fermentors or bioreactors. Bioreactor systems can be classified into four different types: stirred-tank, airlift, microcarrier (e.g., fixed bed bioreactors) and membrane bioreactors (e.g., hollow fiber perfusion bioreactors) (see Figure 3.1). Because of its reliability and experience with the design and scaling up potential, the stirred tank is still the most commonly used bioreactor.

The kinetics of cell growth and product formation will not only dictate the type of bioreactor used, but also how the growth process is run. Three types of fermentation protocols are commonly employed: (1) batch, (2) fed-batch and (3) continuous production protocols. In all cases the cells go through four distinctive phases: lag, exponential growth, stationary and death phase. For further details the reader is referred to Chapter 1 of this book. Animal cells have to be free from undesired microorganisms that may destroy the cell culture or present hazards to the patient. This requires strict sterility measures for both the procedures and materials used (FDA, 1987; Bergemann *et al.*, 1993; Berthold and Walter, 1994).

Examples of animal cells that produce proteins of clinical interest are lymphoblastoid tumor cells (interferon production), melanoma cells (plasminogen activator) and hybridized tumor cells (monoclonal antibodies).

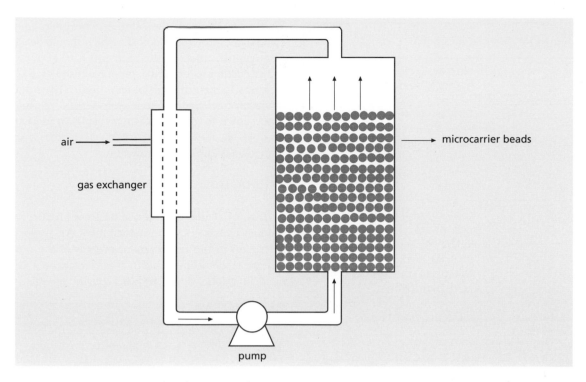

Figure 3.1c. Schematic representation of a fixed bed bioreactor (adapted from Klegerman and Groves, 1992).

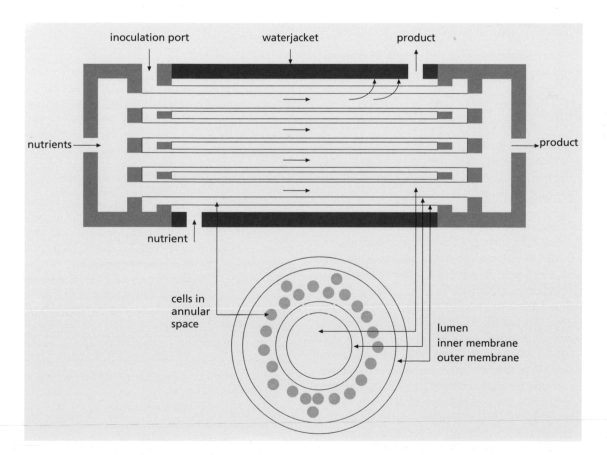

Figure 3.1d. Schematic representation of a hollow fiber perfusion bioreactor (adapted from Klegerman and Groves, 1992).

Type of nutrient	Example(s)
Sugars	glucose, lactose, sucrose, maltose, dextrins
Fat	fatty acids, triglycerides
Water (high quality, sterilized)	water for injection
Amino acids	glutamine
Electrolytes	calcium, sodium, potassium, phosphate
Vitamins	ascorbic acid, α-tocopherol, thiamine, riboflavine, folic acid, pyridoxin
Serum (fetal calf serum, synthetic serum)	albumin, transferrin
Trace minerals	iron, manganese, copper, cobalt, zinc
Hormones	growth factors

Table 3.2. Major components of growth media for mammalian cell structures.

Medium

In order to achieve optimal growth of cells it is of great importance that not only conditions such as pH, oxygen pressure and temperature are chosen and controlled appropriately, but also to provide a medium with the proper nutrients.

The media used for mammalian cell culture are complex and consist of a mixture of diverse components, such as sugars, amino acids, electrolytes, vitamins, fetal calf serum and a mixture of peptones, growth factors, hormones and other proteins (see Table 3.2). Many of these ingredients are preblended either diluted or as homogeneous mixtures of powders. To prepare the final medium, components are dissolved in purified water before sterile filtration. Some supplements, especially fetal calf serum, contribute considerably to the presence of contaminating proteins and may seriously complicate purification procedures. Additionally, the composition of serum is variable; it depends on the individual animal, season of the year, suppliers' treatment, etc. The use of serum may introduce adventitious material such as viruses, mycoplasmas, bacteria, prions and fungi into the culture system (Berthold and

Walter, 1994). Even when sterile, serum may contain substantial quantities of endotoxin which should be eliminated during purification. These problems have been recognized by the customers of media and have stimulated the manufacturers to meet the customers' need. They offer a range of serum-free media. Completely serum-free media have been shown to give satisfactory results in industrial scale production settings in certain cases, for example, in monoclonal antibody production.

Contaminants

Quality is usually measured in terms of product purity and product consistency (reproducibility). An important consideration in the development process of the purification scheme is the ultimate purity that is required. For pharmaceutical applications, product purity mostly is $\geq 99\%$

Origin	Contaminant
Host-related	viruses, bacteria
	host-derived proteins and DNA
	glycosylation variants
	N- and C-terminal variants
	endotoxins (from gram negative bacterial hosts
Product-related	amino acids substitution and deletion
	denatured protein
	conformational isomers
	dimers and aggregates
	disulfide pairing variants
	deamidated species
	protein fragments
Process-related	growth medium components
	purification reagents
	metals
	column materials

Table 3.3. Potential contaminants in recombinant protein products derived from bacterial and non-bacterial hosts.

(Berthold and Walter, 1994; European Communities Guidelines, 1989).

Purification processes should yield potent proteins with well-defined characteristics for human use from which "all" contaminants have been removed. The purity of the drug protein in the final product will therefore largely depend upon the purification technology applied (Sharma, 1986a).

Table 3.3 lists potential contaminants that may be present in recombinant protein products from bacterial and non-bacterial sources. These contaminants can be either host-related, process-related or product-related. In the following sections special attention will be paid to the detection and elimination of contamination by viruses, bacteria, cellular DNA and undesired proteins.

VIRUSES

Viruses, which require the presence of living cells to propagate, are potential contaminants of animal cell cultures and, therefore, of the final product produced by the cells (Arathoon and Birch, 1986). If present, their concentration in the purified product will be very low and it will be difficult to detect them. Moreover, methods to detect these viral contaminants in the cell media, or in the final product are not very well documented (Sharma, 1990). Although viruses such as retrovirus (type B) can be visualized under an electron microscope, a highly sensitive *in vitro* assay for their presence is lacking (Liptrot and Gull, 1991; Zoletto, 1985). The implications of the presence of some viruses (e.g., hepatitis virus) are known (Feinstone *et al.*, 1983; Bouchard *et al.*, 1984; Walter *et al.*, 1991; Marcus-Sekura, 1991) but there are other viruses whose risks can not be

properly judged because of lack of solid experimental data. Some virus infections, such as with parvovirus, can have long latent periods before clinical effects show up. Long-term effects of introducing viruses into a patient treated with a recombinant protein should not be overlooked. The specific virus testing regime required will depend on the cell type used for production (Löwer, 1990; Commission of the European Communities, 1991).

Viruses can be introduced by nutrients or they are generated by an infected production cell line. The most frequent source of virus introduction is animal serum. In addition, animal serum can introduce other unwanted agents such as bacteria, mycoplasmas, fungi and endotoxins. It should be clear that appropriate screening of cell banks and growth medium constituents for viruses and other adventitious agents should be strictly regulated and supervised (Walter *et al.*, 1991; FDA 1993; WHO Technical Report Series 823). There is a trend toward using better defined growth media in which serum levels are significantly reduced.

Column regeneration methods for re-use in purification should be validated for viral removal and inactivation as well. Viruses can be inactivated by physical and chemical treatment of the product. Heat, irradiation, sonication, extreme pH, detergents, solvents, and certain disinfectants can inactivate viruses. These procedures can be harmful to the product as well and should therefore be carefully evaluated and validated (Note for Guidance, 1991; Walter *et al.*, 1992). A number of methods for reducing or inactivating viral contaminants are mentioned in Table 3.4 (Burnouf *et al.*, 1989; Feinstone *et al.*, 1983; Horowitz *et al.*, 1991; Perret *et al.*, 1991; Horowitz *et al.*, 1994).

Category	type	example
Inactivation	heat treatment	pasteurization
	radiation	UV-light
	dehydration	lyophilization
	cross linking agents, denaturating or disrupting agents	β-propiolactone, formaldehyde, NaOH, organic solvents (e.g., chloroform), detergents (e.g. Na-cholate)
	neutralization	specific, neutralizing antibodies
Removal	chromatography	ion-exchange, immuno-affinity chromatography
	filtration	ultrafiltration
	precipitation	cryoprecipitation

Table 3.4. Methods for reducing or inactivating viral contaminants.

BACTERIA

Unwanted bacterial contamination may be a problem for cells in culture. Usually the size of bacteria allows simple sterile filtration to remove the microorganisms. In order to further prevent bacterial contamination during production, the pharmaceuticals used have to be sterilized and the products are manufactured under strict aseptic conditions (FDA, 1987). Additionally, antibiotic agents can be added to the culture media in some cases. In bacterial culture systems the expression systems should then be resistant to the antibiotic agent used (Novitsky and Gould, 1985; Berthold and Walter, 1994). This practice may in itself present problems; firstly by the selection of antibiotic resistant bacteria, and secondly (important from purification viewpoint) because of the persistence of antibiotic residues which are difficult to completely eliminate from the product. Therefore, appropriately designed production plants and extensive quality control systems for added reagents (medium, serum, enzymes, etc.) permitting antibiotic-free operation are preferable (FDA, 1987).

Pyrogens (usually endotoxins of gram-negative bacteria) are potentially hazardous substances (cf. Chapter 4). Humans are sensitive to pyrogen contamination at very low concentrations (picograms per mL). Pyrogens may elicit a strong fever response and can even be fatal. Simple sterile filtration does not remove pyrogens. Removal is complicated further because pyrogens vary in size and chemical composition (Homma et al., 1983; Pearson, 1987). However, sensitive tests to detect and quantify pyrogens are commercially available. Purification schemes usually contain at least one step of ion-exchange chromatography (anionic exchange material) to remove the negatively charged endotoxins (Berthold and Walter, 1994; Nolan et al., 1975).

CELLULAR DNA

The application of continuous cell lines to the production of recombinant proteins might result in the presence of oncogene-bearing DNA-fragments in the final protein product (Walter and Werner, 1993; Löwer, 1990; Bergemann et al., 1993; Smith et al., 1991). A stringent purification protocol that is capable of reducing the DNA content to a safe level is therefore necessary (Berthold and Walter, 1994). There are a number of approaches available to demonstrate that the purification method removes cellular DNA and RNA. One such approach involves incubating the cell line with radiolabeled nucleotides and determining radioactivity in the purified product obtained through the purification protocol. Another method is a dye-binding fluorescence-enhancement assay for nucleotides. If the presence of nucleic

acids persists in a final preparation, then additional steps must be introduced in the purification process. The question about a safe level of nucleic acids in biotech products is difficult to answer, because of lack of relevant know-how. Nevertheless, it is generally agreed that final product contamination by nucleic acids should not exceed 10 pg per dose (WHO, 1996; Kung et al., 1990).

PROTEIN CONTAMINANTS

As mentioned before, trace amounts of 'foreign' proteins may appear in biotech products. These types of contaminants are a potential health hazard because, if present, they may be recognized as antigens by the patient receiving the recombinant protein product. On repeated use the patient may show an immune reaction caused by the contaminant while the protein of interest is performing its beneficial function. In such cases the immunogenicity may be misinterpreted as being due to the recombinant protein itself. Therefore, one must be very cautious in interpreting safety data of a given recombinant therapeutic protein.

Generally, the sources of protein contaminants are the growth medium used, the host proteins of the cells, and ligands from affinity columns used in the purification process. Basis medium is frequently supplemented with physiologically active proteins (e.g., insulin, transferrin, bovine serum albumin) and vitamins for cell propagation as well. As mentioned before in this chapter, the use of serum-free media is favored for the large scale manufacturing of pharmaceutical proteins, but biological parameters like insufficient cell growth and productivity are still significant barriers to the extensive use of well-defined serum-free media.

Among the host derived contaminant, the host species' version of the recombinant protein could be present (WHO, 1987). As these proteins are similar in structure, it is possible that undesired proteins are co-purified with the desired product. For example, urokinase is known to be present in many continuous cell lines. The synthesis of highly active biological molecules such as cytokines by hybridoma cells, might be another concern (FDA, 1990; Schindler and Dinarello, 1990). Depending upon their nature and concentration these cytokines might enhance the antigenicity of the product.

'Known' or expected contaminants should be monitored at the successive stages in a purification process by suitable in-process controls, e.g., sensitive immunoassay(s). Tracing of the many 'unknown' cell-derived proteins is more difficult. When developing a purification process other, more general, analyses are usually used e.g., SDS-PAGE in combination with various staining techniques (Bergemann et al., 1993; Per et al., 1989).

Downstream Processing

Introduction

Recovering a biological reagent from a cell culture supernatant is one of the critical parts of the manufacturing procedure for biotech products. Often the product is available in a very dilute form (for actual cell systems 10–200 mg/L, up to as high as 500–800 mg/l for advanced (mammalian) cell systems) (Berthold and Walter, 1994; Garnick *et al.*, 1988). Typically, a concentration step is required to reduce handling volumes for further purification. Usually, the product subsequently undergoes a series of purification steps, the first one to capture and initially purify; the second one to remove the bulk of the contaminants including DNA, and a final step to remove all trace contaminants and variant forms of the molecule. After purification, the bulk product undergoes a series of steps, including formulation and sterilization to obtain the product in its required stable form. Formulation aspects will be dealt with in Chapter 4.

When designing a purification protocol, the possibility for scaling up should be considered carefully. A process that has been designed for small quantities may not be suitable for large quantities. At commercial production scale, the requirements for purity are equal to laboratory separations, but the desired recovery level is higher since the yield will determine the overall economics of the process.

Developing a downstream process (i.e. the isolation and purification of the desired product) to recover a biological protein in large quantities occurs in two stages: *design* and *scale-up*.

Separating a product protein from impurities requires a series of purification steps (*process design*), each removing some of the impurities and bringing the product closer to its final specification. In general, the starting feed stream contains cell debris and/or whole-cell particulate material which must be removed. Defining the major contaminants in the starting material is helpful in the downstream process design. This includes detailed information on the source of the material (e.g., bacterial or mammalian cell culture) and major contaminants (e.g., albumin or product analogs). Moreover, physical characteristics of the product (thermal stability, isoelectric point, molecular weight, hydrophobicity, density, specific binding properties) largely determine the process design. The risk of microbial (cross) contamination can be minimized by introducing separate production facilities ('closed systems') for cell-containing and cell-free operations.

Processes used for large scale productions should be reproducible and reliable (Johansson *et al.*, 1988). Both protein and non-protein contaminants, such as pyrogenic endotoxins, DNA, viruses, etc. that could negatively affect the health of patients must be removed from the product.

Methods used for recovery may expose the protein molecules to high physical stress (e.g., high temperatures and extreme pH) which may alter the protein's properties leading to appreciable loss in protein activity. Any substance that is used by injection must be sterile and "free" from pyrogens, i.e., below a certain level (i.e. the pyrogen concentration must be under a certain level depending on the product (limits are stated in the individual monographs which are to be consulted, e.g., European Pharmacopoeia, 1997)). This necessitates aseptic techniques and procedures throughout with clean air and microbial control of all materials and equipment (FDA, 1987). During validation of the purification process it must also be demonstrated that potential viral contaminants can be removed (Walter *et al.*, 1992). The purification matrices should be at least sanitizable or, better, autoclavable. For depyrogenation, the purification material must withstand either extended dry heat at 180°C or treatment with 1–2 M sodium hydroxide (for further information see Chapter 4). If any material in contact with the product inadvertently releases compounds, these leachables must be analyzed and their removal by subsequent purification steps must be demonstrated during process validation (European Community Guidelines, 1989). Finally, as stated before, DNA contamination of the product should be reduced to an acceptable level.

Scale-up is the term used to describe a number of processes employed in converting a laboratory procedure into an economical, industrial process. During the scale-up phase, the process moves from the laboratory through the pilot plant and finally to the production plant. The objective of scale-up is to produce a product of high quality at a competitive price. Since costs of downstream processing can be as high as 50 to 80% of the total cost of a product, practical and economical ways of purifying the product should be used. Superior protein purification methods hold the key to a strong market position (Wheelwright, 1993).

Basic operations required for a downstream purification process used for macromolecules from biological sources are shown in Figure 3.2. As mentioned before, the design of downstream processing protocols is highly product dependent. Therefore, each product requires a specific multistage purification procedure (Sadana, 1989). The basic scheme as represented in Figure 3.2 becomes complex. A typical example of a process flowchart for the downstream processing is shown Figure 3.3. This scheme represents the processing of a glycosylated recombinant interferon (about 28 kD) produced in mammalian cells. The intention of the individual unit operations are described (Berthold and Walter, 1994).

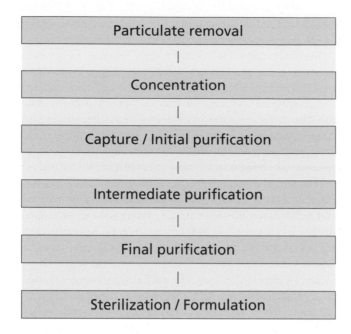

Figure 3.2. Basic operations required for the purification of a biopharmaceutical macromolecule.

A wide range of purification methods is now available, and new techniques are continuously added to this arsenal. A number of methods are available to separate proteins on the basis of a wide variety of different physicochemical criteria such as size, charge, hydrophobicity and solubility (Table 3.5). Detailed information about some separation and purification methods commonly used in purification schemes follows below.

Filtration/Centrifugation

Products from biotechnological industry have to be separated from biological systems that contain suspended particulates, including whole cells, lysed cell material, and fragments of broken cells generated when cell breakage has been necessary to release intracellular products. Most downstream processing flow sheets will therefore include at least one unit-operation for the removal ("clarification") or concentration, just the opposite, of particulates. Most frequently used methods are centrifugation and filtration techniques (e.g., ultrafiltration, diafiltration and microfiltration). The effectiveness of such methods is highly dependent on the physical nature of the particulate material and of the product.

FILTRATION

Filtration can be used to concentrate the biomass prior to further purification. Several filtration systems have been developed for separation of cells from media, the most

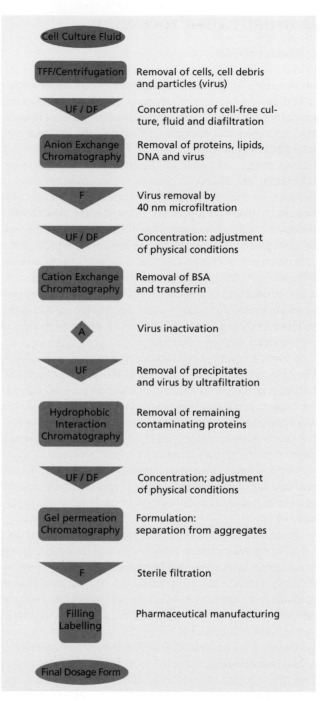

Figure 3.3. Downstream processing of a glycosylated recombinant interferon, describing the purpose of the inclusion of the individual unit operations. (TFF: Tangential Flow Filtration, UF: Ultrafiltration, DF: Diafiltration, A: Adsorption; adapted from Berthold and Walter, 1994).

successful being tangential flow systems where high shear across the membrane surface limits fouling, gel layer formation and concentration polarization. In ultrafiltration, mixtures of molecules of different molecular dimensions are separated by passage of a dispersion under pressure across a membrane with a defined pore size (Minton, 1990). In general, little purification can be achieved by ultrafiltration, because of the relatively large pore size distribution of the membranes. However, this technique is widely used to concentrate macromolecules or viruses, and also to change the aqueous phase in which the particles are dispersed or in which molecules are dissolved (diafiltration) to one required for the subsequent purification step.

CENTRIFUGATION

Subcellular particles and organelles, suspended in a viscous liquid (for example the particles produced when cells are disrupted by mechanical procedures) are difficult to separate either by using one fixed centrifugation step or by filtration. But, they can be isolated efficiently by centrifugation at different speeds. For instance nuclei can be obtained at $400 \times g$ for 20 minutes, while plasma membrane vesicles are pelleted at higher centrifugation rates and longer centrifugation times (fractional centrifugation).

Buoyant density centrifugation can be useful for separation of particles as well. This technique uses a viscous fluid with a continuous gradient of density in a centrifuge tube. Particles and molecules of various densities within the density range in the tube will cease to move when the isopycnic region has been reached. The different fractions can then be recovered by carefully siphoning the fluid or allowing it to flow through a hole made in the bottom of the tube. Both continuous (fluid densities gradually changing within a range) and discontinuous (stepwise changing fluid densities) density gradient centrifugation are used in buoyant density centrifugation.

For application on industrial scale the development of centrifuges which are steam sterilizable (and expensive as well) may be very useful. However, before routine use these methods should be validated extensively (reliability and reproducibility) (Walter and Werner, 1993; European Community Guidelines, 1989).

Precipitation

The solubility of a particular protein depends on the physicochemical environment, e.g., pH, ionic species and ionic strength of the solution (cf. Chapter 4). A slow continuous increase of the ionic strength (of a protein mixture) will selectively drive proteins out of solution. This phenomenon is known as 'salting-out'. A wide variety of agents, with different 'salting out' potencies are available. Chaotropic series with increasing 'salting out' effects of negatively (I) and positively (II) charged ions are given below (von Hippel et al., 1964):

$I - SCN^-, I^-, ClO_4^-, NO_3^-, Br^-, Cl^-, CH_3COO^-, PO_4^{3-}, SO_4^{2-}$

$II - Ba^{2+}, Ca^{2+}, Mg^{2+}, Li^+, Cs^+, Na^+, K^+, Rb^+, NH_4^+$

Ammonium sulfate is highly soluble in cold aqueous solutions and is frequently used in 'salting-out' purification.

Another method to precipitate proteins is to use water-miscible organic solvents (change in the dielectric constant). Examples of precipitating agents are polyethylene glycol, trichloracetic acid, chitosan and non-ionic polyoxyethylene detergents (Cartwright, 1987; Homma et al., 1993; Terstappen et al., 1993). Precipitation is a scalable, simple and a relatively economical procedure for recovery of a product from a dilute feed stream. It has been widely used for the isolation of proteins from culture supernatants. Unfortunately, most bulk precipitation methods provide very little in the way of purification, which make these methods not very attractive for the large scale purification of recombinant proteins. Additionally, they introduce extraneous components which must later be eliminated. Furthermore, large quantities of precipitates may be difficult to handle. Despite these limitations, recovery by precipitation has been used with considerable success for some products.

Chromatography

INTRODUCTION

The separation of molecules from biological materials often involves the isolation of one particular molecular species from a mixture of compounds with similar properties. Chromatographic techniques (cf. Chapter 2) are very effective in purification procedures (Janson and Hedman, 1982). In chromatography components of a sample are primarily separated based on differences in distribution between two phases, one of which is the stationary phase (mostly a solid phase) while the other moves (this mobile phase may be liquid or gaseous). In practice almost all stationary phases (fine particles) are packed into a column (provides a large surface area) over which the mobile phase is passed.

Downstream purification protocols usually have at least two to three chromatography steps. Chromatographic methods used in purification procedures of biotech products are listed in Table 3.5 and will be briefly discussed in the following sections.

CHROMATOGRAPHIC STATIONARY PHASES

Chromatographic procedures often represent the rate-limiting step in the overall downstream processing. An important primary factor governing the rate of operation is the mass transport into the pores of conventional packing ma-

Separation technique	Mode/Principle	Separation based on
Membrane separation	microfiltration ultrafiltration dialysis	size size size
Centrifugation	isopycnic banding non-equilibrium settling	density density
Extraction	fluid extraction liquid/liquid extraction	solubility partition, change in solubility
Precipitation	fractional precipitation	change in solubility
Chromatography	ion-exchange gel filtration affinity hydrophobic interaction adsorption	charge size specific ligand-substrate interaction hydrophobicity covalent/noncovalent binding

Table 3.5. Frequently used separation processes and their physical basis.

terials. Adsorbents employed include inorganic materials such as silica gels, hydroxyapatite, various metal oxides (alumina, glass beads), silica gels and polymers (cross-linked dextrans, cellulose, agarose). The separation occurs by differential interaction of sample components with the chromatographic medium. Ionic groups such as amines and carboxylic acids, dipolar groups such as carbonyl functional groups, and hydrogen bond-donating and accepting groups control the interaction of the sample components with the stationary phase and functional groups slow down the elution rate if interaction occurs.

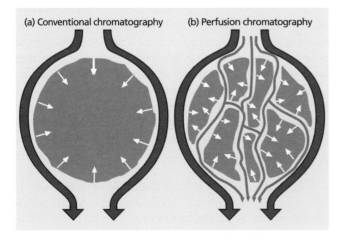

Figure 3.4. The structure of conventional chromatographic particles (a) and perfusion or flow-through chromatographic particles (b) (from Fulton, 1994).

Chromatographic stationary phases for use on a large-scale have improved considerably over the last decade. Hjerten *et al.* (1993) reported on the use of compressed acrylamide-based polymer structures. These materials combine relatively fast separations with good chromatographic performance. Another approach to the problems associated with mass transport in conventional systems is to use chromatographic particles that contain some large 'through pores' in addition to conventional pores (see Figure 3.4). These flow-through or 'perfusion chromatography' media enable faster convective mass transport into particles and allow operation at much higher speeds without loss in resolution or binding capacity (Afeyan *et al.*, 1989; Fulton, 1994). Another development is the design of spirally wrapped columns containing the adsorption medium. This configuration permits high throughput, high capacity and high capture efficiency (Cartwright, 1987).

The ideal stationary phase for protein separation should possess a number of characteristics, among which are high mechanical strength, high porosity, no non-specific interaction between protein and the support phase, high capacity, biocompatibility and high stability of the matrix in a variety of solvents. The latter is especially true for columns used for the production of clinical materials which need to be cleaned, depyrogenized, disinfected and sterilized at regular intervals. High-Performance Liquid Chromatography (HPLC) systems fulfil many of these criteria. Liquid phases should be carefully chosen to minimize loss of biological activity resulting from the use of some organic solvents. In HPLC small pore size stationary phases that are incompressible are used. These particles are small, rigid and regularly sized (to provide a high surface area). The mobile liquid phase is forced under high pressure through the column material. Reversed-phase HPLC systems, using less polar stationary phases than the mobile phases can be effectively integrated into large-scale purification schemes of proteins and can serve both as a means of concentration and purification (Benedek and Swadesh, 1991).

Fast Protein Liquid Chromatography (FPLC) columns operate at relatively low back pressure and can thus be used in equipment constructed from plastics which, unlike conventional stainless steel equipment, resists all buffers likely to be employed in the separation of biomolecules. These columns are commercially available and permit the efficient separations of proteins in a single run. Results can be obtained rapidly and with high resolution. A new development is the use of stainless steel equipment which resists almost all chemicals used in protein purification including disinfection and sterilization media.

Unfortunately, HPLC equipment costs are high and this technology will probably find only limited application in large-scale purification schemes (Strickler and Gemski, 1987; Jungbauer and Wenisch, 1989).

ADSORPTION CHROMATOGRAPHY

In adsorption chromatography (also called 'normal phase' chromatography) the stationary phase is more polar than the mobile phase. The protein of interest selectively binds to a static matrix under one condition and is released under a different condition (Chase, 1988). Adsorption chromatography methods enable high ratios of product load to stationary phase volume, therefore, this principle is economically scalable.

ION-EXCHANGE CHROMATOGRAPHY

Ion-exchange chromatography can be a powerful adsorption step at the beginning of a purification scheme. It can be easily scaled up. Ion-exchange chromatography can be used in a negative mode, i.e. the product flows through the column under conditions that favor the adsorption of contaminants to the matrix, while the protein of interest does not bind (Tennikova and Svec, 1993). The type of the column needed is determined by the protein (e.g., isoelectric point and charge density) to be purified. Anion exchangers bind negatively charged molecules and cation exchangers bind positively charged molecules. In salt-gradient ion-exchange chromatography, the salt concentration in the perfusing elution buffer is continuously or in steps increased. The stronger the binding of an individual protein to the ion exchanger, the later it will appear in the elution buffer. Likewise, in pH-gradient chromatography, the pH is continuously or in steps changed. Here, the protein binds at one pH and is released at a different pH. As a result of the heterogeneity in glycosylation, glycosylated proteins may elute in a relatively broad pH range (up to 2 pH units).

In order to simplify purification, a specific amino acid tail can be added to the protein at the gene level to create a "purification handle". For example, a short tail consisting of arginine residues allows a protein to bind to a cation exchanger under conditions where almost no other cell proteins bind.

(IMMUNO)AFFINITY CHROMATOGRAPHY

Affinity chromatography is based on highly specific interactions between an immobilized ligand and the protein of interest. Affinity chromatography is a very powerful method for the purification of proteins. Under physiological conditions the protein binds to the ligand. Extensive washing of this matrix will remove contaminants and the purified protein can be recovered by the addition of ligands competing for the stationary phase binding sites or by changes in physical conditions (e.g., low or high pH of the eluent) which greatly reduce the affinity. Examples of affinity chromatography include the purification of glycoproteins, which bind to immobilized lectins, and the purification of serine proteases with lysine binding sites, which bind to immobilized lysine. In these cases a soluble ligand (sugar or lysine, respectively) can be used to elute the required product under relatively mild conditions. Another example is the use of the affinity of protein A and protein G for antibodies. Protein A and protein G have a high affinity for the Fc portions of many immunoglobulins from various animals. Protein A and G matrices can be commercially obtained with a high degree of purity. For the purification of hormones or growth factors, the receptors or short peptide sequence that mimic the binding site of the receptor molecule can be used as affinity ligands. Some proteins show highly selective affinity for certain dyes that are commercially available as immobilized ligands on purification matrices. When considering the selection of these ligands for pharmaceutical production, one must realize that some of these dyes are carcinogenic and that a fraction may leach out during operation.

An interesting approach to optimize purification is the use of a gene that codes not only for the desired protein, but also for an additional sequence that facilitates recovery by affinity chromatography. At a later stage the additional sequence is removed by a specific cleavage reaction. This is a complex process which needs additional purification steps.

The specific binding of antibodies to their epitopes is used in immunoaffinity chromatography (Chase, 1993;

Kamihira *et al.*, 1993). These techniques can be applied for purification of both the antigen and the antibody. The antibody can be covalently coupled to the stationary phase and act as the "receptor" for the antigen to be purified. Alternatively, the antigens, or parts thereof, can be attached on the stationary phase for the purification of the antibodies. Immunoaffinity chromatography has several advantages such as high specificity and the combination of concentration and purification in one step.

There are certain disadvantages associated with immunoaffinity methods. The antibody-antigen binding may be very strong, requiring harsh conditions for the separation of the antibody-antigen complex to elute the purified ligand. Under such conditions, sensitive ligands could be harmed (e.g., denaturation of the protein to be purified). This can be alleviated by (1) the selection of antibodies and environmental conditions with high specificity and sufficient affinity to induce an antibody ligand interaction, while the antigen can be released under mild conditions (Jones, 1990), (2) the use of tandem columns to quickly moderate the physical conditions (e.g., pH and ionic strength), (3) the use of a stabilizing recipient solution into which the product is eluted. Another concern is disruption of the covalent bond linking the "receptor" to the matrix. This would result in elution of the entire complex. Therefore, in practice, a further purification step after affinity chromatography as well as an appropriate detection assay (e.g., ELISA) is almost always necessary. On the other hand, improved coupling chemistry that is less susceptible to hydrolysis has been developed to prevent leaching (Knight, 1990).

Scale-up of immunoaffinity chromatography is often hampered by the relatively large quantity of the specific "receptor" (either the antigen or the antibody) that is required and the lack of commercially available, ready-to-use matrices.

Examples of proteins of potential therapeutic value that have been purified using immunoaffinity chromatography are interferons, urokinase, factor VIII:c, erythropoietin, interleukin-2, human factor X, and recombinant tissue plasminogen activator.

HYDROPHOBIC INTERACTION CHROMATOGRAPHY

Under physiological conditions most hydrophobic amino acid residues are located inside the protein core and only a small fraction of hydrophobic amino acids is exposed on the "surface" of a protein. Their exposure is suppressed because of the presence of hydrophilic amino acids that attract large clusters of water molecules and form a "shield". High salt concentrations reduce the hydration of a protein and the surface-exposed hydrophobic amino acid residues

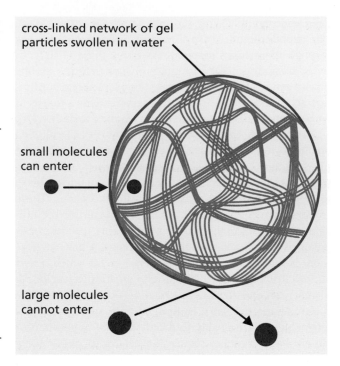

Figure 3.5. Schematic representation of the principle of gel filtration (from James, 1992).

become more accessible. Hydrophobic Interaction Chromatography (HIC) is based on non-covalent and non-electrostatic interactions between proteins and the stationary phase. HIC is a "mild" technique, usually yielding high recoveries of proteins that are not damaged, are folded correctly and are separated from contaminants that are structurally related. HIC is ideally placed in the purification scheme after ion-exchange chromatography, where the protein usually is released in high ionic strength elution media (Heng and Glatz, 1993).

GEL PERMEATION CHROMATOGRAPHY

Gel-permeation or size-exclusion chromatography, also known as gel filtration, separates proteins according to their shape and size (see Figure 3.5). Inert gels with narrow pore-size distributions in the size range of proteins are available. These gels are packed into a column and the protein mixture is then loaded on top of the column and the proteins diffuse into the gel. The smaller the protein, the more volume it will have available to disperse in. Molecules that are larger than the largest pores are not able to penetrate the gel beads and will therefore stay in the void volume of the column. When a continuous flow of buffer passes through the column, the larger proteins will elute first and the smallest molecules last. Gel permeation chromatography is a good alternative to diafiltration for buffer exchange at almost any purification stage and it is often used in laboratory design. At production scale, the use of this technique is usually limited, because of the inherent dilution effect. It is therefore best avoided or used late in the purification process when the protein is available in a highly concentrated form. Gel filtration is very commonly used as the final step in the purification to bring proteins in the appropriate buffer used in the final formulation.

Expanded Beds

As mentioned before, purification schemes are based on multistep protocols. This adds greatly to the overall production costs. Moreover, it can result in significant loss of product. Therefore, there still is an interest in the development of new methods for simplifying the purification process. Adsorption techniques are popular methods for the recovery of proteins and the conventional operating format for preparative separations is a packed column (or fixed bed) of adsorbent. Particulate material, however, can be trapped near the bed, which results in an increase in the pressure drop across the bed and eventually in clogging of the column. This can be avoided by the use of pre-column filters (0.2 μm) to save the column integrity. Another solution to this problem may be the use of expanded beds (Chase and Draeger, 1993; Fulton, 1994), also called fluidized beds (see Figure 3.6). In principle, the use of expanded beds enables clarification, concentration and purification to be achieved in a single step. The concept is to employ a particulate solid-phase adsorbent in an open bed with upward liquid flow. The hydrodynamic drag around the particles tends to lift them upwards, which is counteracted by the gravity because of a density difference between the particles and the liquid phase. The particles remain suspended if particle diameter, particle density, liquid viscosity and liquid density are properly balanced by choosing the correct flow rate. The expanded bed allows particles (i.e., cells) to pass through, whereas molecules in solution are selectively (e.g., by the use of ion-exchange or affinity adsorbents) retained on the adsorbent particles. Feedstocks can be applied to the bed without prior removal of particulate material by centrifugation or filtration. Fluidized beds have been used previously for the industrial scale recovery of antibiotics such as streptomycin and novobiocin (Fulton, 1994; Chase, 1994). Stable, expanded beds can be obtained using simple equipment adapted from that used for conventional, packed bed adsorption and chromatography processes. Ion-exchange adsorbents are likely to be chosen for such separations.

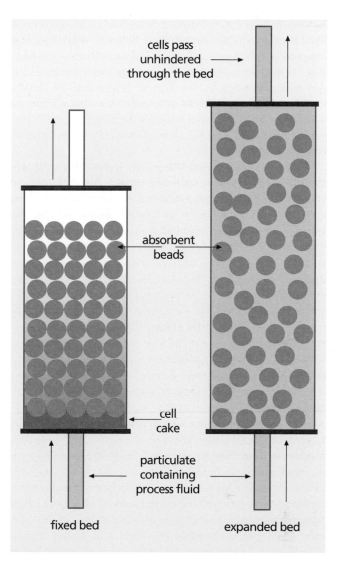

Figure 3.6. Comparison between (a) a fixed bed and (b) an expanded bed (adapted from Chase and Draeger, 1993).

Issues to Consider in Production and Purification of Proteins

N- and C-terminal Heterogeneity

A major problem connected with the production of biotech products is the problem associated with the amino (NH$_2$)-terminus of the protein. Obviously, it is important to develop methods (Christensen *et al.*, 1990) that generate proteins with an NH$_2$-terminus as found in the authentic protein. When the proteins are not produced in the correct way, the final product may be a mixture of several methionyl variants of the protein in question or even contain proteins lacking one or more residues from the amino terminus. This is called the amino terminal heterogeneity. This heterogeneity can also occur in case of recombinant proteins (e.g., α-interferon) that are susceptible to proteases which are either secreted by the host or introduced by serum-containing media. These proteases can clip off amino acids from the C-terminal and/or N-terminal of the desired product (amino- and/or carboxy-terminal heterogeneity) (Garnick *et al.* 1988).

Amino- and/or carboxy-terminal heterogeneity is not desirable since it may cause difficulties in purification and characterization of the proteins. In case of the presence of an additional methionine at the N-terminal end of the protein, its secondary and tertiary structure can be altered. This can affect the biological activity and stability and may make it immunogenic. Moreover, N-terminal methionine and/or "internal" methionine are sensitive to oxidation (Sharma, 1990).

Chemical Modification/Conformational Changes

Although mammalian cells are able to produce proteins that are structurally equal to endogenous proteins, one should remain cautious. Transcripts containing the full-length coding sequence could result in conformational isomers of the protein because of unexpected secondary structures that affect translational fidelity (Sharma, 1990). Another factor to be taken into account is the possible existence of equilibria between the desired form and other forms such as dimers. The correct folding of proteins after biosynthesis is important, because it determines the specific activity of the protein (Berthold and Walter, 1994). Therefore, it is important to determine if all molecules of a given recombinant protein secreted by a mammalian expression system are folded in their native conformation. In some cases it may be relatively easy to detect misfolded structures, in other cases it may be extremely difficult.

Apart from conformational changes, proteins can undergo chemical alterations, such as proteolysis, deamidation, hydroxyl and sulfhydryl oxidations during the purification process. These alterations can result in (partial) denaturation of the protein. Vice versa, denaturation of the protein may cause chemical modifications as well (e.g., as a result of exposure of sensitive groups) (Ptitsyn, 1987).

Glycosylation

Many therapeutic proteins produced by recombinant DNA technology are glycoproteins (Sharma, 1990). The presence and nature of oligosaccharide side chains in proteins affect a number of important characteristics, amongst which the proteins' serum half life, solubility, stability and some-

times even the pharmacological function. As a result, the therapeutic profile may be "glycosylation" dependent. As mentioned previously, protein glycosylation is not directly determined by the DNA sequence. It is an enzymatic modification of the protein after translation, and can depend on the environment in the cell. Although mammalian cells are very well able to glycosylate proteins, it is hard to fully control glycosylation. Carbohydrate heterogeneity is detected by variations in the size of the chain, type of oligosaccharide and sequence of the carbohydrates. This has been demonstrated for a number of recombinant products including interleukin-4, chorionic gonadotropin, erythropoietin and tissue plasminogen activator. Carbohydrate structure and composition in recombinant proteins may differ from their native counterparts, because the enzymes required for synthesis and processing vary in different expression systems (e.g., glycoproteins in insect cells are frequently smaller than the same glycoproteins expressed in mammalian cells) or even from one mammalian system to another.

Proteolytic Processing

Proteases play an important role in processing, maturation, modification, or isolation of recombinant proteins (Sharma and Hopkins, 1981). Proteases from mammalian cells are involved in secreting proteins into the cultivation medium. If secretion of the recombinant protein occurs co-translationally, then the intracellular proteolytic system of the mammalian cell should not be harmful to the recombinant protein. Proteases are released if cells die or break (e.g., during cell break at cell harvest) and undergo lysis. It is therefore important to control growth and harvest conditions in order to minimize this effect. Another source of proteolytic attack is found in the components of the medium in which the cells are grown. For example, serum contains a number of proteases and protease zymogens that may affect the secreted recombinant protein. If present in small amounts, and if the nature of the proteolytic attack on the desired protein is identified, the use of appropriate protease inhibitors to control proteolysis could be considered. It is best to document the integrity of the recombinant protein, after each purification step (cf. Chapter 2).

Proteins become much more susceptible to proteases at elevated temperatures. Purification strategies should be designed such that all the steps can be carried out at 4°C (Sharma, 1986b) if proteolytic degradation will occur.

Protein Inclusion Body Formation

In bacteria normally soluble proteins can form dense, finely granular inclusions within the cytoplasm. These "inclusion bodies" often occur in bacterial cells that overproduce proteins through the use of plasmid expression. The protein inclusions appear in electron micrographs as large, dense bodies often spanning the entire diameter of the cell. Protein inclusions are probably formed by a build-up of amorphous protein aggregates that are held together by covalent and non-covalent bonds. The inability to directly measure inclusion body proteins may lead to the inaccurate assessment of recovery and yield and may cause problems if protein solubility is essential for efficient, large scale purification (Berthold and Walter, 1994). Several schemes for recovery of proteins from inclusion bodies have been described (Krueger *et al.*, 1989). The recovery of proteins from inclusion bodies requires cell breakage, protein sedimentation and pellet washing. Dissolution and refolding (in case the three-dimensional structure is the biologically active form) of inclusion proteins is the next step in the purification scheme. Generally, inclusion proteins dissolve in denaturing agents such as sodium dodecylsulfate (SDS), urea, or guanidine hydrochloride. In cases in which molecules are interlinked by disulfide bonds, the addition of reducing agents may enhance or facilitate the solubilization of protein inclusion bodies. Once the protein is solubilized, conventional chromatographic separations can be used for further purification of the protein.

Aggregate formation at first sight may seem undesirable, but there may also be advantages as long as the protein of interest will unfold and refold properly. Inclusion body proteins can easily be recovered to yield proteins with >50% purity, a substantial improvement over the purity of soluble proteins (sometimes below 1% of the total cell protein). Furthermore, the aggregated forms of the proteins are more resistant to proteolysis (Krueger *et al.*, 1989), because most molecules of an aggregated form are not accessible to proteolytic enzymes. ∎

References

- **Afeyan N, Gordon N, Mazsaroff I, Varady L, Fulton S, Yang Y, Regnier F.** (1989). Flow-through particles of the high-performance liquid chromatographic separation of biomolecules, perfusion chromatography. *J Chromatogr*, 519, 1–29
- **Arathoon WR, Birch JR.** (1986). Large-scale cell culture in biotechnology. *Science*, 232, 1390–1395
- **Benedek K, Swadesh JK.** (1991). HPLC of proteins and peptides in the pharmaceutical industry. In *HPLC in the pharmaceutical industry*, edited by GW Fong, SK Lam. Dekker, New York, pp. 241–302
- **Bergemann K, Walter J, Berthold W.** (1993). Removal of host cell DNA from protein solutions. Validation of Pharmaceuticals and Biopharmaceuticals, Parenteral Drug Associates, Inc. (PDA), 2nd *International Congress*, Basel
- **Berthold W, Walter, J.** (1992). Virus removal and Inactivation. *Biotech Form Europe*, 9
- **Berthold W, Walter J.** (1994). Protein Purification: Aspects of processes for pharmaceutical products. *Biologicals*, 22, 135–150
- **Bouchard L, Gelinas C, Asselin C, Bastin M.** (1984). Tumorogenic activity of Polyoma virus and SV40 DNA's in newborn rodents. *Virology*, 135, 53–64
- **Burnouf T, Dernis D, Michalski C, Goudemand M, Huart JJ.** (1989). Therapeutic advantages of a high purity plasma factor IX concentrate produced by conventional chromatography. *Colloque Inserm*, 175, 25–334
- **Cartwright T.** (1987). Isolation and purification of products from animal cells. *Trends in Biotechnology*, 5, 25–30
- **Chase H, Draeger N.** (1993). Affinity purification of proteins using expanded beds. *J Chromatogr*, 597, 129–145
- **Chase HA.** (1988). Adsorption preparation processes for protein purification. In *Downstream processes: Equipment and techniques*, edited by A Mizrahi. AR Liss, New York, Vol. 8, pp. 163–312
- **Chase HA.** (1994). Purification of proteins by adsorption chromatography in expanded beds. *Tibtech.*, 12, 296–303
- **Christensen T, Dalboge H, Snel L.** (1990). Postbiosynthesis Modification: Human Growth Hormone and Insuline precursors. In *Drug Manufacture Part IV*
- **Commission of the European Communities.** (1989). Guidelines on the Quality, Safety and Efficacy of Medicinal Products for Human Use, 2, *Rules Governing Medicinal Products in the European Community*
- **Commission of the European Communities.** (1989). Guidelines to Good Manufacturing Practice for Medicinal Products, 4, *Rules Governing Medicinal Products in the European Community*
- **Commission of the European Communities.** (1991). Ad Hoc Working Party on Biotechnology/Pharmacy. *Note for Guidance: Validation of Virus Removal and Inactivation procedures*, EC DG III/81 15/89-EN
- **European Pharmacopoeia**, 3rd Edition, 1997
- **FDA, Center for Biologics Evaluation and Research.** (1990). *Cytokine and Growth Factor Pre-Pivotal Trial Information Package with Special Emphasis on Products Identified for Consideration under 21 CFR 312 Subpart E*, Bethesda, MD, USA
- **FDA, Division of Manufacturing and Product Quality.** (1987). *Guidelines on Sterile Drug Product Produced by Aseptic Processing*, Rockville Rike, Bethesda MD, USA
- **FDA, Office of Biologicals Research and Review.** (1993). *Points to consider in the characterization of cell lines used to produce biologicals*, Rockville Rike, Bethesda MD, USA

- **Feinstone SM, Mihalik KB, Kamimura T, Alter HJ, London TW, Purcell RH.** (1983). Inactivation of hepatitis B virus and non-A, non-B hepatitis by chloroform. *Infect Immun*, 41, 816–821
- **Fulton SP.** (1994). Large scale processing of macromolecules. *Current Opinion in Biotechnology*, 5, 201–205
- **Garnick RL, Solli NJ, Papa PA.** (1988). The role of quality control in biotechnology: an analytical perspective. *Anal Chem*, 60, 2546–2557
- **Heng M, Glatz C.** (1993). Charged fusions for selective recovery of ß-galactosidase from cell extract using hollow fiber ion-exchange membrane adsorption. *Biotechnol Bioeng*, 42, 333–338
- **Hippel, van PH, Wong K-Y.** (1964). Neutral salts: the generality of their effects on the stability of macromolecular conformations. *Science*, 145, 577–580
- **Hjerten S, Mohammed J, Nakazato K.** (1993). Improvement in flow properties and pH stability of compressed, continuous polymer beds for high-performance liquid chromatography. *J Chromatogr*, 646, 121–128
- **Homma JY, Kanegasaki S, Lüderitz O, Shiba T, Wertphal O.** (1984). *Bacterial Endotoxin*. Verlag Chemie, Weinheim, New York
- **Homma T, Fuji M, Mori J, Kawakami T, Kuroda K, Taniguchi M.** (1993). Production of cellobiose by enzymatic hydrolysis: removal of ß-glucosidase from cellulase by affinity precipitation using chitosan. *Biotechnol Bioeng*, 41, 405–410
- **Horowitz MS, Bolmer SD, Horowitz B.** (1991). Elimination of disease-transmitting enveloped viruses from human blood plasma and mammalian cell culture products. *Bioseparation*, 1, 409–417
- **Horowitz B, Prince AM, Hamman J, Watklevicz C.** (1994). Viral safety of solvent/detergent-treated blood products. *Blood Coagulation and Fibrinolysis*, 5, S21–S28
- **James AM.** (1992). Introduction fundamental techniques. In *Analysis of Amino Acids and Nucleic Acids*, edited by AM James. Butterworth-Heinemann, Oxford, pp. 1–28
- **Janson, J-C, Hedman P.** (1982). Large-scale chromatography of proteins. In *Advances in Biochemical Engineering*, edited by A Fiechter. Heidelberg, Springer-Verlag
- **Johansson H, Östling M, Sofer G, Wahlsttröm H, Low D.** (1988). Chromatographic equipment for large-scale protein and peptide purification. In *Downstream Processes: Equipment and Techniques*, edited by AR Liss. New York, pp. 127–157
- **Jones K.** (1990). Affinity chromatography, A technology up-date, *Am Biotechnol Lab*, 8, 26–30
- **Jungbauer A, Wenisch E.** (1989). High Performance Liquid Chromatography and related methods in purification of monoclonal antibodies. In *Advances in biotechnological processes*, edited by AR Liss. New York, pp. 161–192
- **Kamihira M, Kaul R, Mattiasson B.** (1993). Purification of recombinant protein A by aqueous two-phase extraction integrated with affinity precipitation. *Biotechnol Bioeng*, 40, 1381–1387
- **Klegerman ME, Groves MJ.** (1992). *Pharmaceutical Biotechnology*. Interpharm Press, Inc., USA
- **Knight P.** (1990). Bioseparations: media and modes. *Biotechnology*, 8, 200
- **Krueger JK, Kulke MH, Schutt C, Stock J.** (1989). Protein inclusion body formation and purification. *Pharmaceutical Technology International*, 48–51
- **Kung VT, Panfili PR, Sheldon EL, King RS, Nagainis PA, Gomez B, Ross DA, Briggs J, Zuk RF.** (1990). Picogram Quantification of Total DNA Using DNA-Binding Proteins in a Silicon Sensor Based System. *Anal Biochem*, 187, 220–227
- **Liptrot C, Gull K.** (1991). Detection of Viruses in Recombinant Cells by Electron Microscopy. In *Animal Cell Technology, Developments, Processes and Products*, edited by RE Spier, JB Griffiths, C MacDonald. Butterworth-Heinemann Ltd, Oxford, 653–656
- **Löwer J.** (1990). Risk of Tumor Induction *in Vivo* by Residual Cellular DNA, Quantitative Considerations. *J Med Virol*, 31, 50–53
- **Marcus-Sekura CJ.** (1991). *Validation and Removal of Human Retroviruses*. Center for Biologics Evaluation and Research, FDA. Bethesda, MD, USA
- **Minton AP.** (1990). Quantitative characterization of reversible molecular associations via analytical centrifugation. *Anal Biochem*, 190, 1–6
- **Nolan JG, McDevitt JJ, Goldmann GS.** (1975). Endotoxin binding by charged and uncharged resin. *Proc Soc Exp Biol Med*, 149, 766–770
- **Note for Guidance.** (1991). *Validation of Virus Removal and Inactivation Procedure*, Ad Hoc Working Party on Biotechnology/ Pharmacy, European Community, DG III/8115/89–EN
- **Novitsky T, Gould MJ.** (1985). Inactivation of Endotoxin by Polymyxin B, Technical Report No. 7, Parenteral Drug Association, Inc., Philadelphia
- **Pearson FC.** (1987). Pyrogens and Depyrogenation, Theory and Practice. In *Aseptic Pharmaceutical Manufacturing*, edited by WP Olson, MJ Groves. Interpharm Press, Inc., Prairie View
- **Per SR, Aversa CR, Sito AF.** (1989). Quantification of Residual DNA in Biological Products. *Clin Chem*, 35, 1859–1860
- **Perret BA, Poorbeik M, Morell A.** (1991). Klinische prüfung von Premogfil M SRK, einem mit monoklonalen antikörpern hochgereinigten gerinningsfaktor VIII-Konzentrat aus human plasma. *Schweiz Med Wochenschr*, 121, 1624–1627
- **Ptitsyn OB.** (1987). Protein folding: Hypothesis and experiments. *J Protein Chem*, 6, 273–293
- **Sadana A.** (1989). Protein inactivation during downstream separation, part I: The Processes. *Biopharm*, 2, 14–25
- **Schindler R, Dinarello CA.** (1990). Ultrafiltration to Remove Endotoxins and other Cytokine-Inducing Materials from Tissue Culture Media and Parenteral Fluids. *Bio Techniques*, 8, 408–413
- **Sharma SK.** (1986a). Endotoxin detection and elimination in biotechnology. *Biotechn Appl Biochem*, 8, 5–22
- **Sharma SK.** (1986b). On the recovery of genetically engineered proteins from E. coli. *Sep Sci Technol*, 21, 701–126

- **Sharma SK, Hopkins TR.** (1981). Recent developments in the activation process of bovine chymotrypsinogen A. *Bioorganic Chem*, 10, 357–374
- **Sharma SK.** (1990). Key issues in the purification and characterization of recombinant proteins for therapeutic use. *Advanced Drug Delivery Reviews*, 4, 87–111
- **Smith KT, Doherty I, Thomas JA, Per SR, Sito AF.** (1991). Quantitation of Residual DNA in Biological Products: New Regulatory Concerns and Methodologies. In *Animal Cell Technology: Developments, Processes and Products*, edited by RE Spier, JB Griffiths, C MacDonald. Butterworth-Heinemann Ltd., Oxford, pp. 696–698
- **Strickler MP, Gemski MJ.** (1987). *Commercial production of monoclonal antibodies*. Marcel Dekker, New York, pp. 217–245
- **Tennikova T, Svec F.** (1993). High Performance Membrane Chromatography: Highly efficient separation method for proteins in ion-exchange, hydrophobic interaction and reversed phase modes. *J Chromatogr*, 646, 279–288
- **Terstappen G, Ramelmeier R, Kula M.** (1993). Protein partitioning in detergent-based aqueous two-phase systems. *J Biotechnol*, 28, 263–275
- **Walter J, Werner RG.** (1993). Regulatory Requirements and Economic Aspects in Downstream processing of Biotechnically Engineered Proteins for Parenteral Application as Pharmaceuticals. In *Downstream Processing, Recovery and Purification of Proteins*, edited by KH Kroner, N Papamichael, H Schütte. A Handbook of Principles and Practice, John Wiley Publishers, Inc., New York
- **Walter J, Werz W, McGoff P, Werner RG, Berthold W.** (1991). Virus Removal/Inactivation in Downstream Processing. In *Animal Cell Technology: Development, Processes and Products*, edited by RE Spier, JB Griffiths, C MacDonald. Butterworth-Heinemann Ltd., Linacre House, Oxford, pp. 624–634
- **Walter K, Werz W, Berthold W.** (1992). Virus Removal and Inactivation, Concept and Data for Process Validation of Downstream Processing. *Biotech Forum Europe*, 9, 560–564
- **Wheelwright SM.** (1993). Designing downstream processing for large scale protein purification. *Biotechnology*, 5, 789–793
- **World Health Organization.** (1987). Acceptability of cell substrates for production of biologicals, Report of a WHO Study Group, *Technical Report Series*, 747, 1–29
- **World Health Organization, Guidelines for assuring the quality of pharmaceutical and biological products prepared by recombinant DNA technology.** *Technical Report Series*, 823, 105–115
- **World Health Organization.** (1996). Expert Committee on Biological Standardization. Requirements for use of animal cells as *in vitro* substrates for the production of biologicals.
- **Zoletto R.** (1985). Parvovirus serologically related to the minute virus of mice (MVM) as contaminant of BHK 21 CL.13 suspension cells. *Dev Biol Stand*, 60, 179–183

Self-Assessment Questions

Question 1:   *Name four different types of bioreactors.*

Question 2:   *Chromatography is an essential step in the purification of biotech products. Name at least 5 different chromatographic purification methods.*

Question 3:   *What are the major safety concerns in the purification of cell-expressed proteins?*

Question 4:   *What are the critical issues in production and purification that must be addressed in process validation ?*

Question 5:   *Mention at least 5 issues to set specifications for before starting the design of cultivation and purification schemes for proteins.*

Answers

Answer   1:   Stirred-tank, Airlift, Microcarrier and Membrane bioreactors.

Answer   2:   Adsorption chromatography, Ion-exchange chromatography, Affinity chromatography, Hydrophobic Interaction Chromatography, Gel permeation or Size-exclusion chromatography.

Answer   3:   Removal of viruses, bacteria, protein contaminants and cellular DNA.

Answer   4:   Procedures should be reliable in generating constant potency and quality of the product and in the removal of viral, bacterial and protein contaminants.

Answer   5:   Grade of purity, pyrogen limit, N- and C-terminal heterogeneity, chemical modification/conformational changes, glycosylation pattern and proteolytic processing, etc.

4 Formulation of Biotech Products, Including Biopharmaceutical Considerations

by: Daan J.A. Crommelin

Introduction

In this Chapter 4 formulation aspects of pharmaceutical proteins will be discussed. Apart from technological questions, biopharmaceutical issues such as the choice of the delivery systems, the route of administration and possibilities for target site specific delivery of proteins are also considered.

Microbiological Considerations

Sterility

Most proteins are administered parenterally and have to be sterile. In general proteins are sensitive to heat and other regularly used sterilization treatments; they cannot withstand autoclaving, gas sterilization, or sterilization by ionizing radiation. Consequently, sterilization of the end product is not possible. Therefore, protein pharmaceuticals have to be assembled under aseptic conditions, following the established and evolving rules in the pharmaceutical industry for aseptic manufacture. The reader is referred to standard textbooks for details (Halls, 1994; Groves, 1988; Klegerman and Groves, 1992).

Equipment and excipients are treated separately and autoclaved, or sterilized by dry heat (> 160°C), chemical treatment or γ radiation to minimize the bioburden. Filtration techniques are used for removal of microbacterial contaminants. Prefilters remove the bulk of the bioburden and other particulate materials. The final 'sterilizing' step before filling the vials is filtration through 0.2 or 0.22 µm membrane filters. Assembly of the product is done in class 100 (maximum 100 particles ≥ 0.5 µm per cubic foot) rooms with laminar air flow that is filtered through HEPA (high efficiency particulate air) filters. Last but not least, the 'human factor' is a major source of contamination. Well-trained operators wearing protective cloths (face masks, hats, gowns, gloves, or head-to-toe overall garments) should operate the facility. Regular exchange of filters, regular validation of HEPA equipment and thorough cleaning of the room plus equipment are critical factors for success.

Viral Decontamination

As recombinant DNA products are grown in micro-organisms, these organisms should be tested for viral contaminants and appropriate measures should be taken if viral contamination occurs. In the rest of the manufacturing process no (unwanted) viral material should be introduced. Excipients with a certain risk factor such as blood derived, human serum albumin should be carefully tested before use and their presence in the formulation process should be minimized (see Chapter 3).

Pyrogen Removal

Pyrogens are compounds that induce fever. Exogenous pyrogens (pyrogens introduced into the body, not generated by the body itself) can be derived from bacterial, viral or fungal sources. Bacterial pyrogens are mainly endotoxins shed from gram negative bacteria. They are lipopolysaccharides. A general structure is shown in Figure 4.1. The basic, conserved, structure in the full array of thousands of different endotoxins is the lipid A-moiety. Another general property shared by endotoxins is their high, negative electrical charge. Their tendency to aggregate and to form large units with M_w of over 10^6 in water and their tendency to adsorb to surfaces indicate that these compounds are amphipatic in nature. They are stable under standard autoclaving conditions, but break down when heated in the dry state. For this reason equipment and container are treated at temperatures above 160°C for prolonged periods (e.g., 30 minutes dry heat at 250°C).

Pyrogen removal of recombinant products derived from bacterial sources should be an integral part of the preparation process. Ion exchange chromatographic procedures (utilizing its negative charge) can effectively reduce endotoxin levels in solution (cf. Chapter 3).

Excipients used in the protein formulation should be essentially endotoxin-free. For solutions Water for Injection (compendial standards) is (freshly) distilled or produced by reverse osmosis. The aggregated endotoxins can not pass through the reverse osmosis membrane. Removal of endotoxins immediately before filling the final container can be accomplished by using activated charcoal or other

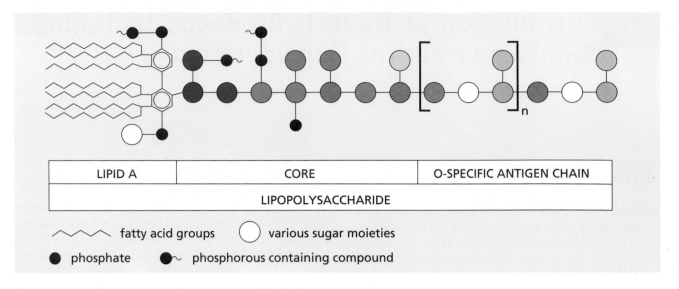

| LIPID A | CORE | O-SPECIFIC ANTIGEN CHAIN |

LIPOPOLYSACCHARIDE

∿∿∿ fatty acid groups   ◯ various sugar moieties
● phosphate   ●∿ phosphorous containing compound

Figure 4.1. Generalized structure of endotoxins. Most properties of endotoxins are accounted for by the active, insoluble 'Lipid A' fraction being solubilized by the various sugar moieties (circles with different colors). Although the general structure is similar, individual endotoxins vary according to their source and are characterized by the O-specific antigenic chain. Adapted from Groves, 1988.

materials with large surfaces offering hydrophobic interactions. Endotoxins can also be inactivated on utensil surfaces by oxidation (e.g., peroxide) or dry heating (e.g., 30 minutes dry heat at 250°C).

Excipients used in Parenteral Formulations of Biotech Products

In a protein formulation one will find, apart from the active substance, a number of excipients selected to serve different purposes. This process of formulation design should be carried out with great care to ensure therapeutically effective and safe products. The nature of the protein (e.g., lability) and its therapeutic use (e.g., multiple injection systems) can make these formulations quite complex in terms of excipient profile and technology (freeze-drying, aseptic preparation). Table 4.1 lists components that can be

- active ingredient
- solubility enhancers
- anti-adsorption and anti-aggregation agents
- buffer components
- preservatives and anti-oxidants
- lyoprotectants/cake formers
- osmotic agents
- carrier system (see later on in this section)

Table 4.1. Components found in parenteral formulations of biotech products. Not necessarily all of the above ● are present in one particular protein formulation.

found in the presently marketed formulations. In the following sections this list will be discussed in more detail.

Solubility Enhancers

Proteins, in particular those that are non-glycosylated, may have a tendency to aggregate and precipitate. Approaches that can be used to enhance solubility include selection of the proper pH and ionic strength conditions. Addition of amino acids such as lysine or arginine (used to solubilize tissue plasminogen activator, t-PA), or surfactants such as sodium dodecylsulfate to solubilize non-glucosylated IL-2 can also help to increase the solubility. The mechanism of action of these solubility enhancers depends on the type of enhancer and the protein involved and is not always fully understood.

Figure 4.2 shows the effect of arginine concentration on the solubility of t-PA (alteplase) at pH 7.2 and 25°C. This figure clearly indicates the dramatic effect of this basic amino acid on the apparent solubility of t-PA.

In the above examples aggregation is physical in nature, i.e. based on hydrophobic and/or electrostatic interactions between molecules. However, aggregation based on the formation of covalent bridges between molecules through disulfide bonds, and ester or amide linkages has been described as well. In those cases proper conditions should be found to avoid these chemical reactions.

Anti-adsorption and Anti-aggregation Agents

Anti-adsorption agents are added to reduce adsorption of the active protein to interfaces. Some proteins tend to expose

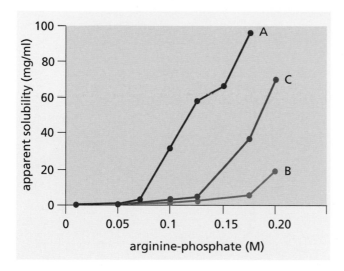

Figure 4.2. Effect of arginine on type I and type II alteplase at pH 7.2 and 25°C. A, type I alteplase; B, type II alteplase; C, 50:50 mixture of type I and type II alteplase. From Nguyen and Ward, 1993.

hydrophobic sites, normally present in the core of the native protein structure when an interface is present. These interfaces can be water/air, water/container wall or interfaces formed between the aqueous phase and utensils used to administer the drug (e.g., catheter, needle). These adsorbed, partially unfolded protein molecules form aggregates, leave the surface, return to the aqueous phase, form larger aggregates and precipitate. As an example, the proposed mechanism for aggregation of insulin in aqueous media through contact with a hydrophobic surface (or water-air interface) is presented in Figure 4.3 (Thurow and Geisen, 1984).

Native insulin in solution is in an equilibrium state between monomeric, dimeric tetrameric and hexameric forms (cf. Chapter 10). The relative abundance of the different aggregation states depends on the pH, insulin concentration, ionic strength and specific excipients (e.g., Zn^{2+} and phenol). It has been suggested that the dimeric form

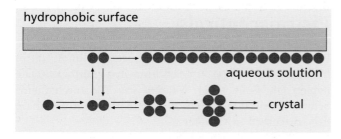

Figure 4.3. Reversible self-association of insulin, its adsorption to the hydrophobic interface and irreversible aggregation in the adsorbed protein film: ● represents a monomeric insulin molecule. Adapted from Thurow and Geisen, 1984.

of insulin adsorbs to hydrophobic interfaces and subsequently forms larger aggregates at the interface. This explains why anti-adhesion agents can also act as anti-aggregation agents. Albumin has a strong tendency to adsorb to surfaces and is therefore added in relatively high concentrations (e.g., 1%) to protein formulations as an anti-adhesion agent. Albumin competes with the therapeutic protein for binding sites and supposedly prevents adhesion of the therapeutically active agent by a combination of its binding tendency and abundant presence.

Insulin is one of the many proteins that can form fibrillar precipitates (long rod-shaped structures with diameters in the 0.1 μm range). Low concentrations of phospholipids and surfactants have been shown to exert a fibrillation-inhibitory effect. The selection of the proper pH can also help to prevent this unwanted phenomenon (Brange and Langkjaer, 1993).

Apart from albumin, surfactants can also prevent adhesion to interfaces and precipitation. These molecules readily adsorb to hydrophobic interfaces with their own hydrophobic groups and render this interface hydrophilic by exposing their hydrophilic groups to the aqueous phase.

Buffer Components

Buffer selection is an important part of the formulation process, because of the pH dependence of protein solubility and physical and chemical stability. Buffer systems regularly encountered in biotech formulations are phosphate, citrate and acetate. A good example of the importance of the i.e.p. (iso-electric point, negative logarithm = pI) is the solubility profile of human growth hormone (hGH, pI around 5) as presented in Figure 4.4.

Even short, temporary pH changes can cause aggregation. These conditions can occur, for example, during the freezing step in the freeze-drying process, when one of the buffer components is crystallizing and the other is not.

In a phosphate buffer, Na_2HPO_4 crystallizes faster than NaH_2PO_4. This causes a pronounced drop in pH during the freezing step. Other buffer components do not crystallize, but form amorphous systems and then pH changes are minimized.

Preservatives and Anti-oxidants

Methionine, cysteine, tryptophan, tyrosine and histidine are amino acids that are readily oxidized (cf. Chapter 2, Table 2.4). Proteins rich in these amino acids are liable to oxidative degradation. Replacement of oxygen by inert gases in the vials helps to reduce oxidative stress. Moreover, the addition of anti-oxidants such as ascorbic acid or sodium formaldehyde sulfoxylate can be considered (Groves, 1988). Interestingly, destabilizing effects on proteins have been described for anti-oxidants as well (Vemuri et al., 1993b).

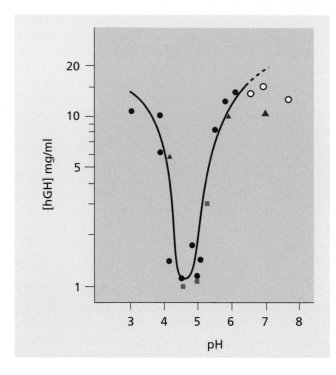

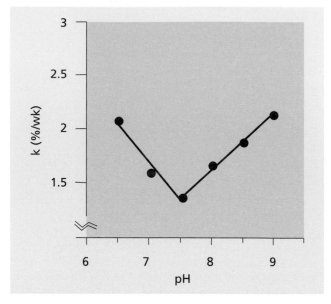

Figure 4.4. A plot of the solubility of various forms of hGH as a function of pH. Samples of hGH were either recombinant hGH (circles), Met-hGH (triangles) or pituitary hGH (squares). Solubility was determined by dialysing an approximately 11 mg/ml solution of each protein into an appropriate buffer for each pH. Buffers were citrate, pH 3-7, and borate, pH 8-9, all at 10 mM buffer concentrations. Concentrations of hGH were measured by UV absorbance as well as by RP-HPLC, relative to an external standard. The closed symbols indicate that precipitate was present in the dialysis tube after equilibration, whereas open symbols mean that no solid material was present, and thus the solubility is at least this amount. From Pearlman and Bewley, 1993.

Figure 4.5. pH stability profile (at 25°C) of monomeric recombinant α_1-antitrypsin (rAAT) by size exclusion-HPLC assay. k = degradation rate constant. Monomeric rAAT decreased rapidly both under acidic and basic conditions. Optimal stability occurred at pH 7.5. Adjusted from Vemuri *et al.*, 1993.

Certain proteins are formulated in containers designed for multiple injection schemes. After administering the first dose, contamination with microorganisms may occur and preservatives are needed to minimize growth. Usually, these preservatives are present in concentrations that are bacteriostatic rather than bactericide in nature. Antimicrobial agents mentioned in the USP XXIII are the mercury-containing phenylmercuric nitrate and thimerosal and p-hydroxybenzoic acids, phenol, benzyl alcohol and chlorobutanol (XXIII/NF 18, 1995; Groves, 1988; Pearlman and Bewley, 1993).

Osmotic Agents

For proteins the regular rules apply for adjusting the tonicity of parenteral products. Saline and mono- or disaccharide solutions are commonly used. These excipients may not be inert; they may influence protein structural stability. For example, sugars and polyhydric alcohols can stabilize the protein structure through the principle of 'preferential exclusion' (Arakawa *et al.*, 1991). These additives enhance the interaction of the solvent (water structure promoters) with the protein and are themselves excluded from the protein surface layer; the protein is preferentially hydrated. This phenomenon can be monitored through an increased thermal stability of the protein. Unfortunately, a strong 'preferential exclusion' effect enhances the tendency of proteins to self-associate.

Shelf Life of Protein Based Pharmaceuticals

Proteins can be stored (1) as an aqueous solution, (2) in freeze dried form, (3) in dried form in a compacted state (tablet) (cf. Table 17.4a, Chapter 17). The mechanisms behind chemical and physical degradation processes have been discussed in Chapter 2.

Stability of protein solutions strongly depends on factors such as pH, ionic strength, temperature, the presence of stabilizers. For example, Figure 4.5 shows the pH dependence of αi-antitrypsin and clearly demonstrates the critical importance of pH on shelf life of proteins.

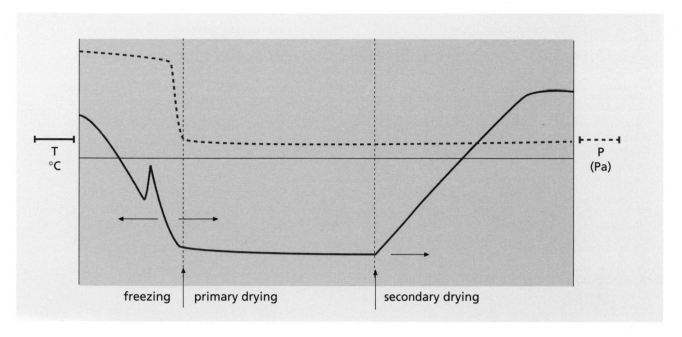

Figure 4.6. Example of a freeze drying protocol for systems with crystallizing water. T = temperature; P = pressure.

Freeze-drying of Proteins

Proteins in solution usually do not comply with the preferred shelf life for industrially produced pharmaceutical products (> 2 years), even when permanently kept under refrigerator conditions (cold chain). The abundant presence of water promotes chemical and physical degradation processes.

Freeze drying may provide the requested stability. During freeze-drying water is removed through sublimation and not by evaporation. Three stages can be discerned in the freeze-drying process: (1) a freezing step, (2) the primary drying step and (3) the secondary drying step (Figure 4.6). Table 4.2 explains what happens during these stages.

Freeze drying of a protein solution without the proper excipients will cause, as a rule, irreversible damage to the protein. Table 4.3 lists excipients typically encountered in successfully freeze dried protein products.

Freezing

In the freezing step (cf. Figure 4.6) the temperature of the aqueous system in the vials is lowered. Ice crystal formation does not start right at the thermodynamic or equilibrium freezing point, but supercooling occurs. That means that crystallization often only occurs when temperatures of −15°C or lower have been reached. During the crystallization step the temperature may temporarily rise in the vial, because of the generation of crystallization heat. During the cooling stage, concentration of the protein and excipients occurs because of the growing ice crystal mass at the expense of the aqueous water phase. This can cause precipitation of one or more of the excipients, which may consequently result in pH shifts (see above and Figure 4.7) or ionic strength changes. It may also induce protein denaturation. Cooling of the vials is done through lowering the temperature of the shelf. Selecting the proper cooling scheme for the shelf — and consequently vial — is impor-

---

Freezing
The temperature of the product is reduced from ambient temperature to a temperature below the eutectic temperature (T_e), or below the glass transition temperature (T_g) of the system. A T_g is encountered if amorphous phases are present.

Primary drying
Crystallized and water not bound to protein/excipient is removed by sublimation. The temperature is below the T_e or T_g; the temperature is for example -40 °C and reduced pressures are used.

Secondary drying
Removal of water interacting with the protein and excipients. The temperature in the chamber is kept below T_g and rises gradually, e.g., from -40 °C to 20 °C.

Table 4.2. Three stages in the freeze drying process of protein formulations.

• bulking agents: mannitol/glycine	reason: elegance/blowout prevention*
• collapse temperature modifier: dextran, albumin/gelatine	reason: increase collapse temperature
• lyoprotectant: sugars, albumin	reason: protection of the physical structure of the protein**

* Blowout is the loss of material taken away by the water vapor that leaves the vial. It occurs when little solid material is present in the vial.
** Mechanism of action of lyoprotectant is not fully understood. Factors that might play a role are:
(1) lyoprotectants replace water as stabilizing agent (water replacement theory),
(2) lyoprotectants increase the Tg of the cake/frozen system
(3) lyoprotectants will absorb moisture from the stoppers
(4) lyoprotectants slow down the secondary drying process and minimize the chances for overdrying of the protein. Overdrying might occur when residual water levels after secondary drying become too low. Pikal (Pikal, 1990b) considers the chance for overdrying 'in real life' small.

Table 4.3. Typical excipients in a freeze-dried protein formulation.

tant as it dictates the degree of supercooling and ice crystal size. Small ice crystals are formed by fast cooling, large crystals by lower cooling rates. Small ice crystals are requested for porous solids and fast sublimation rates (Pikal, 1990a).

If the system does not (fully) crystallize but forms an amorphous mass upon cooling, the temperature in the 'freezing stage' should drop below T_g, the glass transition temperature. In amorphous systems the viscosity changes dramatically in the temperature range around the T_g: a 'rubbery' state exists above and a glass state below the T_g.

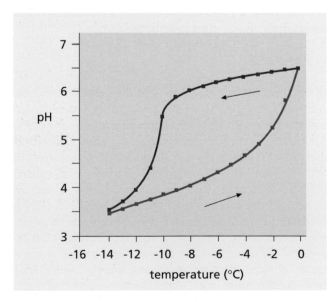

Figure 4.7. Thawing/cooling; ■ = thawing ■ = cooling. The effect of freezing on the pH of a citric acid-disodium phosphate buffer system. Cited in Pikal, 1990a.

At the start of the primary drying stage no 'free and fluid' water should be present in the vials. Minus forty degrees Celsius is a typical freezing temperature before sublimation is initiated through pressure reduction (Pikal, 1990a).

Primary Drying

In the primary drying stage (cf. Figure 4.6) sublimation of the water mass in the vial is initiated by lowering down the pressure. The water vapor is collected on a condenser, with a (substantially) lower temperature than the shelf with the vials. Sublimation costs energy (about 2500 kJ/gram ice). Temperature drops are avoided by the supply of heat from the shelf to the vial. Thus, the shelf is heated during this stage.

Heat is transferred to the vial through (1) direct shelf-vial contact (conductance), (2) radiation and (3) gas-conduction (Figure 4.8). Gas conduction depends on the pressure: if one selects relatively high gas pressures, heat transport is promoted because of a high conductivity. But, it reduces mass transfer, because of a low driving force: the pressure between equilibrium vapor pressure at the interface between the frozen mass/ dried cake and the chamber pressure.

During the primary drying stage one transfers heat from the shelf through the vial bottom and through the frozen mass to the interface frozen mass/dry powder, to keep the sublimation process going. During this drying stage the vial content should never reach or exceed the eutectic temperature or glass transition temperature range. Typically a safety margin of 2–5°C is used, otherwise the cake will collapse. Collapse causes a strong reduction in sublimation rate and poor cake formation. Heat transfer resistance

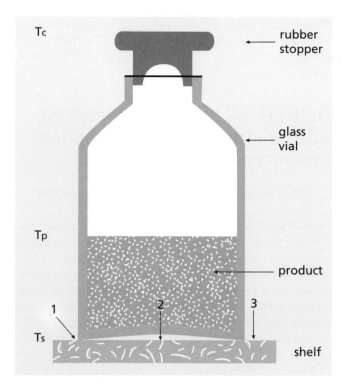

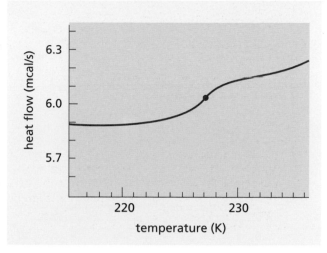

Figure 4.9. Differential scanning calorimetry heating trace for a frozen solution of sucrose and sodium chloride, showing the glass transition temperature of the freeze concentrate at 227 K. For pure freeze-concentrated sucrose, $T_g = 241$ K (1 cal = 4.2 J). From Franks *et al.*, 1991.

Figure 4.8. Heat transfer mechanisms during the freeze drying process:
1. direct conduction via shelf and glass at points of actual contact,
2. gas conduction: contribution heat transfer via conduction through gas between shelf and vial bottom,
3. radiation heat transfer. Ts = shelf temperature, Tp = temperature sublimating product, Tc = temperature condensor. Ts > Tp > Tc.

decreases during the drying process as the transport distance is reduced by the retreating interface. With the mass transfer resistance (transport of water vapor), however, the opposite occurs. Mass transfer resistance increases during the drying process as the dry cake becomes thicker.

The above described situation makes it clear that parameters such as chamber pressure and shelf heating are not necessarily constant during the primary drying process. They should be carefully chosen and adjusted as the drying process proceeds.

The eutectic temperature or glass transition temperature are parameters of great importance to develop a rationally designed freeze-drying protocol. Information about these parameters can be obtained by microscopic observation of the freeze-drying process, differential scanning calorimetry (DSC), or electrical resistance measurements.

An example of a DSC scan providing information on the T_g is presented in Figure 4.9 (Franks *et al.*, 1991). T_g strongly depends on the composition of the system: excipients and water content. Lowering the water content of an amorphous system causes the T_g to shift to higher temperatures (Pikal, 1990a).

Secondary Drying Stage

When all frozen or amorphous water that is non-protein and non-excipient bound is removed, the secondary drying step starts (Figure 4.6). The end of the primary drying stage is reached when product temperature and shelf temperature become equal, or when the partial water pressure drops (Pikal, 1990a). As long as the 'non-bound' water is being removed, the partial water pressure almost equals the total pressure. In the secondary drying stage the temperature is slowly increased to remove 'bound' water; the chamber pressure is still reduced. The temperature should stay all the time below the collapse/eutectic temperature, which continues to rise when residual water contents drop. Typically, the secondary drying step ends when the product has been kept at 20°C for some time. The residual water content is a critical, endpoint indicating parameter. Values as low as 1% residual water in the cake have been recommended. Figure 4.10 (Pristoupil, 1985; Pikal, 1990a) exemplifies the decreasing stability of freeze dried hemoglobin with increasing residual water content.

The stability of freeze dried proteins in the presence of reducing lyoprotectants such as glucose and lactose can be affected by the occurrence of the Maillard reaction: amino groups of the proteins react with the lyoprotectant in the dry state and the cake color turns yellow-brown. The use of non-reducing sugars can be considered to solve this problem (Pikal, 1990a).

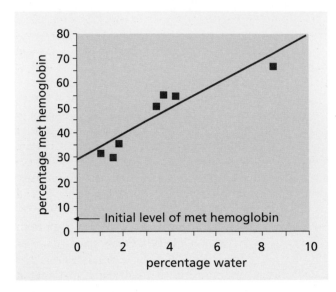

Figure 4.10. The effect of residual moisture on the stability of freeze-dried hemoglobin (~6%) formulated with 0.2 M sucrose; decomposition to met hemoglobin during storage at 23°C for 4 years. From Pikal, 1990a. Data reported by Pritoupil *et al.*, 1985.

Other Approaches to Stabilize Proteins

Compacted forms of proteins are being used for certain veterinary applications, e.g., for sustained release of growth hormones. The pellets should contain as few additives as possible. They can be applied subdermally or intramuscularly when the compact pellets are introduced by compressed air-powered rifles into the animals (Klegerman and Groves, 1992).

Delivery of Proteins: Routes of Administration and Absorption Enhancement

The Parenteral Route of Administration

Parenteral administration is here defined as administration via those routes where a needle is used, including intravenous, intramuscular, subcutaneous and intraperitoneal injections. More information on the pharmacokinetic behaviour of recombinant proteins is provided in Chapter 5. It suffices here to state that the blood half-life of biotech products can vary over a wide range. For example, the circulation half-life of tissue plasminogen activator (t-PA) is a few minutes, while monoclonal antibodies reportedly have half-lives of a few days. Obviously, one reason to develop modified proteins through site directed mutagenesis is to enhance circulation half-life. A simple way to expand the mean residence time for short half-life proteins is to switch from intravenous to intramuscular or subcutaneous administration. One should realise that by doing that, changes in disposition may occur, with a significant impact on the therapeutic performance of the drug. These changes are

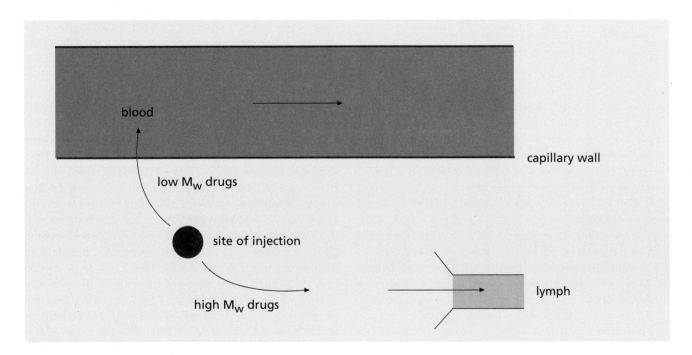

Figure 4.11. Routes of uptake of s.c. or i.m. injected drugs.

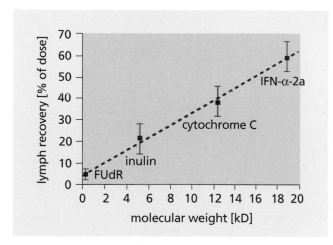

Figure 4.12. Correlation between the molecular weight and the cumulative recovery of rIFN α-2a (M_W 19 kD), cytochrome c (M_W 12.3 kD), inulin (M_W 5.2 kD), and FUDR (M_W 256.2 kD) in the efferent lymph from the right popliteal lymph node following s.c. administration into the lower part of the right hind leg of sheep. Each point and bar shows the mean and standard deviation of three experiments performed in separate sheep. The line drawn is the best fit by linear regression analysis calculated with the four mean values. The points have a correlation coefficient r of 0.998 ($p < 0.01$). From Supersaxo et al., 1990.

related to: (1) the prolonged residence time at the i.m. or s.c. site of injection compared to i.v. administration and the enhanced exposure to degradation reactions (peptidases), and (2) differences in disposition.

Regarding point 1: Prolonged residence time at the i.m. or s.c. site of injection. For instance, diabetics can become 'insulin resistant' through high tissue peptidase activity (Maberly et al., 1982). Other factors that can contribute to absorption variation are related to local blood flow: differences in exercise level of the muscle at the injection site and also massage and heat at the injection site play a role. The state of the tissue, e.g., the occurrence of pathological conditions may be important as well.

Regarding point 2: Differences in disposition. Upon administration, a major fraction of the protein can be transported to the blood through the lymphatics and does not enter the blood circulation through the capillary wall at the site of injection (Figures 4.11, 4.12). The fraction taking this lymphatic route is molecular weight dependent (Supersaxo et al., 1990).

The Oral Route

Oral delivery of protein drugs would be preferable, because it is patient friendly and no medical professional

intervention is necessary to administer the drug. Oral bioavailability, however, is usually very low. Two main reasons for this failure of uptake can be discerned: (1) protein degradation in the GI-tract, (2) poor permeability in case of a passive transport process.

Regarding point 1: Protein degradation in the GI-tract. The human body has developed a very efficient system to break down proteins in our food to amino acids, or di- or tri-peptides. These building stones for body proteins are actively absorbed to be utilized wherever necessary in the body. In the stomach pepsins, a family of aspartic proteases, are secreted. They are particularly active between pH 3 and 5 and lose activity at higher pH values. Pepsins are endo-peptidases (capable of cleaving peptide bonds distant from the ends of the peptide chain) and they preferentially cleave peptide bonds between two hydrophobic amino acids. Other endopeptidases are active in the gastro-intestinal tract at neutral pH values: e.g., trypsin, chymotrypsin and elastase. They have different peptide bond cleavage characteristics that more or less complement each other. Exopeptidases, proteases degrading peptide chains from their ends, are present as well. Examples are carboxypeptidase A and B. In the lumen the proteins are cut into fragments. These fragments are effectively further broken down to amino acids, di- and tri-peptides by brush border and cytoplasmic proteases of the enterocytes.

Regarding point 2: Permeability. High molecular weight molecules are poor penetrators of the intact and mature epithelial barrier, if diffusion is the sole driving force for mass transfer. Proteins are no exception to this rule. Active transport of intact therapeutic recombinant proteins over the GI-epithelium has not yet been described.

The above analysis leads to the conclusion that, unfortunately, nature does not allow us to utilize the oral route of administration for therapeutic proteins, if high (or at least constant) bioavailability is required.

For the category of oral vaccines, however, the above mentioned hurdles of degradation and permeation are not necessarily prohibitive. For oral immunization only a (small) fraction of the antigen (protein) has to reach its target site to elicit an immune response. The target cells are lymphocytes and antigen presenting accessory cells located in Peyer's patches (Figure 4.13). The B lymphocyte population includes cells that produce secretory IgA antibodies.

These Peyer's patches are macroscopically identifiable follicular structures located in the wall of the gastro-intestinal tract. Peyer's patches are overlaid with microfold (M) cells that separate the luminal contents from the lymphocytes. These M cells have little lysosomal degradation capacity and allow for antigen sampling by the underlying lymphocytes. Moreover, mucus producing goblet cell density is reduced over Peyer's patches. This reduces mucus production and facilitates access to the M cell surface for luminal contents (Jani et al., 1992; Roitt et al., 1993). Attempts to

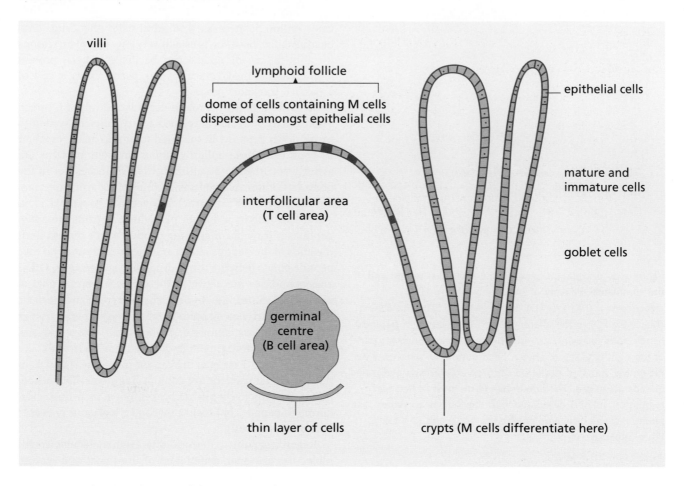

Figure 4.13. Schematic diagram of the structure of intestinal Peyer's patches. M-cells within the follicle-associated epithelium are enlarged for emphasis. From O'Hagan, 1990.

improve antigen delivery and to enhance the immune response are made by utilizing microspheres, liposomes or modified live vectors, such as attenuated bacteria and viruses (Eldridge *et al.*, 1990; Holmgren *et al.*, 1989).

Alternative Routes of Administration

Parenteral administration has disadvantages (needles, sterility, injection skills) compared to other possible routes. Therefore, systemic delivery of recombinant proteins by alternative routes of administration for the parenteral route has been studied extensively. The nose, lungs, rectum, oral cavity and skin have been selected as potential sites of application. The potential pros and cons for the different relevant routes have been listed in Table 4.4.

If systemic action is required, the nasal, buccal, rectal and transdermal routes all have been shown to be of little clinical relevance, if simple protein formulations without an absorption enhancing technology are used. In general, bioavailability is too low! The pulmonary route may be the exception to this rule (Table 4.5, from Patton *et al.*, 1994).

Therefore, different approaches have been evaluated to increase bioavailability via these alternative, (non-parenteral) routes of administration. The goal is to develop a system that temporarily decreases the absorption barrier resistance with minimum and acceptable safety concerns. The mechanistic background of these approaches has been given in Table 4.6. Up until now no products utilizing one of these approaches have successfully passed clinical test programs. Safety concerns are an important hurdle. Questions center around the specificity and reversibility of the protein permeation enhancing effect and the toxicity (Zhou and Li Wan Po, 1991a; Zhou and Li Wan Po, 1991b).

Examples of Absorption Enhancing Effects

In the following paragraphs the 'state of the art' of this important issue: absorption enhancement and non-parenteral administration of recombinant proteins, will be dealt with. A number of typical examples will be shown.

An example of the (apparently complex) relationship between nasal bioavailability of some peptide and protein

Route	+ = relative advantage, - = relative disadvantage

Nasal (Edman and Björk, 1992)

+ easily accessible, fast uptake, proven track record with a number of 'conventional' drugs, probably lower proteolytic activity than in the GI tract, avoidance of first pass effect, spatial containment of absorption enhancers is possible
- reproducibility (in particular under pathological conditions), safety (e.g., ciliary movement), low bioavailability for proteins

Pulmonary (Patton and Platz, 1992)

+ relatively easy to access, fast uptake, proven track record with 'conventional' drugs, substantial fractions of insulin are absorbed, lower proteolytic activity than in the GI tract, avoidance of hepatic first pass effect, spatial containment of absorption enhancers (?)
- reproducibility (in particular under pathological conditions, smokers/non-smokers), safety (e.g., immunogenicity), presence of macrophages in the lung with high affinity for particulates

Rectal (Zhou and Li Wan Po, 1991b)

+ easily accessible, partial avoidance of hepatic first pass, probably lower proteolytic activity than in the upper parts of the GI tract, spatial containment of absorption enhancers is possible, proven track record with a number of 'conventional' drugs
- low bioavailability for proteins

Buccal (Zhou and Li Wan Po, 1991b)(Ho et al., 1992)

+ easily accessible, avoidance of hepatic first pass, probably lower proteolytic activity than in the lower parts of the GI tract, spatial containment of absorption enhancers is possible, option to remove formulation if necessary
- low bioavailability of proteins, no proven track record yet (?)

Transdermal (Cullander and Guy, 1992)

+ easily accessible, avoidance of hepatic first pass effect, removal of formulation if necessary is possible, spatial containment of absorption enhancers, proven track record with 'conventional' drugs, sustained/controlled release possible
- low bioavailability of proteins

Table 4.4. Alternative routes of administration to the oral route for biopharmaceuticals.

Molecule	Mw kD	#AA	absolute bioavailability (%)
α-interferon	20	165	> 56
PTH-84	9	84	> 20
PTH-34	4.2	34	40
calcitonin (human)	3.4	32	17
calcitonin (salmon)	3.4	32	17
glucagon	3.4	29	< 1
somatostatin	3.1	28	< 1

PTH = recombinant human parathyroid hormone
# AA = number of amino acids

Table 4.5. Absolute bioavailability of a number of proteins (intratracheal vs intravenous) in rats (adapted from Patton *et al.*, 1994).

drugs, their molecular weight and the presence of the absorption enhancer glycocholate is presented in Table 4.7 (Zhou and Li Wan Po, 1991b).

Another example is presented in Figure 4.14 (Björk and Edman, 1988) where degradable starch microspheres loaded with insulin were used and where changes in glucose levels were monitored after nasal administration to rats.

In these examples, the effect of the presence of the absorption enhancers is clear. Major issues now being addressed are: reproducibility, effect of pathological conditions (e.g., rhinitis) on absorption and safety aspects on chronic use. Interestingly, absorption enhancing effects were shown to be species dependent. Pronounced differences in effect were observed, e.g., between rats and rabbits.

With iontophoresis a transdermal electrical current is induced by positioning two electrodes on different places

Classified according to proposed mechanism of action

-increase the permeability of the absorption barrier:

* addition of fatty acids/phospholipids, bile salts, enamine derivatives of phenylglycine, ester and ether type (non)-ionic detergents, saponins, salicylate derivatives, derivatives of fusidic acid or glycyrrhizinic acid, or methylated β cyclodextrins

* through iontophoresis,

* by using liposomes

- decrease peptidase activity at the site of absorption and along the 'absorption route':
aprotinin, bacitracin, soybean tyrosine inhibitor, boroleucin, borovaline

- enhance resistance against degradation by modification of the molecular structure

- prolongation of exposure time (e.g., bio-adhesion technologies)

Table 4.6. Approaches to enhance bioavailability of proteins (adapted from Zhou and Li Wan Po, 1991a).

Molecule	# AA	Bioavailability (%)	
		without	*with glycocholate*
glucagon	29	< 1	70-90
calcitonin	32	< 1	15-20
insulin	51	< 1	10-30
met-hGH*	191	< 1	7-8

* cf. chapter 5, Growth Hormones

Table 4.7. Effect of glycocholate (absorption enhancer) on nasal biovailability and molecular weights of some proteins and peptides (adapted from Zhou and Li Wan Po, 1991b).

on the skin (Figure 4.15). This current induces a migration of (ionized) molecules through the skin. Delivery depends on the current (on/off, pulsed/direct, wave shape), pH, ionic strength, molecular weight, charge on the protein and temperature. The protein should be charged over the full thickness of the skin (pH of hydrated skin depends on the depth and varies between pH 4 (surface) and pH 7.3), which makes proteins with pI values outside this range prime candidates for iontophoretic transport. It is not clear whether there are size restrictions (protein Mw) for ionto-phoretic transport. Only potent proteins, however, will be successful candidates. With the present technology, the

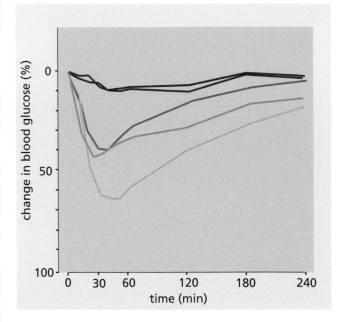

Figure 4.14. Change in blood glucose in rats after intranasal administration of insulin.
— Soluble insulin 2.0 IU/kg i.n.
— Soluble insulin 0.25 IU/kg i.v.
— Degradable starch microspheres-insulin 0.75 IU/kg i.n.
— Degradable starch microspheres-insulin 1.70 IU/kg i.n.
— Empty degradable starch microspheres 0.5 mg/kg i.n.
Discussed by Edman and Björk (Edman and Björk, 1992).

protein flux through the skin is in the 10 $\mu g/cm^2/hr$ range (Sage *et al.*, 1995).

In Figure 4.16 the plasma profile of growth hormone releasing factor, GRF (44 amino acids, Mw 5 kD after s.c., i.v. and iontophoretic transdermal delivery to hairless guinea pigs is presented. A prolonged appearance in the plasma can be observed. Iontophoretic delivery offers interesting opportunities, if pulsed delivery of the protein is required. The device can be worn permanently and only switched on over the desired periods of time, thus simulating pulsatile secretion of endogenous hormones such as growth hormone and insulin (Lee *et al.*, 1991)

Delivery of Proteins: Approaches for Rate Controlled and Target Site Specific Delivery by the Parenteral Route

Presently used therapeutic proteins widely differ in their pharmacokinetic characteristics (cf. Chapter 5). If they are endogenous active agents such as insulin, tissue plasminogen activator, growth hormone, erythropoetin, interleukins or

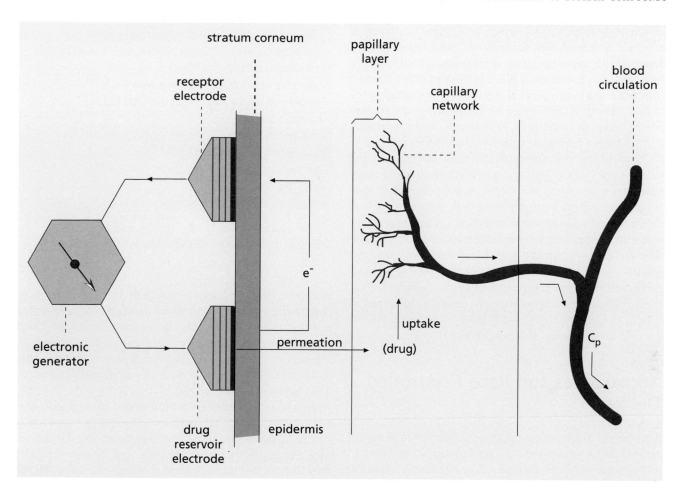

Figure 4.15. Diagrammatic illustration of the transdermal iontophoretic delivery of peptide and protein drugs across the skin. Adapted from Chien, 1991.

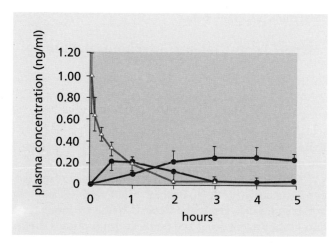

Figure 4.16. Plasma concentration versus time profiles after subcutaneous, intravenous and iontophoretic transdermal administration of GRF (1–44) to hairless guinea pigs.
●—●: Iontophoresis (1 mg/g; 0.17 mA/cm²; 5 cm² patch).
●—●: Subcutaneous (10 μg/kg; 0.025 mg/ml). △—△: Intravenous (10 μg/kg; 0.025 mg/nl). From Kumar *et al.*, 1992.

factor VIII, it is important to realize why, when and where they are secreted. There are three different fashions in which cells can communicate with each other: the endocrine, paracrine and autocrine fashion (Table 4.8).

Endocrine hormones:
a hormone secreted by a distant cell to regulate cell functions distributed widely through the body. The blood stream plays an important role in the transport process

Paracrine acting mediators:
the mediator is secreted by a cell to influence surrounding cells, short range influence

Autocrine acting mediators:
the agent is secreted by a cell and affects the cell by which it is generated, (very) short range influence.

Table 4.8. Communication between cells: chemical messengers.

The dose-response relationship of these mediators is often not S-shaped, but, for instance, bell-shaped: at high doses the therapeutic effect disappears (cf. Chapter 5). Moreover, the presence of these mediators may activate a complex cascade of events that needs to be carefully controlled. Therefore, key issues for their therapeutic success are: (1) access to target cells, (2) retention at the target site and (3) proper timing of delivery (Tomlinson, 1987).

In particular, for the paracrine and autocrine acting proteins, site specific delivery can be highly desirable, because otherwise side effects will occur outside the target area. Severe side effects were reported with cytokines such as tumor necrosis factor and interleukin-2. Their occurrence limits the therapeutic potential of these compounds. Therefore, the delivery of these proteins at the proper site, rate and dose is a crucial part in the process of the design and development of these compounds as a pharmaceutical entity. In the following sections first (1) concepts developed to control the release kinetics and later (2) concepts for site directed drug delivery will be discussed.

Approaches for Rate Controlled Delivery

Rate control can be achieved by several different technologies similar to those used for 'conventional' drugs. Insulin provides an excellent example. A spectrum of options is available and accepted: different types of suspensions and continuous infusion systems are marketed (see Chapter 10).

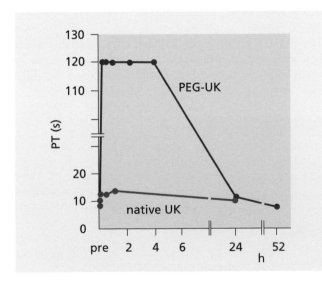

Figure 4.17. Influence of chemical grafting of polyethylene glycol (PEG) on the ability of urokinase (UK) to affect the prothrombin time (PT) *in vivo* in beagles with time. Through Tomlinson, 1987.

Rate control through open loop type approach
- continuous infusion with pumps: mechanically or osmotically driven
input: constant/pulsatile/wave form
- implants: biodegradable polymers, lipids
input: limited control
Rate control through closed loop approach/feed back system
- biosensor-pump combination
- self regulating system
- encapsulated secretory cells

Table 4.9. Controlled release systems for parenteral delivery.

Moreover, chemical approaches can be used to change protein characteristics. Polyoxyethyleneglycol-attachment to proteins changes their circulation half-life in the blood dramatically. An example of this approach is shown in Figure 4.17. Chemical modification of proteins for pharmacokinetic purposes is dealt with in more detail later on in this chapter (Chapter 5).

As a rule, proteins are administered in aqueous solution. Only recombinant vaccines and most insulin formulations are delivered as (colloidal) dispersions. At the present time, no other protein drugs than insulin are routinely, clinically applied through some form of controlled release system (cf. Chapter 10) other than through continuous infusion. As experience with biotech drugs grows, more advanced technologies will definitely be introduced to optimize the therapeutic benefit of the drug. Table 4.9 lists some of the technologically feasible options. They will be briefly touched upon below.

Open Loop Systems: Mechanical Pumps

Mechanically driven pumps are common tools to administer drugs intravenously in hospitals (continuous infusion, open loop type). They are available in different kinds of sizes/prices, portable or not, inside/outside the body, etc. Table 4.10 presents a check list with issues to be considered when selecting the proper pump.

Continuous infusion and release control of a drug does not necessarily imply a constant input rate. Pulsatile or variable-rate delivery is the desired mode of input for a number of protein drugs and for these drugs pumps should provide flexible input rate characteristics. Insulin is a prime example of a protein drug, where there is a need to adjust the input rate to the needs of the body and today by far most experience with pump systems in an ambulatory setting has been gained with this drug. The pump system may fail because of energy-failure, problems with the syringe,

The pump must deliver the drug at the prescribed rate(s) for extended periods of time. It should
- have a wide range of delivery rates
- ensure accurate, precise and stable delivery
- contain reliable pump and electrical components
- contain drugs compatible with pump internals
- provide simple means to monitor the status and performance of the pump

The pump must be safe. It should
- have a biocompatible exterior if implanted
- have overdose protection
- show no leakage
- have a fail-safe mechanism
- have sterilizable interiors and exteriors (if implantable)

The pump must be convenient. It should
- be reasonably small in size and inconspicuous
- have a long reservoir life
- be easy to program

Table 4.10. Listing the characteristics of the ideal pump (Banerjee *et al.*, 1991).

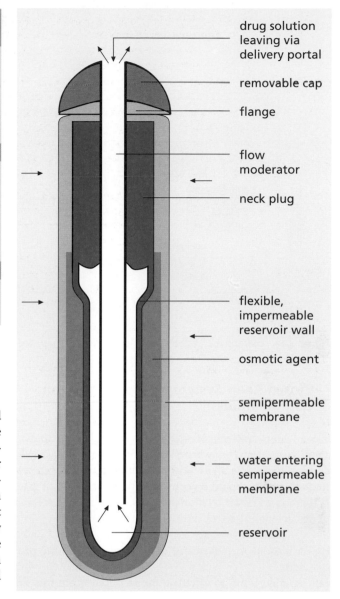

Figure 4.18. Cross-section of functioning Alza Alzet osmotic minipump. Through Banerjee *et al.*, 1991.

Labels: drug solution leaving via delivery portal; removable cap; flange; flow moderator; neck plug; flexible, impermeable reservoir wall; osmotic agent; semipermeable membrane; water entering semipermeable membrane; reservoir

accidental needle withdrawal, leakage of the catheter and problems at the injection or implantation site (Banerjee *et al.*, 1991). Moreover, long-term drug stability may become a problem. The protein should be stable at 37°C or ambient temperature (internal and external device, respectively) between two refills. Finally, even with high tech pump systems, the patient still has to collect data to adjust the pump rate. This implies invasive sampling from body fluids on a regular basis followed by calculation of the required input rate. This problem would be solved when the concept of closed loop systems would be realized: feed back systems (see below).

Open Loop Systems: Osmotically Driven Systems

The subcutaneously implantable, osmotic minipump developed by ALZA (Alzet minipump, Figure 4.18 (Banerjee *et al.*, 1991)) has proven to be useful in animal experiments where continuous, constant infusion is required over prolonged periods of time. The rate determining process is the influx of water through the rigid, external semipermeable membrane. The incoming water empties the drug containing reservoir (solution or dispersion) surrounded by a flexible impermeable membrane. The release rate depends on the characteristics of this semipermeable membrane and on osmotic pressure differences over this membrane

(osmotic agents inside the pump). Zero-order kinetics exist as long as the osmotic pressure difference over the semipermeable membrane is maintained constant.

The protein solution (or dispersion) must be physically and chemically stable at body temperature over the full term of the experiment. Moreover, the protein solution must be compatible with the pump parts to which it is exposed. A limitation of the system is the fixed release rate, which is not always desired (see above). These devices have not been used currently on a regular basis in the clinic.

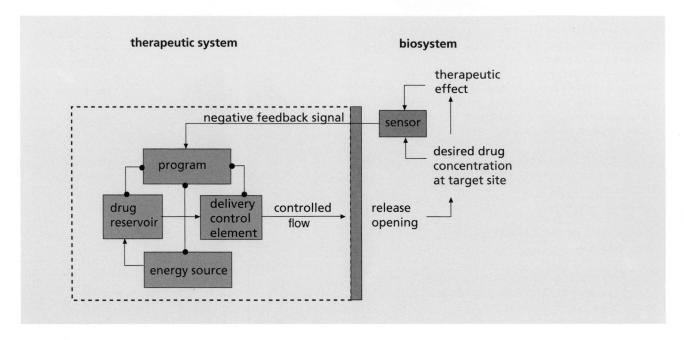

Figure 4.19. Therapeutic system with closed control loop. From Heilman, 1984.

Closed Loop Systems: Biosensor-pump Combinations

Closed loop systems. If input rate control is desired to stabilize a certain body function, then this function should be monitored. Via an algorithm and connected pump settings this data should be converted into a drug input rate. If there is a known relationship between plasma level and pharmacological effect these systems contain:

(1) a biosensor, measuring the plasma level of the protein,
(2) an algorithm, to calculate the required input rate for the delivery system,
(3) a pump system, able to administer the drug at the required rate over prolonged periods of time.

The concept of a closed loop delivery of proteins (see Figure 4.19) still has to overcome many conceptual and practical problems. Not always a simple relationship between plasma level and therapeutic effect exists (see Chapter 5). There are many exceptions known to this rule, e.g., 'hit and run' drugs can have long lasting pharmacological effects after only a short exposure time. Also, drug effect-blood level relationships may be time-dependent, e.g., because of down regulation of relevant receptors on prolonged stimulation. Finally, if circadian rhythms exist, these will be responsible for variable PK/PD relationships as well.

If the above expressed PK/PD concerns do not apply, as with insulin, technical problems form the second hurdle in the development of closed loop systems. It has not been possible yet to design biosensors that work reliably *in vivo* over prolonged periods of time. Biosensor stability, robustness and absence of histological reactions still pose problems (See also Chapter 6).

Protein Delivery by Self-regulating Systems

Apart from the design of biosensor-pump combinations two other developments should be mentioned when discussing closed loop approaches: self-regulating systems and encapsulated secretory cells. At the present time both concepts are still under development.

In self-regulating systems drug release is controlled by stimuli in the body. By far most of the research is focused on insulin release as a function of local glucose concentrations in order to stabilize blood glucose levels in diabetics. Two approaches for controlled drug release are being followed: (1) competitive desorption, and (2) enzyme-substrate reactions. The competitive desorption approach is schematically depicted in Figure 4.20.

It is based on the competition between glycosylated-insulin and glucose for concanavalin (Con A) binding sites. Con A is a plant lectin with a high affinity for certain sugars. Con A attached to sepharose beads and loaded with glycosylated-insulin (a bio-active form of insulin) is

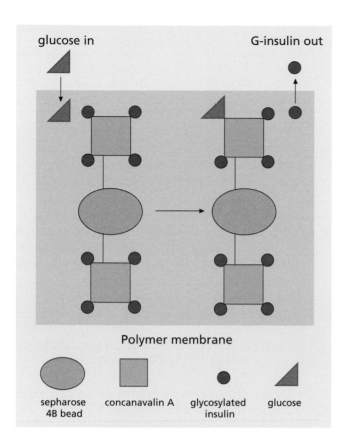

glucose in

G-insulin out

Polymer membrane

| sepharose 4B bead | concanavalin A | glycosylated insulin | glucose |

Figure 4.20. Schematic design of the Con A immobilized bead/G (glycosylated)-insulin/membrane self-regulating insulin delivery system. From Kim *et al.*, 1990.

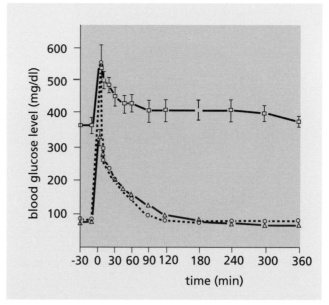

Figure 4.21. Peripheral blood glucose profiles of dogs administered bolus dextrose (500 mg/kg) during an intravenous glucose tolerance test. Normal dogs (O) had an intact pancreas, diabetic dogs (□) had undergone total pancreatectomy, and implant dogs (Δ) had been intraperitoneally implanted with a cellulose pouch containing a Con A-G-insulin complex. Blood glucose at t = −30 minutes shows the overnight fasting level 30 minutes prior to bolus injection of dextrose. Through Heller, 1993.

implanted, e.g., in a pouch with a semipermeable membrane: permeable for insulin and glucose, but impermeable for the sepharose beads carrying the toxic Con A. An example of the performance of a Con A-glycosylated-insulin complex in pancreatectomized dogs is given in Figure 4.21.

Enzyme-substrate reactions to regulate insulin release from an implanted reservoir are all based on pH drops occurring when glucose is converted to gluconic acid in the presence of the enzyme glucose oxidase. This pH drop then induces changes in the structure of acid-sensitive delivery devices such as acid sensitive polymers, which start releasing insulin, lowering down the glucose concentration, and consequently increasing the local pH and 'closing the reservoir' (Heller, 1993).

Protein Delivery by Microencapsulated Secretory Cells

The idea to use implanted, secretory cells to administer therapeutic proteins was launched long ago. A major goal has been the implantation of Langerhans cells in diabetics to restore their insulin production in a bio-feedback fashion. These implanted secretory cells should be protected from the body environment as rejection processes would immediately start, if imperfectly matched cell material is used. Besides, it is desirable to keep the cells from migrating in all different directions. If genetically modified cells are used, safety issues would be even more strict. Therefore, (micro)encapsulation of the secretory cells has been proposed (Figure 4.22).

Thin (wall thickness in μm range), robust, biocompatible and permselective polymeric membranes have been designed for these (micro)capsules. The membrane should ensure transport of nutrients (in general low M_w) from the outside medium to the encapsulated cells to keep them in a physiological, 'healthy' state and, on the other hand, prohibit induction of undesirable immunological responses (rejection process). For instance, antibodies (M_w >150 kD) and cells belonging to the immune system (e.g., lymphocytes) should not be able to reach the encapsulated cells. The polymer membrane should have a cut off between 50 and 150 kD, the exact number still being a matter of debate. In the case of insulin the membrane is permeable for this

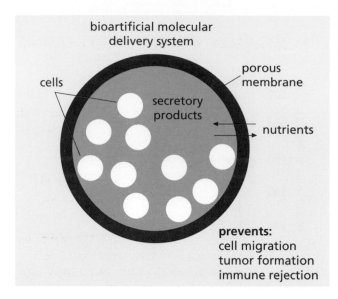

Figure 4.22. Schematic illustration of a 'bioartificial molecular delivery system'. Secretory cells are surrounded by a semi-permeable membrane prior to implantation in host tissue. Nutrients and secretory products passively diffuse through pores in the encapsulating membrane powered by concentration gradients. The use of a membrane that excludes the humoral and the cellular components of the host immune system allows immunologically incompatible cells to survive implantation without the need to administer immunosuppressive agents. Extracellular matrix material may be included depending upon the requirements of the encapsulated cells. From Tresco, 1994.

relatively small sized hormone (5.4 kD) and for glucose ('indicator' molecule), which is essential for proper bio-feedback processes. Successful studies in diabetic animals were performed. Promising clinical data has been reported with human secretory islet cells encapsulated in alginate based microspheres (Shoon-Shiong *et al.*, 1994; Tresco, 1994; Uludag *et al.*, 1993).

Site Specific Delivery (Targeting) of Protein Drugs

Why are we still not able to beat life threatening diseases such as cancer with our current arsenal of drugs? Causes of failure can be summarized as follows (Crommelin *et al.*, 1992) :

1)   The active compound never reaches the target site, because it is rapidly eliminated in intact form from the body through the kidneys, or it is inactivated through metabolic action, e.g., in the liver.

* an active moiety	for: therapeutic effect
** a carrier	for: (metabolic) protection, changing the disposition of the drug
*** a homing device	for: specificity, selection of the assigned target site

Table 4.11. Components for targeted drug delivery (carrier-based).

2)   Only a small fraction of the drug reaches the target site. By far the largest fraction of the drug is distributed over non-target organs, where they exert side effects; in other words: accumulation of the drug at the target site is the exception and not the rule.

3)   Many drug molecules (in particular high M_w and hydrophilic molecules, i.e. many proteins) do not enter cells easily. This poses a problem, if intracellular delivery is required for their therapeutic activity.

Drug targeting is the concept where attempts are made to increase the therapeutic index of drugs:

(1)   by specific delivery of the active compound at its site of action, and

(2)   to keep it there until it has been inactivated and detoxified.

Targeted drug delivery should maximize the therapeutic effect and avoid toxic effects elsewhere. The basics of the concept of drug targeting were defined already in the early days of this century by Paul Ehrlich. But, only in the last decade substantial progress has been made to implement this site specific delivery concept. Recent progress can be ascribed to: (1) the rapidly growing number of technological options (e.g., safe carriers) for drug delivery. Moreover, (2) many new insights were gained into the pathophysiology of diseases at the cellular and molecular level, including the presence of cell specific receptors and homing devices to target to them (e.g., monoclonal antibodies) and, finally, (3) the nature of the anatomical and physiological barriers that hinder easy access to target sites was revealed. Site specific delivery systems that are presently in different stages of development consist, in general, of three functionally separate units (Table 4.11).

Nature has provided us with antibodies, which exemplify a class of natural drug targeting devices. In an antibody molecule one can recognize a homing device part (antigen binding site) and 'active' parts. These active parts in the molecule are responsible for participating in the complement cascade, or induce interactions with monocytes

1. Drugs with high total clearance are good candidates for targeted delivery.

2. Response sites with a relatively small blood flow require carrier-mediated transport.

3. Increases in the rate of elimination of free drug from either central or response compartments tend to increase the need for targeted drug delivery; this also implies a higher input rate of the drug-carrier conjugate to maintain the therapeutic effect.

4. For maximizing the targeting effect, the release of drug from the carrier should be restricted to the response compartment.

Table 4.12. Pharmacokinetic considerations related to protein targeting.

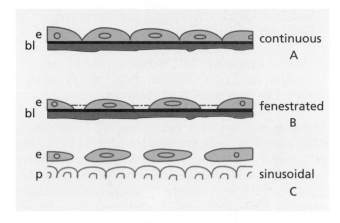

Figure 4.23. Schematic illustration of the structure of different classes of blood capillaries. A. Continuous capillary. The endothelium is continuous with tight junctions between adjacent endothelial cells. The subendothelial basement membrane is also continuous. B. Fenestrated capillary. The endothelium exhibits a series of fenestrae which are sealed by a membranous diaphragm. The subendothelial basement membrane is continuous. C. Discontinuous (sinusoidal) capillary. The overlying endothelium contains numerous gaps of varying size enabling materials in the circulation to gain access to the underlying parenchymal cells. The subendothelial basement is eigher absent (liver) or present as a fragmented interrupted structure (spleen, bone marrow). The fenestrae in the liver are about 0.1–0.2 µm; the pores between the endothelial cells and those in the basement membrane outside liver, spleen and bone marrow are much smaller. bl: basement membrane. From Poste, 1985.

when antigen is bound. The rest of the molecule can be considered as carrier (cf. Chapter 13).

Most of the drug (protein) targeting work is done with delivery systems that are designed for parenteral and, more specifically, intravenous delivery. Only a limited number of papers has dealt with the pharmacokinetics of the drug targeting process (Hunt *et al.*, 1986). From these kinetic models a number of conclusions could be drawn for situations where targeted delivery is, in principle, advantageous (Table 4.12).

The potential and limitations of carrier-based, site specific drug delivery systems for proteins will be briefly discussed. The focus will be on concepts where monoclonal antibodies are being used. They can be used (1) as such (also in Chapter 13), or (2) in modified form when antibodies are conjugated with an active moiety, or (3) attached to drug laden colloidal carriers such as liposomes.

Two terms are regularly used in the context of targeting: passive and active targeting. With passive targeting the 'natural' disposition pattern of the carrier system is utilized for site specific delivery. For instance, particulate carriers circulating in the blood (see below) are often rapidly taken up by macrophages in contact with the blood circulation and accumulate in liver (Kupffer cells) and spleen. Active targeting is the concept where attempts are made to change the natural disposition of the carrier by some sort of homing device or homing principle to select one particular tissue or cell type.

Anatomical, Physiological and Pathological Considerations Relevant for Protein Targeting

Carrier mediated transport in the body depends on the physico-chemical properties of the carrier: its charge,

molecular weight/size, surface hydrophobicity and the presence of ligands for interaction with surface receptors (Crommelin and Storm, 1990). If a drug enters the circulation and the target site is outside the blood circulation, the drug has to pass through the endothelial barrier. Figure 4.23 gives a schematic picture of the capillary wall structures (under physiological conditions) present at different locations in the body.

Figure 4.23 shows a diagram of intact endothelium under normal conditions. Under pathological conditions, such as those encountered in tumors and inflammation sites, endothelium can differ considerably in appearance and endothelial permeability may be widely different from that in 'healthy' tissue. e.g., particles with sizes up to 0.1 µm can enter tumor tissue as was demonstrated with long circulating, colloidal carrier systems (long circulating liposomes). On the other hand, necrotic tissue can also hamper access to tumor tissue (Jain, 1987). In conclusion, the body is highly compartmentalized; it should not be considered as one big pool without internal barriers for transport.

Soluble Carrier Systems for Targeted Delivery of Proteins

(MONOCLONAL) ANTIBODIES (MAB) AS TARGETED THERAPEUTIC AGENTS: HUMAN AND HUMANIZED ANTIBODIES

Antibodies are 'natural targeting devices'. Their homing ability is combined with functional activity. MAb can affect the target cell function upon attachment. Complement can be bound via the Fc receptor and subsequently cause lysis of the target cell. Alternatively, certain Fc receptor-bearing killer cells can induce 'antibody dependent, cell mediated cytotoxicity' (ADCC), or contact with macrophages can be established. Moreover, metabolic deficiencies can be induced in the target cells through a blockade of certain essential cell surface receptors by MAb. Structural aspects and therapeutic potential of MAb are dealt with in detail in Chapter 13.

A problem that occurs when using murine antibodies for therapy is the production of human anti-mouse (HAMA) antibodies after administration. HAMA induction may prohibit further use of these therapeutic MAb by neutralizing the antigen binding site; anaphylactic reactions are relatively rare. Concurrent administration of immunosuppressive agents can be considered as a strategy to minimize side effects.

There are several other ways to cope with this immunogenicity problem. These are dealt with in more detail in Chapter 13. Here, a brief summary of the options relevant for protein targeting suffices. First of all, the use of F(ab')$_2$ or F(ab') fragments (Figure 4.24) avoids raising an immune response against the Fc part. But, the development of humanized or human MAb minimizes the induction of HAMA even further. For humanization of MAb several options can be considered. One can build chimeric (partly human, partly murine) molecules consisting of a human Fc part and a murine Fab part, with the antigen binding sites or, alternatively, only the six complementarity determining regions (CDR) of the murine antibody can be grafted in a human antibody structure. CDR grafting minimizes the exposure to murine material.

Completely human MAb can be produced by transfecting human antibody genes into mouse cells, which subsequently produce the human MAb. Alternatively, transgenic mice can be used (cf. Chapter 6). These approaches reduce the immunogenicity compared to the existing generation of murine MAb. But, even with all these human or humanized MAb, anti-idiotypic immune responses against the binding site structure of the MAb can not be excluded (cf. Chapter 12) (Crommelin et al., 1992; Crommelin and Storm, 1990).

BISPECIFIC ANTIBODIES

To enhance the therapeutic potential of antibodies, bispecific antibodies have been designed. Bispecific antibodies are manufactured from two separate antibodies to create a molecule with two different binding sites (Fanger and Guyre, 1991). Bispecific MAb bring target cells or tissue (one antigen binding site) in contact with other structures (second antigen binding site). This second antigen binding site can bind to effector cells via cytotoxicity triggering molecules on, for instance, T cells, NK (natural killer) cells, or macrophages and trigger cytotoxicity.

Bispecific antibodies have been used experimentally in the clinic, for instance, to direct intraperitoneally injected autologous T-lymphocytes, stimulated with recombinant interleukin-2, to intraperitoneally located ovarian carcinoma cells. This MAb combines an antigen binding site for a carcinoma-surface antigen with an antigen binding site with T cell affinity. The MAb are in vitro incubated with the stimulated T-lymphocytes prior to intraperitoneal injection (De Leij et al., 1990; Crommelin and Storm, 1990).

IMMUNOCONJUGATES: COMBINATIONS BETWEEN AN ANTIBODY AND AN ACTIVE COMPOUND

In many cases antibodies alone or bispecific antibodies have been shown to lack sufficient therapeutic activity. To

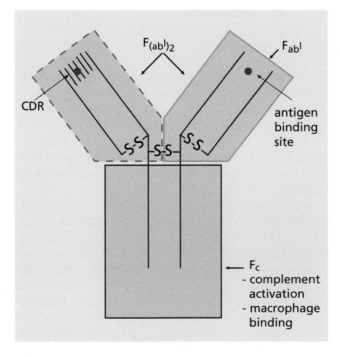

Figure 4.24. Highly simplified IgG1 structure; CDR = complementarity determining region.

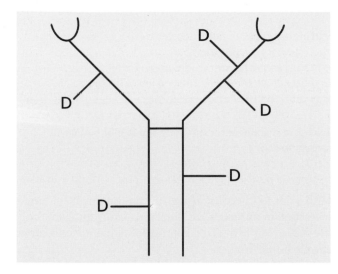

Figure 4.25. A schematic view of an immunoconjugate (D = drug molecules covalently attached to antibody fragments).

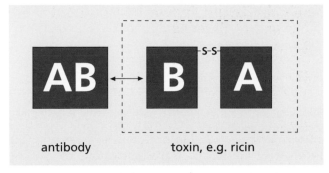

Figure 4.26. Immunotoxins are composed of antibody molecules connected to a toxin, e.g. ricin. Both the integral ricin molecule has been used as well as the A-chain alone. AB = antibody; A and B stand for the A and B chain of the ricin toxin, respectively (not in the list of abbreviations).

enhance their activity, conjugates of MAb and drugs have been designed. These efforts mainly focus on the treatment of cancer and no products have reached the market yet (Crommelin and Storm, 1990). To test the concept of immunoconjugates, a wide range of drugs has been covalently bound to antibodies and has been evaluated in animal tumor models. As only a limited number of antibody molecules can bind to the target cells, only conjugation of highly potent drugs will lead to sufficient therapeutic activity. Table 4.13 lists a number of potential problems encountered with immunoconjugates (Crommelin et al., 1992).

Cytostatics with a high intrinsic cytotoxicity are needed (see above). Because the kinetic behavior of an active compound is strongly affected by the conjugating antibody, not only existing cytostatics, but also active compounds that were never used before as drugs, because of their high toxicity, should now be re-considered (e.g., proteins such as toxins).

1. Covalent binding of the protein to the antibody can change the cytotoxic potential of the drug and decrease the affinity of the MAB for the antigen

2. The stability of the conjugate in vivo can be insufficient; fragmentation will lead to loss of targeting potential

3. The immunogenicity of the MAB and toxicity of the protein involved can change dramatically

Table 4.13. Potential problems encountered with immunoconjugates (Crommelin et al., 1992).

Immunoconjugated toxins are now tested as chemotherapeutic agents to treat cancer (immunotoxins). Examples of the toxin family are: ricin, abrin and diphteria toxin. These proteins are extremely toxic; they block enzymatically intracellular protein synthesis at the ribosomal level. Ricin (M_w 66 kD) consists of an A and a B chain, that are linked through a cystin bridge. The A chain is responsible for blocking protein synthesis at the ribosomes. The B chain is important for cellular uptake of the molecule (endocytosis) and the intracellular trafficking.

In animal studies with immuno-conjugated ricin only a small fraction of these immunotoxins accumulates in tumor tissue (e.g., 1%). A major fraction still ends up in the liver, the main target organ for 'natural' ricin. Moreover, in clinical phase I studies (to assess the safety of the conjugates) the first generation of immunoconjugates turned out to be immunogenic. Now attempts are being made to adapt the ricin molecule (e.g., by genetic engineering) so, that liver targeting is being minimized. This can be done by blocking (removing or masking) on the ricin molecule ligands for galactose receptors on hepatocytes. Besides, murine MAb can be replaced by human or humanized MAb (see above) (Ramakrishnan, 1990).

Potential Pitfalls in Tumor Targeting

Upon intravenous injection only a small fraction of the homing device-carrier-drug complex is sequestered at the target site. Apart from the compartmentalisation of the body (see above: anatomical and physiological hurdles) and consequently the carrier-dependent barriers that result, several other factors account for this lack of target site accumulation (Table 4.14).

How successful are MAb in discriminating target cells (tumor cells) from non-target cells? And, do all tumor cells

1. Tumor heterogeneity	
2. Antigen shedding	
3. Antigen modulation	

Table 4.14. Factors that interfere with successful targeting of proteins to tumor cells.

1. size
2. charge
3. surface hydrophilicity
4. presence of homing devices on their surface
5. exchange of constitutive parts with blood components

Table 4.15. Parameters controlling the fate of particulate carriers *in vivo*.

expose the tumor associated antigen? These questions are still difficult to answer (Hellström *et al.*, 1987). Tumor cell-surface specific molecules used for homing purposes are often differentiation antigens on the tumor cell wall. These structures are not unique as they occur in a lower density level on non-target cells as well. Therefore, the target site specificity of MAb raised against these structures is more quantitative than qualitative in nature.

Another category of tumor associated antigens are the clone specific antigens. They are unique for the clone forming the tumor. However, the practical problem when focusing on clone specific antibodies for drug targeting is that each patient probably needs a tailor-made MAb.

The surface 'make up' of tumor cells in a tumor or a metastasis is not constant; neither in time nor between cells in the same tumor. There are many subpopulations of cells and they express different surface molecules. This heterogeneity means that not all cells in the tumor will interact with one, single targeted conjugate. Antigen shedding and antigen modulation are two other ways tumor cells can avoid recognition. Shedding of antigens means that antigens are released from the surface. They can then interact with circulating conjugates outside the target area, form an antigen-antibody complex and neutralize the homing potential of the conjugates before the target area has been reached. Finally, antigen modulation can occur upon binding of MAb to the cell surface antigen. Modulation is the phenomenon that upon endocytosis of the (originally exposed) surface antigen-immunoconjugate complex, some of these antigens are not exposed anymore on the surface; there is no replenishment of endocytosed surface antigens.

What strategies can be implemented to solve problems related to tumor cell heterogeneity, shedding and modulation? (1) Cocktails of different MAb attached to the toxin can be used. (2) Another approach is to give up to strive for complete target cell specificity and induce so-called 'bystander' effects. Then, the targeted system is designed in such a way that the active part is released from the conjugate after reaching a target cell, but before the antigen-conjugate complex has been taken up (is endocytosed) by the target cell. (3) Not all surface antigens show shedding or modulation. If these phenomena occur, other antigen/MAb combinations should be selected that do not demonstrate these effects. (4) At the present, injection of free

MAb prior to injection of the immunoconjugate is under investigation to neutralize 'free' circulating antigen; then, the subsequently injected conjugate should not encounter shedded, free antigen.

In conclusion, targeted (modified) MAb and MAb-conjugates are now studied to assess their value in fighting life-threatening diseases such as cancer. During the last decade, technology has evolved fast; many different new options became available. Lack of detailed pathophysiological and cell biological knowledge about the behavior of, for instance, tumors slows down progress. It is even possible that the whole concept of MAb-(conjugates) will turn out to be only of limited therapeutic value, because of problems such as tumor cell heterogeneity, poor access to tumors and immunogenicity concerns.

Colloidal Particulate Carrier Systems for Targeted Delivery of Proteins

A wide range of carrier systems in the colloidal size range (diameters up to a few micrometers) has been proposed for protein targeting. Examples are: liposomes, biodegradable polycyanoacrylate nanoparticles, albumin microspheres, polylactic acid microspheres, low density lipoproteins (LDL). Upon entering the bloodstream after i.v. injection, it is difficult for many of these particulate systems to pass through epithelial and endothelial membranes in healthy tissue, as the size cut off for permeation through these multilayered barriers is around 20 nm (excluding the liver, see above Figure 4.23). Parameters that control the fate of particulate carriers *in vivo* are listed in Table 4.15.

As a rule, cells of the mononuclear phagocyte system (MPS), e.g., macrophages, recognize stable, colloidal particulate systems (< 5 µm) as 'foreign body like structures' and phagocytose them. Thus, the liver and spleen, organs rich in blood circulation exposed macrophages, take up the majority of these particulates (Tomlinson, 1987; Crommelin and Storm, 1990). Larger (> 5 µm) intravenously injected particles tend to form emboli in lung capillaries on their first encounter with this organ.

Liposomes have gained considerable attention among the colloidal particulate systems proposed for site specific drug delivery of proteins. Liposomes are vesicular struc-

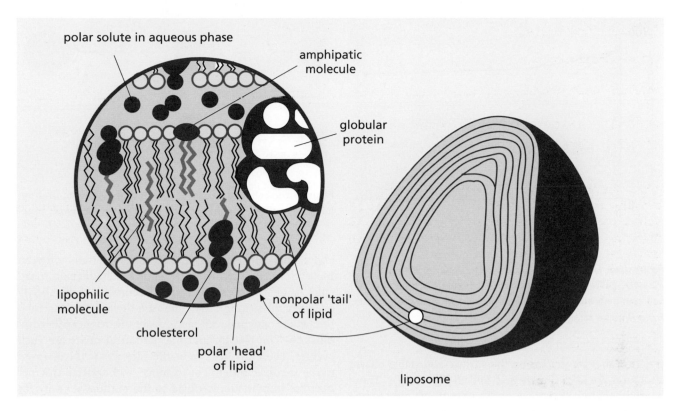

Figure 4.27. An artist's view of what a multilamellar liposome looks like. The lamellae are bilayers of (phospho)lipid molecules with their hydrophobic tails oriented inwards and their polar heads directed to, and in contact with, the aqueous medium. The bilayer may accomodate lipophilic drugs inside. Hydrophilic drugs will be found in the aqueous core and in between the bilayers. Depending on their hydrophilic/hydrophobic balance and tertiary structure proteins and peptides will be found in the aqueous phase, at the bilayer-water interface, or inside the lipid bilayer. Adapted from Fendler, 1980.

tures based on (phospho) lipid bilayers surrounding an aqueous core. The main component of the bilayer usually is phosphatidylcholine.

By selecting their bilayer constituents and one of the many preparation procedures described, liposomes can be made varying in (a) size between 30 nm (e.g., by extrusion or ultrasonication) and 10 μm, and (b) charge (by incorporation of negatively or positively, cf. Chapter 7, charged lipid), and (c) bilayer rigidity (by selecting special phospholipids or adding lipids such as cholesterol). Liposomes can carry their pay-load (proteins) either in the lipid core of the bilayer through partitioning, or attached to the bilayer or physically entrapped in the aqueous phase. To make liposomes target site specific (except for passive targeting to liver (Kupffer cells) and spleen macrophages) homing devices are covalently coupled to the outside bilayer leaflet (Toonen and Crommelin, 1983). In Table 4.16 three (relative) advantages of liposomes over other particulate systems are given.

After injection 'standard' liposomes stay in the blood circulation only for a short time. They are taken up by macrophages in liver and spleen, or they degrade by ex-

change of bilayer constituents with blood constituents. Liposome residence time in the blood circulation can be extended to many hours and even days, if polyoxyethylene

Liposomes stand out among other particulate carrier systems, because of:

1. their relatively low toxicity, existing safety record and experience with marketed, intravenously administered liposome products (e.g., amphotericin B, doxorubicin, daunorubicin) (Storm et al., 1993)

2. the presence of a relatively large aqueous core, which is essential to stabilize the structural features of many proteins

3. the possibility to manipulate release characteristics of liposome associated proteins and to control disposition in vivo by changing preparation techniques and bilayer constituents (Crommelin and Schreier, 1994).

Table 4.16.

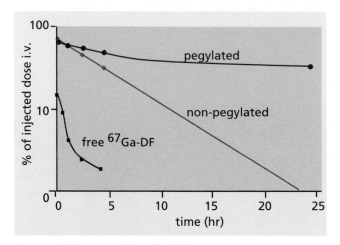

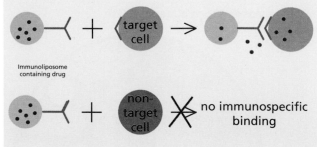

Figure 4.29. Schematic representation of the concept of drug targeting with immunoliposomes. From Nässander *et al.*, 1990.

Figure 4.28. Comparison of the blood levels of free label, ^{67}Ga-DF, gallium-desferal with ^{67}Ga-DF laden pegylated (PEG) and non-pegylated liposomes upon i.v. administration in rats. From Woodle *et al.*, 1990.

(PEG) chains are grafted on the surface and stable bilayer structures are used (Figure 4.28 and cf. Figure 4.17). These long circulating liposomes apparently are able to escape macrophage uptake for prolonged periods of time and are sequestered in other organs than liver and spleen alone, e.g., tumors and inflamed tissues.

The accumulation of protein laden liposomes in macrophages (passive targeting) offers interesting therapeutic opportunities. Liposome encapsulated lymphokines and 'microbial' products, e.g., interferon-γ or muramyltripeptide-phosphatidylethanolamine (MTP-PE), respectively, can activate macrophages and enable them to kill micrometastases, or help to stimulate immune reactions. Moreover, reaching macrophages may help us to more effectively fight macrophage located microbial, viral or bacterial diseases than with our present approaches (Emmen and Storm, 1987; Crommelin and Schreier, 1994).

Several attempts have been made to sequester immunoliposomes (i.e., antibody (fragment)-liposome combinations) at predetermined sites in the body. Here the aim is active targeting to the desired target site instead of passive targeting to macrophages. The concept is schematically presented in Figure 4.29.

When designing immunoliposomes, antibodies or antibody-fragments are covalently bound to the surface of liposomes through lipid anchor molecules (Toonen and Crommelin, 1983). Just like liposomes, immunoliposomes have poor access to target sites outside the blood circulation after intravenous injection. Reason is the high resistance against liposome penetration through the endothelial lining at target sites and their relatively short circulation time. Therefore, target sites should be sought in the blood circulation (red blood cells, thrombi, lymphocytes, or endothelial cells exposing (under stress) certain adhesion molecules, e.g., ICAM-1, intercellular cell adhesion molecule) (Vingerhoeds *et al.*, 1994; Crommelin *et al.*, 1995).

Other interesting target sites are those located in cavities, where one can locally administer the drug-carrier combination. The bladder and the peritoneal cavity are such cavities. These cavities can be the sites where the diseased tissue is concentrated. For instance, with ovarian carcinomas the tumors are confined to the peritoneal cavity for most of their lifetime. After intraperitoneal injection of immunoliposomes directed against human ovarian carcinomas in athymic, nude mice, a specific interaction between immunoliposomes and the human ovarian carcinoma was observed (Nässander and colleagues) (Figure 4.30).

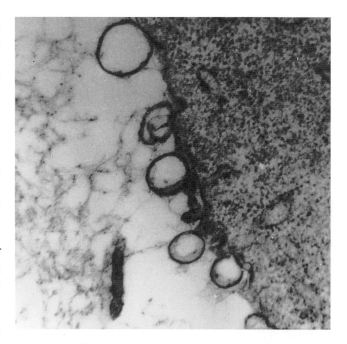

Figure 4.30. Electromicrograph showing immunoliposomes (vesicular structures) attached to human ovarian carcinoma cells (see text above).

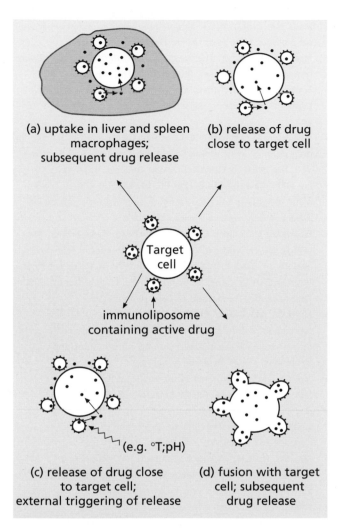

(a) uptake in liver and spleen macrophages; subsequent drug release

(b) release of drug close to target cell

Target cell

immunoliposome containing active drug

(e.g. °T;pH)

(c) release of drug close to target cell; external triggering of release

(d) fusion with target cell; subsequent drug release

Figure 4.31. Several pathways of drug internalisation after immunospecific binding of the immunoliposomes to the appropriate target cell. From Peeters *et al.*, 1987.

Attaching an immunoliposome to target cells usually does not induce a therapeutic effect *per se*. After establishment of an immunoliposome-cell interaction the protein drug has to exert its action on the cell. To do that, the protein has to be released in its active form. There are several pathways proposed to reach this goal (Figure 4.31) (Peeters *et al.*, 1987).

When the immunoliposome-cell complex encounters a macrophage, the cells plus adhering liposome are probably phagocytosed and enter the macrophage (option a). Subsequently, the liposome associated protein drug can be released. As this will most likely happen in the 'hostile' lysosomal environment, little intact protein will become available. In the situation depicted in Figure 4.31 option b, the drug is released from the adhering immunoliposomes in the close proximity of the target cell. In principle, release rate control is achieved by selecting the proper liposomal bilayers with delayed or sustained drug release characteristics. A third approach is depicted as option 3c: drug release is induced from liposomal bilayers by external stimuli (local pH change or temperature change). Finally, one can envision that immunoliposomes can be built with intrinsic fusogenic potential which is only activated upon attachment of the carrier to the target cell. This exciting option d, Figure 4.31, resembles the behavior of certain viruses. However, this complicated technology is still in an early stage of development (Crommelin *et al.*, 1992).

Perspectives for Targeted Protein Delivery

Protein targeting strategies have been developing at a rapid pace. A new generation of homing devices (target cell specific monoclonal antibodies) and a better insight in the anatomy and physiology of the human body, also under pathological conditions, have been critical factors to achieve this success. A much better picture has emerged not only about the potentials, but also the limitations of the different targeting approaches.

Very little attention has been paid to typically pharmaceutical aspects of advanced drug delivery systems such as immunotoxins and immunoliposomes. These systems are now produced on a lab scale and their therapeutic potential is currently under investigation. If therapeutic benefits have been clearly proven in preclinical and early clinical trial, then scaling up, shelf life and quality assurance issues (e.g., reproducibility of technology, purity of the ingredients) will still require considerable attention. ∎

References

- **Arakawa T, Kita Y, Carpenter, JF.** (1991). Protein-solvent interactions in pharmaceutical formulation. *Pharmaceutical Research*, 8, 285–291

- **Banerjee PS, Hosny EA, Robinson JR.** (1991). Parenteral delivery of peptide and protein drugs. In *Peptide and protein drug delivery*, edited by VHL Lee. New York: Marcel Dekker, Inc., pp. 487–543

- **Björk E, Edman P.** (1988). Characterization of degradable starch microspheres as a nasal delivery system for drugs. *Int J Pharm*, 62, 187–192

- **Brange J, Langkjaer L.** (1993). Insulin structure and stability. In *Stability and characterization of protein and peptide drugs. Case histories*, edited by YJ Wang, R Pearlman. New York: Plenum Press, Inc., pp. 315–350

- **Chien YW.** (1991). Transdermal route of peptide and protein drug delivery. In *Peptide and protein drug delivery*, edited by VHL Lee. New York: Marcel Dekker, Inc., pp. 667–689

- **Crommelin DJA, Bergers J, Zuidema J.** (1992). Antibody-based drug targeting approaches: perspectives and challenges. In *Medicinal chemistry for the 21st century*, edited by CG Wermuth, N Koga, H König, BW Metcalf. Oxford: Blackwell Scientific Publications, pp. 351–365

- **Crommelin DJA, Scherphof G, Storm G.** (1995). Active targeting with particulate carrier systems in the blood compartment. *Adv Drug Delivery Reviews*, 17, 49–60

- **Crommelin DJA, Schreier H.** (1994). Liposomes. In *Colloidal drug delivery systems*, edited by J Kreuter. New York: Marcel Dekker, Inc., pp. 73–190

- **Crommelin DJA, Storm G.** (1990). Drug Targeting. In *Comprehensive Medicinal Chemistry*, edited by PG Sammes, JD Taylor. Oxford: Pergamon Press, pp. 661–701

- **Cullander C, Guy RH.** (1992). Transdermal delivery of peptides and proteins. *Advanced Drug Delivery Reviews*, 8, 291–329

- **De Leij L, De Jonge MWA, Ter Haar J, Spakman H, De Vries E, Willmese P, Mulder NH, Berendsen H, Elias M, Smit Sibinga C, De Lau W, Tax W, The TH.** (1990). Bispecific monoclonal antibody (BIAB) retargeted cellular therapy for local treatment of cancer patients. In *From Clone to Clinic*, edited by DJA Crommelin, H Schellekens. Dordrecht: Kluwer Academic, pp. 159–165

- **Edman P, Björk E.** (1992). Nasal delivery of peptide drugs. *Advanced Drug Delivery Reviews*, 8, 165–177

- **Eldridge JH, Hammond CJ, Meulbroek JA, Staas JK, Giley RM, Tice TR.** (1990). Controlled vaccine release in the gut-associated lymphoid tissues. I. Orally administered biodegradable microspheres target the Peyer's patches. *J Controlled Release*, 11, 205–214

- **Emmen F, Storm G.** (1987). Liposomes in the treatment of infectious diseases. *Pharm Weekblad Sci Ed*, 9, 162–171

- **Fanger MW, Guyre PM.** (1991). Bispecific antibodies for targeted cellular cytotoxicity. *TIBTECH*, 9, 375–380

- **Fendler JH.** (1980). Optimizing drug entrapment in liposomes. Chemical and biophysical considerations. In *Liposomes in biological systems*, edited by G Gregoriadis, AC Allison. Chichester: Wiley J & Sons, Ltd., pp. 87

- **Franks F, Hatley RHM, Mathias SF.** (1991). Materials science and the production of shelf-stable biologicals. *Pharmaceutical Technol Int*, 3

- **Groves M.** (1988). *Parenteral Technology Manual*. Buffalo Grove, Il: Interpharm Press, Inc.

- **Halls NA.** (1994). *Achieving sterility in medical and pharmaceutical products*. New York: Marcel Dekker, Inc.

- **Heilmann K.** (1984). *Therapeutic systems. Rate controlled delivery: concept and development*. Stuttgart: G. Thieme Verlag

- **Heller J.** (1993). Polymers for controlled parenteral delivery of peptides and proteins. *Advanced Drug Delivery Reviews*, 10, 163–204

- **Hellström KE, Hellström I, Goodman GE.** (1987). Antibodies for drug delivery. In *Controlled drug delivery*, edited by JR Robinson, VHL Lee. New York: Marcel Dekker, Inc., pp. 623–653

- **Ho NFH, Barsuhn CL, Burton PS, Merkle HP.** (1992). Mechanistic insights to buccal delivery of proteinaceous substances. *Advanced Drug Delivery Reviews*, 8, 197–235

- **Holmgren J, Clemens J, Sack D, Sanchez J, Svennerholm AM.** (1989). Development of oral vaccines with special reference to cholera. In *Topics in Pharmaceutical Sciences 1989*, edited by DD Breimer, DJA Crommelin, KK Midha. The Hague: International Pharmaceutical Federation (F.I.P.), pp. 297–311

- **Hunt CA, MacGregor RD, Siegel RA.** (1986). Engineering targeted *in vivo* drug delivery. I. The physiological and physicochemical principles governing opportunities and limitations. *Pharm Research*, 3, 333–344

- **Jain RK.** (1987). Transport of molecules in the tumor interstitium: a review. *Cancer Research*, 47, 3039–3051

- **Jani PU, Florence AT, McCarthy DE.** (1992). Further histological evidence of the gastrointestinal absorption of polystyrene nanospheres in the rat. *Int J Pharm*, 84, 245–252

- **Kim SW, Pai CM, Makino K, Seminoff LA, Holmberg DL, Gleeson JM, Wilson DA, Mack EJ.** (1990). Self-regulated glycosylated insulin delivery. *J Controlled Release*, 11, 193–201

- **Klegerman ME, Groves MJ.** (1992). *Pharmaceutical biotechnology: Fundamentals and essentials*. Buffalo Grove, IL: Interpharm Press, Inc.

- **Kumar S, Char H, Patel S, Piemontese D, Malick, AW, Iqbal K, Neugroschel E, Behl CR.** (1992). *In vivo* transdermal iontophoretic delivery of growth hormone releasing factor GRF (1–44) in hairless guinea pigs. *J Controlled Release*, 18, 213–220

- **Lee VHL, Dodda-Kashi S, Grass GM, Rubas W.** (1991). Oral route of peptide and protein drug delivery. In *Peptide and protein drug delivery*, edited by VHL Lee. New York: Marcel Dekker, Inc., pp. 691–738

- **Maberly GF, Wait GA, Kilpatrick JA, Loten EG, Gain KR, Stewart RDH, Eastman CJ.** (1982). Evidence for insulin degradation by muscle and fat tissue in an insulin resistant diabetic patient. *Diabetologica* (23), 333–336

- **Nässander UK, Storm G, Peeters PAM, Crommelin DJA.** (1990). Liposomes. In *Biodegradable Polymers as Drug Delivery Systems*, edited by M Chasin, R Langer. New York: Marcel Dekker, pp. 261–33

- **O'Hagan DT.** (1990). Intestinal translocation of particulates — implications for drug and antigen delivery. *Advanced Drug Delivery Reviews*, 5, 265–285

- Nguyen TH, Ward C. (1993). Stability characterization and formulation development of alteplase, a recombinant tissue plasminogen activator. In *Stability and characterization of protein and peptide drugs. Case histories*, edited by YJ Wang, R Pearlman. New York: Plenum Press, Inc., pp. 91–134
- Patton JS, Platz RM. (1992). Pulmonary delivery of peptides and proteins for systemic action. *Advanced Drug Delivery Reviews*, 8, 179–196
- Patton JS, Trinchero P, Platz RM. (1994). Bioavailability of pulmonary delivered peptides and proteins: α-interferon, calcitonins and parathyroid hormones. *J Controlled Release*, 28, 79–85
- Pearlman R, Bewley TA. (1993). Stability and characterization of human growth hormone. In *Stability and characterization of protein and peptide drugs. Case histories*, edited by YJ Wang, R Pearlman. New York: Plenum Press, Inc., pp. 1–58
- Peeters PAM, Storm G, Crommelin DJA. (1987). Immunoliposomes *in vivo*: state of the art. *Advanced Drug Delivery Reviews*, 1, 249–266
- Pikal MJ. (1990a). Freeze-drying of proteins. Part I: Process Design. *BioPharm*, 3, 18–27
- Pikal MJ. (1990b). Freeze-drying of proteins. Part II: Formulation selection. *BioPharm*, 3, 26–30
- Poste G. (1985). Drug targeting in cancer therapy. In *Receptor-mediated targeting of drugs*, edited by G Gregoriadis, G Poste, J Senior, A Trouet. New York: Plenum Press, Inc., pp. 427–474
- Pristoupil TI. (1985). Haemoglobin lyophilized with sucrose: effect of residual moisture on storage. *Haematologia*, 18, 45–52
- Ramakrishnan S. (1990). Current status of antibody-toxin conjugates for tumor therapy. In *Targeted therapeutic systems*, edited by P Tyle, BP Ram. New York: Marcel Dekker, Inc., pp. 189–213
- Roitt IM, Brostoff J, Male DK. (1993). *Immunology*, third edition, Mosby, St. Louis, MO
- Sage BH, Bock CR, Denuzzio JD, Hoke RA. (1995). Technological and developmental issues of iontophoretic transport of peptide and protein drugs. In *Trends and future perspectives in peptide and protein drug delivery*, edited by VHL Lee, M Hashida, Y Mizushima. Chur: Harwood Academic Publishers GmbH, pp. 111–134
- Soon-Shiong P, Heintz RE, Merideth N, Yao QX, Yoa Z, Zheng T, Murphy M, Moloney MK, Schmehl M, Harris M, Mendez R, Mendez R, Sandford PA. (1994). Insulin independence in a type 1 diabetic patient after encapsulated islet transplantation. *Lancet*, 343, 950–951
- Storm G, Oussoren C, Peeters PAM, Barenholz YB. (1993). Tolerability of liposomes *in vivo*. In *Liposome Technology*, edited by G Gregoriadis. Boca Raton: CRC Press, Inc., pp. 345–383
- Storm G, Nässander U, Vingerhoeds MH, Steerenberg PA, Crommelin DJA. (1994) Antibody-targeted liposomes to deliver doxorubicin to ovarian cancer cells. *J Liposome Research*, 4, 641–666
- Supersaxo A, Hein WR, Steffen H. (1990). Effect of molecular weight on the lymphatic absorption of water-soluble compounds following subcutaneous administration. *Pharm Research*, 7, 167–169
- Thurow H, Geisen K. (1984). Stabilization of dissolved proteins against denaturation at hydrophobic interfaces. *Diabetologica*, 27, 212–218
- Tomlinson E. (1987). Theory and practice of site-specific drug delivery. *Adv Drug Del Reviews*, 1, 87–198
- Toonen P, Crommelin DJA. (1983). Immunogobulins as targeting agents for liposome encapsulated drugs. *Pharm Weekblad Sci Ed*, 16, 269–280
- Tresco PA. (1994). Encapsulated cells for sustained neurotransmitter delivery to the central nervous system. *J Controlled Release*, 28, 253–258
- Uludag H, Kharlip L, Sefton MV. (1993). Protein delivery by microencapsulated cells. *Adv Drug Delivery Reviews*, 10, 115–130
- Vemuri S, Yu CT, Roosdorp N. (1993a). Formulation and stability of recombinant α-antitrypsin. In *Stability and characterization of protein and peptide drugs. Case histories*, edited by YJ Wang, R Pearlman. New York: Plenum Press, Inc., pp. 263–286
- Vemuri S, Yu CT, Roosdorp N. (1993b). Formulation and stability of recombinant α1–antitrypsin. In *Stability and characterization of protein and peptide drugs. Case histories*, edited by YJ Wang, R Pearlman. New York: Plenum Press, Inc., pp. 263–286
- Vingerhoeds MH, Storm G, Crommelin DJA. (1994). Immunoliposomes *in vivo*. *Immunomethods*, 4, 259–272
- Woodle M, Newman M, Collins L, Redemann C, Martin F. (1990). Improved long-circulating (Stealth®) liposomes using synthetic lipids. *Proc Int Symp Control Rel Bioactive Mater*, 17, 77–78
- USP XXIII/NF 18. (1995). United States Pharmacopeial Convention, Inc. Rockville, MD
- Zhou XH, Li Wan Po A. (1991a). Peptide and protein drugs: I. Therapeutic applications, absorption and parenteral administration. *Int J Pharm*, 75, 97–115
- Zhou XH, Li Wan Po A. (1991b). Peptide and protein drugs: II. Non-parenteral routes of delivery. *Int J Pharm*, 75, 117–130

Self-Assessment Questions

Question 1: *How does one sterilize biotech products for parenteral administration?*

Question 2: *A pharmaceutical protein which is poorly water soluble around its i.e.p. has to be formulated as an injection. What conditions would one select to produce a water soluble, injectable solution?*

Question 3: *Why are most of the biotech proteins to be used in the clinic formulated in freeze dried form? Why is, as a rule, the presence of lyoprotectants required? Why is it important to know the glass transition temperature or eutectic temperature of the system?*

Question 4: *Why is it not necessarily wise to work at the lowest possible chamber pressures?*

Question 5: *Why are (with the exception of oral vaccines) no oral delivery systems for proteins available?*

Question 6: *What alternative route of administration to the parenteral route would be the first to look into if a systemic therapeutic effect is pursued and if one does not wish to exploit absorption enhancing technologies?*

Question 7: *If one considers to use the iontophoretic transport route for protein delivery, what are the variables to be considered?*

Question 8: *What are the differences between the endocrine, paracrine and autocrine way of cell communication? Why is information on the way cells communicate important in the drug formulation process?*

Question 9: *A company decides to explore the possibility to develop a feed back system for a therapeutic protein. What information should be available to estimate the chances for success?*

Question 10: *Why is the selection of the dimensions of a colloidal particulate carrier system for targeted delivery of a protein of utmost importance?*

Question 11: *Design a targeted, colloidal carrier system and a protocol for its use to circumvent the three hurdles to achieve successful treatment of solid tumors (mentioned in Table 4.14).*

Question 12: *What are the options to induce therapeutic actions upon attachment of immunoliposomes to (tumor) target cells.*

Answers

Answer 1: Through aseptic manufacturing protocols; filtration through 0.2 or 0.22 μm pore filters plays an important role in reducing the degree of contamination of the protein solutions.

Answer 2: One has to go through the items listed in Table 4.1. As the aqueous solubility is probably pH dependent, information on the preferred pH ranges should be collected. If necessary, solubility enhancers (e.g., lysine, arginine and/or surfactants) and stabilizers against adsorption/aggregation should be added. 'As a last resort', one might consider carriers such as liposomes.

Answer 3: Chemical and physical instability of proteins in aqueous media is usually the reason to dry the protein solution.
Freeze-drying is then the preferred technology, as other drying techniques do not give rapidly reconstitutable dry forms for the formulation, and/or because elevated temperatures necessary for drying jeopardise the integrity of the protein.
One should not exceed the glass transition/eutectic temperature as otherwise collapse of the cake can be observed. Collapse reduces the drying rate and collapsed material does not rapidly dissolve upon adding water for reconstitution.

Answer 4: Because gas conduction (one of the three heat transfer routes) depends on pressure and is reduced when the pressure is.

Answer 5: Because of the hostile environment in the GI tract regarding protein stability and the poor absorption characteristics of proteins (high molecular weight/often hydrophilic).

Answer 6: The pulmonary route

Answer 7: Physical characteristics of the protein and medium, such a molecular weight, i.e.p., ionic strength, pH. And, in addition, electrical current options (pulsed, permanent, wave shape) and desired dose level/pattern (pulsed/constant/variable).

Answer 8: See Table 4.8. This information is important because in particular with paracrine and autocrine acting proteins targeted delivery should be considered to minimise unwanted side effects.

Answer 9:
 - The desired pharmacokinetic profile (e.g., information on the PK/PD relationship/circadian rhythm)
 - Chemical and physical stability of the protein on long-term storage at body/ambient temperature
 - Availability of a bio-sensor system (stability *in vivo*, precision/accuracy)
 - Availability of a reliable pump system (see Table 4.10)

Answer 10: The body is highly compartmentalised and access to target sites inside and outside the blood circulation is highly dependent on the size of the carrier system involved (and other factors: presence of diseased tissue, and surface characteristics such as charge, hydrophobicity/hydrophilicity, ligands).

Answer 11: The selection should be based on the induction of bystander effects, 'cocktails' of homing devices (e.g., monoclonal antibodies), selection of non-modulating receptors and non-shedding receptors. Neutralisation of free, shedded tumor antigens with free, non-conjugated monoclonal antibodies by injection of these free antibodies before the administration of ligand-carrier-drug combinations would be an approach to avoid neutralization of the carrier-homing device combination by shedded antigen.

Answer 12: Figure 4.31 gives an overview of these options.

5 Pharmacokinetics and Pharmacodynamics of Peptide and Protein Drugs

by: Rene Braeckman

Introduction

Pharmacokinetics is the study of the rate processes that are responsible for the time course of the level of an exogenous compound in the body. The processes involved are absorption (A), distribution (D), metabolism (M), and excretion (E) (Figure 5.1). The pharmacokinetics of peptides, peptoids, proteins and other biotechnology products are an important factor in their pharmacodynamics, i.e., the time course of their pharmacological effect. Therefore, knowledge of the pharmacokinetics and pharmacodynamics of a pharmaceutical drug in humans and laboratory animals is required when selecting dose levels and dose regimens. Similarly, the toxicokinetics (pharmacokinetics in toxicology studies, including higher doses than used clinically) and toxicodynamics (time course of undesired effects) are important for the design of toxicology studies (dose levels and dose regimens) as well as in determining safety margins and extrapolating toxicological data to humans.

In this chapter, the pharmacokinetics (PK) of protein therapeutics will be described, followed by an introduction of the complex relationship with the pharmacodynamic (PD) effect, and how PK and PD can be influenced by plasma protein binding. Furthermore, interspecies extra-

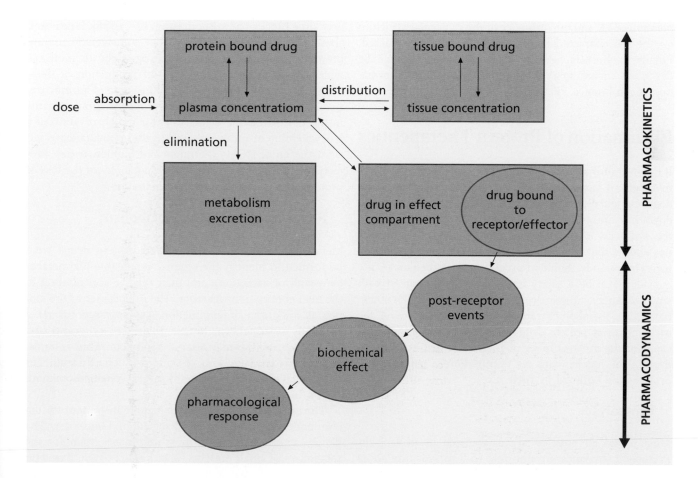

Figure 5.1. Physiological scheme of pharmacokinetic and pharmacodynamic processes.

M$_W$	Site of elimination	Dominating clearance mechanism	Determinant factor
< 500	blood liver	extracellular hydrolysis passive lipoid diffusion	
500 - 1,000	liver	carrier-mediated uptake passive lipoid diffusion	structure lipophilicity
1,000 - 50,000	kidney	glomerular filtration	M$_W$
50,000 - 200,000	kidney liver	receptor-mediated endocytosis receptor-mediated endocytosis	sugar, charge
200,000 - 400,000		opsonization	α_2-macroglobulin, IgG
> 400,000		phagocytosis	particle aggregation

Table 5.1. Clearance mechanisms for peptides and proteins as a function of molecular weight (M$_w$). Other determining factors are size, charge, lipophilicity, functional groups, sugar recognition, vulnerability for proteases, aggregation to particles, formation of complexes with opsonisation factors, etc. The indicated mechanisms overlap, and fluid-phase endocytosis can in principle occur across the entire M$_w$ range (after Meijer and Ziegler, 1993).

polation of PK and the influence of the molecular structure on the PK characteristics of proteins will be discussed. Finally, the immunogenicity of protein therapeutics will be described, including a discussion on how antibody formation can influence PK and PD.

Elimination of Protein Therapeutics

It is commonly accepted that peptide and protein drugs are metabolized through identical catabolic pathways as endogenous and dietary proteins. Generally, proteins are broken down into amino acid fragments that can be re-utilized in the synthesis of endogenous proteins. Although history has shown that proteins can be powerful and potentially toxic compounds, their end-products of metabolism are not considered to be a safety issue. This is in contrast with small organic synthetic drug molecules from which potentially toxic metabolites can be formed. The study of the metabolism of protein drugs is also very complicated because of the great number of fragments that can be produced. The mechanisms for elimination of peptides and proteins are outlined in Table 5.1.

Proteolysis

Most if not all proteins are catabolized by proteolysis. Proteolytic enzymes are not only widespread throughout the body, they are also ubiquitous in nature, and therefore the potential number of catabolism sites on any protein is

very large (Bocci, 1987; Bocci, 1990; Lee, 1988). It has been shown for interferon-γ (INF-γ) that truncated forms are present in the circulation after dosing of rhesus monkeys with rIFN-γ. The rate and extent of production of these metabolites may be dependent on the route of administration. This, and the cross-reactivity of these degraded forms in the ELISA may be responsible for the observation of a bioavailability of more than 100% after subcutaneous administration of rIFN-γ (Ferraiolo and Mohler, 1992). Proteolytic activity in tissue may be responsible for the loss of protein after subcutaneous administration.

Renal Excretion and Metabolism

Metabolism studies of peptide and protein drugs were performed to identify the organs responsible for metabolism (and/or excretion), and their relative contribution to the total elimination clearance. The importance of the kidney as an organ of elimination was assessed for rIL-2 (Gibbons *et al.*, 1995), M-CSF (Bauer *et al.*, 1994) and rIFN-γ (Mordenti *et al.*, 1992) in nephrectomized animals. The relative contributions of renal and hepatic clearances to the total plasma clearance of several other proteins are shown in Figure 5.2.

The different renal processes that are important for the elimination of proteins are depicted in Figure 5.3. The kidney appears to be the most dominant organ for the catabolism of small proteins (Maack *et al.*, 1979). Based on the observation that only trace amounts of albumin pass the glomerulus, it is believed that macromolecules have to

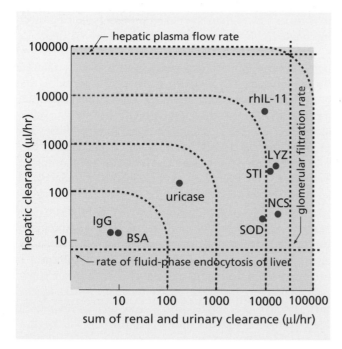

Figure 5.2. Hepatic and renal clearances of proteins in mice. LYZ: lysozyme, STI: soy bean trypsin inhibitor, NCS: neocarzinostatin, SOD: superoxide dismutase, IgG: immunoglobulin G, BSA: bovine serum albumin, rhIL-11: recombinant human interleukin-11. From Takagi *et al.* (Takagi *et al.*, 1995).

bc smaller than 68 kD to undergo glomerular filtration (Takakura *et al.*, 1990). Although this rule of thumb is usually true, it is the effective molecular radius that determines the degree of sieving by the glomerulus (Figure 5.4) (Rabkin and Dahl, 1993). The glomerular barrier is also charge selective: the clearance of anionic molecules is impaired relative to that of neutral molecules, and the clearance of cationic macromolecules is enhanced. The influence of charge on glomerular filtration is especially important for molecules with a radius greater than 2.0 nm (Maack *et al.*, 1985).

After glomerular filtration, complex polypeptides and proteins are actively re-absorbed by the proximal tubulus by endocytosis and then hydrolyzed within the cell to peptide fragments and amino acids (Maack *et al.*, 1985; Wall and Maack, 1985). The amino acids are returned to the systemic circulation. Consequently, only small amounts of intact protein are detected in the urine. For example, cathepsin D, a major renal protease, is responsible for the hydrolysis of IL-2 in the kidney (Ohnishi *et al.*, 1989).

Small linear peptides such as angiotensin and bradykinin are subjected to intraluminal metabolism. They are hydrolyzed by enzymes in the luminal brush membrane of the proximal tubules and the amino acids are subsequently transported through the cells into the systemic circulation (Carone and Peterson, 1980).

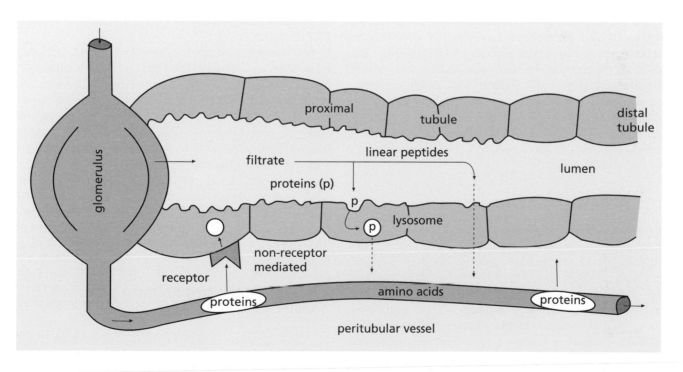

Figure 5.3. Pathways of renal elimination of proteins, including glomerular filtration, catabolism at the luminal membrane, tubular absorption followed by intracellular degradation, and postglomerular peritubular uptake followed by intracellular degradation. From Rabkin and Dahl, 1993.

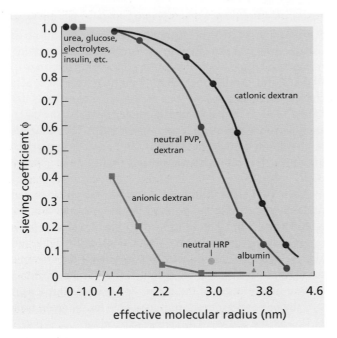

Figure 5.4. Glomerular sieving curves of several macromolecules. The different sieving coefficients reflect the influence of size, charge, and rigidity of molecules. HRP: horseradish peroxidase. From Arendshorst and Navar (Arendshorst and Navar, 1988).

Peritubular extraction of proteins from the postglomerular capillaries and intracellular catabolism is another renal mechanism of elimination (Rabkin and Kitaji, 1983). This route of elimination was demonstrated for IL-2, insulin (Hellfritzsch *et al.*, 1988; Rabkin *et al.*, 1984), calcitonin, parathyroid hormone, vasopressin and angiotensin II (Maack *et al.*, 1979). It is believed that the peritubular pathway exists mainly for the delivery of certain hormones to their site of action, i.e., to the receptors on the contraluminal site of the tubular cells.

Hepatic Metabolism

Besides proteolytic enzymes and renal catabolism, the liver has also been shown to contribute significantly to the metabolism of protein therapeutics. The rate of hepatic catabolism, which determined in part the elimination half-life, is largely dependent on the presence of specific amino acid sequences in the protein (Meijer and Ziegler, 1993). Long-lived proteins are mainly degraded by lysosomal digestion. Proteolysis is started by endopeptidases (mainly cathepsin D) that act on the middle part of the proteins. Oligopeptides as the result of the first step are further degraded by exopeptidases. The resulting amino acids and dipeptides re-enter the metabolic pool of the cell (Meijer and Ziegler, 1993). The hepatic metabolism of glycoproteins

may occur slower than the naked protein because protecting oligosaccharide chains need to be removed first.

Before intracellular hepatic catabolism, proteins and peptides need to be transported from the blood stream to the hepatocytes. Cyclosporins are cyclic peptides that permeate the hepatocyte membrane by simple non-ionic passive diffusion because of their highly hydrophobic characteristics (Ziegler *et al.*, 1988). For larger peptides and proteins, there is a multitude of energy-dependent, carrier-mediated transport processes available for cellular uptake. Yet another possibility is receptor-mediated endocytosis, such as for insulin and epidermal growth factor (EGF) (Burwen and Jones, 1990; Kim *et al.*, 1988; Sugiyama and Hanano, 1989). For glycoproteins, if a critical number of exposed sugar groups (mannose, galactose, fucose, N-acetylglucosamine, N-acetylgalactosamine, or glucose) is exceeded, receptor-mediated endocytosis through sugar-recognizing receptors is an efficient hepatic uptake mechanism (Meijer and Ziegler, 1993). Low density lipoprotein receptor-related protein (LRP) is a member of the low-density lipoprotein (LDL) receptor family responsible for endocytosis of several important lipoproteins, proteases, and protease-inhibitor complexes in the liver and other tissues (Strickland *et al.*, 1995). Examples of proteins and protein complexes for which hepatic uptake is mediated by LRP are tissue type plasminogen activator (t-PA), urokinase type plasminogen activator (u-PA), complexes of t-PA and u-PA with plasminogen activator inhibitor type I (PAI-1), tissue factor pathway inhibitor (TFPI), and thrombospondin (TSP).

Receptor-mediated uptake of protein drugs by hepatocytes followed by intracellular metabolism causes sometimes dose-dependent plasma disposition curves due to the saturation of the active uptake mechanism at higher doses. As an example, EGF administered at low doses (50 µg/kg and lower) to rats showed an elimination clearance proportional to hepatic blood flow, since the systemic supply of drug to the liver is the rate limiting process for elimination. At high doses (>200 µg/mL), the hepatic clearance is saturated, and extrahepatic clearance by other tissues is the dominant factor in the total plasma clearance. At intermediate doses of EGF, both hepatic blood flow and EGF receptors responsible for the active uptake affect the total plasma clearance (Murakami *et al.*, 1994).

Receptor-Mediated Elimination by Other Cells

For small synthetic drugs, the fraction of the dose bound to receptors at each moment after administration is usually negligible, and receptor-binding is reversible mostly without internalization of the receptor-drug complex. For protein drugs, however, a substantial part of the dose may be bound to the receptor, and receptor-mediated uptake by

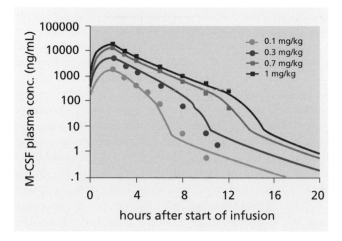

Figure 5.5. Observed and predicted plasma concentration-time profiles of M-CSF after 2-hour intravenous infusions of 0.1–1 mg/kg in cynomolgus monkeys. A two-compartmental pharmacokinetic model with a linear clearance pathway and a parallel Michaelis-Menten elimination pathway was used.

specialized cells followed by intracellular catabolism may play an important part in the total elimination of the drug from the body. A derivative of granulocyte colony-stimulating factor (G-CSF), nartograstim, and most likely G-CSF itself, is taken up by bone marrow through a saturable receptor-mediated process (Kuwabara *et al.*, 1995). It has been demonstrated for M-CSF that besides the linear renal elimination pathway, there is a saturable non-linear elimination pathway that follows Michaelis-Menten kinetics (Bartocci *et al.*, 1987; Bauer *et al.*, 1994). The importance of the non-linear elimination pathway was demonstrated by a steeper dip in the plasma concentration profile at lower M-CSF concentrations (Figure 5.5). At higher levels, linear renal elimination was dominant, and the non-linear pathway was saturated. The non-linear pathway could be blocked by coadministration of carrageenan, a macrophage inhibitor, indicating that receptor-mediated uptake by macrophages was likely responsible for the non-linear elimination (Bauer *et al.*, 1994). This is especially relevant since M-CSF stimulates the proliferation of macrophages. It is also possible that the receptor-mediated uptake and the effect of M-CSF are closely linked. Indeed, it was observed that after chronic administration of M-CSF the non-linear elimination was probably induced by autoinduction since M-CSF increases circulating levels of macrophages. Although autoinduction and consequently accelerated metabolism of most drugs is related to a loss of the pharmacological effect, for M-CSF it may be an indication of sustained pharmacodynamic activity. Similar kinetics were observed for other hematopoietic stimulating factors such as granulocyte-CSF (G-CSF) (Tanaka and Kaneko,

1991) and granulocyte macrophage-CSF (GM-CSF) (Petros *et al.*, 1992).

Distribution of Protein Therapeutics

Because of the large size of proteins, their apparent volume of distribution is usually relatively small. The initial volume of distribution after intravenous injection is approximately equal to or slightly higher than the total plasma volume. The total volume of distribution is generally twice or less than twice the initial volume of distribution. Although this is sometimes interpreted as a low tissue penetration, it is difficult to generalize. Indeed, adequate concentrations may be reached in a single target organ because of receptor mediated uptake, while the contribution to the total volume of distribution may be rather small. Biodistribution studies with the measurement of the protein drug in tissues are necessary to establish tissue distribution. Because of the difficulty of performing biodistribution studies, the intensity and duration of the pharmacological effects of the drug are sometimes used as an indirect measurement of drug levels in a target organ or tissue.

Biodistribution studies are usually performed with radiolabeled compounds. Biodistribution studies are imperative for small organic synthetic drugs since long residence times of the label in certain tissues may be an indication of tissue accumulation of potentially toxic metabolites. Because of the possibility of re-utilization of amino acids from protein drugs in endogenous proteins, such a safety issue does not exist. Therefore, biodistribution studies for protein drugs are usually performed to assess drug targeting to specific tissues, or to detect the major organs of elimination (usually kidneys and liver).

If the protein contains a suitable amino acid such as tyrosine or lysine, an external label such as ^{125}I can be chemically coupled to the protein (Ferraiolo and Mohler, 1992). Although this is easily accomplished and a high specific activity can be obtained, the protein is chemically altered. Therefore, it may be better to label proteins and other biotechnology compounds by introducing radioactive isotopes during their synthesis by which an internal atom becomes the radioactive marker. For recombinant proteins, this can be accomplished by growing the production cell line in the presence of amino acids labeled with ^{3}H, ^{14}C, ^{35}S, etc. This method is not routinely used because of the prohibition of radioactive contamination of fermentation equipment. Moreover, internally labeled proteins may be less desirable than iodinated proteins because of the potential for re-utilization of the radiolabeled amino acid fragments in the synthesis of endogenous proteins and cell structures. Irrespective of the labeling method, but more so for external labeling, the labeled product should have demonstrated physicochemical and biological properties identical to the unlabeled molecule (Bennett and McMartin, 1979).

In addition, as for all types of radiolabeled studies, it needs to be established whether the measured radioactivity represents intact labeled protein, or radiolabeled metabolites, or the liberated label. Trichloro-acetic acid- precipitable radioactivity is often used to distinguish intact protein from free label or low-molecular-weight metabolites, which appear in the supernatant. Proteins with re-utilized labeled amino acids and large protein metabolites can only be distinguished from the original protein by techniques such as PAGE, HPLC, specific immunoassays, or bioassays. This discussion implies also that the results of biodistribution studies with autoradiography can be very misleading. Although autoradiography is becoming more quantitative, one never knows what is being measured qualitatively without specific assays. It is therefore sometimes better to perform biodistribution studies by collection of the tissues, and the specific measurement of the protein drug in the tissue homogenate.

A method was developed to calculate early-phase tissue uptake clearances based on plasma and tissue drug measurements during the first 5 minutes after intravenous administration (Kim *et al.*, 1988). The short time interval has the advantage that metabolism and the tissue efflux clearance presumably can be ignored. As an example, with this method, dose-independent (non-saturable) uptake clearance values were observed for a recombinant derivative of hG-CSF, nartograstim, for kidney and liver (Kuwabara *et al.*, 1995). In contrast, a dose-dependent reduction in the uptake clearance by bone marrow with increasing doses of nartograstim was observed. These findings suggested that receptor mediated endocytosis of the G-CSF receptor in bone marrow may participate in the non-linear properties of nartograstim. Since G-CSF is one of the growth factors that stimulates the proliferation and differentiation of neutropoietic progenitor cells to granulocytes in bone marrow, the distribution aspects of nartograstim into bone marrow are especially relevant for the pharmacodynamics. In addition, since G-CSF and nartograstim are catabolized in the bone marrow cells after receptor-mediated uptake, the biodistribution into bone marrow is also a pathway for elimination of these molecules. Unlike for classical small synthetic drugs, it is not uncommon for biotechnology derived drugs that biodistribution, pharmacodynamics, and elimination are closely connected.

Besides receptor-mediated uptake into target organs and tissues, other proteins, or macromolecules in general, distribute into tissues in more non-specific ways. It was demonstrated in at least one study with tumor-bearing mice that high total systemic exposure of target-non-specific macromolecules was the most important factor determining the extent of tissue uptake (Takakura *et al.*, 1990) (cf. Chapter 4). Consequently, molecules with physicochemical characteristics that minimize hepatic and renal elimination clearances showed the highest tumoral exposure. Compounds with relatively low molecular weights (approximately 10 kD) or positive charges were rapidly eliminated and showed lower tumor radioactivity accumulation; large (>70 kD) and negatively charged compounds (carboxymethyl dextran, BSA, mouse IgG) showed prolonged retention in the circulation, and high tumoral levels. A typical example is the murine urokinase (muPA) EGF-like domain peptide of 48 amino acids, muPA(1–48). This peptide is a urokinase receptor antagonist under consideration as an anticancer drug since urokinase has been implicated in invasive biological processes such as tumor metastasis, trophoblast implantation, and angiogenesis. Scientists at Chiron have fused muPA(1–48) to the human IgG constant region. The fused molecule (IgG-muPA(1–48)) retained its activity of inhibition of the murine UPA receptor, but has a much longer *in vivo* elimination half-life (79 versus 0.5 hr; Figure 5.6). The half-life increase was due to both a decrease in elimination clearance (4.3 versus 95 mL/hr/kg) and an increase in the peripheral volume of distribution (434 versus 43 mL/kg). Although the fused molecule was substantially larger, tissue distribution increased, possibly because of substantial tissue binding. This is in contrast with some polyethylene glycol-modified (Pegylated) molecules such as PEG IL-2 (polyethylene glycol-modified interleukin-2) for which size increase resulted in a smaller distribution volume compared with the original molecule (see below).

As discussed earlier (Figure 4.12), biodistribution into the lymphatics after subcutaneous (s.c.) injection deserves special attention since it is a rather unique transport pathway for macromolecules. Following s.c. administration, the drug can be transported to the systemic circulation by absorption into the blood capillaries or by the lymphatics. Since the permeability of macromolecules through the capillary wall is low, they were found to enter blood indirectly through the lymphatic system (Supersaxo *et al.*, 1988; Supersaxo *et al.*, 1990). Compounds with a molecular weight larger than 16 kD are absorbed mainly (>50%) by the lymphatics, while compounds smaller than 1 kD are hardly absorbed by the lymphatics at all (Figure 4.12).

Pharmacodynamics of Protein Therapeutics

Although the time course of the compound at the receptor or effector site is the desired knowledge to predict or ex-

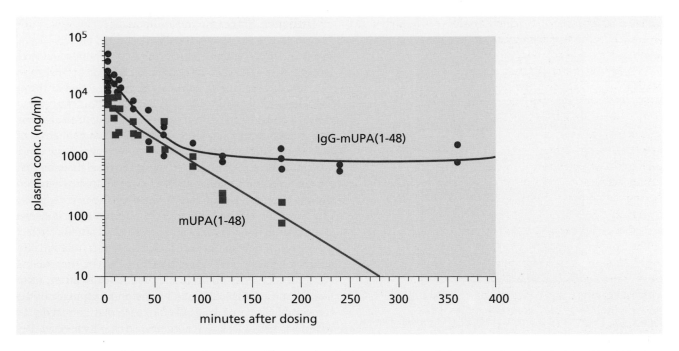

Figure 5.6. Fusion of the murine urokinase EGF-like peptide of 48 amino acids with human IgG (IgG-mUPA(1-48)) resulted in a much longer half-life than the original peptide (mUPA(1-48)). The data were modeled according to a linear compartmental model.

plain the pharmacodynamics (PD), accurate drug level data at that site are difficult to obtain. In most cases, pharmacokinetic (PK) data are limited to plasma concentration data. Pharmacokinetic models are widely used to describe and predict the time course of the drug in plasma and tissues. These models include compartmental models and physiological models.

During the last decade, the application of PD models for *in vivo* effect data has increased tremendously (Girard *et al.*, 1990). In addition, the PD models have been linked to PK models, and this approach has made integrated PK/PD analysis possible. PK/PD modeling has been reviewed extensively for small drug molecules (Colburn and Blue, 1992; Derendorf and Hochhaus, 1995; Holford, 1990; Kroboth *et al.*, 1991; Schwinghammer and Kroboth, 1988; Steimer *et al.*, 1993), but relatively few publications are available for proteins, or biotechnological therapeutics in general (Colburn, 1991). PD models are based on the law of mass action of drug-receptor interaction, classically called the occupancy theory (Kenakin, 1993). These models that express the effect as a function of drug concentration are known for a long time from the classical *in vitro* pharmacological experiments wherein receptors in organ baths or tissue strips were exposed to a drug concentration. A similar situation occurs *in vivo* when the effect concentration is the concentration in plasma, an effect compartment or biophase (Holford and Sheiner, 1981a).

Direct Effects

Sometimes, the effect concentration in the PD model equations can be set equal to the plasma concentration when there is a direct relationship between the plasma drug concentration and the pharmacological effect. These are the direct effect PK/PD models. Figure 5.7 shows an example of a PK/PD model wherein the effect is directly related to the concentration in the central compartment (the plasma concentration). Any appropriate compartmental model, or other PK model that predicts the plasma concentration-time curve can be used. In the direct effect PK/PD models, the effect-time profile follows the plasma-concentration profile, and the maximum effect occurs at the time of the peak plasma concentration.

A typical example is the thrombolytic effect of tissue factor pathway inhibitor (TFPI). The increase of the prothrombin time (PT) during continuous infusion of *E. Coli* derived recombinant human TFPI in a 2–week toxicology study in cynomolgus monkeys was directly related to the TFPI plasma concentrations (Figure 5.8) (Childs *et al.*, 1996). The PD model equation is

$$E = E_o + S\ C$$

where E is the effect (PT); E_o is the baseline effect (predose PT), C is the TFPI plasma concentration, and S is the slope

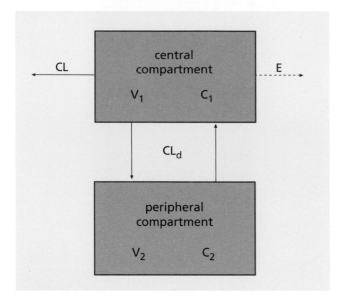

Figure 5.7. Example of a direct effect PK/PD model. The PK model is a typical two-compartmental model with a linear elimination clearance from the central compartment (CL) and a distributional clearance (CL_d). C_1 and C_2 are the concentrations in the central and peripheral compartments, and V_1 and V_2 are their respective apparent volumes of distribution. The effect (E) is a function of C_1.

of the effect-concentration curve. The slope represents the sensitivity of the effect or the potency, i.e., change in PT (in sec) per unit change of concentration (µg/mL). An integrated PK/PD analysis according to a two-compartmental PK model and a direct effect PD model explained the observed data.

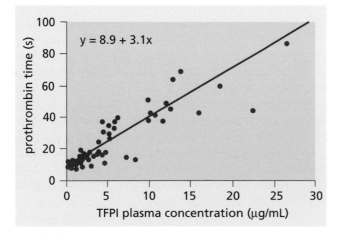

Figure 5.8. Direct relationship of the increase in prothrombin time (PT) and the plasma concentrations of TFPI after continuous i.v. infusion of TFPI in cynomolgus monkeys.

Indirect Effects

For most effects after administration of peptides and proteins, however, no such direct relationship can be observed. In a lot of cases, the maximum effect is reached at times later than the maximum plasma concentration, and sometimes, a considerable effect can still be measured at times where the plasma drug levels have fallen below the limit of detection. The temporal differences between drug exposure and onset/duration of effect has created the idea that for peptides and proteins, there is no relationship between plasma drug levels and effect. The opposite is true: if the effect is drug related, there must be a relationship between plasma drug concentrations and the time course of effect intensity. A plot of the concentration-effect relationship from non-steady state conditions, i.e., when the plasma concentrations rise and fall, such as following an i.v. infusion or an extravascular dose, is a helpful diagnostic of the temporal features of drug effect. In such plots, effect delays manifest themselves as (counterclockwise) hysteresis. Delays caused between the appearance of drug in plasma and the appearance of the pharmacodynamic response, by processes such as distribution into the biophase or cascade-type post-receptor events (Figure 5.1) may cause counterclockwise hysteresis. The relationship can be described by more complicated combined PK/PD models. Two basic approaches are available. The first one is the family of PK/PD link models, the second approach uses the indirect effect PK/PD models.

PK/PD Link Models

The temporal delay of the effect appearance and duration in the PK/PD link models is explained by a distributional delay (Holford and Sheiner, 1981b). In this case, drug concentrations in a slowly equilibrating tissue compartment with plasma are directly related to the effect intensity. Since the peak level of drug in the biophase is reached later than the time of the peak plasma concentration, the peak effect also occurs later than the plasma peak level. Although theoretically the biophase drug concentration may equal the drug concentration in a peripheral compartment, it rarely happens that a peripheral pharmacokinetic compartment acts as the biophase or effect compartment. More often the biophase is a small part of a pharmacokinetic compartment that from a pharmacokinetic point of view cannot be distinguished from other tissues within that compartment. Compartmental modeling with plasma concentration-time data is just not sensitive enough to isolate the biophase as a separate compartment without the availability of measured drug concentration data in the biophase. The solution to this problem has been to postulate a hypothetical effect compartment linked to the central

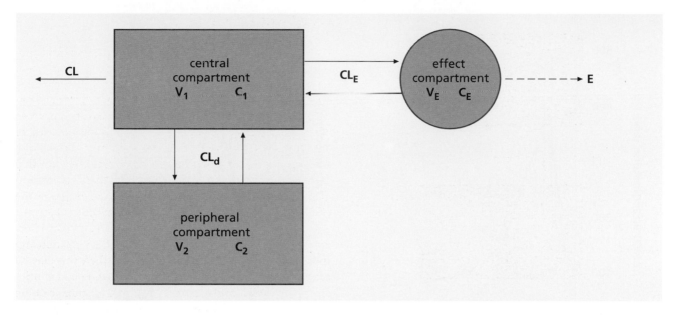

Figure 5.9. Example of a typical PK/PD link model. A hypothetical effect compartment is linked to the central compartment of a two-compartmental pharmacokinetic model. The concentration in the effect compartment (C_E) drives the intensity of the pharmacodynamic effect (E). CL_E is the linear clearance for distribution of drug to the effect compartment and elimination from the effect compartment. V_E is the apparent volume of distribution in the effect compartment. All PK parameters are identical to those used in Figure 5.7.

compartment (or to a peripheral compartment in some cases) (Figure 5.9). Drug distributes into the effect compartment (this is the link) but since the amount of drug in the effect compartment is rather small, no actual mass transfer is implemented in the pharmacokinetic part of the PK/PD model. The drug concentration in the effect compartment is then plugged into the pharmacodynamic part of the PK/PD model. Although this PK/PD model is constructed with tissue distribution as the reason for the delay in effect, the distribution clearance to the effect compartment can be interpreted as including other reasons of delay, such as transduction processes and secondary post receptor events. The hypoglycemic effect of insulin has been modeled by this type of PK/PD model (Hooper, 1991; Woodworth *et al.*, 1994). Figure 5.10 shows the mean serum concentration profile of insulin after a single s.c. injection of 10 U in 10 volunteers, and the corresponding effect measured as the glucose infusion rate to maintain an euglycemic state. Figure 5.11 shows the hysteresis in the effect-concentration relationship, and how a typical sigmoidal effect-concentration curve is obtained with the hypothetical effect concentration from a one-compartmental PK/PD link model (Woodworth *et al.*, 1994).

Indirect Effect Models

Another and better approach to include effect delays in PK/

PD modeling based on post receptor events has been the indirect effect models (Dayneka *et al.*, 1993; Jusko and Ko, 1994; Nagashima *et al.*, 1968; O'Reilly and Levy, 1970). In this modeling approach, the observed effect is an indirect effect, i.e., is not the primary effect, but rather a consequence of rate-limiting transduction and other post receptor events. In the simplest indirect effect model, the effect is maintained by a balance of two processes (Figure 5.12), which together form the biosignal flux. The first process is the production of the effect, determined by a zero-order production rate. The second process is the decrease or disappearance of the effect by a first-order dissipation rate. In a normal (predose; no drug present) situation, both processes are in equilibrium and homeostasis of the effect is maintained (baseline effect). Drug effect is caused by stimulation or inhibition of either the production or disappearance rate. The degree of stimulation or inhibition is determined by the plasma concentration. This type of model was recently applied to model the effects of IL-2 treatment in HIV patients (Piscitelli *et al.*, 1996). The PK model for IL-2 included two compartments with a time-varying serum clearance, which was related to concentrations of the soluble IL-2 receptor (sIL2R). Increasing circulating sIL2R levels were used as a surrogate marker for the upregulation of the cell-based IL-2 receptor, which causes probably an increase of the receptor-mediated clearance of IL-2 after chronic dosing. Indirect PK/PD models with IL-2 stimula-

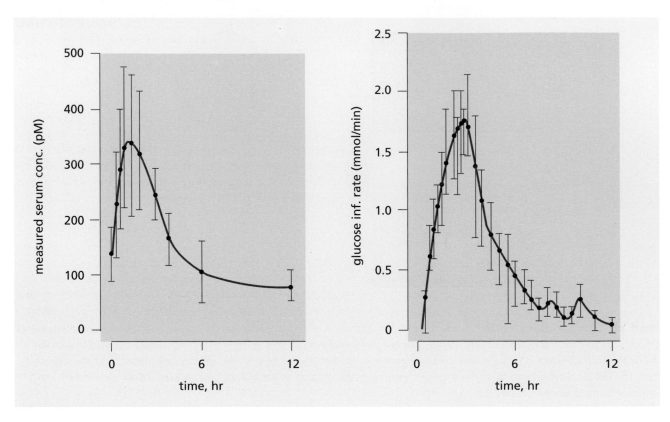

Figure 5.10. Mean measured serum insulin concentrations after a single 10-U subcutaneous dose of regular insulin in 10 volunteers (left panel); corresponding glucose infusion rates needed to maintain euglycemia (right panel). From Woodworth *et al.* (Woodworth *et al.*, 1994).

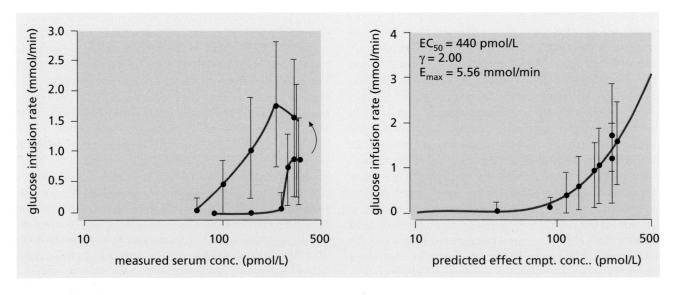

Figure 5.11. Relationship between the glucose infusion rate to maintain euglycemia versus serum insulin concentrations after a single subcutaneous dose of 10 U regular insulin in 10 volunteers (left panel). The time-dependent hysteresis, which is an indication of the indirect nature of the effect, is indicated by the arrow. The right panel shows the sigmoidal relationship between the effect and the predicted effect compartment (cmpt.) concentration, demonstrating the collapse of the hysteresis loop. From Woodworth *et al.* (Woodworth *et al.*, 1994).

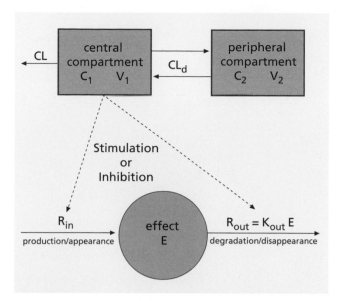

Figure 5.12. Pharmacodynamic indirect effect model wherein the effect is maintained by equilibrium between a zero-order appearance rate, R_{in}, and a first-order disappearance rate, R_{out}. A drug effect is caused by stimulation or inhibition of R_{in} or R_{out}. The degree of stimulation or inhibition is dependent on the plasma drug concentration. The PD parameters are R_{in}, K_{out} (the first order rate constant for effect disappearance), EC_{50} (the concentration that produces 50% of maximum inhibition or stimulation), and E_{max} (the maximum inhibition or stimulation). The pharmacokinetic model is identical to the one presented in Figure 5.7.

tion of the formation rates were used for sIL2R as well as for the serum levels of tissue necrosis factor-α, which were increased by IL-2.

Complex PK/PD Models

Many protein therapeutics have multiple and/or biphasic responses, which are indirect in nature. In some cases, more complicated PK/PD models based on the basic models described above are necessary. An example is the model that was developed to explain the effects of subcutaneous PEG IL-2 (polyethylene glycol-modified interleukin-2) in rats. An early moderate decrease of the number of blood lymphocytes was followed by a pronounced increase of the blood lymphocyte count. The model (Figure 5.13) describes the production of lymphocytes in tissues, after which they traffic into the blood pool, followed by trafficking out of blood and subsequent degradation. The indirect, but relatively early decrease of the number of blood lymphocytes after PEG IL-2 administration is caused by a stimulation of the lymphocyte traffic out of blood. The indirect, delayed increase of the blood lymphocytes is modeled by a stimu-

lation of the production rate of lymphocytes. The effect delay relative to the maximum plasma levels of PEG IL-2 is caused by distributional and post receptor events through three delay compartments. An additional delay is caused by the fact that the lymphocytes need to travel from their site of production to blood before an increase can be measured. Figure 5.14 does not only demonstrate the goodness-of-fit of the modeling, but also shows that the blood lymphocyte increase on Day 3 post dosing occurs after most of the PEG IL-2 is eliminated. PK/PD models like this one link the effect to drug exposure in a quantitative way, which allows extrapolations to other dose levels and routes of administration. It is obvious that a better understanding of the receptor-mediated and post receptor transduction mechanisms of protein drugs may contribute to the creation of representative and useful PK/PD models.

The stimulation of erythropoiesis by recombinant human erythropoietin (EPO) therapy in patients with uremic anemia, was analyzed with a different PD model (Uehlinger et al., 1992). The model assumes a linear stimulatory effect of EPO on the production rate of red blood cells, as measured by hematocrit. In the first stage (Figure 5.15), EPO increases the hematocrit because red cells are produced at an increased rate and none of the newly produced red cells die yet. However, after reaching one life span, the red cells start dying at the increased rate they were produced and a new steady state is reached. Although the effect of EPO is almost immediate after dosing initiation, it takes time to develop fully. This is an alternate mechanism responsible for the appearance of hysteresis in concentration-effect curves.

Dose-Response and Concentration-Response Curves

PK/PD modeling is especially useful in Phase II studies wherein the relationship between dose (and/or concentration) and response for new drug candidates needs to be established. The outcome from these studies does not only convince the sponsors and the regulatory agencies of an existing drug effect, but also assists in the selection of the optimal dose for Phase III trials. For many biotechnology-derived drugs, the Phase II trial was non-existent or too small (one dose level for example) to design a successful or optimal Phase III trial. To complicate this matter even more, it is believed that biotechnology drugs (and potentially all types of drugs) sometimes show bell-shaped dose-response curves, i.e., there is a dose that gives a maximum response, and any increase beyond this dose level results in a further decrease of the response. As an example, lower doses of rINF-γ in multiple myeloma patients seemed to induce a greater increase in natural killer activity than higher doses (Einhorn et al., 1982).

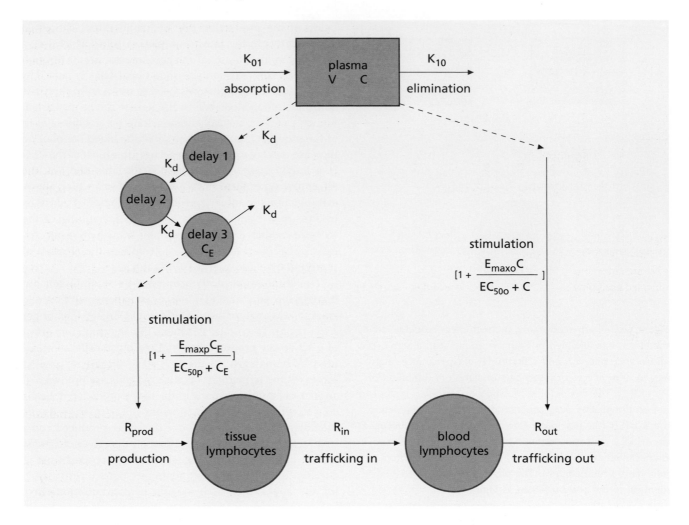

Figure 5.13. PK/PD model for changes in blood lymphocytes after sc administration of PEG IL-2 in rats. The PK model is a one-compartmental model with first-order absorption (rate constant K_{01}) and elimination (rate constant K_{10}). PEG IL-2 stimulates the trafficking out of blood and/or catabolism of lymphocytes (first-order rate R_{out}) according to an E_{max} model (parameters E_{maxo} and EC_{50o}), which is a function of the PEG IL-2 plasma concentration (C). The delayed increase of blood lymphocytes is modeled in two consecutive ways: 1. Three delay compartments with first-order input and output rates (rate constant K_d) resembling distribution and transduction delays; 2. Stimulation of lymphocyte production in tissues according to an E_{max} model (parameters E_{maxp} and EC_{50p}), which is a function of the effect concentration C_E. Tissue lymphocytes traffic into the blood pool (first-order rate R_{in}).

Protein Binding of Protein Therapeutics

The binding of drugs to circulating plasma proteins can influence both the distribution and elimination of drugs, and consequently their pharmacodynamics. Since it is generally accepted for small drug molecules, including small proteins, that only the unbound drug molecules can pass through membranes, distribution and elimination clearances of total drug are usually smaller than those of free drug. Accordingly, the activity of the drug is more closely related to the unbound drug concentration than to the total plasma concentration. For other protein drugs, however, plasma binding proteins may act as facilitators of cellular uptake processes, especially for drugs that pass membranes by active processes. When a binding protein facilitates the interaction of the protein therapeutic with receptors or other cellular sites of action, the amount of bound drug influences the pharmacodynamics directly.

Numerous examples of binding proteins have been reported for proteins: IGF-I and IGF-II (insulin like growth factor), t-PA, growth hormone, DNase (Mohler *et al.*, 1993), nerve growth factor, etc. (Mohler *et al.*, 1992). Some pro-

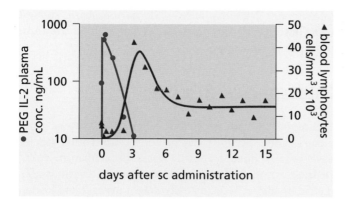

Figure 5.14. PEG IL-2 pharmacokinetics and pharmacodynamics (changes in blood lymphocyte count) after subcutaneous administration of 10 MIU/kg in rats, modeled according to the PK/PD model depicted in Figure 5.13.

teins have their own naturally occurring binding proteins which bind the protein specifically. As an example, six specific binding proteins are identified for IGF-I, denoted as IGFBP-1 to IGFBP-6 (Baxter, 1993; Clemmons, 1993).

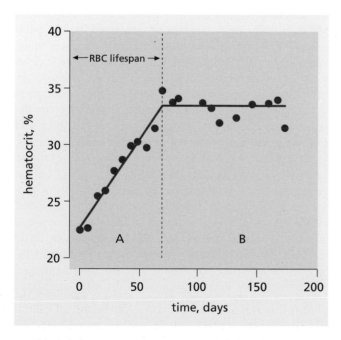

Figure 5.15. Hematocrit (Hct) in an uremic patient on a constant EPO dose of 3 × 4000 U/week. Stage A: Hct increases because EPO stimulates erythrocyte production and none of the newly formed red cells are old enough to die; Stage B: EPO maintains increased red cell production, but red cells die at a faster rate since newly formed cells from Stage A exceed their average life span. Consequently a new steady state is reached. From Uehlinger et al. (Uehlinger et al., 1992).

The IGFBPs are high affinity, soluble carrier proteins that transport IGF-I (and IGF-II) in the circulation (Clemmons, 1993). IGFBP-3 appears to be the most important binding protein for IGF-I since it is the most abundant in serum and tissues. At least 95% of the total serum concentration of IGF-I is bound to IGFBP-3 (Baxter and Martin, 1989). IGFBP-3 seems to act as a reservoir for IGF-I, and as such to protect the organism against acute insulin-like hypoglycemic effects. Indeed, the hypoglycemic effect is related to the free IGF-I plasma concentration. In this case, the binding protein limits the accessibility of IGF-I to receptors since all binding proteins have substantially higher affinities for IGF-I than the IGF receptors (Clemmons et al., 1992). In contrast, the delayed, indirect effects of IGF-I, such as its anabolic effects, may be related to the bound IGF-I levels. This is supported by evidence that the IGFBPs may play an active role in the interaction with target cells, and may act as facilitators for the delivery of IGF-I to certain receptors (Clemmons, 1993). One example is the demonstration that the affinity of the binding protein for IGF-I (IGFBP-6) at the cell surface is lower than in solution, which would make it easier for IGF-I to leave its association with the binding protein and to engage in binding with a cell-based receptor. As such, the IGFBPs may act as inhibitors for certain IGF-I effects, and as stimulators for other IGF-I effects.

It is demonstrated that the elimination half-life of bound IGF-I is significantly prolonged relative to that of free IGF-I (Cohen and Nissley, 1976; Mohler et al., 1992; Zapf et al., 1986). This suggests that unbound IGF-I is only available for elimination by routes such as glomerular filtration and peritubular extraction. The binding proteins for IGF-I are also responsible for the complicated pharmacokinetic behavior of IGF-I. The IGFBPs can be saturated at high IGF-I plasma concentrations, typically reached after therapeutic administration of IGF-I. At high doses, the binding proteins saturate and leave a larger proportion of free protein available for elimination. Additionally, the nonlinear pharmacokinetics of IGF-I are complicated by the fact that the concentrations and relative ratios of the IGFBPs change with time during chronic dosing. The binding proteins are also very different between species, which makes interspecies scaling of the IGF-I pharmacokinetics for IGF-I impossible.

Another example is growth hormone (GH), for which a specific high-affinity binding protein homologous with the extracellular domain of the growth hormone receptor is present in human plasma (Herington et al., 1986; Leung, 1987). At least two GH-binding proteins (GHBP) have been identified in plasma with respectively high and low binding affinities for GH (Mohler et al., 1992). GHBP binds about 40–50% of circulating GH at low GH concentrations of about 5 ng/mL (Baumann et al., 1988a). At higher circulating GH levels, the binding proteins become saturated

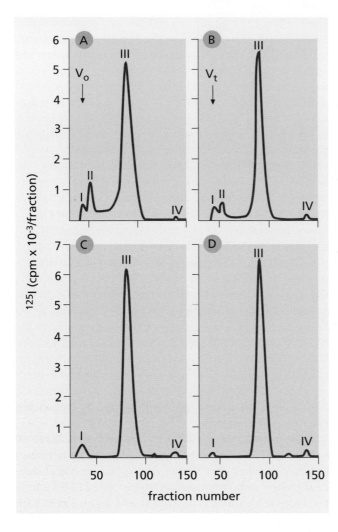

Figure 5.16. Gel filtration profiles of ^{125}I-hGH in plasma on Sephadex G-100. V_o and V_t are the void and total volumes, respectively. A. Blank plasma with endogenous level of hGH only; B. 126 ng/mL hGH added; C. 10 µg/mL hGH added; D. Tracer only (no plasma). Peak III corresponds to monomeric hGH; peak II and the plateau region between peaks II and III refer to the plasma-bound hGH; peak IV is free iodide. Higher hGH concentrations saturate the binding proteins as peak II becomes smaller relative to peak III (C versus B versus A). From Clemmons (Clemmons, 1993).

(Figure 5.16). The clearance of bound GH is about ten-fold slower than that of free GH (Baumann *et al.*, 1988b). Consequently, the binding proteins prolong the elimination half-life of GH, and as a result, enhance or prolong its activity. On the other hand, plasma binding of GH prevents access of free GH to its receptors, and this could decrease its activity (Mohler *et al.*, 1992).

Other protein therapeutics seem to bind to circulating proteins in a more non-specific way. As an example, a recombinant derivative of hG-CSF, nartogastrim, showed 92% binding in rat plasma, presumably to albumin (Kuwabara *et al.*, 1995).

Interspecies Scaling

Techniques for the prediction of pharmacokinetic parameters in one species from data derived from other species have been applied for many years (Boxenbaum, 1986; Dedrick, 1973). Such scaling techniques use various allometric equations based on body weight using the following allometric equation:

$$P = a.W^b$$

where P is the pharmacokinetic parameter being scaled, W is the body weight, a is the allometric coefficient, and b is the allometric exponent. Although a and b are specific constants for any compound and for each pharmacokinetic parameter, the exponent b seems to average around 1 for volume terms such as the volume of distribution and 0.75 for rates such as elimination and distribution clearances. Since the elimination half-life of any drug is proportional to the volume of distribution and inversely proportional to the elimination clearance, b is about 0.25 for elimination half-lives. Allometric scaling of pharmacokinetic parameters has been difficult for small synthetic drug molecules, especially for those drugs with a high hepatic clearance and quantitative and/or qualitative interspecies differences in metabolism. In contrast, the biochemical and physiological processes that are responsible for the pharmacokinetic fate of biologics such as peptides and proteins are better conserved across mammalian species. As such, allometric scaling for those compounds has been more reliable and accurate (Mordenti *et al.*, 1991). It is our experience that the systemic exposure in humans of proteins that follow linear pharmacokinetics can be predicted within a factor of two from pharmacokinetic data obtained from 3 to 4 animal species. As a typical example, we could scale the pharmacokinetic parameters for IL-2 and PEG IL-2, as demonstrated in Figure 5.17, for the elimination clearance. Notice that the regression lines for both compounds are parallel, which is expected if PEGylation decreases the clearance to the same degree in all species.

A helpful, although potentially less accurate prediction can be made based on pharmacokinetic data from one species to another based on the average allometric exponents for volumes and clearances for other compounds. Interspecies scaling is helpful in the prediction of doses for animal models of disease, toxicology studies, and for the first human studies. Indeed, if the efficacious concentration of a protein drug is known from *in vitro* studies, one might predict the dose needed to reach these levels in an

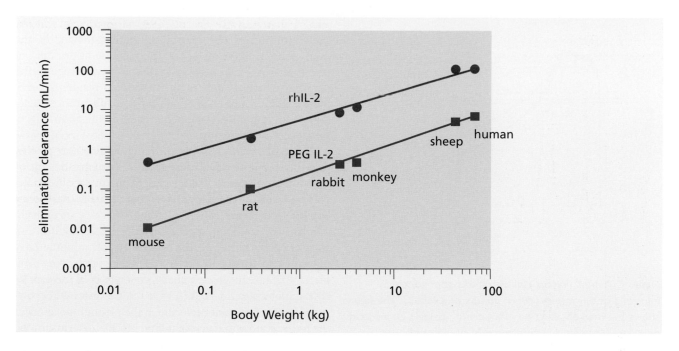

Figure 5.17. Allometric interspecies scaling of the elimination clearance of IL-2 and PEG IL-2.

animal efficacy or toxicology model when pharmacokinetic data are known from another species. Similarly, if an estimation of the maximum tolerated exposure can be made, allometric scaling may be helpful to determine the highest dose in toxicology studies. The dose that results in efficacious concentrations may be taken as the lowest dose in the toxicology studies. Additionally, the efficacious dose in humans can be estimated from the animal pharmacokinetic data, and, as a rule, the starting dose in the first human study (dose-escalation study) is smaller by a factor of two or more, based on safety considerations.

It needs to be emphasized that allometric scaling techniques are useful tools for the prediction of doses used in dose-ranging studies, but they can never replace such studies. The advantage of including such dose prediction in the protocol design of dose-ranging studies is that a smaller number of doses needs to be tested before finding the final dose level. Interspecies dose predictions simply narrow the range of doses in the initial pharmacological efficacy studies, the animal toxicology studies, and the human safety and efficacy studies.

Heterogeneity of Protein Therapeutics

The identity, purity and potency of small synthetic drugs can be demonstrated analytically, and consequently, they are usually completely defined in terms of their chemical structure. Peptides, proteins, and other biotechnologically derived compounds are usually more complex compounds, and it is generally not possible to define them as discrete chemical entities with unique compositions. As described in Chapter 2, the physicochemical and biochemical characteristics of proteins are not only dependent on the amino acid sequence (primary structure), but also on the shape and folding (secondary and tertiary structures), and the relationship between the protein molecules themselves, such as the formation of aggregates (quaternary structure). Biotechnologically derived and endogenous proteins may be heterogeneous at each structural level. For natural IFN-γ, for example, six naturally occurring C-terminal sequences have been identified (Pan *et al.*, 1987; Rinderknecht and Burton, 1985; Rinderknecht *et al.*, 1984).

In addition, post-translational modifications of proteins, such as the degree of glycosylation of amino acid residues, may be different. As an example, the degree of glycosylation of GM-CSF and M-CSF, as for all proteins, differs according to the cell lines used for production: non-glycosylated in bacterial cell lines such as *E. Coli*, moderately glycosylated in yeast, and heavily glycosylated in mammalian cell lines (see Chapter 3). Receptor binding studies with GM-CSF have shown that the receptor affinity decreases with an increase of the level of glycosylation (Stoudemire, 1992).

Another classical example is recombinant human tissue-plasminogen activator (t-PA). Although the active enzyme was first derived from *E. coli* cultures, this cell line lacks several desirable biological activities, such as glyco-

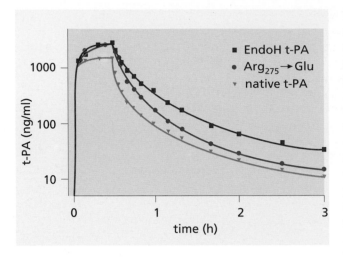

Figure 5.18. t-PA plasma concentrations after 30-min IV infusions of 0.6 mg/kg t-PA in groups of 4 rabbits. The figure shows the marked effect on clearance of a single amino acid mutation (Arg$_{275}$->Glu) or of removal of high mannose carbohydrate at Asn$_{114}$ by the enzyme endoglycosidase H (EndoH t-PA), as compared to native t-PA. From Tanswell (Tanswell, 1992).

sylation ability and the ability to form the correct three-dimensional t-PA structure. Finally, recombinant t-PA was cloned into a Chinese hamster ovary (CHO) cell line. These mammalian cells carried out the glycosylation, disulfide bond formation, and proper folding similar to human cells (Ogez *et al.*, 1991).

Chemical Modifications of Protein Therapeutics

Besides the mostly unwanted heterogeneity of protein drugs introduced by the manufacturing process, other chemical modifications of protein and peptide drugs are intentional to obtain molecules with specified characteristics. Variant proteins can be engineered that differ from natural proteins by exchange, deletion, or insertion of single amino acids, or longer sequences up to entire domains. Small changes in the chemical structure of proteins may cause differences in pharmacokinetics and pharmacodynamics. In addition, mutations may affect glycosylation patterns and conformational changes, which in turn may affect clearance and receptor interactions. A single amino acid mutation in t-PA or the removal of carbohydrate on a single amino acid in t-PA resulted in plasma concentration profiles that were very different from natural t-PA (Figure 5.18) (Tanswell, 1992).

Modification of peptide and protein drugs with the

aim of changing the pharmacological activity may at the same time affect the pharmacokinetic behavior of the molecules. In other instances, the increase of duration of response may be exclusively attributed to a change in the pharmacokinetics such as an increase in residence time. Such modifications include amino acid substitution, deletions and additions, cyclization, drug conjugation, glycosylation or deglycosylation, etc.

The elimination half-life of many peptide and protein drugs is rather small. Consequently, frequent dosing or continuous infusion is necessary to maintain efficacious plasma levels of the drug. Several approaches have been applied to decrease the elimination clearance of biotechnological drugs. One approach is chemical modification such as PEGylation, i.e., the attachment of monomethoxy polyethylene glycol polymer (PEG) to the protein. An example is PEG IL-2, which usually consists of a mixture of rhIL-2 molecules (M_w 15 kD) with 1 to 5 or more PEG polymers attached to each molecule at the ε-amino portions of the lysine residues. The production process determines the average number of PEG residues attached, but any process results in a mixture. With each PEG addition, the molecular weight increases with about 7 kD, but because of the attraction of water molecules, the hydrodynamic size increases even more (95–250 kD). Increasing the degree of PEGylation decreases the elimination clearance and the volume of distribution (Figure 5.19). Since the elimination clearance usually decreases relatively more than the decrease in volume of distribution, the elimination half-life of PEG IL-2 is longer than for IL-2. Based on the relationship between elimination clearance and effective molecular weight, it is possible to calculate the optimal degree of PEGylation to obtain the desired systemic exposure (Bauer *et al.*, 1992; Knauf *et al.*, 1988).

The effect of prosthetic sugar groups on elimination and targeting is illustrated by the comparison of the pharmacokinetics of native glucose-oxidase (GO), deglycosylated GO (dGO), and galactosylated GO (gGO) in mice (Demignot and Domurado, 1987). A saturable mechanism was responsible for GO and dGO uptake by mononuclear phagocytes, although there was a substantial difference in elimination half-life (10 min. for GO; 100 min. for dGO). In contrast, gGO had a half-life of 4 min. and was taken up preferably by hepatocytes, presumably through hepatic galactose receptors. This is an example where receptor-mediated endocytosis through sugar-recognizing receptors is an efficient hepatic uptake mechanism for glycoproteins. However, when terminal sialic acid residues on the carbohydrate moieties of glycoproteins shield the receptor-binding sugars, hepatic receptor-mediated endocytosis is lower than for the desialylated analogues (Meijer and Ziegler, 1993). This has been demonstrated for rEPO and rGM-CSF (Cumming, 1991). The protection by sialic residues appears to be a natural mechanism essential for the normal

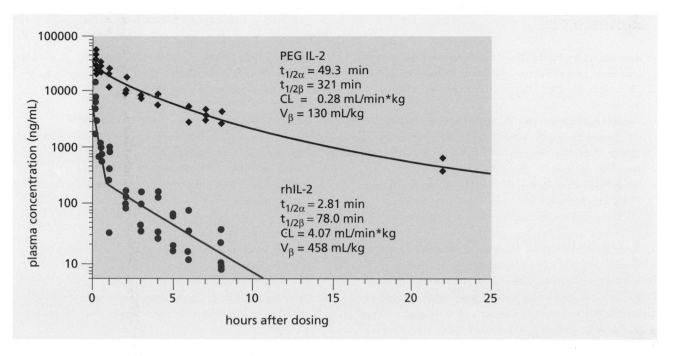

Figure 5.19. Pharmacokinetics of recombinant human interleukin-2 (rhIL-2) and its PEGylation form (PEG IL-2) in rats after IV bolus administration of 0.25 mg/kg. The data were described by a linear two-compartmental pharmacokinetic model.

survival of enzymes, acute-phase proteins (such as α_1-acid glycoprotein), and most plasma proteins of the immune system.

Immunogenicity

Antibody formation is often observed after chronic dosing of human proteins in animal studies, but is also occurring in clinical studies. Immunogenicity can be a problem in the study of protein drugs since the presence of antibodies can complicate the interpretation of preclinical and clinical studies by inactivating (neutralizing) the biological activity of the protein drug. Additionally, protein-antibody complex formation may affect the distribution, metabolism, and elimination of the protein drug. Neutralizing antibodies may inactivate the biological activity of the protein by blocking its active site or by a change of the tertiary structure by steric effects. Antibodies are most likely to be induced when the protein is foreign to the host. Examples of such situations are when mouse-derived monoclonal antibodies are administered to humans, or when human recombinant proteins are tested for safety in animals. Extravascular injections (e.g., s.c., i.m.) are also more likely to stimulate antibody production than intravenous administrations, presumably because of the higher degree of protein precipitation and aggregation at the injection site. This was demonstrated for IL-2 (Krigel *et al.*, 1988) and INF-β (Konrad *et al.*, 1987; Larocca *et al.*, 1989).

Antibodies may directly neutralize the activity of the protein. If neutralization occurs, it indicates that at least some fraction of the antibody population binds at or near the active site, which blocks activity (Working, 1992). Irrespective of the neutralizing capabilities of the antibodies formed, they may also indirectly affect the efficacy of a protein drug by changing its pharmacokinetic profile. Elimination clearances of protein drugs may be either increased or decreased by antibody formation and binding. An increase of the clearance is observed if the protein-antibody complex is eliminated more rapidly than the unbound protein (Rosenblum *et al.*, 1985). This may occur when high levels of the protein-antibody complex stimulate its clearance by the reticuloendothelial system (Sell, 1987). In other situations, the serum concentration of a protein can be increased if binding to an antibody slows down its rate of clearance, because the protein-antibody complex is eliminated slower than the unbound protein (Working, 1992). In this case, the complex may act as a depot for the protein and, if the antibody is not neutralizing, a longer duration of the pharmacological action may occur.

Both an increased and decreased clearance is possible for the same protein, dependent on the dose level administered. At low doses, protein-antibody complexes delay clearance because their elimination is slower than the unbound protein. In contrast, at high doses, higher levels of protein-antibody complex result in the formation of aggregates, which are cleared more rapidly than the unbound protein. ∎

References

- **Arendshorst WJ, Navar LG.** (1988). Renal circulation and glomerular hemodynamics. In *Diseases of the kidney*, edited by RW Schrier and CW Gottschalk. Little, Brown, Boston, pp. 65–117
- **Bartocci A, Mastrogiannis DS, Migliorati G, Stockert RJ, Wolkoff AW, Stanley ER.** (1987). Macrophages specifically regulate the concentration of their own growth factor in the circulation. *Proc Natl Acad Sci USA*, 84, 6179–6183
- **Bauer RJ, Gibbons JA, Bell DP, Luo Z-P, Young JD.** (1994). Nonlinear pharmacokinetics of recombinant human macrophage colony-stimulating factor (M-CSF) in rats. *J Pharmacol Exper Ther*, 268, 152–158
- **Bauer RJ, Winkelhake JL, Young JD, Zimmerman RZ.** (1992). Protein drug delivery by programmed pump infusion: Interleukin-2. In *Therapeutic proteins. Pharmacokinetics and pharmacodynamics*, edited by AHC Kung, RA Baughman, JW Larrick. WH Freeman and Company, New York, pp. 239–253
- **Baumann G, Amburn K, Shaw MA.** (1988a). The circulating growth hormone (GH)-binding protein complex: A major constituent of plasma GH in man. *Endocrinology*, 122, 976–984
- **Baumann G, Shaw MA, Buchanan TA.** (1988b). *In vivo* kinetics of a covalent growth hormone-binding protein complex. *Metabolism*, 38, 330–333
- **Baxter RC.** (1993). Circulating binding proteins for the insulin-like growth factors. *Trends Endocrinol Metab*, 4, 91–96
- **Baxter RC, Martin JL.** (1989). Structure of the Mr 140,000 growth hormone-dependent insulin-like growth factor binding protein complex: determination by reconstitution and affinity labeling. *Proc Natl Acad Sci USA*, 86, 6898–6902
- **Bennett HPJ, McMartin C.** (1979). Peptide hormones and their analogues: distribution, clearance from the circulation, and inactivation *in vivo*. *Pharmacol Reviews*, 30, 247–292
- **Bocci V.** (1987). Metabolism of anticancer agents. *Pharmacol Ther*, 34, 1–49
- **Bocci V.** (1990). Catabolism of therapeutic proteins and peptides with implications for drug delivery. *Adv Drug Del Rev*, 4, 149–169
- **Boxenbaum H.** (1986). Time Concepts in Physics, Biology and Pharmacokinetics. *Journal of Pharmaceutical Sciences*, 75, 1053–1062
- **Burwen SJ, Jones AL.** (1990). Hepatocellular processing of endocytosed proteins. *J Electron Microsc Tech*, 14, 140–151
- **Carone FA, Peterson DR.** (1980). Hydrolysis and transport of small peptides by the proximal tubule. *Am J Physiol*, 238, F151–F158
- **Childs A, Grevel J, Baron DA, Reynolds DL, McCabe RD, Burton EG, Johnson DE, Braeckman RA.** (1996). Population PK/PD of tissue factor pathway inhibitor (TFPI) in cynomolgus monkeys during a 14-day toxicity study. *Fund Appl Toxicol*, 30, 104
- **Clemmons DR.** (1993). IGF binding proteins and their functions. *Molecular Reproduction and Development*, 35, 368–375
- **Clemmons DR, Dehoff MH, Busby WH, Bayne ML, Cascieri MA.** (1992). Competition for binding to IGFBP-2, 3, 4 and 5 by the insulin-like growth factors and IGF analogs. *Endocrinology*, 132, 890–895
- **Cohen KL, Nissley SP.** (1976). The serum half-life of somatomedin activity: Evidence for growth hormone dependence. *Acta Endocrinol*, 83, 243–258
- **Colburn WA.** (1991). Peptide, peptoid, and protein pharmacokinetics/pharmacodynamics. In *Peptides, peptoids, and proteins. Pharmacokinetics and pharmacodynamics*, edited by PD Garzone, WA Colburn, M Mokotoff. Harvey Whitney Books, Cincinnati, pp. 93–115
- **Colburn WA, Blue JW.** (1992). Using pharmacokinetics and pharmacodynamics to direct pharmaceutical research and development. *Applied Clinical Trials*, 1, 42–46
- **Cumming DA.** (1991). Glycosylation of recombinant protein therapeutics: control and functional implications. *Glycobiology*, 1, 115–130
- **Dayneka NL, Garg V, Jusko WJ.** (1993). Comparison of Four Basic Models of Indirect Pharmacodynamic Responses. *Journal of Pharmacokinetics and Biopharmaceutics*, 21, 457–478
- **Dedrick RL.** (1973). Animal Scale-Up. *Journal of Pharmacokinetics and Biopharmaceutics*, 1, 435–461
- **Demignot S, Domurado D.** (1987). Effect of prosthetic sugar groups on the pharmacokinetics of glucose-oxidase. *Drug design and delivery*, 1, 333–348
- **Derendorf H, Hochhaus G.** (1995). Handbook of Pharmacokinetic/Pharmacodynamic Correlation. In *Handbooks of Pharmacology and Toxicology*, edited by MA Hollinger. CRC Press, London
- **Einhorn S, Ahre A, Blomgren H, Johansson B, Mellstedt, H, Strander H.** (1982). Interferon and natural killer activity in multiple myeloma. Lack of correlation between interferon-induced enhancement of natural killer activity and clinical response to human interferon-α. *Int J Cancer*, 30, 167–172
- **Ferraiolo BL, Mohler MA.** (1992). Goals and analytical methodologies for protein disposition studies. In *Protein pharmacokinetics and metabolism*, edited by BL Ferraiolo, MA Mohler, CA Gloff. Plenum Press, New York
- **Gibbons JA, Luo Z-P, Hannon ER, Braeckman RA, Young JD.** (1995). Quantitation of the renal clearance of interleukin-2 using nephrectomized and ureter-ligated rats. *J Pharmacol Exp Ther*, 272, 119–125
- **Girard P, Nony P, Boissel JP.** (1990). The place of simultaneous pharmacokinetic pharmacodynamic modeling in new drug development: trends and perspectives. *Fundamental and Clinical Pharmacology*, 4, 103s–115s
- **Hellfritzsch M, Nielsen S, Christensen EI, Nielsen JT.** (1988). Basolateral tubular handling of insulin in the kidney. *Contrib Nephrol*, 68, 86–91

- **Herington AC, Ymer S, Stevenson J.** (1986). Identification and characterization of specific binding proteins for growth hormone in normal human sera. *J Clin Invest*, 77, 1817–1823
- **Holford NHG.** (1990). Concepts and usefulness of pharmacokinetic-pharmacodynamic modelling. *Fundamental and Clinical Pharmacology*, 4, 93s–101s
- **Holford NHG, Sheiner LB.** (1981a). Pharmacokinetic and Pharmacodynamic Modeling *in Vivo*. *Critical Reviews in Bioengineering*, 5, 273–322
- **Holford NHG, Sheiner LB.** (1981b). Understanding the Dose-Effect Relationship: Clinical Application of Pharmacokinetic-Pharmacodynamic Models. *Clinical Pharmacokinetics*, 6, 429–453
- **Hooper S.** (1991). Pharmacokinetics and Pharmacodynamics of Intravenous Regular Human Insulin. In *Pharmacokinetics and Pharmacodynamics. Peptides, Peptoids, and Proteins*, edited by PD Garzone, WA Colburn, M Mokotoff. Harvey Whitney Books, Cincinnati, OH, pp. 128–137
- **Jusko WJ, Ko HC.** (1994). Pharmacodynamics and Drug Action. Physiologic Indirect Response Models Characterize Diverse Types of Pharmacodynamic Effects. *Clinical Pharmacology and Therapeutics*, 56, 406–419
- **Kenakin T.** (1993). Drug-Receptor Theory. In *Pharmacologic Analysis of Drug-Receptor Interaction*, edited by T Kenakin. Raven Press, New York, pp. 1–38
- **Kim DC, Sugiyama Y, Satoh H, Fuwa T, Iga T, Hanano M.** (1988). Kinetic analysis of *in vivo* receptor-dependent binding of human epidermal growth factor by rat tissues. *J Pharm Sci*, 77, 200–207
- **Knauf MJ, Bell DP, Hirtzer P, Luo Z-P, Young JD, Katre NV.** (1988). Relationship of effective molecular size to systemic clearance in rats of recombinant interleukin-2 chemically modified with water-soluble polymers. *J Biological Chem*, 263, 15064–15070
- **Konrad M, Childs A, Merigan T, Bordon E.** (1987). Assessment of the antigenic response in humans to a recombinant mutant interferon β. *J Clin Immunol*, 7, 365–375
- **Krigel RL, Padavic-Shaller KA, Rudolph AR, Litwin S, Konrad M, Bradley EC, Comis RL.** (1988). A Phase I study of recombinant interleukin-2 plus recombinant β-interferon. *Cancer Res*, 48
- **Kroboth PD, Schmith VD, Smith RB.** (1991). Pharmacodynamic Modelling — Application to New Drug Development. *Clinical Pharmacokinetics*, 20, 91–98
- **Kuwabara T, Uchimura T, Takai K, Kobayashi H, Kaboyashi, S, Sugiyama Y.** (1995). Saturable uptake of a recombinant human granulocyte colony-stimulating factor derivative, nartograstim, by the bone marrow and spleen of rats *in vivo*. *J Pharmacol Exper Ther*, 273, 1114–1122
- **Larocca AP, Leung SC, Marcus SG, Colby CB, Borden EC.** (1989). Evaluation of neutralizing antibodies in patients treated with recombinant interferon-β$_{ser}$. *J Interferon Res*, 9(Suppl. 1), S51–S60
- **Lee VHL.** (1988). Enzymatic barriers to peptide and protein absorption. *CRC Crit Rev Ther Drug Carrier Syst*, 5, 69–97
- **Leung DW.** (1987). Growth hormone receptor and serum binding: Purification, cloning and expression. *Nature*, 330, 537–543
- **Maack T, Johnson V, Kau ST, Figueiredo, J, Sigulem D.** (1979). Renal filtration, transport, and metabolism of low-molecular weight protein: a review. *Kidney Int*, 16, 251–270
- **Maack T, Park CH, Camergo MJF.** (1985). Renal filtration, transport, and metabolism of proteins. In *The kidney: Physiology and pathophysiology*, edited by DW Seldin and G Giebisch. Raven Press, New York, pp. 1173–1803
- **Meijer DKF, Ziegler K.** (1993). Mechanisms for the hepatic clearance of oligopeptides and proteins. In *Biological barriers to protein delivery*, edited by KL Audus, TJ Raub. Plenum Press, New York, pp. 339–408
- **Mohler MA, Cook JE, Lewis D, Moore J, Sinicropi D, Championsmith A, Ferraiolo B, Mordenti J.** (1993). Altered pharmacokinetics of recombinant human deoxyribonuclease in rats due to the presence of a binding protein. *Drug Metabol Dispos*, 21, 71–75
- **Mohler MA, Cook JE, Baumann G.** (1992). Binding proteins of protein therapeutics. In *Protein pharmacokinetics and metabolism*, edited by BL Ferraiolo, MA Mohler, CA Gloff. Plenum Press, New York, pp. 35–71
- **Mordenti J, Chen SA, Moore JA, Ferraiolo BL, Green JD.** (1991). Interspecies Scaling of Clearance and Volume of Distribution Data for Five Therapeutic Proteins. *Pharmaceutical Research*, 8, 1351–1359
- **Mordenti J, Chen SC, Ferraiolo BL.** (1992). Pharmacokinetics of interferon-γ. In *Therapeutic proteins. Pharmacokinetics and pharmacodynamics*, edited by AHC Kung, RA Baughman, JW Larrick. WH Freeman and Company, New York, pp. 187–199
- **Murakami T, Misaki M, Masuda S, Higashi Y, Fuwa T, Yata N.** (1994). Dose-dependent plasma clearance of human epidermal growth factor in rats. *J Pharm Sci*, 83, 1400–1403
- **Nagashima R, O'Reilly RA, Levy G.** (1968). Kinetics of pharmacologic effects in man: The anticoagulant action of warfarin. *Clinical Pharmacology and Therapeutics*, 10, 22–35
- **O'Reilly RA, Levy G.** (1970). Kinetics of the anticoagulant effect of bishydroxycoumarin in man. *Clinical Pharmacology and Therapeutics*, 11, 378–384
- **Ogez JR, van Reis R, Paoni N, Builder SE.** (1991). Recombinant human tissue-plasminogen activator: biochemistry, pharmacology, and process development. In *Peptides, peptoids, and proteins*, edited by PD Garzone, WA Colburn, M Mokotoff. Harvey Whitney Books, Cincinnati, pp. 170–188
- **Ohnishi H, JTY Chan, Lin KK, Lee H, Chu TM.** (1989). Role of the kidney in metabolic change of interleukin-2. *Tumor Biol*, 10, 202–214
- **Pan Y-CE, Stern AS, Familletti PC, Khan FR, Chizzonite R.** (1987). Stuctural characterization of human interferon γ. *Eur J Biochem*, 166, 145–149
- **Petros WP, Rabinowitz J, Stuart AR, Gilbert CJ, Kanakura Y, Griffin JD, Peters WP.** (1992). Disposition of recombinant human granulocyte-macrophage colony-stimulating factor in patients receiving high-dose chemotherapy and autologous bone marrow support. *Blood*, 80, 1135–1140

- **Piscitelli SC, Forrest A, Vogel S, Metcalf J, Baseler M, Stevens, R, Kovacs JA.** (1996). A novel PK/PD model for infused interleukin-2 (IL-2), in HIV-infected patients. In *Ninety-Seventh Annual Meeting of the American Society for Clinical Pharmacology and Therapeutics*. Lake Buena Vista, Florida, pp. 152
- **Rabkin R, Dahl DC.** (1993). Renal uptake and disposal of proteins and peptides. In *Biological barriers to protein delivery*, edited by KL Audus, TJ Raub. Plenum Press, New York, pp. 299–338
- **Rabkin R, Kitaji J.** (1983). Renal metabolism of peptide hormones. *Mineral Electrolyte Metab*, 9, 212–226
- **Rabkin R, Ryan MP, Duckworth WC.** (1984). The renal metabolism of insulin. *Diabetologica*, 27, 351–357
- **Rinderknecht E, Burton LE.** (1985). Biochemical characterization of natural and recombinant IFN-γ. In *The biology of the interferon system 1984*, edited by H Kirchner, H Schellekens. Elsevier, Amsterdam, pp. 397–402
- **Rinderknecht E, O'Connor BH, Rodriguez H.** (1984). Natural human interferon-γ: complete amino acid sequence and determination of sites of glycosylation. *J Biol Chem*, 259, 6790–6797
- **Rosenblum MG, Unger BW, Gutterman JU, Hersh EM, David GS, Fincke JM.** (1985). Modification of human leucocyte interferon pharmacology with monoclonal antibody. *Cancer Res*, 45, 2421–2424
- **Schwinghammer TL, Kroboth PD.** (1988). Basic Concepts in Pharmacodynamic Modeling. *Journal of Clinical Pharmacology*, 28, 388–394
- **Sell S.** (1987). *Immunology, immunopathology and immunity*. Elsevier, Amsterdam
- **Steimer J-L, Ebelin M-E, Van Bree J.** (1993). Pharmacokinetic and Pharmacodynamic data and models in clinical trials. *European Journal of Drug Metabolism and Pharmacokinetics*, 18, 61–76
- **Stoudemire JB.** (1992). Pharmacokinetics and metabolism of hematopoietic proteins. In *Protein pharmacokinetics and metabolism*, edited by BL Ferraiolo, MA Mohler, CA Gloff. Plenum Press, New York, pp. 189–222
- **Strickland DK, Kounnas MZ, Argraves WS.** (1995). LDL receptor-related protein: a multiligand receptor for lipoprotein and proteinase catabolism. *Faseb J*, 9, 890–898
- **Sugiyama Y, Hanano M.** (1989). Receptor-mediated transport of peptide hormones and its importance in the overall hormone disposition in the body. *Pharm Res*, 6, 192–202
- **Supersaxo A, Hein W, Gallati, H, Steffen H.** (1988). Recombinant human interferon α-2a: delivery to lymphoid tissue by selected modes of application. *Pharm Res*, 5, 472–476
- **Supersaxo A, Hein WR, Steffen H.** (1990). Effect of molecular weight on the lymphatic absorption of water-soluble compounds following subcutaneous administration. *Pharm Res*, 7, 167–169
- **Takagi A, Masuda H, Takakura, Y, Hashida M.** (1995). Disposition characteristics of recombinant human interleukin-11 after a bolus intravenous administration in mice. *J Pharmacol Exper Ther*, 275, 537–543
- **Takakura Y, Fujita T, Hashida M, Sesaki H.** (1990). Disposition characteristics of macromolecules in tumor-bearing mice. *Pharm Res*, 7, 339–346
- **Tanaka H, Kaneko T.** (1991). Pharmacokinetics of recombinant human granulocyte colony-stimulating factor in the rat. *Drug Metabol Dispos*, 19, 200–204
- **Tanswell P.** (1992). Tissue-type plasminogen activator. In *Therapeutic proteins. Pharmacokinetics and pharmacodynamics*, edited by AHC Kung, RA Baughman, JW Larrick. WH Freeman and Company, New York, pp. 255–281
- **Uehlinger DE, Gotch FA, Sheiner LB.** (1992). A pharmacodynamic model of erythropoietin therapy for uremic anemia. *Clinical Pharmacology and Therapeutics*, 51, 76–89
- **Wall DA, Maack T.** (1985). Endocytic uptake, transport, and catabolism of proteins by epithelial cells. *Am J Physiol*, 248, C12–C20
- **Woodworth JR, Howey DC, Bowsher RR.** (1994). Establishment of time-action profiles for regular and NPH insulin using pharmacodynamic modeling. *Diabetes Care*, 17, 64–69
- **Working PK.** (1992). Potential effects of antibody induction by protein drugs. In *Protein pharmacokinetics and metabolism*, edited by BL Ferraiolo, MA Mohler, CA Gloff. Plenum Press, New York, pp. 73–92
- **Zapf J, Hauri C, Waldvogel, M, Froesch ER.** (1986). Acute metabolic effects and half-lives of intravenous insulin-like growth factor I and II in normal and hypophysectomized rats. *J Clin Invest*, 77, 1768–1775
- **Ziegler K, Polzin G, Frimmer M.** (1988). Hepatocellular uptake of cyclosporin A by simple diffusion. *Biochim Biophys Acta*, 938, 44–50

Self-Assessment Questions

Question 1: *What are the major elimination pathways for protein drugs after administration?*

Question 2: *Which pathway of absorption is rather unique for proteins after s.c. injection?*

Question 3: *Explain counterclockwise hysteresis in plasma concentration-effect plots.*

Question 4: *What is the role of plasma binding proteins for natural proteins?*

Question 5: *How do the sugar groups on glycoproteins influence hepatic elimination of these glycoproteins?*

Question 6: *In which direction might elimination clearance of protein drug change when antibodies are produced after chronic dosing with protein drugs? Why?*

Answers

Answer 1: Proteolysis, glomerular filtration followed by tubular reabsorption and catabolism, renal peritubular absorption followed by catabolism, receptor-mediated endocytosis followed by metabolism in the liver and possibly other cells.

Answer 2: Biodistribution from the injection site into the lymphatics.

Answer 3: Counterclockwise hysteresis is an indication of the indirect nature of the effects seen for many protein drugs. It can be explained by delays between the appearance of drug in plasma and the appearance of the pharmacodynamic response, by processes such as distribution into the biophase or cascade-type post-receptor events.

Answer 4: Plasma proteins may act as circulating reservoirs for the proteins that are their ligands. Consequently, the protein ligands may be protected from elimination and distribution. In some cases, protein binding may protect the organism from undesirable, acute effects; in other cases, receptor binding may be facilitated by the binding protein.

Answer 5: In some cases, the sugar groups are recognized by hepatic receptors (galactose by the galactose receptor, for example), facilitating receptor-mediated uptake and metabolism. In other cases, sugar chains and terminal sugar groups (terminal sialic acid residues, for example) may shield the protein from binding to receptors and hepatic uptake.

Answer 6: Clearance may increase or decrease by binding to antibodies. A decrease of clearance occurs when the antibody-protein complex is eliminated slower than free drug. An increase of clearance occurs when the protein-antibody complex is eliminated more rapidly than the unbound protein, such as when reticuloendothelial uptake is stimulated by the complex.

6 Additional Biotechnology-Related Techniques

by: Robert D. Sindelar

Introduction

The techniques made available by advances in molecular biology and biotechnology that have provided currently approved therapeutic agents generally fall into two broad areas: recombinant DNA (rDNA) technology, and hybridoma techniques (to produce monoclonal antibodies). A wealth of additional and innovative biotechnologies, however, have been and will continue to be developed in order to enhance pharmaceutical research. These additional biotechnology-related techniques are improving the very competitive process of drug discovery and development of new medicinal agents and diagnostics. Some of the techniques described in this chapter are both well-established and commonly used applications of biotechnology producing potential therapeutic products now in clinical trials. Still more applications are evolving as you read this text. Techniques such as the polymerase chain reaction (PCR), genetically engineered animals (including transgenic animals and knockout mice), protein engineering, peptide chemistry and peptidomimetics, nucleic acid technologies (including antisense technology, aptamer technology and ribozyme catalysis), catalytic antibodies, the emerging field of glycobiology, and biosensors are directly influencing the pharmaceutical sciences and are well positioned to impact significantly modern pharmaceutical care. These "additional techniques in biotechnology and molecular biology" are being rapidly exploited to bring new drugs to market.

It is not the intention of this author to detail each and every biotechnology technique exhaustively, since numerous specialized resources already meet that need. Rather, this chapter will illustrate and enumerate various additional biotechnologies that should be of key interest to pharmacy students, practicing pharmacists and pharmaceutical scientists because of their impact on many aspects of pharmacy.

Polymerase Chain Reaction

Authors Hoekstra and Smeekens provide an introduction to the polymerase chain reaction (PCR) in Chapter 1. As described, PCR, the *in vitro* gene amplification technique invented by Chemistry 1993 Nobel Prize recipient Kary Mullis, has found many applications including those in genetic research (i.e., genomic cloning, RNA analysis, and

Method [1]	Template	Thermostable enzyme(s)
Basic PCR	DNA	DNA polymerase
RT-PCR	RNA	Reverse transcriptase and DNA polymerase
TAS	RNA	Reverse transcriptase and RNA polymerase
LCR	DNA	DNA ligase
G-LCR	DNA	DNA ligase and DNA polymerase
AG-LCR	RNA	Reverse transcriptase and DNA ligase
OLA	DNA	DNA ligase

Table 6.1. Some examples of modified PCR and related methodologies. [1] Key abbreviations: PCR = polymerase chain reaction; RT-PCR = reverse transcription PCR; TAS = transcription-based amplification system; LCR = ligation chain reaction; G-LCR = gap LCR; AG-LCR = asymmetric gap LCR; OLA = oligonucleotide ligation assay.

in vitro mutagenesis, etc.), clinical diagnosis, forensic science and molecular archaeology/paleontology (Innis *et al.*, 1990; Arnheim and Erlich, 1992). In the dozen years since the first report of PCR amplification, the technology has continued to evolve with the discovery of new thermostable polymerases, the development of improved PCR protocols and the introduction of alternative amplification methods. Of particular importance to our study of additional technologies are continual improvements and modifications to the basic PCR methodology (Innis *et al.*, 1995) and related protocols. Several examples have been selected solely to illustrate the on-going development of PCR methodology. While the selected examples will be introduced only very briefly, differences to the basic PCR methodology will be indicated and references for further reading will be provided. Table 6.1 provides a list of the templates and enzymes involved in some examples of modified PCR and related methodologies. Numerous sources of PCR and related protocols are available (Ausubel *et al.*, 1995; McPherson *et al.*, 1995; Clapp, 1996; Harwood, 1996; White, 1997).

Basic PCR Methodology

To properly understand the modified PCR technologies dealt with in the next section, it is essential that the reader has a full understanding of the basic PCR technology first introduced in Chapter 1. For convenience the basic PCR protocol is here given again in some more detail.

As already described (see Chapter 1), the PCR methodology (Newton, 1995) involves a repetitive series of temperature cycles with each cycle composed of three stages (see Figure 6.1): Stage 1) Denaturation, a very brief heating period (>91°C, ˜1 min.) causing strand separation of the DNA template containing the target DNA sequence (into the sense and the antisense strand); Stage 2) Annealing (also called Primer Binding), the specific, synthesized oligonucleotide primer strands complementary to the DNA flanking the target sequence of interest are annealed at the 3′ ends of each separated strand pointing toward each other (much lower temperature, ˜1 min.); and Stage 3) Extension, the DNA polymerase catalyzed synthesis (at ˜72°C, ˜1.5 min.) of a complementary copy to each strand of the sense and antisense sequence, in effect, extends each chain. Since multiple copies of the specific, synthesized oligonucleotide primer strands are present during the process, continuous cycling significantly amplifies the DNA. During PCR, one cycle doubles the number of target DNA molecules. The newly synthesized extended strand products can themselves anneal to the opposite strand primer and serve as the template for another round of amplification extensions utilizing additional copies of the primer strands. A logarithmic growth in product results since two cycles increase the number of DNA copies 4 times, 3 cycles 8 times, 10 cycles

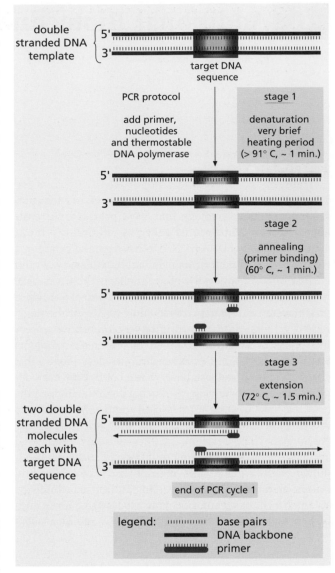

Figure 6.1. Schematic representation of one cycle of PCR: stages 1, 2 and 3.

1, 024 times and 30 cycles 1, 073, 741, 824, etc. Numerous variations of PCR have been developed to improve efficiency and decrease errors.

Some Examples of Modified PCR and Related Methodologies

A quick examination of the clinical diagnostic literature provides the names of numerous examples of variations to the basic PCR methodology that pharmacists and pharmaceutical scientists may often encounter (Table 6.1). An example is reverse transcription PCR (RT-PCR; also called reverse transcriptase PCR, RNA-PCR, and RNA phenotyping) (Innis *et al.*, 1995; Larrick and Siebert, 1995). The basic

PCR protocol allows for the amplification of DNA, but does not allow for RNA amplification. PCR has been extended to include RNA as the target template by the methodology of RT-PCR. The RT-PCR protocol utilizes a thermoactive reverse transcriptase enzyme for preparing a complementary DNA copy (known as cDNA) of a target template mRNA molecule and is coupled to the tremendous DNA amplification of PCR (by DNA polymerase). This provides an invaluable technology for cloning, detecting gene expression, and diagnosing various genetic diseases and infectious agents.

Transcription-based amplification system (TAS) is another DNA amplification system requiring fewer cycles to generate millions of copies of the target DNA from an RNA template (Gingeras et al., 1990; Kwoh and Kwoh, 1990). The DNA can then be analyzed by standard DNA techniques. This methodology is ideally suited for a convenient, very sensitive DNA assay such as in the detection of HIV (Kwoh et al., 1989; Davis et al., 1990).

A powerful PCR-related detection and alternative amplification method growing in clinical importance is the ligation chain reaction (LCR) (Barany, 1991a). While PCR is a DNA amplification method involving DNA polymerase, the key element of the LCR procedure is the use of a thermostable ligase enzyme. An advantage of LCR over PCR is that LCR methodology is exceptionally good at detecting single base pair differences of gene mutants. Variations of the LCR methodology include "gap LCR" (G-LCR) and "asymmetric gap LCR" (AG-LCR) (Barany, 1991b; Marshall et al., 1994; Abravaya et al., 1995). The entire protocol can be easily automated and coupled with PCR (Wilson et al., 1994), thus providing a powerful diagnostic tool with widespread application to the detection of infectious disease organisms as well as DNA point mutations (i.e., as found in genetic disease or cancer) (Lee, 1993; Landegren, 1993; Laffler et al., 1993; De-Barbeyrac et al., 1995; Miyashita et al., 1996). LCR can detect DNA in samples containing as few as 200-300 molecules. G-LCR has an increased sensitivity to be able to detect as few as 5 target molecules. AG-LCR, because of the reverse transcriptase-containing protocol, can detect as few as 20 RNA molecules.

Oligonucleotide ligation assay (OLA) is a sensitive detection method for mutated genes developed by Landegen and co-workers (Landegen et al., 1988; Stone et al., 1995; Delahunty et al., 1996). In standard PCR, the specific, synthesized oligonucleotide primer strands (a pair) complementary to the DNA flanking the target sequence of interest are annealed at the 3' ends of each separated strand. Many copies of the primer pairs are used to obtain logarithmic amplification. In the OLA method, only one copy of a synthesized oligonucleotide primer pair is used resulting in a linear increase in product. OLA can be automated and can be coupled with an amplification method such as PCR (Kwok et al., 1992; Eggerding, 1995).

Genetically Engineered Animals

For thousands of years, man has selectively bred animals and plants either to enhance or to create desirable traits in numerous species. The explosive development of recombinant DNA technology and other molecular biology techniques have made it possible to engineer species possessing particular unique and distinguishing genetic characteristics. The genetic material of an animal can be manipulated so that extra genes may be inserted (transgenes), replaced (i.e., human gene homologues coding for related human proteins), or deleted (knockout). A greater understanding of specific gene regulation and expression will contribute to important new discoveries made in relevant animal models. Such genetically altered species have found utility in a myriad of research and potential commercial applications (Cuthbertson and Klintorth, 1988; Hanahan, 1989; Isola and Gordon, 1991).

Engineered animal models are proving invaluable to pharmaceutical research since small animal models of disease are often poor mimics of that disease in human patients. Genetic engineering can predispose an animal to a particular disease under scrutiny and the insertion of human genes into the animal can initiate the development of a more clinically-relevant disease condition. For example, Muller and co-workers (Muller et al., 1988) have reported on the high incidence of induction of mammary adenocarcinoma (breast cancer) in genetically engineered mice bearing the activated c-neu oncogene. Also, it is possible to screen potential drugs in vivo against a human receptor inserted into an animal model. Table 6.2 provides a list of some selected examples of genetically engineered animal disease models.

Transgenic Animals

Transgenic animals contain either foreign DNA (a transgene) which has been incorporated into their genome or endogenous genomic DNA that has had its molecular structure manipulated (Cuthbertson and Klintorth, 1988; Hanahan, 1989; Isola and Gordon, 1991; Lodish et al., 1995). It is important to distinguish clearly between transgenic animals and gene therapy (see Chapter 7). Technically speaking, the introduction of foreign DNA sequences into a living cell is called gene transfer. Thus, one method to create a transgenic animal involves gene transfer (transgene incorporated into the genome). Gene therapy is also a gene transfer procedure and, in a sense, produces a transgenic human. In transgenic animals, however, the foreign gene is transferred indiscriminately into all cells, including germ line cells. The process of gene therapy differs generally from transgenesis since it involves a transfer of the desired gene in such a way that involves only specific somatic and hematopoietic cells, and not germ cells.

Genetic engineering	Gene [a]	Disease model
knockout	apolipoprotein E	atherosclerosis [1]
knockout	glucocerebrosidase	Gaucher's disease [2]
knockout	HPRT	Lesch-Nyhan syndrome [3]
knockout	human CFTR	cystic fibrosis [4]
knockout	p53	cancer suppressor gene deletion [5]
transgene	c-neu oncogene	cancer [6]
transgene	c-myc oncogene	cancer [7]
transgene	growth hormone	dwarfism [8]
transgene	H-ras oncogene	cancer [9]
transgene	histocompatibility antigens	autoimmunity [10]
transgene	HIV tat	Kaposi sarcoma [11]
transgene	human APP	Alzheimer's disease [12]
transgene	human β-globin	thalassemia [13]
transgene	human CD4 expression	HIV infection [14]
transgene	human β-globin mutant	sickle cell anemia [15]
transgene	human CETP	atherosclerosis [16]
transgene	LDL receptor	hypercholesterolemia [17]

Table 6.2. Some selected examples of genetically engineered animal disease models. a. Key abbreviations: APP = amyloid precursor protein; CETP = cholesterol (cholesteryl) ester transfer protein; CFTR = cystic fibrosis transport regulator; HIV = human immunodeficiency virus; HPRT = hypoxanthine phosphoribosyl transferase; LDL = low-density lipoprotein; 1. See Zhang *et al*. 1992; 3. See Isola and Gordon 1991; 4. See Collins and Wilson 1992; 5. See Donehower *et al*. 1992; Lane 1993; 6. See Muller *et al*. 1988; 7. See Leder *et al*. 1986; 8. See Cuthbertson and Klintworth 1988; 8. See Andes *et al*. 1987; 10. See Hanahan 1990; 11. See Hanahan 1989; 12. See Quon *et al*. 1991; 13. See Isola and Gordon 1991; 14. See Gillespie *et al*. 1993; 15. See Greaves *et al*. 1990; 16. See Hayek *et al*. 1991, Marotti *et al*. 1993, Breslow 1994; 17. See Isola and Gordon 1991.

While the mouse has been the most studied animal species, transgenic technology has been applied to cattle, fish, goats, poultry, rabbits, rats, sheep, swine, and various lower animal forms. Transgenic animals have already made valuable research contributions to studies involving regulation of gene expression, the function of the immune system, genetic diseases, viral diseases, cardiovascular disease, and the genes responsible for the development of cancer. Each of these applications is used in the drug discovery and development process.

Production of Transgenic Animals by DNA Microinjection and Random Gene Addition

The production of transgenic animals has most commonly involved the microinjection (also called gene transfer) of 100–200 copies of exogenous transgene DNA into the larger, more visible male pronucleus (as compared to the female pronucleus) of a recipient fertilized embryo (see Figure 6.2). The transgene contains both the DNA encod-

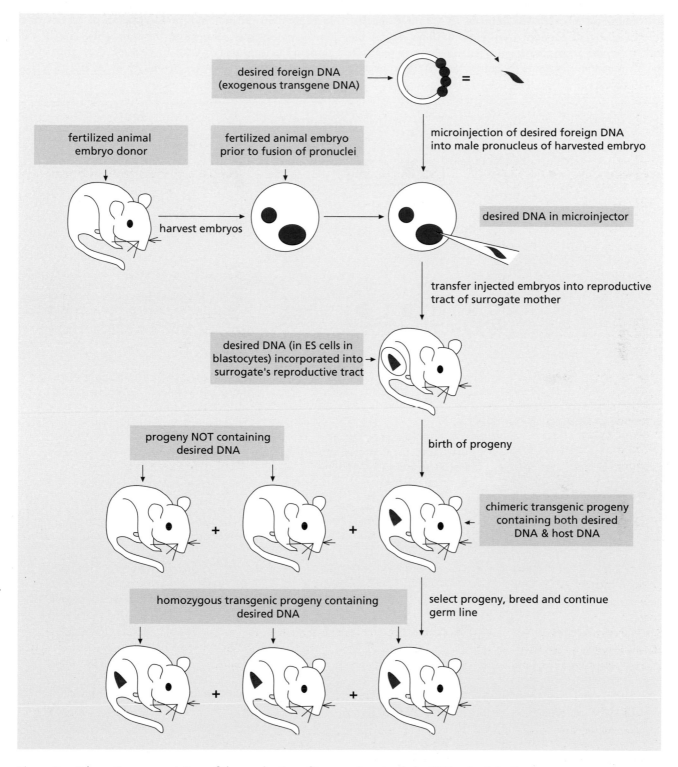

Figure 6.2. Schematic representation of the production of transgenic animals by DNA microinjection.

ing for the desired target amino acid sequence along with regulatory sequences that will mediate the expression of the added gene. The microinjected eggs are then implanted into the reproductive tract of a female and allowed to de-velop into embryos. The foreign DNA generally becomes randomly inserted at a single site on just one of the host chromosomes (i.e., the founder transgenic animal is heterozygous). Thus each transgenic founder animal (positive transgene incorporated animals) is a unique species. Interbreeding of founder transgenic animals where the transgene was incorporated into germ cells may result in the birth of a homozygous progeny provided the transgene incorporation did not induce a mutation of an essential endogenous gene. All cells of the transgenic animal will contain the transgene if DNA insertion occurs prior to the first cell division. However, usually only 20%-25% of the

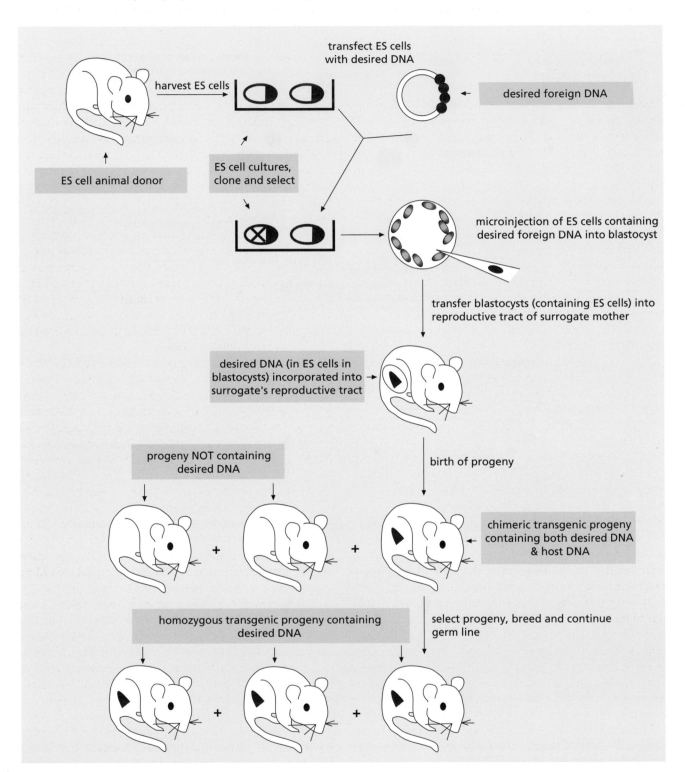

Figure 6.3. Schematic representation of the production of transgenic animals by pluripotent embryonic stem cell methodology.

offspring contain detectable levels of the transgene. Selection of neonatal animals possessing an incorporated transgene can readily be accomplished either by the direct identification of specific DNA or mRNA sequences or by the observation of gross phenotypic characteristics.

PRODUCTION OF TRANSGENIC ANIMALS BY HOMOLOGOUS RECOMBINATION IN EMBRYONIC STEM CELLS

Transgenic animals can also be produced by the *in vitro* genetic alteration of pluripotent embryonic stem cells (ES cells) (see Figure 6.3) (Sedivy and Joyner, 1992). ES cell technology is more efficient at creating transgenics than microinjection protocols. ES cells, a cultured cell line derived from the inner cell mass (blastocyst) of a mouse blastocyte (early preimplantation embryo), are capable of having their genomic DNA modified while retaining their ability to contribute to both somatic and germ cell lineages. The desired gene is incorporated into ES cells by one of several methods such as microinjection. This is followed by introduction of the genetically modified ES cells into the blastocyst of an early preimplantation embryo, selection and culturing of targeted ES cells which are transferred subsequently to the reproductive tract of the surrogate host animal. The resulting progeny is screened for evidence that the desired genetic modification is present and selected appropriately. In mice, the process results in approximately 30% of the progeny containing tissue genetically derived from the incorporated ES cells. Interbreeding of selected founder animals can produce species homozygous for the mutation.

Non-homologous recombination readily occurs if the desired DNA is introduced into the ES cell genome randomly by a gene recombination process that does not require any sequence homology between genomic DNA and the foreign DNA. A significant advance in the production of transgenic animals in ES cells is the advent of homologous recombination techniques. Homologous recombination, while much more rare than non-homologous recombination, can be favored when the researcher carefully designs the transferred DNA to have sequence homology to the endogenous DNA at the desired integration site and also carefully selects the transfer vector conditions. Homologous recombination at a precise chromosomal position provides an approach to very subtle genetic modification of an animal or can be used to produce knockout mice (to be discussed later). A modification of the procedure involves the use of hematopoietic bone marrow stem cells rather than pluripotent embryonic stem cells. The use of ES cells results in changes to the whole germ line, while hematopoietic stem cells modified appropriately are expected to repopulate a specific somatic cell line or lines (more similar to gene therapy).

PROTEIN PRODUCTION IN TRANSGENIC ANIMALS

The techniques to produce transgenic animals have been used to develop animal strains that secrete important proteins in milk. During such large animal "gene farming, " the transgenic animals serve as bioreactors to synthesize recoverable quantities of therapeutically useful proteins. Among the advantages of expressing protein in animal milk is that the protein is generally produced in sizable quantities and can be harvested manually or mechanically by simply milking the animal. Protein purification from the milk requires the usual separation techniques described in Chapter 3. In general, recombinant genes coding for the desired protein product are fused to the regulatory sequences of the animal's milk-producing genes. The animals are not endangered by the insertion of the recombinant gene. The logical fusion of the protein product gene to the milk-producing gene targets the transcription and translation of the protein product exclusively in mammary tissues normally involved in milk production and does not permit gene activation in other, non-milk producing tissues in the animal. Transgenic strains are established and perpetuated by breeding the animals since the progeny of the original transgenic animal (founder animal) usually also produce the desired recombinant protein.

Yields of protein pharmaceuticals produced transgenically are expected to be 10–100 times greater than those achieved in recombinant cell culture (Thayer, 1996). Protein yields in transgenic animals are generally good [conservative estimates of 1 gram/Liter (g/L) with a 30% purification efficiency] with milk yield from various species per annum estimated at: cow = 10, 000 L; sheep = 500 L; goat = 400 L; and pig = 250 L (Rudolph, 1995). The company PPL Therapeutics has estimated that the cost to produce human therapeutic proteins in large animal bioreactors could be as much as 75% less expensive than cell culture. In addition, should the desired target protein require post-translational modification, the large mammals used in milk production of pharmaceuticals would be a bioreactor capable of adding those groups (unlike a recombinant bacterial culture).

Some examples of human proteins under development in the milk of transgenic animals (See Table 6.3) include the anti-clotting protein antithrombin III, clotting Factor VIII, clotting Factor IX, tissue plasminogen activator (tPA), lactoferrin and monoclonal antibodies against colon cancer (Rudolph, 1995). The first ever clinical trial of a recombinant product isolated from the milk of transgenic animals was initiated by Genzyme Transgenics in the Fall, 1996. Apart from the production of pharmaceuticals, research is underway to produce various nutraceuticals (specialty nutritional products) in genetically engineered animal systems.

An innovative use of transgenics for the production of useful proteins is the generation of clinically transplan-

Species	Protein product	Potential Indication(s)
cow	collagen	burns, bone fracture
cow	human fertility hormones	infertility
cow	human serum albumin	surgery, burns, shock, trauma
cow	lactoferrin	bacterial GI infection
goat	α-1-anti-protease inhibitor	inherited deficiency
goat	α-1-antitrypsin	antiinflammatory
goat	anti-thrombin III	associated complications from genetic or acquired deficiency
goat	human fertility hormones	infertility
goat	human serum albumin	surgery, burns, shock, trauma
goat	LAtPA[1]	venous status ulcers
goat	monoclonal antibodies	colon cancer
goat	tPA[1]	myocardial infarct, pulmonary embolism
pig	Factor IX	hemophilia
pig	Factor VIII	hemophilia
pig	fibrinogen	burns, surgery
pig	human hemoglobin	blood replacement for transfusion
pig	protein C	deficiency, adjunct to tPA
sheep	α-1-antitrypsin	antiinflammatory
sheep	Factor IX	hemophilia
sheep	fibrinogen	burns, surgery
sheep	protein C	deficiency, adjunct to tPA

Table 6.3. Some examples of human proteins under development in the milk of transgenic animals (data from Rudolph 1995)[1]. Abbreviations: tPA = tissue plasminogen activator, LAtPA = long acting tissue plasminogen activator.

table transgenic animal organs. Several research groups in academia and industry have pioneered the transgenic engineering of animals (especially pigs) expressing both human complement inhibitory proteins as well as key human blood group proteins (antigens) (Fodor *et al.*, 1994, Tsuji *et al.*, 1994). Cells, tissues and organs from these double transgenic animals appear to be very resistant to the humoral immune system mediated reactions of both primates and humans. These findings begin to pave the way for potential xenograft transplantation of animal components into humans with a lessened chance of acute rejection.

EXAMPLES OF TRANSGENIC ANIMAL MODELS OF HUMAN DISEASE IN DRUG DISCOVERY AND DEVELOPMENT

The number of examples of transgenic animal models of human disease useful in drug discovery and development efforts is growing rapidly. Swanson and colleagues have reviewed a number of these models, and the author recommends this source to the reader (Swanson *et al.*, 1994). Such models have potential to increase the efficiency and decrease the cost of drug discovery and development by reducing the time it takes to move a medicinal agent from discovery into clinical trials. Also, transgenic animal models are proving to be more clinically-relevant systems to explore drug lead development; two interesting examples are in the areas of cardiovascular medicine and oncology. An exciting application of a transgenic animal model useful in the study of a human disease is the transgenic mouse engineered to contain the human enzyme cholesterol (cholesteryl) ester transfer protein (CETP) (Hayek *et al.*, 1993; Marotti *et al.*, 1993). This plasma enzyme facilitates the exchange of cholesterol ester and triglycerides between lipoproteins. CETP is believed to be atherosclerotic since CETP activity leads to a decrease in HDL-cholesterol and an increase in LDL-cholesterol. This animal model can serve as an *in vivo* bioassay system for the evaluation of potential inhibitors of human CETP as anti-atherosclerotics. Also, a number of animal models for the development of cancer have been created. Transgenic incorporation of oncogenes such as H-*ras* (Andes *et al.*, 1987) and c-*myc* (Leder *et al.*, 1986) have resulted in animal models with a high incidence of tumor growth that may prove useful in the search for novel cancer chemotherapeutics. Some additional selected areas using transgenic animal technology in pharmaceutical research include Alzheimer's disease, autoimmunity, dwarfism, HIV infection, hypercholesterolemia, Kaposi sarcoma, sickle cell anemia, and thalassemia (see Table 6.2).

Knockout Mice

While a mouse carrying an introduced transgene is called a transgenic mouse, transgenic technologies can also produce a knockout animal (mice are the most studied animal species). A knockout mouse, also called a gene knockout mouse or a gene-targeted knockout mouse, is an animal in which an endogenous gene (genomic wild-type allele) has been specifically inactivated by replacing it with a null allele (Lodish *et al.*, 1995). A null allele is a nonfunctional allele of a gene generated by either deletion of the entire gene or mutation of the gene resulting in the synthesis of an inactive protein. Recent advances in intranuclear gene targeting and embryonic stem cell technologies as described

above are expanding the capabilities to produce knockout mice routinely for studying certain human genetic diseases or elucidating the function of a specific gene product.

The procedure for producing knockout mice basically involves a four-step process. A null allele (i.e., knockout allele) is incorporated into one allele of murine ES cells. Incorporation is generally quite low, approximately one cell in a million has the required gene replacement. However, the process is designed to impart neomycin and ganciclovir resistance only to those ES cells in which homologous gene integration has resulted. This facilitates the selection and propagation of the correctly engineered ES cells. The resulting ES cells are then injected into early mouse embryos creating chimeric mice (heterozygous for the knockout allele) containing tissues derived from both host cells and ES cells. The chimeric mice are mated to confirm that the null allele is incorporated into the germ line. The confirmed heterozygous chimeric mice are bred to homogeneity producing progeny that are homozygous knockout mice.

For example, knockout mice have been engineered that have extremely elevated cholesterol levels while being maintained on normal chow diets due to their inability to produce apolipoprotein E (apo E) (Zhang *et al.*, 1992; Breslow 1994). Apo E is the major lipoprotein component of very low density lipoprotein (VLDL) responsible for liver clearance of VLDL. These engineered mice are being examined as animal models of atherosclerosis useful in cardiovascular drug discovery and development. Table 6.2 provides a list of some additional selected examples of knockout mouse disease models.

The knockout mouse is becoming the basic tool for researchers to determine gene function *in vivo*. High-throughput DNA sequencing efforts, positional cloning programs, and novel ES cell-based gene discovery research all exploit the knockout mouse as their laboratory.

Transgenic Animal Patents

The importance of genetically engineered animals is vividly emphasized by the events that have resulted due to animal patents. A number of moral/ethical and economic issues were raised when the United States Patent and Trademark Office (PTO) announced on April 7, 1987 that higher animals were patentable subject matter (Fox, 1993; Lesser, 1995). This PTO Commissioner announcement was a direct result of the explosive development of transgenic technology. While 10 countries tacitly allow animal patents, only the United States expressly permits them. Also, 54 countries have exclusionary language concerning the patenting of animals. An "Onco-mouse", the c-*myc* transgenic mouse mentioned earlier in this chapter, became the first patented, commercially marketed animal on April 12, 1988 (Ezzell, 1988). The development of potentially patentable, transgenic animals especially in the areas of human disease models and pharmaceutical protein production has raised broad-based current concerns in various segments of society.

Genetic Ablation

Genetic ablation, also called cell ablation and genetic amputation, is another genetic engineering technique used to suppress selectively the growth of a specified cell line or cell type in an animal rather than suppress the activity of an individual gene (O'Kane and Moffat, 1992). The transgene inserted into the animal is under the control of a gene promoter that is known to be active only in a certain cell population. This promoter would regulate the expression of a cytotoxic protein (such as the A chain of diphtheria toxin) that would therefore destroy only the targeted cell line or type. For example, genetic ablation suppresses choroidal melanocytes during a study of malignancies of the eye originating in the retinal pigment of transgenic mice (Mintz and Klein-Szanto, 1992).

Protein Engineering

Recombinant DNA technology has made it possible to engineer specifically altered or new and novel protein molecules possessing tailored chemical and biological characteristics. Termed protein engineering, the deliberate design and construction of unique proteins with enhanced or novel molecular properties is a result of specifying the exact amino acid sequence (protein primary structure) of that protein (Oxender, 1985; Oxender, 1986; Winnacker and Huber, 1988; Oxender and Fox, 1987; Narang, 1990; Richardson and Richardson, 1990; Cleland and Craik, 1996). As described in Chapter 2, the primary structure affects the protein's conformation. The conformation of each and every amino acid component present in the protein influences the protein's complex three-dimensional structure. The conformational preference of the protein chain residues determines the protein's secondary structure including α-helices and β-sheets or reverse turns. The local secondary structures are folded into three-dimensional tertiary structures made up of domains. The domains are not only structural units, but are also functional units often containing intact ligand binding (in a receptor) or enzyme catalytic sites. Thus, protein engineering provides an approach to modify a native protein's structure specifically or to create a unique, new protein with a particular structure. Protein engineering has numerous powerful theoretical and practical implications for examining protein structure and function, probing enzyme mechanisms, investigating protein folding and conformation, studying protein stability, introducing detectable groups into proteins as an analytical tool, and producing improved second generation tailored biopharmaceuticals (Fothergill-Gilmore, 1993).

Production of Engineered Proteins

Protein variants have been prepared by many different approaches. Direct chemical synthetic routes for small proteins with modified amino acid sequences have been devised using either wet chemical (solution chemistry) or solid support (chemistry occurring while reactants attached to resin beads) techniques (Parish and McPherson, 1987). Peptide synthesizers have been designed to automate the process. Parish and McPherson as well as Dugas provide useful overviews of the chemistry of protein engineering (site-directed mutagenesis) (Parish and McPherson, 1987; Dugas, 1989a).

The synthesis of gene fragments coding for the mutation(s) is another approach to produce engineered proteins (Zoller and Smith, 1983; Zoller and Smith, 1984; Kunkel, 1985; Rossi and Zoller, 1987). Completely synthetic genes of as many as 100 nucleotides coding for the desired mutation can be inserted into a gene of a prokaryotic (such as Phage M13) or eukaryotic expression vector. The resulting mutant gene (hybrid gene) is then cloned and expressed producing the engineered protein. The genetic route to engineered proteins is limited to the repertoire of the 20 natural amino acids. The purely chemical route allows for the introduction of alternative structures (e.g., non-natural amino acids) in the peptide chain (see section "Peptide Chemistry and Peptidomimetics").

Site-Directed Mutagenesis

Site-Directed Mutagenesis (also called site-specific mutagenesis) is a protein engineering technique allowing specifically (site-direct) alteration (mutation) of the primary amino acid sequence of proteins to create new chemical entities. Mutagenesis at a single amino acid position in an engineered protein is called a point mutation. Therefore, site-directed mutagenesis techniques can aid in the examination at the molecular level of the 3-D structure and function of interesting proteins.

Figure 6.4 suggests possible theoretical mutations of the active site of a model serine protease enzyme that could be engineered to probe the mechanism of action of the enzyme. Structure B of Figure 6.4 represents a theoretical mutation to illustrate the technique. Craik and co-workers have actually tested the role of the aspartic acid residue in the serine protease catalytic triad Asp, His, and Ser. They replaced Asp [102] (carboxylate anion side chain) of trypsin with Asn (neutral amide side chain) by site-directed mutagenesis and observed a pH dependent change in the catalytic activity compared to the wild-type parent serine protease (see Figure 6.4, structure C) (Craik et al., 1987).

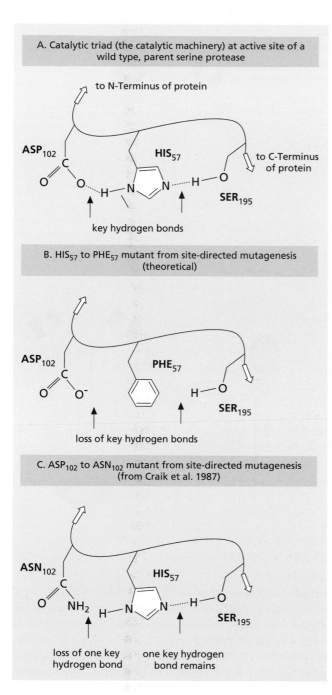

A. Catalytic triad (the catalytic machinery) at active site of a wild type, parent serine protease

B. HIS$_{57}$ to PHE$_{57}$ mutant from site-directed mutagenesis (theoretical)

C. ASP$_{102}$ to ASN$_{102}$ mutant from site-directed mutagenesis (from Craik et al. 1987)

Figure 6.4. Some possible site-directed mutations of the amino acids composing the catalytic triad of a serine protease: influence on key hydrogen bonding.

Applications of this approach to improving the activity, affinity and specificity of useful biopharmaceuticals are far too numerous to be described in detail in this chapter. Livingston and Venuti nicely review second generation recombinant therapeutic proteins (Livingston, 1989; Venuti, 1990). Some examples cited include tissue plasminogen activator, human growth hormone, antibodies and immuno-

conjugates, soluble receptors, interleukin 2, interferons, growth factors, tumor necrosis factor, insulin and factor VIII (see Chapters 8–16).

Site-directed mutagenesis can alter the stability of the "wild type" parent protein. A protein's chemical stability increases by replacing reactive amino acids in the parent with residues that resist reaction. Also, physical stability improves with the introduction of amino acids that contribute to a protein's conformational stability (i.e., introduce site mutations that create new intramolecular hydrogen bonds or disulfide bridges).

Enzyme Engineering

Enzyme engineering is the application of protein engineering techniques to enzymatic molecules. Enzyme engineering can optimize catalytic reactions, improve an enzyme's function under abnormal conditions and enhance the catalytic reaction of unnatural substrates.

An exciting application of protein engineering is the preparation of enzymes that have improved catalytic activity and stability in organic solvents, rather than requiring an aqueous environment. Site-directed mutagenesis replaces hydrophilic, charged amino acids and hydrogen bonding residues at the surface of the enzyme with amino acids that stabilize the conformational stability of the protein at the organic solvent – protein surface interface.

While enzyme engineering is a powerful technique, it is difficult to engineer, via site-directed mutagenesis, a new catalytic function into an existing enzyme because of the precise spatial arrangement required for the catalytic functional groups at the active site. Fusion molecules, however, are examples of protein engineered products that may possess more than one activity or property (see below).

Fusion Proteins

Using ligation chemistry to fuse the gene coding region for one protein with that of another protein, researchers have created chimeric proteins that combine the properties and activities of the two individual parents. The molecule created is called a fusion protein. Fusion proteins contain portions or the entire amino acid sequences of both parent proteins. Fusion proteins have found use in improving the gene expression of a target protein, creating molecules with additive biological activities, and assessing the structure-activity relationships of regions in a protein important to its function. Some examples will be discussed below.

Gene expression of therapeutically useful proteins (or any protein) may be facilitated by creating a fusion protein as an intermediate (Goeddel *et al.*, 1979). Human recombinant proinsulin is expressed highly by cloning a fusion gene consisting of the codes for both proinsulin and the enzyme β-galactosidase. After recovering the fusion protein from *E. coli* culture, cleavage of the methionine peptide bond linking the two proteins with the chemical cyanogen bromide yields the free proinsulin (cf. Chapter 1).

Ligation chemistry can create DNA coding for fusion molecules with additive properties in comparison to the individual parent proteins. For example, Pixykine is a fusion protein resulting from protein engineering containing portions of both granulocyte-macrophage colony stimulating factor (GM-CSF) and interleukin-3 (IL-3). It displays the hematopoietic activities of both parent proteins. Also, numerous fusion proteins have been created that contain a toxin fused to another protein. As described in Chapter 18, the IL-2 fusion protein DAB_{389} IL-2 (also called IL-2 fusion toxin) is a recombinant protein consisting of amino acid residues 2-133 of human IL-2 (the IL-2 residues replace the amino acids of the receptor-binding domain of the native diphtheria toxin) "fused" to the first 389 amino acid residues of diphtheria toxin (catalytic and lipophilic domains) (VanderSpek *et al.*, 1993). Many additional variations of diphtheria toxin-containing fusion proteins have been engineered including DAB_{389} CD4 (containing amino acids 1-178 contained in the V1 and V2 domains of human CD4; studied for the treatment of chronically HIV-infected cells), DAB_{389} IL-4 (linked to interleukin 4; treatment of myeloma and Kaposi's sarcoma), DAB_{389} IL-6 (linked to interleukin 6; therapy of autoimmune diseases and cancer), DAB_{389} EGF (containing the amino acid sequence of epidermal growth factor; prevention of restenosis), and DAB_{389} hGM-CSF (fused peptide sequence of human GM-CSF; potential as an antileukemic agent).

A pharmaceutically important application of protein engineering is the production of chimeras to examine the structure-activity relationships of a protein. An example is the engineering of humanized monoclonal antibodies (MAbs) (described in detail in Chapter 13). These altered MAbs are prepared by expressing a chimeric antibody gene containing the code for both human and murine portions of the resulting antibody protein. The differences between species in the structure-activity relationships and the structure-function relationships of these chimeric antibodies can be examined by studying properties such as antigen specificity, affinity, and avidity (Pluckthun, 1992).

Antibody Engineering

The application of protein engineering to the synthesis of new antibodies is called antibody engineering (Winter and Milstein, 1991; Adair, 1992; Wright *et al.*, 1992). The production of humanized antibodies is one example of the application of antibody engineering.

Immunoadhesins are antibody engineered fusion proteins containing the immunoglobulin Fc effector domain and a molecule that will adhere specifically to other target molecules. Examples include the replacement of the

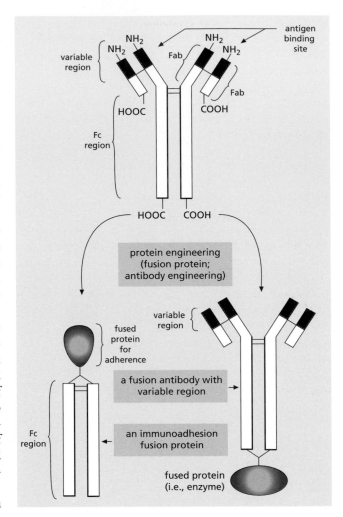

Figure 6.5. Protein engineering (antibody engineering) to produce fusion antibodies.

variable region of an antibody with either the helper T-cell CD4 surface protein or tumor necrosis factor receptor (see Figure 6.5). These immunoadhesins would retain the antibody's Fc effector region (see Chapter 13), but would display specificity for HIV or tumor necrosis factor, respectively. Alternatively, a fused protein can be produced that consists of an antibody with an intact variable region to recognize and bind a specific target (i.e., an antifibrin antibody) along with an enzyme (i.e., tissue plasminogen activator) resulting in a more specific and potent agent (i.e., a fibrin specific thrombolytic agent).

3-D Structures of Engineered Proteins: Protein X-Ray Crystallography, Nuclear Magnetic Resonance Spectroscopy and Protein Modeling

A variety of techniques can produce structural information about the engineered protein. Among the techniques available, only protein X-ray crystallography and nuclear magnetic resonance (NMR) spectroscopy have routinely the ability to determine directly the experimental three-dimensional arrangement of atoms comprising the protein at atomic resolution. A computer can be used for protein modeling, when insufficient quantities of the engineered protein are available, or if X-ray crystallography and NMR are not amenable.

PROTEIN X-RAY CRYSTALLOGRAPHY

Protein X-ray crystallography is a tremendously powerful technique (Hendrickson, 1987; Abraham, 1989; Ducruis and Giege, 1992; McRee, 1993). Following formation of appropriate crystals of the protein, an X-ray diffraction pattern is obtained for the crystal. An electron density map is derived from the diffraction data, which subsequently provides the atom positions in the protein. While the X-ray structure obtained is a structure averaged over all of the mutant protein molecules found in the crystal (various subtle conformational differences among chemically identical molecules of the engineered protein), the technique provides a look at the spatial arrangement of the protein's atoms. Molecular interactions (i.e., ligand-protein binding) and the mechanism of catalytic reactions can be studied at the molecular level. Protein X-ray crystallography is limited by the availability of appropriate crystals for analysis, the inability to get most hydrogen positional information, and the fact that the X-ray structure represents a crystal structure which is not necessarily equal to a solution structure. The cover of this book shows a picture of an X-ray analysis-based structure of part of a Fab' molecule and the interacting antigen (a peptide).

NUCLEAR MAGNETIC RESONANCE (NMR) SPECTROSCOPY

The explosive concurrent development of nuclear magnetic resonance (NMR) techniques and molecular biology has led to an increased study of the three-dimensional structure and dynamics of proteins in solution (Wüthrich, 1986; Markley, 1987; Jefson, 1988; Archer et al., 1996; Craik, 1996). Like X-ray crystallography, NMR spectroscopy generates information directly about the proximity of atoms and about the lifetimes of the through-space interactions of those atoms. Significant advantages of the protein NMR approach over X-ray crystallography include its ability to study proteins in solution, to obtain structural information about dynamic (flexible) portions of the molecule and to look specifically at hydrogen atoms. X-ray crystallography, unlike NMR, provides spatial information about all non-hydrogen atoms. Figure 6.6 provides an example of the differences between structures resulting from both X-ray

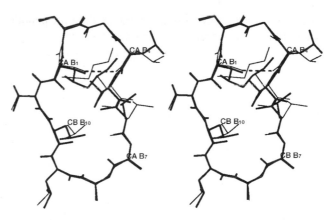

Figure 6.6. An example of the differences between structures produced from both X-ray crystallography and NMR studies. The stereoscopic figure shows the superposition of both the X-ray crystallographic-generated (thinner lines) and NMR-generated structure (thicker lines) of the cyclic peptide immunosuppressive cyclosporin A bound to the protein cyclophilin. The dashed line represents the unique intramolecular hydrogen bond. To simplify the visualization, computer graphics techniques were used to remove the atoms of the protein from the figure. Note the strong similarity in the two different structures. The differences in some side chains may reflect the limits of the methods or resolution. (Reprinted with permission from Ke H, Mayrose D, Belshaw PJ, Alberg DG, Schreiber SL, Chang ZY, Etzkorn FA, Ho S, Walsh CT. (1994). Crystal structures of cyclophilin A complexed with cyclosporin A and N-methyl-4-[(E)-2-butenyl]-4, 4-dimethylthreonine cyclosporin A. *Structure*, **2**, 33–44; Current Biology Ltd.)

crystallographic and NMR spectroscopic studies. The figure shows the superposition of both the X-ray crystallographic-generated and NMR-generated structure of the cyclic peptide immunosuppressant cyclosporin A bound to the protein cyclophilin (Ke et al., 1994). To simplify the visualization, computer graphics techniques were used to remove the atoms of the protein from the figure. Note the strong similarity in the two different structures.

The NOESY method of two-dimensional NMR is commonly used to determine the distance between hydrogens in a protein structure. NOESY is the 2-D equivalent of the transient nuclear Overhauser effect (nOe) that indirectly extracts some inter-hydrogen distance information from the structure if the hydrogens lie sufficiently close to each other. Figure 6.7 shows two typical NOESY 2-D NMR spectra. The example selected examines the difference between two mutants of bovine pancreatic trypsin inhibitor, Y21A[14-38]$_{Abu}$ and Y23A[14-38]$_{Abu}$, each with tyrosine replaced by alanine, at the 21 and 23 positions, respectively (Barbar et al., 1996). Interpretion of the contours of the spectra

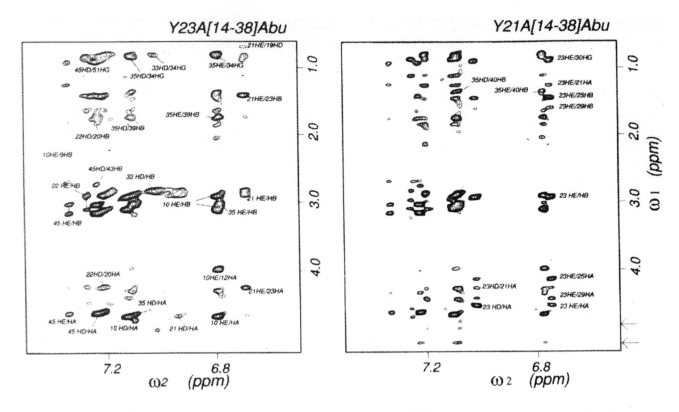

Figure 6.7. Two typical NOESY 2-D NMR spectra. The spectra examine the difference between two mutants of bovine pancreatic trypsin inhibitor, Y21A[14-38]$_{Abu}$ and Y23A[14-38]$_{Abu}$, each with tyrosine replaced by alanine at the 21 and 23 positions respectively. In Y21A[14-38]$_{Abu}$, only the cross peaks that are different from Y23A[14-38]$_{Abu}$ are labeled. (Reprinted with permission from Barbar E, Barany G, Woodward C. (1996). Unfolded BPTI variants with a single disulfide bond have diminished non-native structure distant from the crosslink. *Folding & Design*, **1**, 65–76; Current Biology Ltd.)

provides information about the interatomic distances in solution of particular hydrogens. This in turn suggests the solution conformation of the molecules. Protein NMR, however, is limited by the size of the protein (no greater than 25–30 kD).

PROTEIN MODELING

Protein modeling (in the broader sense, molecular modeling) is a collection of computer techniques, including computer graphics, computational chemistry, statistical methods and database management, applied to the description, analysis, and prediction of protein structures and protein properties (Karplus, 1987; Brooks *et al.*, 1988; Garnier, 1990; Kurtz, 1992; Veerapandian, 1995). Protein folding (including prediction of 3-D structures), dynamics simulations, protein function and protein-molecule (ligand, DNA, protein, etc.) interactions are some of the problems that are being studied currently by protein modeling. Protein modelers often study products from protein engineering. The 3-D protein structures used in modeling are frequently derived from X-

ray crystallography and NMR analyses. When structures are not available from these structural techniques, either *de novo* methods or homology modeling approaches must be used (Greer *et al.*, 1994). *De novo* methods involve the prediction of secondary protein structure from an analysis of the amino acid sequence. Homology modeling uses the known structures of homologous or similar proteins as 3-D templates on which one constructs the framework of the protein being studied. Validation of the computer model resulting from either of these methods with experimental observations is necessary. The success rate for homology approaches (ascertained by comparing a protein's homology modeled structure with its X-ray crystallography determined structure) has limited their broader use.

Peptide Chemistry and Peptidomimetics

Peptide chemistry and biology have become very popular fields of study since the discovery that a large number

Peptide hormone	# Amino acids
angiotensin II	8
β-endorphin	31
bradykinin	9
cholecystokinin	33
dynorphin B	17
endothelin-1	21
gastrin	17
leu-enkephalin	5
met-enkephalin	5
neurotensin	13
somatostatin	14
substance P	11
tuftsin	4

Table 6.4. Some endogenous peptide hormones, neurotransmitters and chemical mediators.

Peptide	Selected indication
Calcitonin	postmenopausal osteoporosis
Chorionic gonadotropin	induction of ovulation
Corticotropin (adrenocorti-cotropic hormone, ACTH)	test of adrenocortical function
Glucagon	hypoglycemia
Octreotide acetate (a pepti-domimetic of the peptide hormone somatostatin)	symptomatic treatment of cancer patients
Oxytocin	initiate/intensify uterine contractions
Vasopressin	diabetes insipidus

Table 6.5. Some selected therapeutically used peptides.

of hormones, neurotransmitters and other endogenous chemical mediators are peptides (some examples are listed in Table 6.4). Peptide receptors are attractive targets in drug discovery and design efforts. Thus, both peptides and proteins have the potential to be developed into useful therapeutic agents (see Table 6.5 for a selection of therapeutically useful peptide pharmaceuticals). Peptides, like the larger proteins, may be produced by various genetic methods (as described for proteins in Chapter 1 and earlier in this chapter). For smaller molecules, however, chemical synthesis is quite viable. Both classical solution methods and newer solid phase approaches based on the technique originally developed by Merrifield technique (the chemistry occurs while the growing peptide chain is anchored onto a polymeric bead) have been applied to the synthesis of thousands of peptides of diverse structure (Atherton and Sheppard, 1989; Gutte, 1995). Peptides of 50 amino acids or greater are synthesized by automated solid phase peptide synthesizers.

Despite their achievable synthesis, peptides suffer from a number of characteristics that make them less suitable as drugs than the classical small organic molecule agents.

In most cases, peptide pharmaceuticals are characterized by low oral bioavailability, poor passage through the blood-brain barrier (for CNS targeted peptides), metabolic instability catalyzed by endogenous peptidases (hydrolysis of the amide bond), and rapid urinary and biliary excretion (Luthman and Hacksell, 1996). Also, the inherent flexibility of peptide molecules allow them to adopt multiple, low energy conformations or shapes. This property permits a peptide drug to interact with several different similar peptide receptors. Such a lack of selectivity at target receptor sites causes side effects and low affinity. Numerous peptide modifications have been studied to overcome the limitations that make peptides poorly suited as drugs (Farmer, 1980; Morgan and Gainor, 1989; Goodman and Ro, 1995; Luthman and Hacksell, 1996; Nakanishi and Kahn, 1996).

Peptidomimetics

The isolation and structure elucidation of two endogenous morphine-like pentapeptides, leu-enkephalin and met-enkephalin, formally introduced the study of peptidomimetics (Hughes et al., 1975). Morphine, a narcotic alkaloid, and the enkephalins were conclusively demonstrated to elicit their analgesia by binding to the same opioid receptor. Therefore, morphine acts as a narcotic analgesic because it is a nature-synthesized mimic of the endogenous pentapeptides.

Peptidomimetics (sometimes called peptide mimetics and nonpeptide mimetics) are defined as "structures which

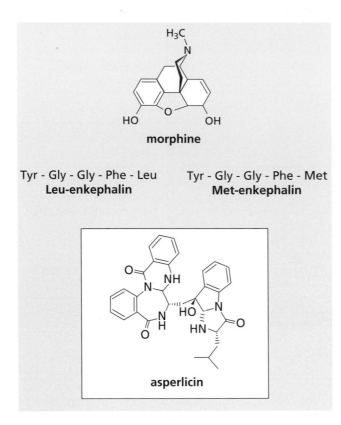

Figure 6.8. Discovery of peptidomimetics: opioid pentapeptides and the CCK antagonist asperlicin.

serve as appropriate substitutes for peptides in interactions with receptors and enzymes. The mimetic must possess not only affinity, but also efficacy or substitute function" (Morgan and Gainor, 1989). Numerous additional reviews on the topic are available (Gante *et al.*, 1994; Giannis and Kolter, 1993; Goodman and Ro, 1995; Luthman and Hacksell, 1996; Nakanishi and Kahn, 1996).

There are a number of approaches to the discovery of peptidomimetics that interact with specific peptide receptors. An empirical approach to peptidomimetic discovery is the screening of pure compound libraries and complex mixtures (from natural product extracts, microbial fermentations or combinatorial chemistry) (Gallop *et al.*, 1994). A screening success was the discovery of the potent cholecystokinin (CCK) receptor antagonist asperlicin (Figure 6.8) from a fermentation and the subsequent medicinal chemistry development of additional agents (Evans *et al.*, 1986; Wiley and Rich, 1993). This nonpeptide natural product containing a 1,4-benzodiazepine moiety acts as a peptidomimetic antagonist at a receptor for a neuroactive peptide ligand (CCK). Computer-aided molecular modeling is often used to design enhanced analogs (exhibiting improved affinity and selectivity) of the lead molecule discovered via such an empirical approach.

"Pseudopeptide" Peptidomimetic Approach

The peptidomimetic approach known as pseudopeptides is an attempt to improve the biostability of peptides (Spatola, 1983; Hirschmann *et al.*, 1995). Numerous pseudopeptides (also called amide bond surrogates) have been prepared that substitute an amide bond bioisostere for the amide peptide bond. A bioisostere is a replacement of an atom or groups of atoms while retaining a broadly similar bioactivity. Examples of some bioisosteric peptide bond replacements are shown in Figure 6.9 (Luthman and Hacksell, 1996). This type of substitution changes the backbone of the peptide and may alter its conformation. For example, the α-carbon-α-carbon distance in a normal dipeptide with a *trans*-peptide bond is 3.8 angstroms (Å). For the methylenethio bioisostere it is 4.2 Å while the methyleneoxy analog distance is 3.7 Å, similar to the parent structure (Morgan and Gainor, 1989) (Figure 6.9). Bioisosteric pseudopeptides do exhibit decreased endogenous peptidase-mediated hydrolysis, however, many still suffer from insufficient oral bioavailability. An interesting amide bond bioisostere is the tetrazole analog (a five-membered ring with four nitrogens, see Figure 6.9) that also serves to restrict the backbone conformation of the peptide amide bond to the *cis*-orientation (see Chapter 2).

Conformationally-Constrained Peptides

The introduction of local conformational constraints into a peptide's backbone and/or α-carbon side chain groups (the R-group attached to the α-carbon of the amino acid residues; i.e., R = –CH$_3$ in alanine and R = –CH$_2$OH in serine, etc.) may result in improved receptor selectivity. Decreased conformational flexibility leads to fewer possible multiple receptor interactions. Also, local conformational constraints may decrease a peptide's biodegradation (Liskamp, 1994). Examples of various types of conformationally-restricted analogs are shown in Figure 6.10. Global conformation may be restricted by cyclizing the peptide through several methods (examples of global conformational contraints are shown in Figure 6.11).

Backbone modifications include the introduction of carbon-carbon double bonds (olefinic analogs) and rings (benzene, carbohydrates, lactams, and azoles) (Hirschmann *et al.*, 1993; Graf von Roedern and Kessler, 1994; Borg *et al.*, 1995). The olefinic analog modified peptides have one less amide bond than the parent peptide, thus restricting conformation and increasing lipophilicity. Replacing a peptide amide bond with an *ortho*-substituted benzene ring results in a *cis*-amide mimic, while a β-D-glucose scaffold provides a *trans*-amide mimic with less conformational flexibility. The lactam (a cyclic amide) and the azole (five-membered ring with at least one nitrogen) modifications

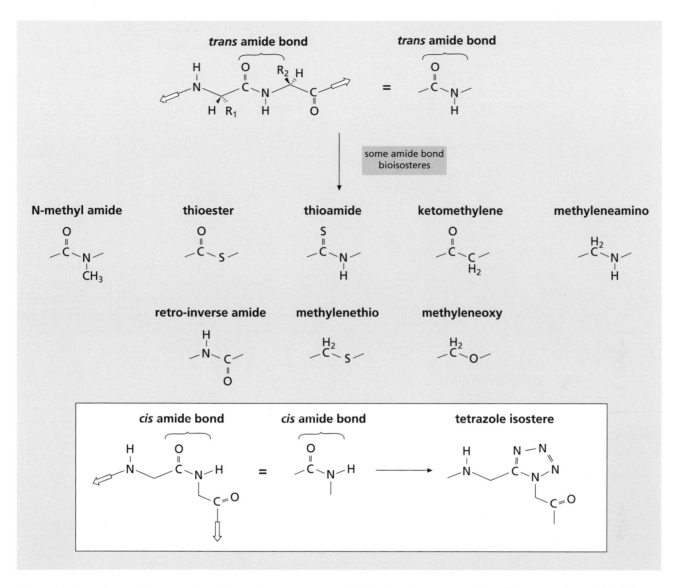

Figure 6.9. Pseudopeptides: examples of some bioisosteric peptide bond replacements (adapted from Goodman and Ro 1995 and Luthman and Hacksell 1996).

restrict the conformation of the chain with a *trans*-amide configuration.

The backbone of a peptide may be covalently linked to a portion of an α-carbon side chain thus fixing the local conformational orientation of both to each other. More global conformational restrictions may be made by cyclization of the peptide through the formation of a disulfide bond, joining two α-carbon side chains or cyclizing the backbone (Hruby, 1982; Gilon *et al.*, 1991).

Rational Design of Peptidomimetics

The rational design of peptidomimetics and other analogs of bioactive peptides and proteins often requires techniques previously described for protein engineering (molecular biology, X-ray crystallography, NMR spectroscopy and computer-aided molecular modeling) to model the 3-D orientation of the amino acid residues (Adang *et al.*, 1994). Using these techniques, one can approach the challenging design of peptidomimetics by mimicry of the molecular architecture created by nature such as α-helices (with α-helix initiators), β-sheets (with β-sheet inducers), and reverse turns (β-turns with β-turn mimetics and γ-turns with γ-turn mimetics) (Boyle *et al.*, 1994). A selected example of each is shown in Figure 6.12. The biologically important functional groups (the pharmacophore) present on the α-carbon side chains of the peptide residues must be held in the requisite spatial orientation when a peptidomimetic is

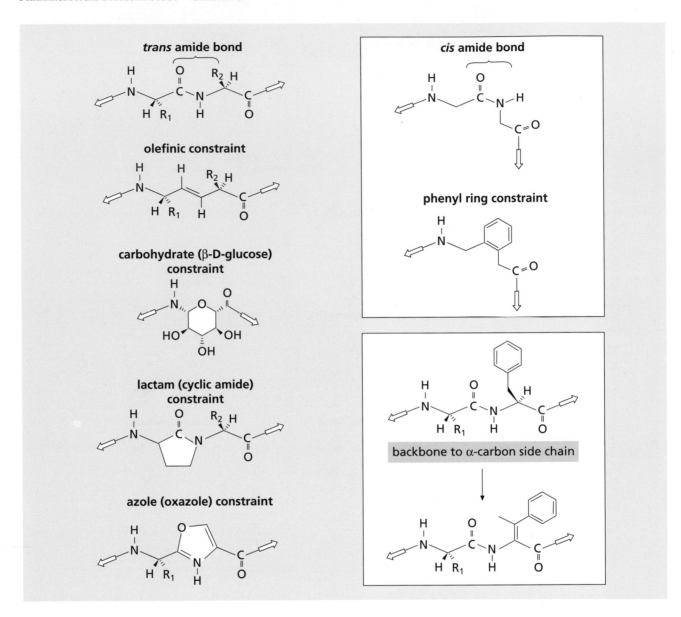

Figure 6.10. Examples of local conformational constraints of peptide backbone and α-carbon side chain groups: olefinic analog, rings, and backbone-α-carbone side chain link.

designed. A careful combination of key secondary structural unit inducers along with scaffolds to hold the pharmacophoric groups in the proper orientation should provide a compound possessing the desired biological activity without the bioavailability, biostability, and selectivity concerns (Kahn, 1993).

Nucleic Acid Technologies

Nucleic acid technologies encompass all the techniques based on oligonucleotides and their analogs including gene therapy (Ramabhadran, 1994). Nucleic acids are polymers of nucleotides. While early nucleic acid technology targeted genetic deficiency diseases with replacement gene therapy (discussed in detail in Chapter 7), antisense and triplex technologies, aptamer technology and the study of ribozymes have become dominant themes in many research and development laboratories around the world. Tremendous effort has been spent the last few years to develop oligonucleotides and oligonucleotide analogs into useful therapeutic products. The Pharmaceutical Research and Manufacturers of America recently listed six oligonucleotide drugs being studied in Phase I-Phase III clinical trials (The Pharmaceutical Research and Manufacturers of America, 1996).

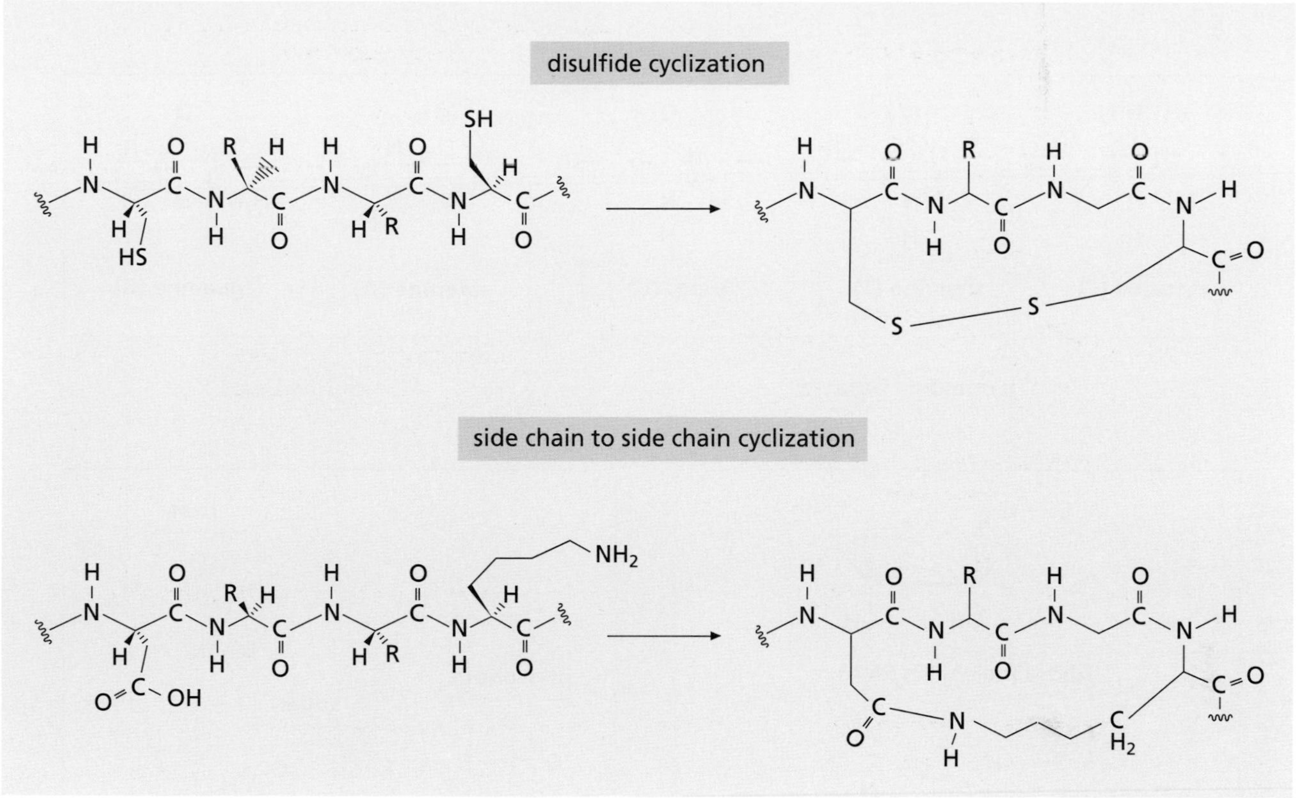

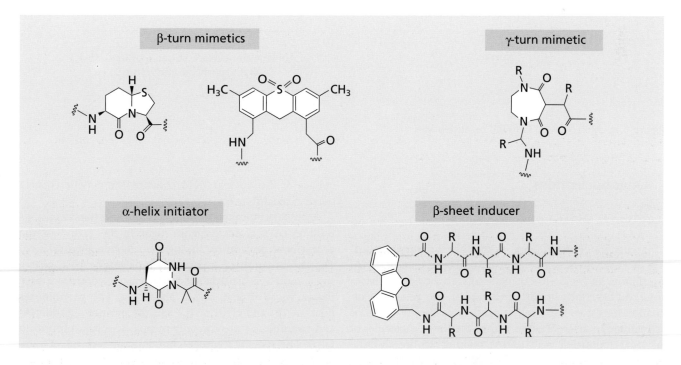

Figure 6.11. Examples of global conformational constraints: disulfide cyclizations and side chain to side chain cyclization.

Figure 6.12. Examples of rationally designed peptidomimetics by mimicry of the molecular secondary structure.

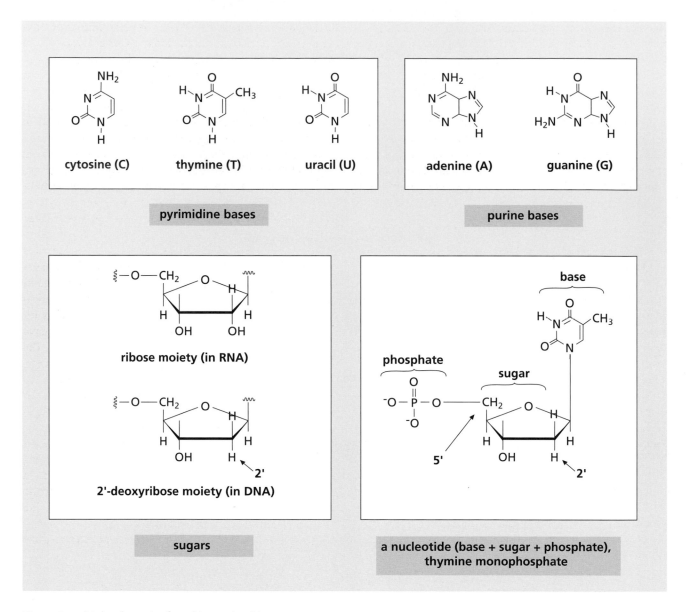

Figure 6.13. Molecular units found in nucleotides.

Oligonucleotides

BIOCHEMISTRY

Oligonucleotides (or "oligos" as they are sometimes called) are short polymeric segments of deoxyribonucleic acid (DNA) or ribonucleic acid (RNA), generally 100 or fewer bases long. As described briefly in Chapter 1, the genetic information necessary for a cell to synthesize specific proteins is retained in discrete genes within the linear molecules of 2'-deoxyribonucleic acid (DNA) making up the chromosomes in the cell nucleus. The genes consist of double helical strands of DNA. The exact nucleic acid base se-

quence of the nuclear DNA contains the genetic code to make a specific protein.

Each base is linked through a phosphate bond at the 5'-position of a 2'-deoxyribose sugar to the 3'-end of the deoxyribose portion on the next nucleotide (Figure 6.13). The combination of a pyrimidine or purine base plus a sugar moiety is a nucleoside, while a nucleotide is a base plus a sugar moiety and a phosphate. The pyrimidines thymine (T) and cytosine (C) and the purines adenine (A) and guanine (G) are the only nucleic acid bases found in DNA. The specific hydrogen bonding interactions of complementary bases on each oligodeoxyribonucleotide strand (A only with T, G only with C) hold the two strands of DNA together to form double-helical DNA with the sugar-phosphate backbones directed toward the outside (see Chapter 1). Oligodeoxyribonucleotides are also called oligodeoxynucleotides and ODNs. In oligoribonucleotides, the pyrimidine base uracil (U) is substituted for T and hydrogen bonds with A.

The nomenclature for oligonucleotides follows a consistent pattern. For a monomer, dimer, trimer up to a decamer, the names would be mononucleotide, dinucleotide, trinucleotide, etc. Beyond that, the name of an oligonucleotide is given by its length as a number followed by "-mer". Thus a 21-base containing oligonucleotide would be a 21-mer (twenty one-mer).

PHYSICOCHEMICAL PROPERTIES OF OLIGONUCLEOTIDES

Normal oligodeoxyribonucleotides and oligoribonucleotides containing the five bases, unmodified sugars and the phosphate group are limited in their potential therapeutic applications because they are highly susceptible to rapid degradation by structurally nonspecific intracellular nucleases (Stein and Narayanan, 1996). Upon hydrolysis, the resulting smaller oligos and nucleotide pieces are not expected to retain their previous biological activity, nor specificity. Also, each of the phosphate groups of the oligonucleotide phosphate-sugar backbone (chemically, a phosphodiester linkage) possesses a negative charge preventing passive diffusion through cellular and nuclear membranes (Stein and Narayanan, 1996). Numerous modifications of the parent oligonucleotide structure have been undertaken to circumvent the degradation and cellular permeation limitations. Natural oligonucleotides have been shown to accumulate in cells by receptor-mediated endocytosis. This process, however, is not very efficient. Microinjection and liposome encapsulation appear to be the most effective routes of administration of normal and modified oligonucleotides (Stein and Narayanan, 1996).

CHEMISTRY AND MODIFICATIONS

Both oligodeoxyribonucleotides and oligoribonucleotides can be readily prepared through automated chemical synthesis or genetic methods (such as enzymatic syntheses utilizing DNA polymerase or RNA polymerase, respectively). The recent availability of chemically pure, short fragments of DNA have permitted the crystallization and x-ray crystallographic structural analysis of nucleic acids, thus offering a "look" at these molecules at the atom level. Research contributions to oligonucleotide synthesis and structural chemistry have aided the search for useful, modified molecules (Cook, 1991).

Chemical manipulation of the oligonucleotides by substituting more nuclease resistant and lipophilic groups for the negatively charged oxygen on the phosphodiester linkages results in a series of modified oligonucleotides with improved physiochemical properties (Miller and Ts'o, 1988; Matteucci and Bischofberger, 1991; Milligan et al., 1993; Crooke, 1995a; Crooke, 1995b). Figure 6.14 illustrates chemical changes of a parent oligonucleotide structure resulting in phosphorothioate, alkyl phosphonate and phosphoamidate analogs, each possessing an additional chiral center (on the phosphorus atom, Lebedev and Wickstrom, 1996). These chemical changes increase lipophilicity and decrease nuclease hydrolysis. For example, the parent oligonucleotide half-life of 1 hour is increased to more than 24 hours by preparing the phosphorothioate derivative (Iverson, 1991; Akhtar and Juliano, 1992; Crooke, 1992a; Murray and Crockett, 1992). Neutral derivatives such as the alkyl phosphonates cross the blood-brain barrier. Achiral formacetal 3'–5' linkers have also been prepared, exhibiting an added advantage in not creating additional chiral centers that make purification difficult (Thayer, 1990). Additional modifications include changes to the heterocyclic bases and extensive derivatization of the ribose moiety (Matteucci, 1996). Replacement of the hydroxyl group (-OH) at the 2'-position of oligoribonucleotides by a methoxyl group ($-OCH_3$) helps to overcome some of the physiochemical hurdles. Pendant cap groups are added to the 5'-terminal end of the oligonucleotide to increase nuclease resistance.

A peptide nucleic acid (PNA) is a more recent variation of the phosphate-sugar backbone of oligonucleotides (Nielsen, 1996). A PNA is a DNA/RNA mimic with a pseudopeptide backbone holding the pyrimidine and purine bases in their proper spatial arrangement. Aminoethyl glycine (gly-NH-CH_2-CH_2-gly) units serve as the backbone of the polymer. These highly modified oligonucleotide analogs have improved physicochemical characteristics.

Antisense Technology and Triplex Technology

NORMAL CELL ACTIVITY: DNA MAKES RNA MAKES PROTEIN

As well described in Chapter 1, during the normal process of transcription, the double-stranded DNA separates into two strands, the sense DNA strand (coding strand or plus strand) and the antisense DNA strand (template strand or minus strand). The antisense DNA strand then serves as the template for the mRNA responsible for the code for protein synthesis in the ribosome. The sense DNA strand may infrequently also code for RNA and this molecule is called antisense RNA. Antisense sequences were first described as a naturally occurring event in which an endogenous antisense RNA is formed complementary to a cellular mRNA resulting in a repressor of gene expression (Murray and Crockett, 1992; Bains, 1993).

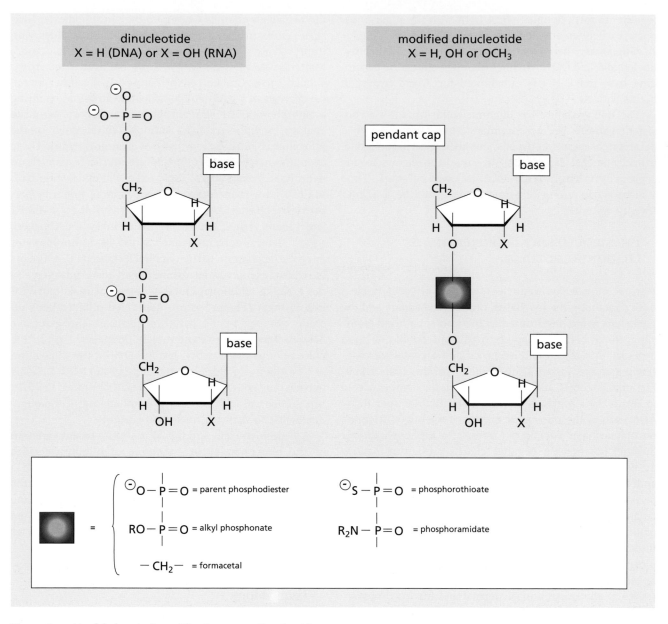

Figure 6.14. Useful chemical modifications to a dinucleotide.

RATIONALE FOR ANTISENSE TECHNOLOGY

The discovery that nature can regulate gene expression, and thus protein synthesis, using antisense RNA suggested that exogenous antisense oligonucleotides might also be useful in regulating gene expression. Antisense oligonucleotide interactions occur when the bases of the synthetic, specifically designed antisense oligonucleotide sequence align in a precise, sequence-specific manner with a complementary series of bases in the target mRNA (Figure 6.15) (Miller and Ts'o, 1988; Matteucci and Bischofberger, 1991; Crooke, 1992a; Murray and Crockett, 1992; Milligan

et al., 1993; Crooke, 1995a; Crooke, 1995b; Tidd, 1996; Kool, 1996). The potential antisense oligonucleotide drug is chemically modified in one or more ways as described earlier.

Antisense oligonucleotide interruption of the flow of genetic information may occur at the mRNA level in the cytoplasm or by interacting with the mRNA precursor in the nucleus. Antisense RNA would be oligoribonucleotides that are complementary for the mRNA sequence that is targeted. Antisense DNA would be single stranded oligodeoxyribonucleotides that are, again, complementary to mRNA. There are several mechanisms by which antisense

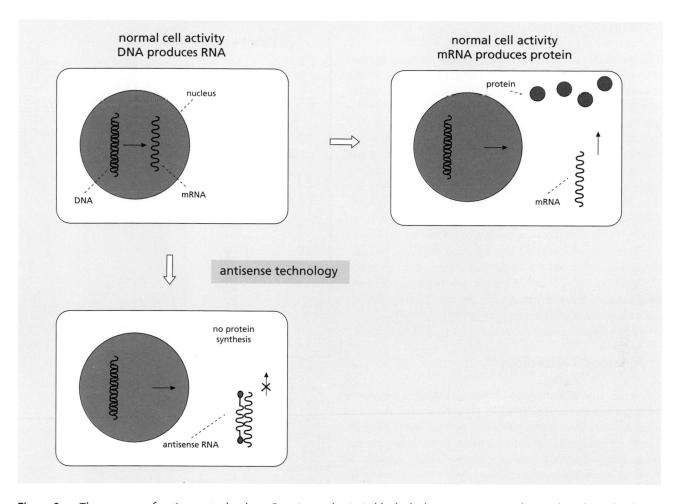

Figure 6.15. The process of antisense technology. Protein synthesis is blocked when an antisense oligonucleotide molecule binds to messenger RNA.

molecules ultimately disrupt gene expression and thus protein synthesis. A transient inhibition may occur by masking the ribosome binding site on mRNA preventing protein synthesis. A permanent inhibition may result from cross-linking the oligonucleotide to the target mRNA. The most important mechanism, however, appears to be through the action of an enzyme found in most cells, ribonuclease H (RNase H), which recognizes the DNA-RNA duplex (antisense DNA interacting with mRNA) or RNA-RNA duplex (antisense RNA interacting with mRNA), disrupts the base pairing, and digests the RNA-part of the double helix. Inhibition of gene expression occurs since the digested mRNA is no longer competent for translation and resultant protein synthesis.

THERAPEUTIC ANTISENSE MOLECULES

While most traditional drug molecules illicit their effect by interacting with an important enzyme or protein receptor (thus defining a receptor loosely to mean any target molecule with which a drug interacts to produce an effect rather than a strict pharmacological definition for receptor reserved for the agonist or antagonist interactions of the regulatory type), antisense technology involves the blocking of genetic messages to stop the production of disease-producing proteins at the source (Agrawal, 1996). Antisense oligonucleotide genetic-code blocking drugs might control disease by inhibiting deleterious or malfunctioning genes, differing from gene therapy which inserts needed genetic information (see Chapter 7). As stated earlier, six oligonucleotide drugs are being studied in Phase I-Phase III clinical trials (The Pharmaceutical Research and Manufacturers of America, 1996). Among the potential therapeutic targets under examination in the current clinical trials are cancer including chronic myelogenous leukemia (CML) in accelerated phase or blast crisis, HIV infection and AIDS, cytomegalovirus (CMV) retinitis in AIDS patients, and inflammatory diseases.

TRIPLEX TECHNOLOGY

The general term "antigene nucleic acids" has been applied to any oligonucleotides that bind to single-stranded or double stranded DNA. An antigene nucleic acid approach related to antisense technology is triple helix (triplex) technology in which short oligodeoxyribonucleotides of 15-27 nucleotides in length can bind sequence-specifically to complementary segments of duplex DNA (Dervan, 1989; Matteucci and Bischofberger, 1991; Helene *et al.*, 1992). The resulting triple helices inhibit DNA replication, thus blocking genetic information flow at the information processing level. While antisense RNA drugs would have to inhibit thousands of copies of the synthesized target mRNA present in a cell, triplex inhibition of transcription requires the inactivation of only one or possibly two copies of the genomic DNA found in each cell. Even though triple helices have been known for over 30 years, modern oligonucleotide chemistry has provided the opportunity to synthesize selectively the required specific sequences in sufficient yield.

Aptamer Technology

Aptamers are single-stranded or double-stranded sequences of oligonucleotides that bind to proteins (rather than nucleic acids) or other small molecules (Ellington and Szostak, 1990). From the Latin *apto* meaning to fit, aptamers are being studied as potential therapeutic agents capable of binding to proteins such as transcription factors and thus blocking gene expression and protein synthesis. Laboratory studies have identified specific oligonucleotide sequences that bind to the NF-κB transcription factor in B- and T-cells, the adenosine deaminase enhancer in T-cells and human thrombin (Stull and Szoka, 1995). Currently, to this author's knowledge, there are no aptamer drugs in clinical trials.

Ribozymes

Ribozymes are catalytic RNAs which cleave covalent bonds, generally degrading a target RNA (for reviews applicable to pharmaceutical research and applications see: Christoffersen and Marr, 1995; Krueger, 1995; Rossi, 1995; Stull and Szoka, 1995; Usman and McSwiggen, 1995). Until the discovery in the mid-1980s of these self-cleaving and splicing RNAs, proteins were thought to be the only types of molecules capable of functioning as biocatalysts. Cech and Altman received the Nobel prize for their co-discovery of ribozymes (Kruger *et al.*, 1982; Guerrier-Takada *et al.*, 1983). There are a number of structurally complex ribozymes that have been isolated, including group I intron, group II intron, RNAse P and VS RNA. Pharmaceutical research has centered on

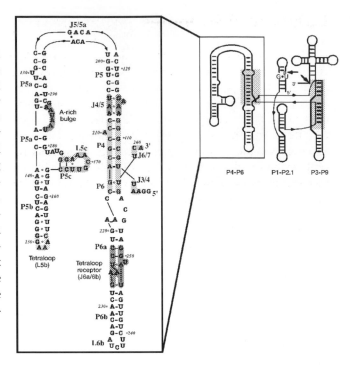

Figure 6.16. The P4-P6 domain of the *Tetrahymena thermophilia* group I self-splicing intron is shown in schematic representation (Cate *et al.*, 1996). Helical regions are numbered sequentially through the sequence; P, paired region; J, joining region. Arrows indicate 5' and 3' splice sites. (Reprinted with permission from Cate JH, Gooding AR, Podell E, Zhou K, Golden BL, Kundrot CE, Cech TR, Doundna JA. (1996). Crystal Structure of a group I Ribozyme Domain: Principles of RNA Packing. *Science*, 273, 1678–1685; American Association for the Advancement of Science.)

three structurally-smaller ribozymes for adaptation; the hammerhead, hairpin and HDV ribozymes. A schematic representation of a group I intron ribozyme is shown in Figure 6.16 (Cate *et al.*, 1996).

Again, modern oligonucleotide chemistry or various genetic techniques have provided the opportunity to engineer selectively the required specific ribozyme sequences in sufficient yield. While still a research technology, ribozymes have the potential to be powerful therapeutic agents directed specifically against viral RNA or cancer cell RNA, leaving the patient's normal RNA untouched. Cancer-causing oncogene transcripts (such as in the *ras* oncogene) and the RNA retrovirus HIV-1 are particularly attractive therapeutic targets. A catalytic ribozyme drug would contain a nucleotide sequence that targets a highly conserved nucleotide region in the RNA of the target cell, thus providing specificity.

Catalytic Antibodies (Abzymes)

A prime example of research at the interface of chemistry and immunology is the development of catalytic antibodies (Lerner *et al.*, 1991; Baird and McLafferty, 1993). Catalytic antibodies or "abzymes" have been considered as a new class of designer enzymes catalyzing reactions for which no natural enzyme exists. Catalytic antibody technology is another example of antibody engineering. Numerous recent reviews and key papers are available to provide an excellent overview of this field and serve as the sources for the discussion that follows (Tramontano *et al.*, 1986; Jacobs *et al.*, 1987; Krafft and Wang, 1990; Lerner *et al.*, 1991; Benkovic, 1992; Schultz and Lerner, 1993; Stewart *et al.* 1993; Webb, 1993; Scanlan, 1995).

Antibodies

Antibody (immunoglobulin) structure and function are described in more detail in Chapter 13 (as an introduction to monoclonal antibodies). Immunoglobulins are structurally highly variable multifunctional glycoproteins produced by the immune system of vertebrates for the eradication of invading microorganisms. Each chemically distinct antibody molecule is able to bind to particular molecular configurations on the invading microorganism (antigen) that stimulated their biosynthesis. A variable region on the antibody provides for the generation of an infinite diversity of antigen recognition (Davies and Chacko, 1993; Jefferis, 1994). Essentially, an antibody can be considered to contain "programmable" chemical binding sites.

Catalysis

Benkovic provides an excellent review of the historical development of catalytic antibodies (Benkovic, 1992). Nearly 50 years ago, Nobel Laureate Linus Pauling suggested that an enzymatic reaction accelerates if the catalytic site is more structurally complementary to the high-energy transition state of the reaction than to its substrate or product ground states. The transition state is a transitory structural entity created from the substrate and present at the energy barrier for the reaction (Jencks, 1969). The better the complementarity between the enzyme and the transition state, the lower the activation energy for the transformation, and thus, the faster the reaction.

While an antibody is a soluble protein capable of ligand-specific binding, the ligand is bound in its low energy ground state. Therefore, normal antibodies lack catalytic activity. Jencks first directly hypothesized the concept of catalytic antibodies in 1969 when he suggested that immunoglobulin proteins that selectively form tight interactions with the transition states of reactions would be catalytic (Jencks, 1969).

The development of hybridoma technology (see Chapter 13) and also protein engineering (earlier in this chapter) provides the ability to produce homogeneous, monoclonal antibodies and modified antibodies in the quantities necessary to reproducibly purify potential abzymes and characterize their properties. The result was the independent production of antibodies with catalytic activity by the Lerner (Tramontano *et al.*, 1986) and Schultz groups (Pollack *et al.*, 1986) in 1986.

Chemistry of Catalytic Antibodies

Since antibodies bind selectively to the antigens that stimulated their synthesis, the key to the production of a catalytic antibody is using a carefully designed, stable transition state analog as the antigen; actually as a hapten. The small molecule is not capable itself to produce an antibody, but is when attached to a larger carrier molecule. A catalytic antibody can be prepared to accelerate a chemical reaction if: 1) the reaction mechanism is well understood, including knowledge of the structure of the high energy transition state; 2) a stable, structurally similar analog of the transition state can be synthesized (the hapten); and 3) sufficient antibodies can be raised to the hapten attached to a carrier used for immunization (generally of mice). Hybridoma techniques are used to fuse the polyclonal catalytic antibody-producing murine spleen cells (from a hapten-carrier immunized mouse) with murine myeloma cells (cf. Chapter 1). Following screening, selection and cloning, monoclonal catalytic antibodies are synthesized. Newer methods of production include the use of phage libraries (see Chapter 13). The antibody so produced would have high affinity for the transition state mimic and thus also the transition state of the studied reaction. The newly generated catalytic antibody should accelerate the transformation of substrate to product. Because antibodies against nearly any molecule (stable transition state analog) can be generated, catalytic antibody technology provides a powerful tool to improve rates of chemical reactions and cause reactions that might possibly not occur otherwise.

Chemists, using carefully designed transition state mimics, have developed general strategies to induce catalytic activity into antibody binding sites by introducing reactive nucleophilic, electrophilic, acidic, or basic groups precisely in complementary key locations optimal for binding the transition state and catalyzing the reaction with the substrate. Accelerations in ester hydrolysis reaction rates of 6×10^6 have been observed for some reactions.

The literature reports a wide range of reactions catalyzed by abzymes. Many early experiments focused on antibodies produced to catalyze ester and amide hydrolysis reactions (esterase-like and amidase-like activities). The stable transition state analog was generally a phosphorus-containing molecule that resembled the tetrahedral transition state of

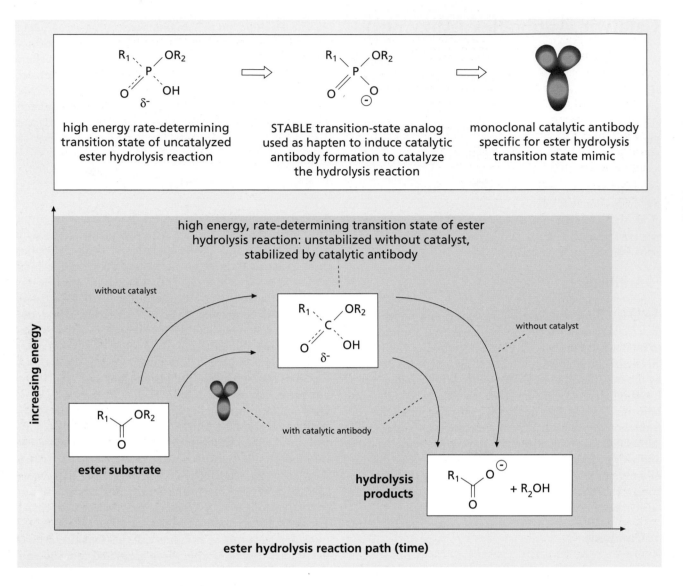

Figure 6.17. Catalytic antibodies produced to catalyze ester hydrolysis reactions. The stable transition state mimic is a phosphorus-containing molecule that resembles the tetrahedral transition state of esters when they are hydrolyzed.

esters or amides when they are hydrolyzed (for an illustration, see Figure 6.17). The three-dimensional information contained in crystal structures (determined to a resolution of 2.5 Å and 3 Å) of catalytic antibody Fab fragments with esterase-like activity may provide greater insight into the nature of antibody-derived catalysis (Golinelli-Pimpaneau et al., 1994; Zhou et al., 1994). In addition to ester and amide hydrolyses/transacylations, reactions examined include enantioselective reactions (creating chiral products), proton transfers, Claisen rearrangements, β-eliminations, bimolecular amide bond formation, lactone ring formation, redox reactions and Diels-Alder reactions. The diversity of reactions is probably limited only by the chemist's imagination and their understanding of reaction mechanisms.

Limitations

There are a number of limitations that affect the general applicability of catalytic antibody technology. One limitation of the antibody catalysts is that they only function in predominantly aqueous environments, similar to enzymes. Organic solvents denature the protein antibodies. Antibody engineering may eventually overcome this limitation. Also, while some tremendous rate enhancements have been noted, many catalytic antibodies are not very efficient.

Potential Pharmaceutical Uses

There are numerous potential pharmaceutical uses of catalytic antibody technology (Krafft and Wang, 1990). Catalytic antibodies may have potential as pharmaceuticals that would enzymatically cleave specific surface proteins or sugars on viruses, or tumor cells thereby disrupting the invaders. Anti-inflammatory abzymes could be generated that break down pro-inflammatory proteins such as certain cytokines. Diagnostic applications may exist where catalytic antibodies are used as biosensors and the resulting enzymatic reaction product(s) are analyzed and quantified. Catalytic antibodies are expected to have better pharmacokinetic and distribution properties than many structurally larger enzymes or enzyme-antibody conjugates (Krafft and Wang, 1990).

Glycobiology

The novel scientific field of glycobiology may be defined most simply as the study of the structure, synthesis and biological role of glycans (may be referred to as oligosaccharides or polysaccharides, depending on size) and glycoconjugates (Rademacher et al., 1988; Welply and Jaworski, 1990; Allen and Kisailus, 1992; Fukuda and Kobata, 1993). Like proteins and nucleic acids, glycans are biopolymers. The building blocks of glycans are simple carbohydrates (called saccharides or sugars) and their derivatives (i.e., amino sugars). The application of glycobiology is sometimes called glycotechnology to distinguish it from biotechnology (referring to glycans rather than proteins and nucleic acids). Glycoconjugates include glycoproteins (predominantly protein), glycolipids and proteoglycans (about 95% polysaccharide and 5% protein). In referring to carbohydrates and glycoconjugates, Borman recently wrote, "The tremendous structural variability of such compounds, the great difficulty of synthesizing them, and the baffling complexity of the life processes in which they are involved have all tended to bog down the process" (Borman, 1996).

While carbohydrate chemistry and biology have been active areas of research for centuries, advances in biotechnology have provided techniques and added energy to the study of glycans (Ginsburg and Robbins, 1981; Sharon and Lis, 1982). The explosive development of biotechnology and molecular biology have provided protein and nucleic acid products for therapy and research. Many of the proteins produced by animal cells contain attached sugar moieties, making them glycoproteins. Bacterial hosts for recombinant DNA could produce the animal proteins with identical or nearly identical amino acid sequences. The bacteria, however, lacked the "machinery" to attach sugar moieties to proteins (a process called glycosylation). Many

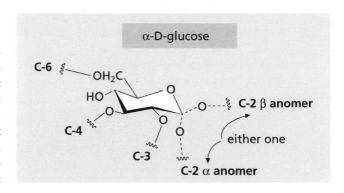

Figure 6.18. Illustration of the common linkage sites to create biopolymers of glucose. Linkages at four positions: C-3, C-4 and C-6 and one of two possible anomeric configurations at C-2 (α and β). The –OH of α-D-glucose would be the C-2 α anomer.

of the non-glycosylated proteins differed in their biological activity as compared to the native glycoprotein. The production of animal proteins that lacked glycosylation provided an unexpected opportunity to study the functional role of sugar molecules on glycoproteins. The result is what is now known as glycobiology. There has been an explosive growth in the literature related to glycobiology. Therefore, this section of Chapter 6 will only very briefly highlight some of the key concepts of glycobiology as they relate to pharmacy and the pharmaceutical sciences.

Basic Principles of Glycobiology

The complexity of the field can best be illustrated by reviewing some basic principles. There are numerous excellent reviews on the basic principles of glycobiology (Berger et al., 1982; Allen and Kisailus, 1992; Fukuda and Kobata, 1993). Oligosaccharides found conjugated to proteins (glycoproteins) and lipids (glycolipids) display a tremendous structural diversity. The linkages of the monomeric units in proteins and in nucleic acids are generally consistent in all such molecules. Glycans, however, exhibit far greater variability in the linkage between monomeric units than that found in the other biopolymers (Rouhi, 1996). As an example, Figure 6.18 illustrates the common linkage sites to create polymers of glucose. Glucose can be linked at four positions: C-2, C-3, C-4 and C-6 and also can take one of two possible anomeric configurations at C-2 (α and β). The effect of multiple linkage arrangements is seen in the estimate of Kobata (Kobata, 1994). He has estimated that for a 10-mer (oligomer of length 10) the number of structurally-distinct linear oligomers for each of the biopolymers is: DNA (with 4 possible bases), 1.04×10^6; protein (with 20 possible amino acids), 1.28×10^{13}; and oligosaccharide (with eight monosaccharide types), 1.34×10^{18}.

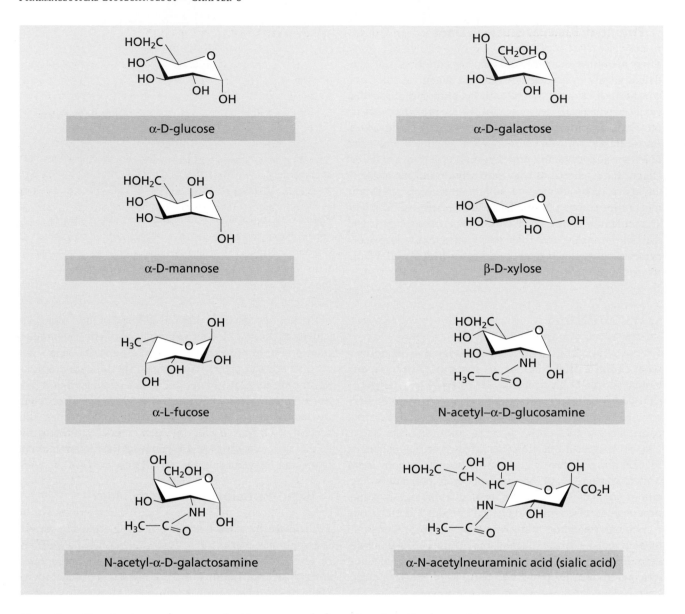

α-D-glucose

α-D-galactose

α-D-mannose

β-D-xylose

α-L-fucose

N-acetyl–α-D-glucosamine

N-acetyl-α-D-galactosamine

α-N-acetylneuraminic acid (sialic acid)

Figure 6.19. The structures of monosaccharides commonly found in eukaryotic glycoproteins.

The structures of monosaccharides commonly found in eukaryotic glycoproteins are shown in Figure 6.19. The glycans of glycoproteins can be divided into two structural types. The O-linked glycans (also called mucins), possessing four different classes of core structure, all contain an N-acetylgalactosamine moiety linked to the hydroxyl group of a serine or a threonine in the protein (Devine and McKenzie, 1992). The N-linked glycans (also called asparagine-linked), all possessing a common pentasaccharide at their core (called the trimannosyl core), contain an N-acetylglucosamine moiety linked to the amide group of an asparagine residue in the protein (Schauer, 1991).

More than 200 glycolipids (called glycosphingolipids) differing in their glycan structure have been isolated and identified from mammalian tissues (Hakomori, 1981; Schnaar, 1991). Also, numerous proteoglycans containing 100–200 monosaccharide residues have been isolated (Ruoslahti, 1988). The proteoglycans are broadly classified in one of six structural groups. These are the chondrotin 4-sulfates, chondrotin 6-sulfates, dermatan sulfates, heparan sulfates, hyaluronic acids and keratan sulfates.

Glycosylation and Biological Activity

Glycosylation affects the biological activity of proteins (West, 1986; Elbein, 1991; Fukuda, 1992; Hart, 1992; Kobata, 1992; Rasmussen, 1992). Many of the therapeutically used recombinant DNA-produced proteins are glycosylated including erythropoietin, glucocerebrosidase and tissue plasminogen activator (Cumming, 1991; Jenkins *et al.*, 1996). Without the appropriate carbohydrates attached, none of these proteins will function therapeutically as does the parent glycoprotein. Glycoforms (variations of the glycosylation pattern of a glycoprotein) of the same protein may differ in physicochemical and biochemical properties. For example, erythropoietin has one O-linked and three N-linked glycosylation sites. The removal of the terminal sugars at each site destroys *in vivo* activity and removing all sugars results in a more rapid clearance of the molecule and a shorter circulatory half-life (Fukuda *et al.*, 1989; Takeuchi *et al.*, 1990). Yet, the opposite effect is observed for the deglycosylation of the hematopoietic cytokine granulocyte-macrophage colony-stimulating factor (GM-CSF) (Donahue *et al.*, 1986; Cebon *et al.*, 1990). In that case, removing the carbohydrate residues increases the specific activity six-fold.

Another example of the role of sugars on biological activity of proteins can be found in the immune system. Immunoglobulin G(IgG) is a glycoprotein containing complex sugar chains (Kobata, 1991). Removal of the galactose residues from IgG results in less effective binding to the first component of the complement cascade. Antigen-antibody complexes activate the complement system; the key component of the activation being the binding of IgG to C1q of complement. Also, N-linked carbohydrates are thought to play an important role in both cellular and humoral immunity (Bradbury and Parish, 1991). Thus, glycosylation patterns of proteins affect the complicated communication network of the immune system.

Sugars linked to proteins can help to shield the surface of a glycoprotein from antibody recognition. Glycosylated recombinant interferon-β from CHO (Chinese hamster ovary) cells and the non-glycosylated form from *E. coli* were found to be immunologically non-identical (Colby *et al.*, 1984).

The Role of Glycosylation in Disease

The sugars of glycoproteins are known to play a role in the recognition and binding of biomolecules to other molecules in disease states such as asthma, rheumatoid arthritis, cancer, HIV-infection, the flu and other infectious diseases (Furukawa *et al.*, 1990; Furukawa and Kobata, 1991; Morikawa *et al.*, 1991; Dabelsteen and Clausen, 1992; Laskey, 1992; Li *et al.*, 1993; Muramatsu, 1993; von Itzstein *et al.*, 1993). A study of which oligosaccharides are involved in the recognition and binding processes associated with a disease state may lead to new molecular targets for possible therapeutic intervention (Musser *et al.*, 1995). Tools such as carbohydrate engineering, carbohydrate analysis and computer-aided molecular modeling will contribute to those efforts.

Cell Adhesion Molecules

Cell-cell interactions, mediated by surface carbohydrates, are essential for the correct assembly of tissues during embryogenesis and in the homeostasis of mature organisms (Brackenbury, 1990). Carbohydrates on the surface of cells can interact with protein receptors on other cells and are responsible for this cell adhesion. For example, this interaction is the basis of the ABO blood group antigen recognition. Two of the main families of cell adhesion molecules (CAMs) are the integrins and the selectins. Among the other major CAM groups (not discussed here) are those of the immunoglobulin superfamily and the cadherins. The discovery of the selectins has sparked a wave of research examining the biology, chemistry and therapeutic potential of adhesion molecules and their processes.

INTEGRINS

The integrins make up a large superfamily of transmembrane heterodimer glycoproteins consisting of an α and a β subunit (Wilcox and Horton, 1994). The specificity of integrin binding among the 20 or more molecules isolated to date appears to stem from an association of a particular α chain with a particular β chain (as many as eight of each identified). Integrin-binding ligands tend to contain the RGD amino acid sequence (Arg-Gly-Asp). Ligands include collagen, fibrinogen, fibronectin, ICAM-1, ICAM-2 (intercellular adhesion molecules 1 and 2), laminin, vitronectin, and von Willebrand factor.

Integrins appear to act as signal transducers across the cell membrane (Wilcox and Horton, 1994). For example, LFA-1 (the integrin $\alpha_L\beta_2$) is inactive in T cells until an antigen is presented by an antigen presenting cell (APC, a B cell or macrophage/monocyte). LFA-1 will then recognize its ligand or counter cell receptor (ICAM-1, on monocytes) and T cell-mediated immunity progresses.

As a result of blood vessel wall injury, integrin $\alpha_{IIb}\beta_3$ (the fibronectin receptor; now more commonly called GpIIb-IIIa) is involved in the initiation of the blood clotting cascade along with platelet aggregation and activation. Fibronectin is the ligand that binds to this integrin, and in a wound cavity provides a temporary scaffolding whereby fibroblasts can more easily commute to the wound site. Other fibronectin receptors (integrins) are located on platelets, which produce fibrinogen, which in turn clogs the area, slows down the migration of fibroblasts, and retards wound healing (Nichols *et al.*, 1994). Preventing or reducing the action of platelets promotes wound healing. Integrelin, in clinical trials for arterial thrombosis, prevents platelet binding to the integrin fibronectin receptor GpIIb-IIIa. It is also in phase III trials for coronary angioplasty and in phase II trials for acute myocardial infarction and unstable angina.

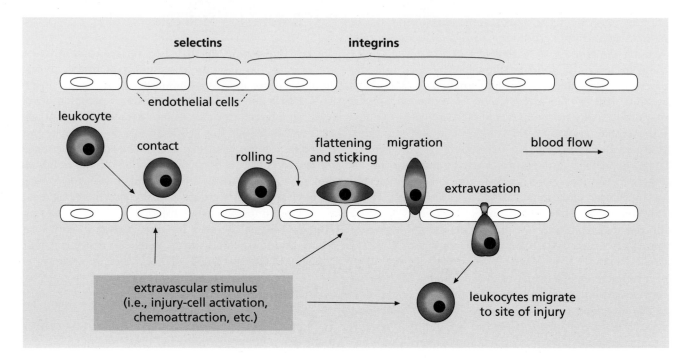

Figure 6.20. Cell adhesion process illustrating role of selectins and integrins. After extravascular activation, leukocytes roll on the endothelial surface of the vessel (selectin driven) until adhesion occurs (integrin driven). Extravasation (migration) of leukocytes out of the vessel and to the site(s) of injury follows.

SELECTINS

Selectins are a family of glycoprotein cell adhesion molecules (Levy *et al.*, 1994). They play a pivotal role in the initial cell-cell interactions involved in leukocyte rolling, platelet binding and passing along neutrophils (and other cell types) to integrins to effect extravasation (migration of cells out of vessel) (see Figure 6.20) (Lawrence and Springer, 1991; Spertini *et al.*, 1992). There are three types of selectins: E-selectin (ELAM-1), P-selectin (GMP-140), and L-selectin (LECAM-1).

E-Selectin is expressed on vascular endothelial cells after activation by different cytokines during inflammation (Bevilacqua *et al.*, 1989). P-Selectin is found on platelets and vascular endothelial cells (Isenberg *et al.*, 1986). It is not induced by cytokines, but is expressed on cell surfaces after stimulation by thrombin or histamine. L-Selectin is expressed on all leukocytes and is definitely involved in inflammation (Butcher, 1991; Spertini *et al.*, 1992).

Circulating leukocyte adhesion is a key step in the inflammatory process (Bevilacqua, 1993; Levy *et al.*, 1994). The selectins may be associated with chronic inflammatory diseases such as arthritis, glomerulonephritis and multiple sclerosis. Also, the selectins may be involved in tumor cell metastasis formation and microbial attachment to cells (Travis, 1993). Thus, the selectins are attractive new targets for drug design. Carbohydrate-based selectin antagonists may have clinical utility in a number of therapeutic areas (Mulligan *et al.*, 1993a; Mulligan *et al.*, 1993b; Levy *et al.*, 1994).

The tetrasaccharide selectin ligand sialyl Lewis X, found on leukocytes and certain cancer cells, appears to play a key role in directing leukocytes to the scene of an inflammatory stimulus. As a ligand for the selectins, sialyl Lewis X acts to facilitate leukocyte adhesion to endothelial cells and may be involved in tumor metastasis formation. Structure-activity relationship studies of sialyl Lewis X are pointed toward the design of potential antagonists to the process (Ohmoto *et al.*, 1996; Hiramatsu *et al.*, 1996).

Biosensors

Biosensors are a class of extremely sensitive and selective sensors that convert a biological action into an electrical signal to detect or quantitively determine a specific compound (Buck *et al.*, 1990; Cass, 1990; Hall, 1990; Scheller and Schubert, 1992; Matthews, 1995). Biosensor technology is the creative synergistic combination of biotechnology, biochemistry, membrane technology and microelectronics. Biosensors are composed of a biological component which recognizes the analyte, and is combined with a transducer

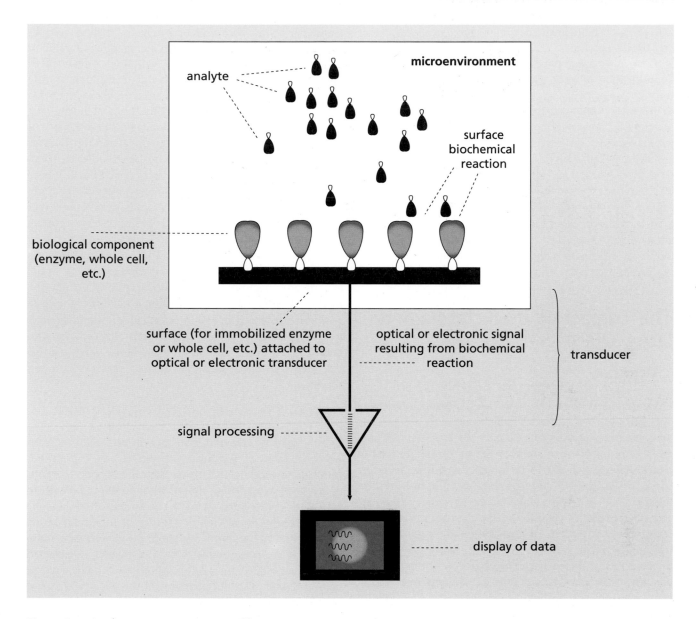

Figure 6.21. A schematic representation of biosensor components.

which translates the recognition event into a signal (see Figure 6.21). The transducer probe may be in contact with the biochemical process directly or through a membrane. The biosensor monitors specific changes in the microenvironment of the system being studied.

The integral biological component is critical to detect selectively particular molecules present in a highly complex mixture. The component can be a native enzyme, engineered enzyme, multienzyme system, antibody, catalytic antibody, antigen, DNA probe, organelle, cell or whole organism, etc. capable of creating a measurable product of, or forming an intermolecular interaction with the molecule(s) being analyzed. The most commonly employed biological component is an immobilized enzyme or microbial cell.

For example, microbial biosensors have been engineered that consist of immobilized whole cells and either an oxygen probe or an electrode. Analyzing compounds of interest is accomplished by either directly measuring microbial respiration or formation of electroactive metabolites (i.e., protons, hydrogen, carbon dioxide, etc.), respectively.

Alberte has stated that biosensors "offer non-conventional, remote real-time or near real-time sensor technologies that embody (1) high signal-to-noise performance, (2) high levels of discrimination, (3) multi-target capabilities, (4) potential expendability, (5) long-term unattended field deployment capabilities and (6) broad ranges in area coverage" (Alberte, 1994). Disadvantages of biosensors include their inability to be steam sterilized, their reaction with products being formed from the biological component and oversensitivity.

Biosensors are applied for the detection, monitoring or quantification of trace chemicals or biologics in the environment or in living systems. The major application area of this biotechnology is in clinical diagnostics. An example of a product being developed is the use of a glucose oxidase-based biosensor as a test for blood glucose levels. Biosensors are also used in drug discovery (Matthews, 1995). Optical biosensors (measuring light at the boundary between media of different refractive index) can provide detailed information on the physiological responses of various cell types to a wide range of receptor specific ligands (agonists and antagonists). They have generated valuable data on the nature of intermolecular interactions in real-time, including on- and off-rates and affinity constants.

The Impact of Biotechnology on Drug Discovery

Overview

Pharmaceutical scientists have taken advantage of every opportunity or technique available to aid in the long, costly drug discovery process (see Chapter 18). In essence, Chapter 6 is an overview of some of the many applications of biotechnology and related techniques useful in drug discovery or design and development. In addition to recombinant DNA and hybridoma technology, the techniques described earlier in Chapter 6 have changed the way drug research is conducted. In a review of the impact of biotechnology on drug discovery, Venuti has suggested that pharmaceutical scientists have refined "without major obstacles" the process that optimizes the pharmacological properties of an identified novel chemical lead (Venuti, 1990; see also Setti and Micetich, 1996).

The polymerase chain reaction, transgenic animal models of human disease, knockout mice, protein engineering and related techniques (including structure determination methods such as X-ray crystallography, NMR and molecular modeling), peptidomimetic modifications, nucleic acid technologies (including antisense technology, aptamer technology and ribozyme catalysis), glycobiology and biosensors have contributed significantly to the drug discovery process.

In Vitro Screening

CONTRIBUTIONS OF BIOTECHNOLOGY

Traditionally, drug discovery programs relied heavily upon random screening followed by analog synthesis and lead optimization. The search for novel, efficacious, and safer medicinal agents is an increasingly costly and complex process. Therefore, any method allowing for a reduction in time and money is extremely valuable. Advances in biotechnology have contributed to a greater understanding of the cause and progression of disease and have identified new therapeutic targets forming the basis of novel drug screens. These advances have facilitated the discovery of new agents with novel mechanisms of action for diseases that were previously difficult or impossible to treat. Recombinant DNA technology has provided the ability to clone, express, isolate and purify receptor enzymes, membrane bound proteins, and other binding proteins in larger quantities than ever before. Instead of using receptors present in animal tissues or partially-purified enzymes for screening, in vitro bioassays now utilize the exact human protein target (Dykes, 1993; Angerhofer and Pezzuto, 1993). Applications of biotechnology to in vitro screening include the improved preparation of: 1) cloned membrane-bound receptors expressed in cell-lines carrying few endogenous receptors; 2) immobilized preparations of receptors, antibodies and other ligand-binding proteins; and 3) soluble enzymes and extracellular cell-surface expressed protein receptors.

HIGH-THROUGHPUT SCREENING (HTS)

Traditional drug research relied heavily on random screening followed by structure-activity studies and lead optimization (Setti and Micetich, 1996; Wermuth, 1996). Libraries of synthetic compounds along with natural products from microbial fermentation, plant extracts, marine organisms and invertebrates provide a diversity of molecular structures to screen randomly. Screening can be made more directed if the compounds to be investigated are selected on the basis of structural information about the receptor or natural ligand. The development of sensitive radioligand binding assays and the access to fully automated, robotic screening techniques have accelerated the screening process.

High-throughput screening (HTS) provides for the bioassay of thousands of compounds in multiple assays (as many as 50) at the same time. The process is automated with robots and utilizes 96-well microtiter plates. Enzyme inhibition assays and radioligand binding assays are the most common biochemical tests employed. In most cases today, biotechnology contributes directly to the understanding, identification and/or the generation of the drug target being screened (e.g., radioligand binding displacement from a cloned protein receptor).

COMBINATORIAL CHEMISTRY

One of the most powerful tools to optimize drug discovery in the 1990's is combinatorial chemistry. The combinatorial approach involves the simultaneous synthesis of

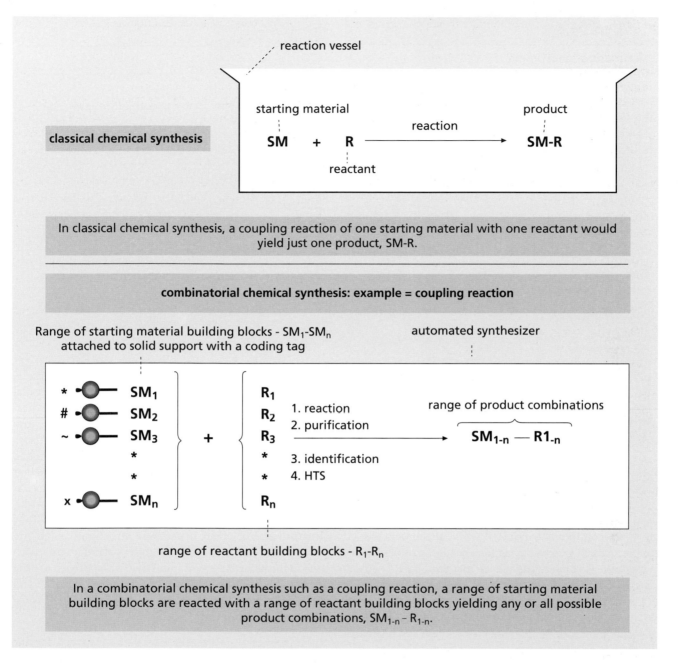

Figure 6.22. A schematic representation of a coupling reaction: difference between classical chemical synthesis and combinatorial chemistry.

hundreds or thousands of related drug candidates (Gallop et al., 1994; Gordon et al., 1994; Ecker and Crooke, 1995; Appell et al., 1996; Baum, 1996; De Witt, 1996; Ferguson et al., 1996; Fenniri, 1996; Mjalli and Harris, 1996). The molecular libraries generated are screened in high-through-put screening assays for the desired activity, and the most active molecules are identified and isolated for further development.

Figure 6.22 provides an illustration of this mix-and-match process in which a simple building block (a starting material such as an amino acid, peptide, heterocycle, other small molecule, etc.) is joined to one or more other simple building blocks in every possible combination. Assigning the task to automated synthesizing equipment results in the rapid creation of large collections or libraries of diverse molecules. The syntheses can take place in solution, but

Compound types
α,β-unsaturated ketones
α-hydroxy acids
acyl piperidines
azoles
β-mercaptoketones
β-turn mimetics
benzisothiazolones
benzodiazepines
biaryls
cyclopentenones
dihydropyridines
γ-butyrolactones
glycosylamines
hydantoins
isoxazoles
isoxazolines
modified oligonucleotides
peptoids
piperazinediones
porphyrins
1,3-propanediols
protease inhibitors
pyrrolidines
sulfamoylbenzamides
tetrahydrofurans
thiazole
thiazolidinones

Table 6.6. A sample of the diversity of compounds capable of being synthesized by combinatorial chemistry methods.

Reaction types
amidation
amide alkylation
cycloaddition
Diels-Alder reaction
enolate alkylation
esterifications
hydroboration
intermolecular cyclization
Michael addition
Mitsunobu reaction
nucleophilic substitution
oxidation
reduction
reductive alkylation
Wittig reaction

Table 6.7. A selection of reactions used in combinatorial chemistry to produce compound libraries.

are more commonly conducted while attached to a solid support (which improves reaction specificity and facilitates compound isolation). Ingenious methods have been devised to direct the molecules to be synthesized, to identify the structure of the products and to isolate compounds. When coupled with high-throughput screening, thousands of compounds can be generated, screened, and evaluated for further development in a matter of weeks.

Building blocks include amino acids, peptides, nucleotides, carbohydrates, and a diversity of small molecule scaffolds or templates. A sample of the diversity of compounds capable of being synthesized by combinatorial chemistry methods is shown in Table 6.6. A selection of reactions used in combinatorial chemistry to produce compound libraries is found in Table 6.7.

Rational Drug Design

Rational drug design or computer-assisted drug design is an iterative process where 3-D structure determination, analysis, design, synthesis and bioassay form a dynamic feedback cycle. To undertake a rational drug design study, a structure for the target receptor (satisfied by the availability of macromolecular crystal structures including recombinant proteins) is required. Biotechnology generally provides the target receptor. *A priori* rational drug design employs the X-ray crystallographic structure to create the initial, structurally novel lead compound with the aid of molecular graphics. A retrospective method, *a posteriori analysis*, rationalizes existing structure-activity relationship data (reflecting ligand binding to the target receptor) with X-ray structure and/or NMR postulating structural design improvements. Rational drug design is a standard approach used in the pharmaceutical industry. This approach to drug design has been reviewed and a number of successful studies could be identified (Greer, 1994; Marshall, 1995; Rondeau and Schreuder, 1996).

Concluding Remarks

Tremendous advances have occurred in biotechnology since Watson and Crick determined the structure of DNA. Improved pharmaceuticals, novel therapeutic agents, unique diagnostic products, and new drug design tools have resulted from the escalating achievements of pharmaceutical biotechnology. While recombinant DNA technology and hybridoma techniques have received "most of the press", a wealth of additional and innovative biotechnologies have been and will continue to be developed in order to enhance pharmaceutical research. The polymerase chain reaction, genetically engineered animals, protein engineering, peptide chemistry and peptidomimetics, nucleic acid technologies, catalytic antibodies, glycobiology, and biosensors are directly influencing the pharmaceutical sciences and are well positioned to significantly impact modern pharmaceutical care. Additional techniques in biotechnology and molecular biology are rapidly improving the competitive process of drug discovery and development of new medicinal agents and diagnostics. Pharmacists, pharmaceutical scientists and pharmacy students should be poised to take advantage of the products and techniques made available by the unprecedented scope and pace of discovery in biotechnology. ∎

Further Reading

- **Borrebaeck CAK.** (1992). *Antibody Engineering: A Practical Guide.* New York, New York: WH Freeman and Company
- **Cohen JS.** (1989). *Oligodeoxynucleotides: Antisense Inhibitors of Gene Expression.* Boca Raton, Florida: CRC Press
- **Dean PM, Jolles G, Newton CG.** (1995). *New Perspectives in Drug Design.* San Diego, California: Academic Press
- **Houdebine LM.** (1997). *Transgenic Animals — Generation and Use.* Amsterdam: Harwood Academic Publishers
- **Innis MA, Gelfand DH, Sninsky JJ.** (1995). *PCR Strategies.* San Diego, California: Academic Press
- **Mayforth RD.** (1993). *Designing Antibodies.* San Diego, California: Academic Press
- **Metcalf BW, Dalton BJ, Poste G.** (1994). *Cellular Adhesion. Molecular Definition to Therapeutic Potential.* New York, New York: Plenum Press
- **Mullis KB, Ferré F, Gibbs RA.** (1994). *The Polymerase Chain Reaction.* Boston, Massachusetts: Birkhäuser
- **Murray JAH.** (1992). *Antisense RNA and DNA.* New York, New York: Wiley-Liss
- **Musser JH.** (1992). Carbohydrates as Drug Discovery Leads. *Ann Rep Med Chem,* 27, 301–310
- **Oxender DL, Fox CF.** (1987). *Protein Engineering.* New York, New York: Alan R. Liss
- **Swanson ME, Grass DS, Ciofalo VB.** (1994). Transgenic and Gene Targeting Technology in Drug Discovery. *Ann Rep Med Chem,* 29, 265–274
- **Turner APF, Karube I, Wilson GS.** (1987). *Biosensors. Fundamentals and Applications.* Oxford, England: Oxford University Press

References

- **Abraham DJ.** (1989). X-Ray Crystallography and Drug Design. In *Computer-Aided Drug Design,* edited by TJ Perun and CL Propst. New York, New York: Marcel Dekker, Inc, pp. 93–132
- **Abravaya K, Carrino JJ, Muldoon S, Lee HH.** (1995). Detection of point mutations with a modified ligase chain reaction (Gap-LCR). *Nucleic Acids Res,* 23, 675–682
- **Adair JR.** (1992). Engineering antibodies for therapy. *Immunol Rev,* 130, 5–40
- **Adang AEP, Hermkens PHH, Linders JTM, Ottenheijm HCJ, van Staveren CJ.** (1994). Case histories of peptidomimetics: progression from peptide to drugs. *Recl Trav Chim Pays-Bas,* 113, 63–78
- **Agrawal A.** (1996). *Antisense Therapeutics.* Totowa, New Jersey: Humana Press
- **Akhtar S, Juliano RL.** (1992). Cellular uptake and intracellular fate of antisense oligonucleotides. *Trends in Cell Biol,* 2, 139–144
- **Alberte RS.** (1994). Biosensor Technologies: Perspectives and Promise. *Naval Res Rev,* 46, 2–3

- **Allen HJ, Kisailus EC.** (1992). *Glycoconjugates: Composition, Structure, and Function.* New York, New York: Marcel Dekker, Inc
- **Andes A-C, Schonenberger C-A, Groner B, Henninghausen L, LeMeur M, Gerlinger P.** (1987). Ha-*ras* Oncogene expression directed by milk protein gene promoter: Tissue specificity, hormonal regulation, and tumor induction in transgenic mice. *Proc Natl Acad Sci USA,* 84, 1299–1303
- **Angerhofer CK, Pezzuto JM.** (1993). Applications of Biotechnology in Drug Discovey and Evaluation. In *Biotechnology and Pharmacy,* edited by JM Pezzuto, ME Johnson, HR Manasse. New York, New York: Chapman & Hall, pp. 312–365
- **Appell KC, Chung TDY, Ohlmeyer MJ, Sigal NH, Baldwin JJ, Chelsky D.** (1996). Biological Screening of a Large Combinatorial Library. *J Biomolecular Screen,* 1, 27–31
- **Archer SJ, Domaille PJ, Laue ED.** (1996). New NMR Methods for Structural Studies of Proteins to Aid Drug Design. *Ann Rep Med Chem* 31, 299–307

- **Arnheim N, Erlich HA.** (1992). PCR Strategy. *Annu Rev Biochem*, 61, 131–156
- **Atherton E, Sheppard RC.** (1989). *Solid Phase Peptide Synthesis, A Practical Approach*. Oxford, England: IRL Press at Oxford University Press
- **Ausubel FM, Brent R, Kingston RE, Moore DD, Seidman JG, Smith JA, Struhl K.** (1995). *Short Protocols in Molecular Biology*, 3rd Ed. New York, New York: Wiley
- **Bains W.** (1993). *Biotechnology from A to Z*. Oxford, England: Oxford University Press, p. 19
- **Baird BA, McLafferty FW.** (1993). Chemistry and Immunology: A Powerful Combination. *Acc Chem Res*, 26, 389–390
- **Barany F.** (1991a). Genetic disease detection and DNA amlification using cloned thermostable ligase. *Proc Natl Acad Sci USA*, 88, 189–193
- **Barany F.** (1991b). The ligation chain assay in the PCR world. *PCR Methods Appl*, 1, 5–16
- **Barbar E, Barany G, Woodward C.** (1996). Unfolded BPTI variants with a single disulfide bond have diminished non-native structure distant from the crosslink. *Folding & Design*, 1, 65–76
- **Baum R.** (1996). Combinatorial Chemistry. *Chem Eng News*, February 12, 28–54
- **Benkovic SJ.** (1992). Catalytic Antibodies. *Annu Rev Biochem*, 61, 29–54
- **Berger EG, Buddecke E, Kamerling JP, Kobata A, Paulson JC, Vliegenthart JFG.** (1982). Structure, biosynthesis and functions of glycoprotein glycans. *Experientia*, 38, 1129–1162
- **Bevilacqua MP.** (1993). Endothelial-leukocyte adhesion molecules. *Annu. Rev. Immunol*, 11, 767–804
- **Bevilacque MP, Stengelin S, Gimbrone MA.** (1989). Endothelial Leukocyte Adhesion Molecule 1: An Inducible Receptor for Neutrophils Related to Complement Regulatory Proteins and Lectins. *Science*, 243, 1160–1165
- **Borg S, Estenne-Bouhton G, Luthman K, Csöregh I, Hesselink W, Hacksell U.** (1995). Synthesis of 1, 2, 4-oxadiazole, 1, 3, 4-oxadiazole, and 1, 2, 4-triazole-derived dipeptidomimetics. *J Org Chem*, 60, 3112–3120
- **Borman S.** (1996). Carbohydrates' Complexities. *Chem Eng News*, September 30, 36–40
- **Boyle S, Guard S, Higginobottom M, Horwell DC, Howson W, McKnight AT, Martin K, Pritchard MC, O'Toole J, Raphy J, Rees DC, Roberts E, Watling KJ, Woodruff GN, Hughes J.** (1994). Rational design of high affinity tachykinin NK₁ receptor antagonists. *Bioorg Med Chem*, 2, 357–370
- **Brackenbury R.** (1990). Cell Adhesion Molecules. *Ann Rep Med Chem*, 25, 235–244
- **Bradbury MG, Parish CR.** (1991). Characterization of lymphocyte receptors for glycosaminoglycans. *Immunology*, 72, 231–238
- **Breslow J.** (1994). Lipoprotein and heart disease: transgenic mice models helping in the search for new therapies. *Bio/Technology*, 12, 665–370
- **Brooks CL, Karplus M, Pettitt M.** (1988). *Proteins – A Theoretical Perspective of Dynamics, Structure, and Thermodynamics*. New York, New York: Wiley-Interscience
- **Buck RP, Hatfield WE, Umana M, Bowden EF.** (1990). *Biosensor Technology*. New York, New York: Dekker
- **Butcher EC.** (1991). Leukocyte-Endotherial Cell Recognition: Three (or more) Steps to Specificity and Diversity. *Cell*, 67, 1033–1036
- **Cass AEG.** (1990). *Biosensors. A Practical Approach*. Oxford, England: IRL Press
- **Cate JH, Gooding AR, Podell E, Zhou K, Golden BL, Kundrot CE, Cech TR, Doundna JA.** (1996). Crystal Structure of a group I Ribozyme Domain: Principles of RNA Packing. *Science*, 273, 1678–1685
- **Cebon J, Nicola N, Ward M, Gardner I, Dempsey P, Layton J, Duhrsen U, Burgess AW, Nice E, Morstyn G.** (1990). Granulocyte-macrophage colony stimulating factor from human lymphocytes. *J Biol Chem*, 265, 4483–4491
- **Christoffersen RE, Marr JJ.** (1995). Ribozymes as Human Therapeutic Agents. *J Med Chem*, 38, 2023–2037
- **Clapp JP.** (1996). *Species Giagnostics Protocols. PCR and Other Nucleic Acid Methods*. Humana Press: Totowa, New Jersey
- **Cleland JL, Craik CS.** (1996). *Protein Engineering. Principles and Practice*. New York, New York: Wiley-Liss
- **Colby CB, Inoue M, Thompson M, Tan YH.** (1984). Immunologic differentiation between E. coli and CHO cell-derived recombinant and natural human β-interferons. *J Immunol*, 133, 3091–3095
- **Collins FS, Wilson JM.** (1992). A welcome animal model. *Nature*, 358, 708–709
- **Cook PD.** (1991). Medicinal chemistry of antisense oligonucleotides – Future opportunities. *Anti-Cancer Drug Design*, 6, 585–607
- **Craik, CS, Roczniak S, Largman C, Rutter WJ.** (1987). The catalytic role of the active site aspartic acid in serine proteases. *Science*, 237, 909–913
- **Craik DJ.** (1996). *NMR in Drug Design*, Boca Raton, Florida: CRC Press
- **Crooke ST.** (1992a). Therapeutic applications of oligonucleotides. *Annu Rev Biochem*, 32, 329–376
- **Crooke ST.** (1992b). Therapeutic applications of oligonucleotides. *Bio/Technology*, 10, 882–886
- **Crooke ST.** (1995a). Oligonucleotide Therapeutics. In *Burger's Medicinal Chemistry, Fifth Edition*, edited by ME Wolff, Vol. 1. New York, New York: John Wiley & Sons, Inc, pp. 863–900
- **Crooke ST.** (1995b). The Future of Antisense Technology. *Pharmaceut News*, 2, 8–11
- **Cumming DA.** (1991). Glycosylation of recombinant protein therapeutics: control and functional implications. *Glycobiology*, 1, 115–130
- **Cuthbertson RA, Klintworth GK.** (1988). Biology of disease: transgenic mice – a goldmine for furthering knowledge in pathobiology. *Lab Invest*, 58, 404–502
- **Dabelsteen E, Clausen H.** (1992). *Carbohydrate Pathology*, APMIS supplement no. 27, vol. 100. Copenhagen, Denmark: Munksgaard Publishers
- **Davies DR, Chacko S.** (1993). Antibody structure. *Acc Chem Res*, 26, 412–427

- Davis GR, Blumeyer K, DiMichele LJ, Whitfield KM, Chappelle H, Riggs N, Gosh SS, Kao PM, Fahy E, Kwoh DY. (1990). Detection of human immunodeficiency virus type I in AIDS patients using amplification-mediated hybridization analyses: reproducibility and quantitative limitations. *J Infect Dis*, 162, 13–20

- De-Barbeyrac B, Rodriguez P, Dutilh B, Le-Roux P, Bebear C. (1995). Detection of *Chlamydia trachomatis* by ligase chain reaction compared with polymerase chain reaction and cell culture in urogenital specimens. *Genitourin Med*, 71, 382–386

- Delahunty C, Ankener W, Deng Q, Eng J, Nickerson DA. (1996). Testing the feasibility of DNA typing for human identification by PCR and an oligonucleotide ligation assay. *Am J Hum Genet*, 58, 1239–1246

- De Witt SH. (1996). Combinatorial Libraries and High-Throughput Synthesis. In *The Practice of Medicinal Chemistry*, edited by CG Wermuth. San Diego, California: Academic Press, pp. 117–134

- Dervan PB. (1989). Oligonucleotide Recognition of Double-helical DNA by Triple-helix Formation. In *Oligodeoxynucleotides: Antisense Inhibitors of Gene Expression*, edited by JS Cohen. Boca Raton, Florida: CRC Press, pp. 197–210

- Devine PL, McKenzie IFC. (1992). Mucins: Structure, function, and associations with malignancy. *BioEssays*, 14, 619–625

- Donahue RE, Wang EA, Kaufman RJ, Foutch L, Leary AC, Witek-Giannetti JS, Metzger M, Hewick RM, Steinbrink DR, Shaw G, Kamen R, Clark SC. (1986). Effects of N-linked carbohydrate on the *in vivo* properties of human GM-CSF. *Cold Spring Harbour Symp Quant Biol*, 51, 685–692

- Donehower LA, Harvey M, Slagle BL, McArthur MJ, Montgomery Jr. CA, Butel JS, Bradley A. (1992). Mice deficient for p53 are developmentally normal but susceptible to spontaneous tumors. *Nature*, 356, 215–221

- Ducruis A, Giege R. (1992). *Crystallization of Nucleic Acids and Proteins – A Practical Approach*. Oxford, England: IHL Press

- Dugas H. (1989a). *Bioorganic Chemistry: A Chemical Approach to Enzyme Action*. New York, New York: Springer-Verlag, pp. 89–96

- Dugas H. (1989b). *Bioorganic Chemistry: A Chemical Approach to Enzyme Action* New York, New York: Springer-Verlag, pp. 85–89

- Dykes CW. (1993). Molecular Biology in the Pharmaceutical Industry. In *Molecular Biology and Biotechnology*, edited by JM Walker and EB Gingold. Cambridge, England: The Royal Society of Chemistry, pp. 164–176

- Ecker DJ, Crooke ST. (1995). Combinatorial drug discovery: which methods will produce the greatest value? *Bio/Technology*, 13, 351–360

- Eggerding FA. (1995). A one-step coupled amplification and oligonucleotide ligation procedure for multiplex genetic typing. *PCR Methods Appl*, 4, 337–345

- Elbein AD. (1991). The role of N-linked oligosaccharides in glycoprotein function. *Trends Biotechnol*, 9, 346–352

- Ellington AD, Szostak JW. (1990). *In vitro* selection of RNA molecules that bind specific ligands. *Nature*, 346, 818–822

- Evans BE, Bock MG, Rittle KE, DiPardo RM, Whitter WL, Veber DF, Anderson PS, Freidinger RM. (1986). Design of potent, orally effective, nonpeptidal antagonists of the peptide hormone cholecystokinin. *Proc Natl Acad Sci USA*, 83, 4918–4922

- Ezzell C. (1988). First ever animal patent issued in United States. *Nature (London)*, 332, 668

- Farmer PS. (1980). Bridging the gap beteen bioactive peptides and nonpeptides: some perspectives in design. *Drug Design*, 10, pp.119–143

- Fenniri H. (1996). Recent Advances at the Interface of Medicinal and Combinatorial Chemistry. Views on Methodologies for the Generation and Evaluation of Diversity and Application to Molecular Recognition and Catalysis. *Curr Med Chem*, 3, 343–378

- Ferguson AM, Patterson DE, Garr CD, Underiner TL. (1996). Designing Chemical Libraries for Lead Discovery. *J Biomolecular Screen*, 1, 65–73

- Fodor WL, William BL, Matis LA, Madri JA, Rollins SA, Knight JW, Velander W, Squinto SA. (1994). Expression of a functional human complement inhibitor in a transgenic pig as a model for the prevention of xenogeneic hyperacute organ rejection. *Proc Natl Acad Sci USA*, 91, 11153–11157

- Fothergill-Gilmore LA. (1993). Recombinant protein technology. In *Protein Biotechnology*, edited by F Franks. Totowa, New Jersey: Humana Press, pp. 467–487

- Fox JL. (1993). Transgenic mice fall far short. *Bio/Technology*, 11, 663

- Fukuda M. (1992). *Cell Surface Carbohydrates and Cell Development*. Ann Arbor, Michigan: CRC Press

- Fukuda M, Kobata A. (1993). *Glycobiology: A Practical Approach*. Oxford, England: IRL Press

- Fukuda MN, Sasaki H, Lopez L, Fukuda M. (1989). Survival of recombinant erythropoietin in the circulation: the role of carbohydrates. *Blood*, 73, 84–89

- Furukawa K, Matsuta K, Takeuchi F, Kosuge E, Miyamoto T, Kobata A. (1990). Kinetic study of a galactosyltransferase in the B cells of patients with rheumatoid arthritis. *Int Immunol*, 2, 105–112

- Furukawa K, Kobata, A. (1991). IgG galactosylation – its biological significance and pathology. *Mol Immunol*, 28, 1333–1340

- Gallop MA, Barrett RW, Dower WJ, Fodor SPA, Gordon EM. (1994). Applications of Combinatorial Technologies to Drug Discovery. 1. Background and Peptide Combinatorial Libraries. *J Med Chem*, 37, 1233–1251

- Gallop MA, Barrett RW, Dower WJ, Fodor SPA, Gordon EM. (1994). Applications of combinatorial technologies to drug discovery. 1. Background and peptide combinatorial libraries. *J Med Chem*, 37, 1233–1251

- Gante J. (1994). Peptidomimetics – tailored enzyme inhibitors. *Angew Chem Int Ed Engl*, 33, 1699–1720

- Garnier J. (1990). Protein structure prediction. *Biochimie*, 72, 513–524

- **Giannis A, Kolter T.** (1993). Peptidomimetics for receptor ligands – Discovery, development, and medical perspectives. *Angew Chem Int Ed Engl*, 32, 1244–1267
- **Gillespie FP, Doros L, Vitale J, Blackwell C, Gosselin J, Snyder BW, Wadsworth SC.** (1993). Tissue-specific expression of human CD4 in transgenic mice. *Mol Cell Biol*, 13, 2952–2958
- **Gilon C, Halle D Chorev M, Selinger Z, Byk G.** (1991). Backbone cyclization: a new method for conferring conformational constraint on peptides. *Biopolymers*, 31, 745–750
- **Gingeras TR, Richman DD, Kwoh DY, Guatelli JC.** (1990). Methodologies for *in vitro* nucleic acid amplification and their applications. *Vet Microbiol*, 24, 235–251
- **Ginsburg V, Robbins P.** (1981). Biology of carbohydrates, vol. 1. New York: J Wiley
- **Goeddel DV, Kleid DG, Bolivar F, Heyneker HL, Yansura DG, Crea R, Hirose T, Kraszewski A, Itakura K, Riggs AD.** (1979). Expression in *Escherichia coli* of chemically synthesized genes for human insulin. *Proc Natl Acad Sci USA*, 76, 106–110
- **Golinelli-Pimpaneau B, Gigant B, Bizebard T, Navaza J, Saludjian P, Zemel R, Tawfik DS, Eshhar Z, Green BS, Knossow M.** (1994). Crystal structure of a catalytic antibody Fab with esterase-like activity. *Structure*, 2, 175–183
- **Goodman M, Ro S.** (1995). Peptidomimetics for Drug Design. In *Burger's Medicinal Chemistry, Fifth Edition*, edited by ME Wolff, Vol. 1. New York, New York: John Wiley & Sons, Inc, pp. 803–861
- **Gordon EM, Barrett RW, Dower WJ, Fodor SPA, Gallop MA.** (1994). Applications of Combinatorial Technologies to Drug Discovery. 2. Combinatorial Organic Synthesis, Library Screening Strategies, and Future Directions. *J Med Chem*, 37, 1385–1401
- **Graf von Roedern E, Kessler H.** (1994). A sugar amino acid as a novel peptidomimetic. *Angew Chem Int Ed Engl*, 33, 687–689
- **Greaves DR, Fraser P, Vidal MA, Hedges MJ, Ropers D, Luzzato L, Grosveld F.** (1990). Transgenic mouse model of sickle cell disorder. *Nature*, 343, 183–185
- **Greer J, Erickson JW, Baldwin JJ, Varney MD.** (1994). Application of the Three-Dimensional Structures of Protein Target Molecules in Structure-Based Drug Design. *J Med Chem*, 37, 1035–1054
- **Guerrier-Takade C, Gardiner K, Marsh T, Pace N, Altman S.** (1983). The RNA moiety of ribonuclease P is the catalytic subunit of the enzyme. *Cell*, 35, 849–857
- **Gutte B.** (1995). *Peptides: Synthesis, Structures, and Applications.* San Diego, California: Academic Press
- **Hakomori S.** (1981). Glycosphingolipids in cellular interaction, differentiation, and oncogenesis. *Annu Rev Biochem*, 50, 733–764
- **Hall EAH.** (1990). *Biosensors.* Buckingham, England: Open University Press
- **Hanahan D.** (1989). Transgenic mice as probes into complex systems. *Science*, 246, 1265–1275
- **Hanahan D.** (1990). Transgenic mouse models of self-tolerance and autoreactivity by the immune system. *Ann Rev Cell Biol*, 6, 493–537
- **Hart GW.** (1992). Glycosylation. *Curr Opin Cell Biol*, 4, 1017–1023
- **Harwood AJ.** (1996). *Basic DNA and RNA Protocols.* Totowa, New Jersey: Humana Press
- **Hayek T, Azrolan N Verdeny RB, Walsh A, Shajek-Shaul J, Agellon LB, Tall AR, Breslo JL.** (1993). Hypertension and cholesteryl ester transfer protein interact to dramatically alter high density lipoprotein levels, particle sizes and metabolism. Studies in transgenic mice. *J Clin Invest*, 92, 1143–1152
- **Helene C, Thuong NT, Harel-Bellan A.** (1992). Control of Gene Expression by Triple Helix-Forming Oligonucleotides. *Ann NY Acad Sci*, 660, 27–36
- **Hendrickson WA.** (1987). X-Ray Diffraction. In *Protein Engineering*, edited by DL Oxender and CF Fox. New York, New York: Alan R. Liss, pp. 5–13
- **Hiramatsu Y, Tsujishita H, Kondo H.** (1996). Studies on Selectin Blocker. 3. Investigation of the Carbohydrate Ligand Sialyl Lewis X Recognition Site of P-Selectin. *J Med Chem*, 39, 4547–4553
- **Hirschmann R, Nicolaou KC, Pietranico S, Leahy EM, Salvino J, Arison B, Cichy MA, Spoors PG, Shakespeare WC, Sprengler PA, Hamley P, Smith III AB, Reisine T, Raynor K, Maechler L, Donaldson C, Vale W, Freidinger RM, Cascieri MR, Strader CD.** (1993). *De novo* design and synthesis of somatostatin non-peptide peptidomimetics utilizing β-D-glucose as a novel scaffolding. *J Am Chem Soc*, 115, 12550–12568
- **Hirschmann R, Smith III AB, Sprengeler PA.** (1995). Some Interactions of macromolecules with Low Molecular Weight Ligands. Recent Advances in peptidomimetic Research. In *New Perspectives in Drug Design*, edited by PM Dean, G Jolles, CG Newton. San Diego, California: Academic Press, pp. 1–14
- **Hruby VJ.** (1982). Conformational restrictions of biologically active peptides via amino acid side chain groups. *Life Sci*, 31, 189–199
- **Hughes J, Smith TW, Kostelitz HW, Fothergill LA, Morgan BA, Morris HR.** (1975). Identification of two related pentapeptides from the brain with potent opiate agonist activity. *Nature*, 258, 577–579
- **Innis MA, Gelfand DH, Sninsky JJ, White TJ.** (1990). *PCR Protocols: A Guide to Methods and Applications.* San Diego, California: Academic Press
- **Innis MA, Gelfand DH, Sninsky JJ.** (1995). *PCR Strategies.* San Diego, California: Academic Press
- **Isenberg WM, McEver RP, Shuman MA, Bainton DF.** (1986). Topographic Distribution of a Granule Membrane Protein (GMP-140) that is Expressed on the Platelet Surface after Activation: an Immunogold-Surface Replica Study. *Blood Cells*, 12, 191–204
- **Isola LM, Gordon JW.** (1991). Transgenic animals: a new era in developmental biology and medicine. In *Transgenic Animals*, edited by NL First and FP Haseltine. Boston, Massachusetts: Butterworth-Heinemann, pp. 3–20
- **Iversen P.** (1991). *In vivo* studies with phosphorothioate oligonucleotides: Pharmacokinetics prologue. *Anti-Cancer Drug Design*, 6, 531–538

- Jacobs J, Schultz PG, Sugasawara R, Powell M. (1987). Catalytic antibodies. *J Am Chem Soc*, 109, 2174–2176
- Jefferis R. (1994). Antibodies. In *The Encyclopedia of Molecular Biology*, edited by J Kendrew. Oxford, England: Blackwell Science Ltd, pp. 54–57
- Jefson M. (1988). Applications of NMR Spectroscopy to Protein Structure Determination. *Ann Rep Med Chem* 23, 275–283
- Jencks WP. (1969). *Catalysis in Chemistry and Enzymology*. New York, New York: McGraw-Hill, p. 268
- Jenkins N, Parekh RB, James DC. (1996). Getting the glycosylation right: Implications for the biotechnology industry. *Nature Biotechnol*, 14, 975–981
- Kahn M. (1993). Peptide secondary structure mimetics: recent advances and future challenges. *Synlett*, 821–826
- Karplus M. (1987). The Prediction and Analysis of Mutant Structures. In *Protein Engineering*, edited by DL Oxender and CF Fox. New York, New York: Alan R. Liss, pp. 35–44
- Ke H, Mayrose D, Belshaw PJ, Alberg DG, Schreiber SL, Chang ZY, Etzkorn FA, Ho S, Walsh CT. (1994). Crystal structures of cyclophilin A complexed with cyclosporin A and N-methyl-4-[(E)-2-butenyl]-4,4-dimethylthreonine cyclosporin A. *Structure*, 2, 33–44
- Kobata A. (1991). Function and pathology of the sugar chains of human immunoglobulin G. *Glycobiology*, 1, 5–8
- Kobata A. (1992). Structures and functions of the sugar chains of glycoproteins. *Eur J Biochem*, 209, 483–501
- Kobata A. (1994). Principles of Glycobiology. In *Tools for Glycobiology*. Oxford, England: Oxford Glycosystems, pp. 3–8
- Kool ET. (1996). Topological modification of oligonucleotides for potential inhibition of gene expression. *Perspectives in Drug Discovery and Design*, 4, 61–75
- Krafft GA, Wang GT. (1990). Catalytic Antibodies: A New Class of Designer Enzymes. *Ann Rep Med Chem*, 25, 299–308
- Krueger RJ. (1995). Ribozymes: RNA as a Therapeutic Agent. *Amer Pharm*, NS35, No. 1, 12–13
- Kruger K, Grabowski PJ, Zaug AJ, Sands J, Gottschling DE, Cech TR. (1982). Self-splicing RNA: autoexcision and autocyclization of the ribosomal RNA intervening sequence of *Tetrahymena*. *Cell*, 31, 147–157
- Kunkel T. (1985). Rapid and efficient site-specific mutagenisis without phenotypic selection. *Proc Natl Acad Sci USA*, 82, 488–492
- Kurtz ID. (1992). Structure-based strategies for drug design and discovery. *Science*, 257, 1078–1082
- Kwoh DY, Davis GR, Whitfield KM, Chappelle HL, DiMichele LJ, Grigeras TR. (1989). Transcription-based amplification system and detection of amplified human immunodeficiency virus type 1 with a bead-based sandwich hybridization format. *Proc Natl Acad Sci USA*, 86, 1173–1177
- Kwoh DY, Kwoh TJ. (1990). Target amplification systems in nucleic acid-based diagnostic approaches. *Am Biotechnol Lab*, 8, 14–25
- Kwok PY, Gremund MF, Nickerson DA, Hood L, Olson MV. (1992). Automatable screening of yeast artificial-chromosome libraries based on the oligonucleotide-ligation assay. *Genomics*, 13, 935–941
- Laffler TG, Carrino JJ, Marshall RL. (1993). The ligase chain reaction in DNA-based diagnosis. *Ann Biol Clin Paris*, 51, 821–826
- Landegren U, Kaiser R, Caskey CT, Hood L. (1988). DNA diagnostics – molecular techniques and automation. *Science*, 242, 229–237
- Landegren U. (1993). Ligation-based DNA diagnostics. *Biassays*, 15, 761–766
- Lane DP. (1993). A death in the life of p53. *Nature*, 362, 786–787
- Larrick JW, Siebert PD. (1995). *Reverse Transcriptase PCR*. London, England: Ellis Horwood
- Lasky LA. (1992). Selectins: interpreters of cell-specific carbohydrate information during inflammation. *Science*, 258, 964–969
- Lawrence MB, Springer TA. (1991). Leukocytes Roll on a Selectin at Physiologic Flow Rates: Distinction from and Prerequisite for Adhesion through Integrins. *Cell*, 65, 859–873
- Lebedev AV, Wickstrom E. (1996). The chirality problem in P-substituted oligonucleotides. *Perspectives in Drug Discovery and Design*, 4, 17–40
- Leder A Pattengale PK, Kuo A, Stewart TA, Leder P. (1986). Consequences of widespread deregulation of the c-*myc* gene in transgenic mice: Multiple neoplasms and normal development. *Cell*, 45, 485–495
- Lee H. (1993). Infectious disease testing by ligase chain reaction. *Clin. Chem*, 4, 1–3
- Lerner RA, Benkovic SJ, Schultz PG. (1991). At the crossroads of chemistry and immunology: catalytic antibodies. *Science*, 252, 659–667
- Lesser W. (1995). Transgenic Animal Patents. In *Molecular Biology and Biotechnology. A Comprehensive Desk Reference*, edited by RA Meyers. New York, New York: VCH Publishers, Inc, pp. 907–910
- Levy DE, Tang PC, Musser JH. (1994). Cell Adhesion and Carbohydrates. *Ann Rep Med Chem*, 29, 215–224
- Li Y, Luo L, Rasool N, Kang CY. (1993). Glycosylation is necessary for the correct folding of human immunodeficiency virus gp120 in CD4 binding. *J. Virol*, 67, 584–588
- Liskamp RMJ. (1994). Conformationally restricted amino acids and dipeptides, (non)peptidomimetics and secondary structure mimetics. *Recl Trav Chim Pays-Bas*, 113, 1–19
- Livingston DJ. (1989). Second Generation Recombinant Therapeutic Proteins. *Ann Rep Med Chem*, 24, 213–221
- Lodish H, Baltimore D, Berk A, Zipursky SL, Matsudaira P, Darnell J. (1995). *Molecular Cell Biology, Third Edition*. New York, New York: Scientific American Books, pp. 293–296
- Lundegren U. (1993). Ligation-based DNA diagnostics. *BioEssays*, 15, 761–766

- **Luthman K, Hacksell U.** (1996). Peptides and Peptidomimetics. In *A Textbook of Drug Design and Development*, edited by P Krogsgaard-Larsen, T Liljefors, U Madsen, 2nd Edition. Amsterdam, The Netherlands: Harwood Academic Publishers GmbH, pp. 386–406

- **Maramatsu T.** (1993). Carbohydrate signals in metastasis and prognosis of human carcinomas. *Glycobiology*, 3, 294–296

- **Markley JL.** (1987). One- and Two-Dimensional NMR Spectroscopic Investigations of the Consequences of Amino Acid Replacement in Proteins. In *Protein Engineering*, edited by DL Oxender and CF Fox. New York, New York: Alan R. Liss, pp. 15–33

- **Marotti KR, Castle CK, Boyle TP, Lin AH, Murray RW, Melchoir GW.** (1993). Severe atherosclerosis in transgenic mice expressing simian cholesteryl ester transfer protein. *Nature*, 364, 73–75

- **Marshall GR.** (1995). Molecular Modeling in Drug Design. In *Burger's Medicinal Chemistry, Fifth Edition*, edited by ME Wolff, Vol. 1. New York, New York: John Wiley & Sons, Inc, pp. 573–659

- **Marshall RL, Laffler TG, Cerney MB, Sustachek JC, Kratochvil JD, Morgan RL.** (1994). Detection of HCV RNA by the asymmetric gap ligase chain reaction. *PCR Methods Appl*, 4, 80–84

- **Matteucci M.** (1996). Structural modifications toward improved antisense oligonucleotides. *Perspectives in Drug Discovery and Design*, 4, 1–16

- **Matteucci MD, Bischofberger N.** (1991). Sequence-defined Oligonucleotides as Potential Therapeutics. *Ann Rep Med Chem*, 26, 287–296

- **Matthews DJ.** (1995). Applications of Biosensor Technology in Drug Discovery. *Ann Rep Med Chem*, 30, 275–283

- **McPherson MJ, Hames BD, Taylor GR.** (1995). *PCR 2. A Practical Approach*, Oxford, England: IRL Press

- **McRee DE.** (1993). *Practical Protein Crystallography*. San Diego, California: Academic Press

- **Miller PS, Ts'o POP.** (1988). Oligonucleotide Inhibitors of Gene Expression in Living Cells: New Opportunities in Drug Design. *Ann Rep Med Chem*, 23, 295–304

- **Milligan JF, Matteucci MD, Martin JC.** (1993). Current Concepts in Antisense Drug Design. *J Med Chem*, 36, 1923–1937

- **Mintz B, Klein-Szanto AJ.** (1992). Malignancy of eye melanomas originating in the retinal pigment epithelium of transgenic mice after genetic ablation of choroidal melanocytes. *Proc Natl Acad Sci USA*, 89, 11421–11425

- **Miyashita N, Matsumoto A, Niki Y, Matsushima T.** (1996). Evaluation of the sensitivity and specificity of a ligase chain reaction test kit for the detection of *Chlamydia trachomatis*. *J Clin Pathol*, 49, 515–517

- **Mjalli AMM, Harris AL.** (1996). Lead Generation Using Combinatorial Chemistry in Drug Discovery. *J Biomolecular Screen*, 1, 17–21

- **Morgan BA, Gainor JA.** (1989). Approaches to the Discovery of Non-Peptide Ligands for Peptide Receptors and Peptidases. *Ann Rep Med Chem*, 24, 243–252

- **Morikawa Y, Moore JP, Wilkinson AJ, Jones IM.** (1991). Reduction in CD4 binding affinity associated with removal of a single glycosylation site in the external glycoprotein of HIV-2. *Virology*, 180, 853–856

- **Muller WJ, Sinn E, Pattengale PK, Wallace R, Leder P.** (1988). Single step induction of mammary adenocarcinoma in transgenic mice bearing the activated c-*neu* oncogene. *Cell*, 54, 105–115

- **Mulligan MS, Lowe JB, Larsen RD, Paulson JC, Zheng ZL, de Frees S, Maemura K, Fukuda M, Ward PA.** (1993b). Protective effects of sialylated oligosaccharides in immune complex-induced acute lung injury. *J Exp Med*, 178, 623–631

- **Mulligan MS, Paulson JC, de Frees S, Zheng ZL, Lowe JB, Ward PA.** (1993a). Protective effects of oligosaccharides in P-selectin-dependent lung injury. *Nature*, 364, 149–151

- **Murray JAH, Crockett N.** (1992). Antisense techniques: an overview. In *Antisense RNA and DNA*, edited by JAH Murray. New York, New York: Wiley-Liss, pp. 1–49

- **Musser JH, Fügedi P, Anderson MB.** (1995). Carbohydrate-based Therapeutics. In *Burger's Medicinal Chemistry, Fifth Edition*, edited by ME Wolff, Vol. 1. New York, New York: John Wiley & Sons, Inc, pp. 901–947

- **Nakanishi H, Kahn M.** (1996). Design of peptidomimetics. In *The Practice of Medicinal Chemistry*, edited by CG Wermuth. San Diego, California: Academic Press, pp. 570–590

- **Narang SA.** (1990). *Protein Engineering, Approaches to the Manipulation of Protein Folding*. Stoneham, Massachusetts: Butterworth Publishers

- **Neilsen PE.** (1996). Peptide nucleic acid (PNA): A new lead for gene therapeutic drugs. *Perspectives in Drug Discovery and Design*, 4, 76–84

- **Newton CR.** (1995). *PCR Essential Data*. New York, New York: John Wiley and Sons

- **Nichols AJ, Vasko JA, Koster PF, Valocik RE, and Samanen JM.** (1994). GPIIb/IIIa Antagonists as Novel Antithrombic Drugs. In *Cellular Adhesion. Molecular Definition to Therapeutic Potential*, edited by BW Metcalf, BJ Dalton and G Poste. New York, New York: Plenum Press, pp. 213–237

- **O'Kane CJ, Moffat KG.** (1992). Selective cell ablation and genetic surgery. *Curr Opin Genet Dev*, 2, 602–60

- **Ohmoto H, Nakamura K, Inoue T, Kondo N, Inoue Y, Yoshino K, Kondo H, Ishida H, Kiso M, Hasegawa A.** (1996). Studies on Selectin Blocker. 1. Structure-Activity Relationships of Sialyl Lewis X Analogs. *J Med Chem*, 39, 41339–1343

- **Oxender DL.** (1985). *Protein Structure, Folding and Design*, Vol. 1. New York, New York: Alan R. Liss

- **Oxender DL.** (1986). *Protein Structure, Folding and Design*, Vol. 2. New York, New York: Alan R. Liss

- **Oxender DL, Fox CF.** (1987). *Protein Engineering*. New York, New York: Alan R. Liss

- **Parish JH, McPherson MJ.** (1987). Chemical and Biochemical Manipulation of DNA and the Expression of Foreign Genes in Micro-organisms. *Nat Prod Rep*, 4, 139–156

- **Pharmaceutical Research and Manufacturers of America.** (1996). *Biotechnology Medicines In Development.* Washington, DC

- **Pluckthun A.** (1992). Mono- and bivalent antibody fragments produced in *Escherichia coli*: engineering, folding and antigen binding. *Immunol Rev*, 130, 151–188

- **Pollack SJ, Jacobs JW, Schultz PG.** (1986). Selective chemical catalysis by an antibody. *Science*, 234, 1570–1573

- **Quon D, Wang Y, Catalano R, Scardina JM, Murakami K, Cordel B.** (1991). Formation of β-amyloid protein deposits in brains of transgenic mice. *Nature*, 352, 239–241

- **Rademacher TW, Parekh RB, Dwek RA.** (1988). Glycobiology. *Annu Rev Biochem*, 57, 785–838

- **Ramabhadran TV.** (1994). *Pharmaceutical Design and Development. A Molecular Biology Approach.* New York, New York: Springer-Verlag, pp. 246–277

- **Rasmussen JR.** (1992). Effect of glycosylation on protein function. *Curr Opin Struct Biol*, 2, 682–686

- **Richardson JS, Richardson DC.** (1990). The *de novo* synthesis of proteins. In *Proteins: Form and Function*, edited by RA Bradshaw and M Purton. Cambridge, England: Elsevier Trends Journal, pp. 173–182

- **Rondeau J-M, Schreuder H.** (1996). The Use of X-ray Structures of Receptors and Enzymes in Drug Discovery. In *The Practice of Medicinal Chemistry*, edited by CG Wermuth. San Diego, California: Academic Press, pp. 485–522

- **Rossi J, Zoller M.** (1987). Site-Specific and Regionally Directed Mutagenesis of Protein-Encoding. In *Protein Engineering*, edited by DL Oxender and CF Fox. New York, New York: Alan R. Liss, pp. 51–63

- **Rossi JJ.** (1995). Therapeutic antisense and ribozymes. *Br Med Bull*, 51, 217–225

- **Rouhi AM.** (1996). Oligosaccharides Coming of Age. *Chem Eng News*, September 23, 62–66

- **Rudolph NS.** (1995). Advances Continue in Production of Proteins in Transgenic Animal Milk. *Genet Eng News*, October 15, 8–9

- **Ruoslahti E.** (1988). Structure and biology of proteoglycans. *Annu Rev Cell Biol*, 4, 229–255

- **Scanlan TS.** (1995). Catalytic Antibodies. *Ann Rep Med Chem*, 30, 255–264

- **Schauer R.** (1991). Biosynthesis and function of N- and O-substituted sialic acids. *Glycobiology*, 1, 449–452

- **Scheller F, Schubert F.** (1992). *Biosensors.* Amsterdam, The Netherlands: Elsevier

- **Schnaar RL.** (1991). Glycosphingolipids in cell surface recognition. *Glycobiology*, 1, 477–485

- **Schuetz EG, Schinkel AH, Relling MV, Schuetz JD.** (1996). P-glycoprotein: a major determinant of rifampicin-inducible expression of cytochrome P450 3A in mice and humans. *Proc Natl Acad Sci USA*, 93, 4001–4005

- **Schultz PG, Lerner RA.** (1993). Antibody Catalysis of Difficult Chemical Transformations. *Acc Chem Res*, 26, 391–395

- **Sedivy JM, Joyner AL.** (1992). *Gene Targeting.* New York, New York: WH Freeman & Co

- **Setti EL, Micetich R.** (1996). Modern Drug Discovery and Lead Discovery: An Overview. *Curr Med Chem*, 3, 317–324

- **Sharon N, Lis H.** (1982). Glycoproteins: research booming on long-ignored ubiquitous compounds. *Mol Cell Biochem*, 42, 167–187

- **Spatola AF.** (1983). Peptide backbone modifications: a structure-activity analysis of peptides containing amide bond surrogates, conformational constraints, and related backbone replacements. In *Chemistry and Biochemistry of Amino Acids, Peptides, and Proteins*, edited by B Weinstein, Vol. VII. New York, New York: Marcel Dekker, pp. 267–357

- **Spertini O, Luscinskas FW, Gimbrone, Jr. MA, Tedder TF.** (1992). Monocyte attachment to activated human vascular endothelium *in vitro* is modulated by leukocyte adhesion molecule-1 (L-selectin) under nonstatic conditions. *J Exp Med*, 175, 1789–1792

- **Stein CA, Narayanan R.** (1996). Antisense oligodeoxynucleotides: Internalization, compartmentalization and non-sequence specificity. *Perspectives in Drug Discovery and Design*, 4, 41–50

- **Stewart JD, Liotta JL, Benkovic SJ.** (1993). Reaction mechanisms displayed by catalytic antibodies. *Acc Chem Res*, 26, 396–404

- **Stone GG, Oberst RD, Hays MP, McVey S, Chengappa MM.** (1995). Combined PCR-oligonucleotide ligation assay for rapid detection of *Salmonella serovars*. *J Clin Microbiol*, 33, 2888–2893

- **Stull RA, Szoka, Jr. FC.** (1995). Antigene, Ribozyme and Aptamer Nucleic Acid Drugs: Progress and Prospects. *Pharmaceut Res*, 12, 465–483

- **Takeuchi M, Takasaki S, Shimada M, Kobata A.** (1990). Role of sugar chains in the *in vitro* biological activity in human erythropoietin produced in recombinant Chinese hamster ovary cells. *J Biol Chem*, 265, 12127–12130

- **Thayer A.** (1996). Firms boost prospects for transgenic drugs. *Chem Eng News*, August 26, 23–24

- **Thayer AM.** (1990) Companies Designing Genetic Code Blocking Drugs To Treat Disease. *Chem Eng News*, December 3, 17–20

- **Tidd DM.** (1996). Specificity of antisense oligonucleotides. *Perspectives in Drug Discovery and Design*, 4, 51–60

- **Tramontano A, Janda KD, Lerner RA.** (1986). Catalytic Antibodies. *Science*, 234, 1566–1570

- **Tramontano A, Janda KD, Lerner RA.** (1986). Chemical reactivity at an antibody binding site elicited by mechanistic design of a synthetic antigen. *Proc Natl Acad Sci*, 83, 6736–6740

- **Travis J.** (1993). Biotech Gets a Grip on Cell Adhesion. *Science*, 260, 906–908

- **Tsuji S, Kaji K, Nagasawa S.** (1994). Decay-accelerating factor on human umbilical vein endothelial cells. *J Immunol*, 152, 1404–1410

- **Tute MS.** (1995). Drug Design: the Present and the Future. *Adv Drug Res*, 26, 45–142

- **Tybulewicz VLJ, Tremblay ML, LaMarca ME, Willemsen R, Zablocka B, Sidransky E, Martin BM, Haung SP, Mintzer KA, Westphal H, Mulligan RC, Ginns EI.** (1992). Animal model for Gaucher's disease from targeted disruption of the mouse glucocerebrosidase gene. *Nature*, 357, 407–410

- **Usman N, McSwiggen JA.** (1995). Catalytic RNA (Ribozymes) as Drugs. *Ann Rep Med Chem*, 30, 285–294

- **VanderSpek JC, Mindell JA, Finkelstein A, Murphy JR.** (1993). Structure/function analysis of the transmembrane domain of DAB_{389}-interleukin-2, an interleukin-2 receptor-targeted fusion toxin. The amphipathic helical region of the transmembrane domain is essential for the efficient delivery of the catalytic domain to the cytosol of target cells. *J Biol Chem*, 268, 12077–12082

- **Veerapandian B.** (1995). Three Dimensional Structure-Aided Drug Design. In *Burger's Medicinal Chemistry, Fifth Edition*, edited by ME Wolff, Vol. 1. New York, New York: John Wiley & Sons, Inc, pp. 303–348

- **Venuti M.** (1990). The Impact of Biotechnology on Drug Discovery. *Ann Rep Med Chem*, 25, 289–298

- **Von Itzstein M, Jin B, Wu W-Y, Kok GB, Pegg MS, Dyason JC, Jin B, Phan TV, Smythe ML, White HF, Oliver SW, Colman PM, Varghese JN, Ryan DM, Woods JM, Bethell RC, Hotham VJ, Cameron JM, Penn CR.** (1993). Rational design of potent sialidase-based inhibitors of influenza virus replication. *Nature*, 363, 418–423

- **Webb EB.** (1993). Monoclonal Antibodies. In *Molecular Biology and Biotechnology*, edited by JM Walker and EB Gingold. Cambridge, England: The Royal Society of Chemistry, pp. 384–385

- **Welply JK, Jaworski E.** (1990). *Glycobiology*. New York, New York: Wiley-Liss

- **Wermuth CG.** (1996). Strategies in the Search for New Lead Compounds or Original Working Hypotheses. In *The Practice of Medicinal Chemistry*, edited by CG Wemuth. San Diego, California: Academic Press, pp. 81–100

- **West CM.** (1986). Current ideas on the significance of protein glycosylation. *Mol Cell Biochem*, 72, 3–20

- **White BA.** (1997). *PCR Cloning Protocols. From Molecular Cloning to Genetic Engineering*, Totowa, New Jersey: Humana Press

- **Wilcox M, Horton MA.** (1994). Integrins. In *The Encyclopedia of Molecular Biology*, edited by J Kendrew. Oxford, England: Blackwell Science Ltd, pp. 552–556

- **Wiley RA, Rich DH.** (1993). Peptidomimetics derived from natural products. *Med Res Rev*, 13, 327–384

- **Wilson WJ, Wiedmann M, Dillard HR, Batt CA.** (1994). Identification of *Erwinia stewartii* by a ligase chain reaction assay. *Appl Environ Microbiol*, 60, 278–284

- **Winnacker E-L, Huber R.** (1988). *Protein Structure and Protein Engineering*. Berlin, Germany: Springer-Verlag

- **Winter G, Milstein C.** (1991). Man-made antibodies. *Nature*, 349, 293

- **Wright A, Shin S-U, Morrison SL.** (1992). Genetically engineered antibodies: Progress and prospects. *Crit Rev Immunol*, 23, 301–321

- **Wüthrich K.** (1986). *NMR of Proteins and Nucleic Acids*. New York, New York: Wiley-Interscience

- **Zhang SH, Reddick RL, Piedrahita JA, Maeda N.** (1992). Spontaneous Hypercholesterolemia and Arterial Lesions in Mice Lacking Apolipoprotein E. *Science*, 258, 468

- **Zhou GW, Guo J, Haung W, Fletterick RJ, Scanlan TS.** (1994). Crystal Structure of a Catalytic Antibody with a Serine Protease Active Site. *Science*, 265, 1059–1064

- **Zoller M, Smith M.** (1982). Oligonucleotide-directed mutagenesis using M13-derived vectors: an efficient and general procedure for the production of point mutations in any fragment of DNA. *Nucleic Acids Res*, 10, 6487–6500

- **Zoller M, Smith M.** (1983). Oligonucleotide-directed mutagenesis of DNA fragments cloned into M13 vectors. *Methods In Enzymology*, 100(B), 468–500

- **Zoller M, Smith M.** (1984). Oligonucleotide-directed mutagenesis: a simple method using two oligonucleotide primers and a single-stranded DNA template. *DNA*, 3, 479–488

Self-Assessment Questions

Question 1:   *What are the three stages of PCR?*
Question 2:   *How does RT-PCR differ from basic PCR?*
Question 3:   *What techniques are variations of the ligation chain reaction (LCR)?*
Question 4:   *Why are engineered animal models valuable to pharmaceutical research?*
Question 5:   *What two techniques are commonly used to produce transgenic animals?*
Question 6:   *What is a knockout mouse?*
Question 7:   *What is site-directed mutagenesis?*
Question 8:   *How does point mutation differ from a site-directed mutation?*
Question 9:   *What are fusion proteins?*
Question 10:   *What structural techniques can provide information about the 3-D structure of a protein?*
Question 11:   *Define the term peptidomimetic.*
Question 12:   *What is the pseudopeptide approach?*
Question 13:   *What are some of the techniques that comprise nucleic acid technology?*
Question 14:   *What chemical modifications have been made to improve the physicochemical properties of oligonucleotides?*
Question 15:   *What are the mechanisms by which antisense oligonucleotides act?*
Question 16:   *What are ribozymes?*
Question 17:   *What are the key technologies that allowed for the development of catalytic antibodies?*
Question 18:   *What is glycobiology?*
Question 19:   *What are some of the diseases that glycosylation may play a role?*
Question 20:   *What are some of the families of cell adhesion molecules?*
Question 21:   *What are biosensors?*
Question 22:   *What is high-throughput screening?*
Question 23:   *What is combinatorial chemistry?*

Answers

Answer 1:   Stage 1) denaturation; Stage 2) annealing (also called primer binding); and Stage 3) extension.

Answer 2:   PCR has been extended to include RNA as the target template by the methodology of RT-PCR; it utilizes a thermoactive reverse transcriptase enzyme for preparing a complementary DNA copy of a target template mRNA molecule and is coupled to the tremendous DNA amplification of PCR.

Answer 3:   One variation of the LCR methodology is gap LCR (G-LCR). Gap LCR has also been modified with the inclusion of the enzyme reverse transcriptase to create "asymmetric gap LCR" (AG-LCR).

Answer 4:   Engineered animal models are proving invaluable since small animal models of disease are often poor mimics of that disease in human patients. Genetic engineering can predispose an animal to a particular disease under scrutiny and the insertion of human genes into the animal can initiate the development of a more clinically-relevant disease condition.

Answer 5:   1) DNA microinjection and random gene addition; and 2) homologous recombination in embryonic stem cells.

Answer 6:   A knockout mouse, also called a gene knockout mouse or a gene-targeted knockout mouse, is an animal in which an endogenous gene (genomic wild-type allele) has been specifically inactivated by replacing it with a null allele.

Answer 7:   Site-directed mutagenesis (also called site-specific mutagenesis) is a protein engineering technique allowing specifically (site-direct) alteration (mutation) of the primary amino acid sequence of proteins to create new chemical entities.

Answer 8: Site directed mutagenesis at a single amino acid position in an engineered protein is called a point mutation.

Answer 9: Fusion proteins contain portions or the entire amino acid sequences of both parent proteins fused together.

Answer 10: Protein X-ray crystallography and nuclear magnetic resonance (NMR) spectroscopy

Answer 11: Peptidomimetic (sometimes called peptide mimetics and nonpeptide mimetics) are defined as structures which serve as appropriate substitutes for peptides in interactions with receptors and enzymes. The mimetic must possess not only affinity, but also efficacy or substitute function.

Answer 12: The pseudopeptide approach is an attempt to improve the biostability of peptides. Numerous pseudopeptides (also called amide bond surrogates) have been prepared that substitute an amide bond bioisostere for the amide peptide bond.

Answer 13: Gene therapy, antisense and triplex technologies, aptamer technology and ribozymes.

Answer 14: Chemical changes resulting in phosphorothioate, alkyl phosphonate, phosphoamidate, and formacetal analogs. Additional modifications include changes to the heterocyclic bases, derivatization of the ribose moiety and pendant cap groups.

Answer 15: There are several mechanisms. A transient inhibition by masking the ribosome binding site on mRNA. A permanent inhibition from cross-linking the oligonucleotide to the target mRNA. The most important mechanism, however, appears to be through the action of RNase H, which recognizes the DNA-RNA duplex or RNA-RNA duplex, disrupts the base pairing, and digests the RNA-part of the double helix.

Answer 16: Ribozymes are catalytic RNAs which cleave covalent bonds, generally degrading a target RNA.

Answer 17: The development of hybridoma technology and also protein engineering provides the ability to produce homogeneous, monoclonal antibodies and modified antibodies in the quantities necessary to reproducibly purify potential abzymes and characterize their properties.

Answer 18: Glycobiology may be defined as the study of the structure, synthesis and biological role of glycans and glycoconjugates.

Answer 19: The sugars of glycoproteins are known to play a role in the recognition and binding of biomolecules to other molecules in disease states such as asthma, rheumatoid arthritis, cancer, HIV-infection, the flu and other infectious disease.

Answer 20: Integrins, selectins, those of the immunoglobulin superfamily and the cadherins.

Answer 21: Biosensors are a class of extremely sensitive and selective sensors that convert a biological action into an electrical signal to determine (qualitatively and/or quantitatively) a specific compound.

Answer 22: High-throughput screening (HTS) provides for the bioassay of thousands of compounds in multiple assays (as many as 50) at the same time. The process is automated with robots and utilizes 96-well microtiter plates. Enzyme inhibition assays and radioligand binding assays are the most common biochemical tests employed.

Answer 23: Combinatorial chemistry is a mix-and-match process in which a simple building block (a starting material such as an amino acid, peptide, heterocycle, other small molecule, etc.) is joined to one or more other simple building blocks in every possible combination. The task is automated and is commonly conducted while attached to a solid support.

7 Gene Therapy

by: Abraham Bout

Introduction

Since the discovery that genetic information of all living organisms is stored as DNA, the knowledge of genetics and molecular biology has grown explosively. The genetic basis of a large number of inherited diseases was identified, and it can be expected that the genes involved in major congenital disorders will be cloned and characterized before the end of this century. Medicine has already benefited from the developments in molecular biology through the generation of diagnostics and pharmaceuticals. Moreover, in the near future we can expect that a greater understanding of diseases at the molecular level will allow us to cure or significantly improve the prognosis of these diseases by introduction of gene(s) into cells of patients: gene therapy, a rapidly growing discipline of medicine.

Gene therapy may be divided into germ-line gene therapy and somatic gene therapy. Germ-line gene therapy aims at the introduction of genes into germ-cells or omnipotent embryonal cells (4–8 cellular stage). For ethical and other reasons, human germ-cell gene therapy is presently not accepted in our society. Somatic gene therapy is the introduction of (a) gene(s) into somatic cells. The ethical considerations of somatic gene therapy have been widely discussed and a consensus emerged which allows to genetically manipulate a patient's somatic cells for the purpose of correcting severe disorders.

All current gene therapy protocols make use of gene addition, where an intact version of a gene is added to the chromosomal DNA of the target cell population of a patient. Therefore, this chapter focuses on gene addition. Before discussing the commonly used gene transfer systems a general overview of gene therapy strategies and diseases that are subject to gene therapy studies is presented.

Ex Vivo versus In Vivo Gene Therapy

Ex Vivo Gene Therapy

Cells from a number of organs and tissues (e.g. skin, hemopoietic system, liver) or from tumors can be removed from the patient and cultured *ex vivo* in the laboratory. During culture, the cells may be provided with a therapeutic gene. This is then followed by reinfusion or reimplantation of the transduced cells into the patient (Figure 7.1a). *Ex vivo* gene therapy is currently the most widely used in clinical trials. In the majority of cases retroviral vectors are used to insert the therapeutic gene into the recipient's cells.

In Vivo Gene Therapy

Other organs (e.g., lung, brain, heart) are less suited for *ex vivo* gene therapy, as culture of the target cells or re-transplantation are not feasible. Then, somatic gene therapy can only be performed by *in vivo* gene transfer, in other words by administering the gene of interest either locally or systemically (Figure 7.1b).

Potential Target Diseases for Gene Therapy

Inherited Disorders

For somatic gene therapy of inherited disorders an intact version of the affected gene is introduced into these cells in which the inadequate expression of the gene is determining the major symptoms of the disease. Because in inherited disorders not all organs are involved (or are not equally involved), somatic gene therapy is aimed at the cells or organ where the disease becomes manifest, such as the hemopoietic system in the case of Adenosine Deaminase (ADA) deficiency, airway epithelium in Cystic Fibrosis (CF), muscle in Duchenne Muscular Dystrophy and liver in Familial Hypercholesterolemia (FH) and Hemophilia. For inherited disorders, stable expression of the introduced genes is required (Figure 7.2a,b). This may be achieved either by integration of the therapeutic gene into the host cell's genome (Figure 7.2a), or by using episomal expression vectors (Figure 7.2b). In the case of integration, the recombinant DNA is duplicated when chromosomal DNA is duplicated in the S-phase of the cell cycle. Episomal vectors that carry an origin of replication, e.g. derived from Epstein-Barr virus, allow the vectors to be maintained

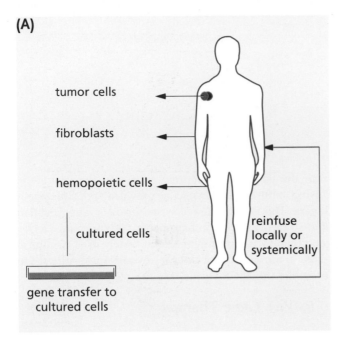

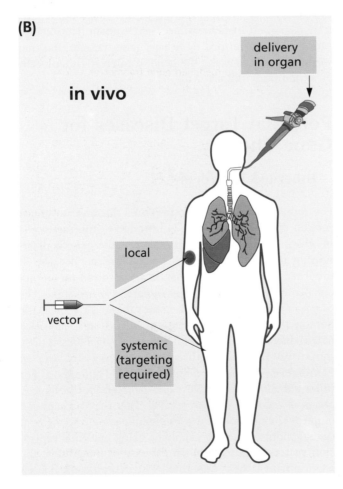

Figure 7.1a,b. Schematic outline of *ex vivo* (A) and *in vivo* (B) gene therapy strategies (courtesy of IntroGene).

episomally (that is: not integrated into the host cell chromosome) at moderate copy numbers. When a sufficiently large number of stem cells are equipped with a new therapeutic gene that is stably expressed, they may provide a life-long correction of the disease. Episomal transfection without an origin of replication (Figure 7.2c) only causes transient transfection. The episomal DNA is lost upon cell division.

Cancer

The most commonly employed approaches for cancer gene therapy include use of (see also Culver and Blaese, 1994):

1. cytokine genes, such as GM-CSF, IFN-γ and interleukins (e.g. IL-2), into cancer cells. These cytokines induce a local inflammatory reaction in the tumor which destroys a significant fraction of the treated tumor. The inflammation in turn induces an anti-tumor cell immune reaction which destroys any surviving malignant cells in the primary tumor as well as in distant metastases (see Figure 7.3).
2. 'suicide genes', such as the Herpes Simplex Virus-thymidine kinase gene (HSV-tk). This enzyme is known to phosphorylate the systemically administered pro-drug ganciclovir (a nucleotide analogue). Phosphorylated ganciclovir is incorporated into DNA of dividing cells, which leads to termination of DNA-chain elongation, resulting in death of the cell. Not all cells within a tumor need to be transduced: cells surrounding a cell that expresses the HSV-tk are also killed after ganciclovir treatment. This is called the bystander effect. The bystander effect may be of different magnitude in different tumors. A current explanation for the bystander effect is that transport of phosphorylated ganciclovir occurs from HSV-tk expressing cells to neighbouring cells through gap-junctions (Figure 7.4).
3. tumor suppressor genes such as p53, which are mutated in a large number of cancers, or antisense genes targeted at oncogenes (for example Ras) to reduce or abolish their expression.
4. protection of hematopoietic stem cells (HSCs) from the toxic effects of chemotherapy by inserting a gene that confers drug resistance, e.g. multiple drug resistance gene MDR-1. The MDR-1 gene has been isolated from drug resistant tumor cells, where it functions by pumping anticancer drugs out of the cell.

Cytokine gene therapy is intended for treatment of both the primary tumor and distant metastases. Suicide and tumor suppressor genes have been designed to mediate direct cytotoxic or antiproliferative effects on the tumor cells, and will only be effective for the treatment of localized tumors. MDR gene therapy is expected to allow cancer patients to

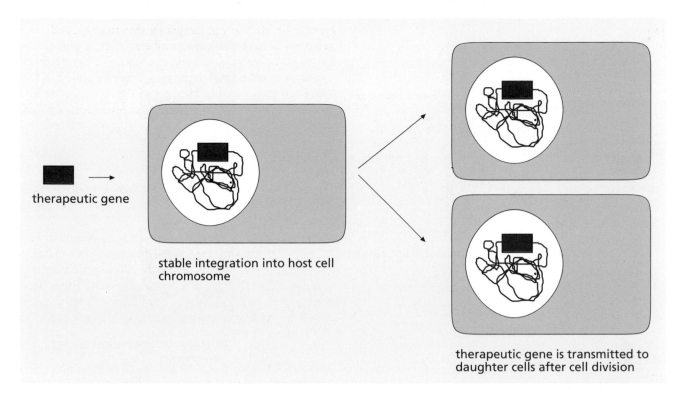

Figure 7.2a. Principles of stable and transient gene transfer. 2a: stable gene transfer is obtained when the therapeutic gene integrates into host cell chromosomal DNA (e.g. retrovirus or adeno-associated virus mediated gene transfer or at low efficiency after non-viral mediated DNA transfer). Therefore, the therapeutic gene is transmitted to progeny cells.

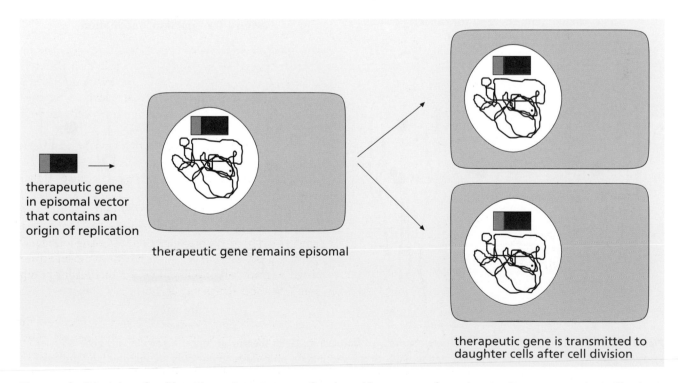

Figure 7.2b. Principles of stable and transient gene transfer. 2b: stable gene transfer and transmittance to progeny cells also occur when episomal vectors containing an origin of replication are used.

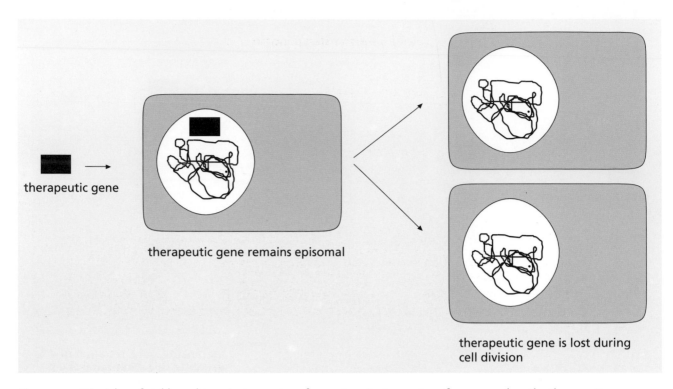

Figure 7.2c. Principles of stable and transient gene transfer. 2c: transient gene transfer occurs when the therapeutic gene remains episomal and is not integrated into the host cell chromosomal DNA. The episomal DNA is lost upon cell division.

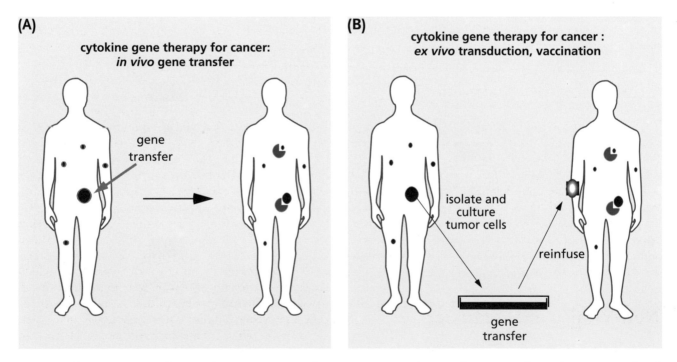

Figure 7.3a,b. Immuno-gene therapy of cancer (courtesy of IntroGene). Gene therapy of cancer e.g. by *in vivo* gene transfer of cytokine genes (3a) or by the *ex vivo* 'vaccination' (3b). In the vaccination procedure, tumor cells are cultured and provided with e.g. a cytokine gene, and retransplanted. Both the *in vivo* and *ex vivo* procedure aim at eliciting an immune response (represented by the green dots) against the cancer cells, which should destroy both the cytokine bearing tumor cells as well as the other non-cytokine bearing tumor cells.

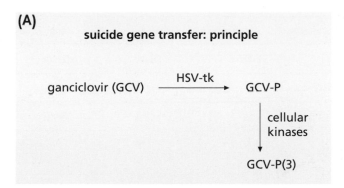

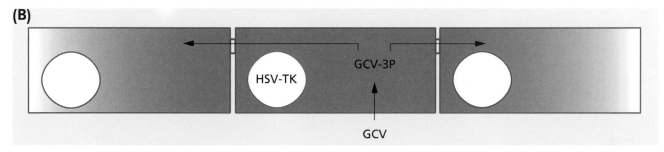

Figure 7.4a,b. Suicide gene therapy of cancer (courtesy of IntroGene). The reaction underlying suicide gene therapy is depicted in (A). The bystander effect is schematically represented in (B). Three cells are presented, of which the middle one is transduced with the HSV-tk gene. When ganciclovir (GCV) is added, it is phosphorylated into the toxic product GCV-P(3). This GCV-P(3) is transported to neighbouring cells through gap junctions.

tolerate higher doses of chemotherapy, thereby increasing the effectivity of the therapy.

Gene Transfer Methods

The method to introduce the genetic material into the target cells of a patient is a key component of every gene therapy protocol. A variety of gene transfer systems are currently employed to insert therapeutic genes into somatic cells. They are divided into viral and non-viral gene transfer methods. The most important methods and their applications will be discussed. Examples of applications are restricted to those that are operational in clinical studies. The characteristics of the different gene transfer systems are summarized in Table 7.1.

Non-Viral Gene Transfer

Methods of Non-Viral Gene Transfer

Non-viral gene transfer systems include injection of naked DNA, particle bombardment and entrapping DNA into liposomes (reviewed by Ledley, 1995). The most straightforward procedure is direct injection of naked plasmid DNA in tissue, which works with reasonable efficiency in muscle and skin. The advantages of such a gene transfer system are clear: it is easy, safe and suited also for the transfer of large gene constructs. Alternatively, naked DNA can be introduced with a 'gene-gun': a high pressure- or electrical discharge device which forces microscopic gold- or tungsten particles coated with DNA into tissues.

A common method of non-viral gene transfer is the administration of liposome-encapsulated DNA (Figure 7.5). DNA molecules (that have a negative charge at neutral pH), are being complexed to cationic liposomes. The liposome/DNA complexes bind to the cell membranes and, in most cases, are internalized into endosomes. Relatively few DNA/plasmid complexes are released into the cytoplasm, enter the nucleus and are expressed (< 0.1%). Several modifications of this system have been made, e.g. by adding peptides or virus shells to the DNA/liposome complex to disrupt the endosomes of the target cells in order to minimize breakdown of the DNA. These modifications resulted in significant improvements in gene transfer efficacy. In addition, antibodies or other proteins have been attached to the complexes for targeting purposes.

Application of Non-Viral Gene Transfer

Direct injection of naked DNA into the pig skin results in transient expression of the recombinant gene by epidermal keratinocytes in the area surrounding the injection site. It

	Retrovirus	Adenovirus	AAV	Naked DNA	Liposome-mediated
Genome transfer	RNA	DNA	DNA	DNA	DNA or RNA
Virus titers	$10^6 - 10^9$/ml	$10^{11} - 10^{12}$/ml	10^{10}/ml	n.a.	n.a.
Purification	difficult	yes	yes	yes	yes
Max. size recombinant gene	8 kb	7.5 kb	5 kb	at least 50 kb	at least 50 kb
In vivo use	no*	yes	yes	yes	yes
Integration	yes	no	yes	low	low
Efficiency	high	very high	moderate	moderate	low
Safety issues	insertional mutagenesis	immune reactions	no known	no known	no known
Non-dividing cells	no	yes	yes	probably	probably
Limitation	cell division needed	transient correction	production is difficult	efficiency is low	efficiency is low

Table 7.1. Characteristics of different methods of gene transfer. * = retrovirus producer cells are used *in vivo*. n.a. = not applicable

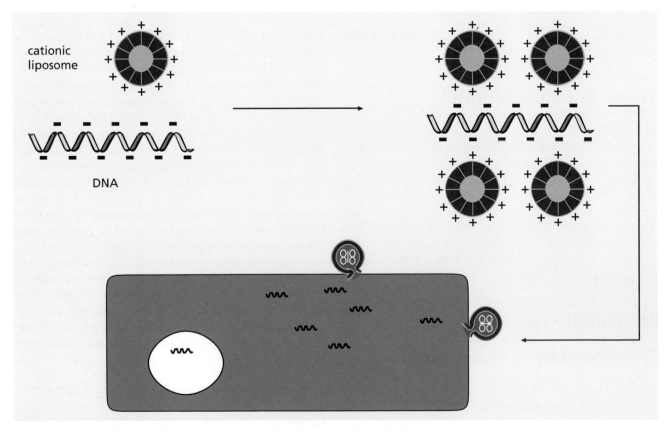

Figure 7.5. Hypothetical model for cationic-liposome mediated gene transfer. Liposomes (positive charge) and DNA (negative charge) form a complex and fuse with the membrane of the target cell, followed by release of DNA into the cell.

has not been applied to humans yet, but potential applications may be found in the treatment of skin disorders and for virus- and cancer vaccinations.

The gene-gun has been used only in pre-clinical studies (Yang and Sun, 1995) and gene transfer and transient expression have been demonstrated in skin, liver and tumors of mice.

Liposome-mediated gene transfer is being used in clinical trials for CF gene therapy and for the treatment of cancer. In both cases the *in vivo* gene transfer approach is used. CF is a recessive, autosomally inherited lethal disorder, caused by mutations in the CFTR (Cystic Fibrosis Transmembrane Conductance Regulator) gene. CFTR codes for a membrane protein acting as a channel that transports chloride. As chloride transport over epithelial membranes is accompanied by water transport, a defect in the CFTR leads to impaired water transport over epithelial membranes, such as airway epithelium. The mucus in lungs of CF patients is therefore strongly dehydrated, causing insufficient muciliary cleaning which leads to recurrent lung inflammations. This lung disease accounts for 95% of morbidity and mortality. Gene therapy of CF aims at introducing a normal version of the CF gene into lungs, in particular airway epithelium. A clinical study has been performed where DNA/liposome mixtures have been instilled into the nose of patients. The rationale for investigating the nasal epithelium is that it manifests the same secretory defect as the respiratory epithelium and is easily accessible for harvesting cells and performing *in vivo* measurements. Transfer of the CFTR gene to epithelial cells was detected and transient partial correction of the chloride transport has been reported. No adverse clinical effects and no histopathological changes in nasal biopsies were observed.

In an ongoing clinical study, liposomes containing a gene encoding a foreign antigen that is expressed on the cell surface, were injected *in vivo* into a tumor (melanoma). The goal is to induce an immune reaction against the modified tumor cells. It is expected that the reaction against the foreign antigen will also elicit an immune reaction against tumor antigens, resulting in a general destruction of tumor cells.

In summary, liposome-mediated gene transfer seems to be safe, but efficiencies are low and expression of the transferred genes is transient. Further studies need to be conducted that deal with improvement of gene transfer efficiency.

Gene Transfer Using Recombinant Viruses (Viral Vectors)

General Requirements

Viruses have a natural capacity to infect cells and deliver their genes very efficiently to the nucleus of the target cells.

In general, viruses have shown much more efficient gene transfer rates than non-viral gene delivery. When viruses are exploited as vehicles for therapeutic genes, they have to meet the following criteria:

1. unlike their wild-type variant, they have to be replication defective to prevent uncontrolled spreading *in vivo*
2. the virus by itself should not possess undesirable properties
3. the viral genome must be able to accommodate the therapeutic gene (size constraints)

Three commonly used viral gene transfer systems (reviewed by Smith, 1995; Jolly, 1994), namely those based on retrovirus, adenovirus and adeno-associated virus, will be discussed in more detail.

Retrovirus Vectors

RETROVIRUS LIFE CYCLE

The most commonly employed retroviral vectors are derived from Murine Leukemia Virus (MuLV). When these viruses are injected in new born rodents, leukemia develops after a latent period. They are not associated with any known pathology in humans.

The retrovirus particle consists of the retrovirus genome, present as two single copy RNA molecules, complexed to the viral core proteins, surrounded by a lipid envelope. The envelope consists of cell membrane derived from the host cell and retroviral 'envelope' proteins.

The first step of the life cycle of retroviruses (Figure 7.6a) consists of recognition of a receptor on the surface of the target cell. Such receptors are transmembrane proteins that have a function in normal cellular metabolism, such as amino acid or phosphate transport. Binding to the receptor triggers fusion of the virus envelope with the host cell's plasma membrane. The recognition of a receptor is mediated by the viral envelope proteins. After penetration of the cell membrane the viral core enters the cytoplasm of the host cell and the single-stranded viral RNA is converted into double-stranded DNA by the viral enzyme reverse transcriptase, which is also packaged in the viral core. Next the retroviral DNA becomes incorporated in the host genome. The retroviral DNA incorporated in the host cell chromosomal DNA is called the provirus. The provirus carries three genes designated *gag*, *pol* and *env*. The *gag* gene codes for the core proteins of the virus which are responsible for the encapsidation of viral genomic RNA and the assembly of the virion. The *pol* gene encodes reverse transcriptase which directs the synthesis of the DNA from the viral RNA. A large part of the *env* (envelope) proteins are located at the surface of the virions and interact with specific cell surface receptors on the target cell membrane. Both proviral termini consist of a non-coding

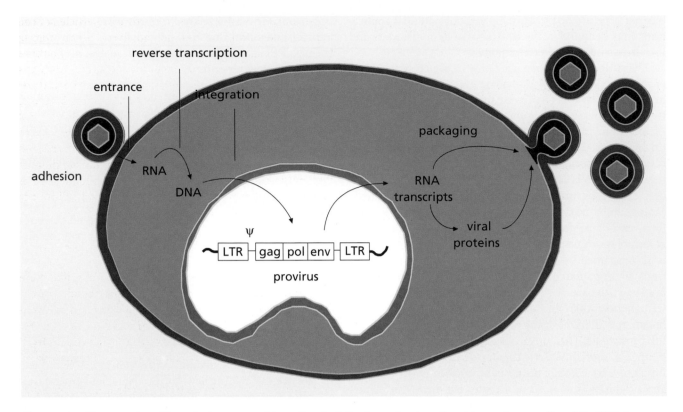

Figure 7.6a. The retrovirus life cycle (courtesy of IntroGene). Following adhesion, the virion enters a cell and its RNA is reverse transcribed into a DNA molecule which is subsequently integrated into the cellular chromosome to form the provirus. Proviral DNA is transcribed and translated into viral proteins which encapsidate full length viral RNA molecules. The encapsidated viral RNA buds from the cell to give progeny virus particles.

sequence, called the Long Terminal Repeat (LTR), that contains sequences that are required for packaging of the RNA genome into virions (so-called packaging signal ψ), promoter and transcription termination sequences and for integration of proviral DNA into the chromosomal DNA of the host (Figure 7.6a).

The provirus remains a stable part of the host cell's genome, so the provirus is transferred to daughter cells following cell division. Transcription and translation of the provirus result in production of the respective retroviral proteins. The envelope proteins are exposed on the host cell membrane. The packaging signal ψ, present on the RNA molecule, is recognized by the retroviral core proteins. They assemble into a new infective virus particle. The retrovirus particles bud from the host cell membrane. The envelope of cellular membrane surrounding the retrovirus core contains retroviral envelope proteins.

RECOMBINANT RETROVIRUS

The specific properties that render retroviruses suitable for foreign gene transfer are: a) they can infect a wide variety of cell types with high efficiency; b) the proviral copy stably integrates into the chromosomal DNA of the cell, thereby warranting life-long correction of the target cell type and its descendants and c) the sequences required for viral replication can be physically separated into cis- and trans-acting elements (see also Figure 7.6b), enabling generation of replication defective recombinant retroviruses. Recombinant retrovirus systems consist of two building blocks, a retroviral vector (to transfer the gene to the "target" cell) and a retrovirus packaging cell (only needed to produce replication defective virus, the vector).

Based on the knowledge of the location of the packaging signal, so-called packaging cell lines for defective viruses have been designed (Valerio, 1992). Packaging cells synthesize all of the proteins encoded by the genes *gag*, *pol* and *env*. These polypeptides are required for the production of viable virus particles and for integration in the host cells genome. By removing the packaging signal ψ and other cis-acting sequences from the viral RNAs, these packaging cells are engineered to express all viral proteins without producing infectious viruses themselves. Most of the currently used packaging cells are based on mouse 3T3 fibroblasts.

Retroviral vectors are recombinant DNA molecules that carry the foreign therapeutic gene(s), the packaging signal

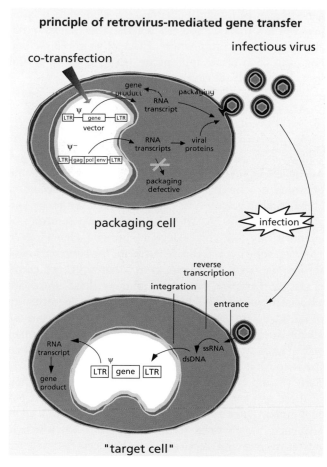

principle of retrovirus-mediated gene transfer

Figure 7.6b. A retrovirus packaging cell at work (courtesy of IntroGene). The packaging cell by itself produces all of the viral proteins, but generates no viable virus particles. A retroviral shuttle vector carrying all of the in-cis requirements as well as the gene(s) of interest is introduced into the packaging cell, e.g. by physical transfection procedures. Transcripts from the shuttle vector can be packaged by the virus proteins present and form infectious virus. The recombinant retroviruses are replication defective such that they can only undergo one cycle of infection.

ψ and at each end a long terminal repeat (LTR). The left LTR functions as the promoter, but optionally, other promoter elements may be introduced in the vector. These sequences are the minimal requirements for retroviral vectors and in between the two LTRs they leave space to accommodate foreign DNA up to approximately 8 kb.

When retroviral vector DNA is introduced into packaging cells e.g. by means of transfection (Figure 7.6b), a RNA copy is generated, which is subsequently packaged into infectious particles by the viral proteins produced by the packaging cell. The newly generated virus particles are released in the culture medium. Using this procedure, virus producing cell lines can be derived that produce

approximately 0.1 to 1 functional retrovirus particle per cell per hour, resulting in recombinant virus titers ranging from ±10³ up to ±10⁷ infectious particles per mL of culture medium. When the culture medium containing the virus particles is harvested and added to cells that have to be genetically corrected, the recombinant retrovirus is able to infect such cells, reverse transcribe its RNA into DNA and integrate as a provirus into the target cell's genome. Since the vector does not contain the viral genes, it can not replicate, which is considered to be a prerequisite in gene therapy procedures. In this way, a recombinant gene is integrated and expressed in the target cell and will lead to correction of its disorder.

APPLICATION OF RETROVIRAL VECTORS

Retroviruses are produced by packaging cells that have been transfected with a retroviral vector containing the therapeutic gene. The recombinant retroviruses are continuously produced by the packaging cells and released into the culture medium. It is difficult to purify the viruses from the medium because of instability of the retrovirus particles.

Therefore, retroviruses are used predominantly in *ex vivo* gene therapy protocols (see e.g., Anderson, 1992; Miller, 1992). Cells that have to be provided with a therapeutic gene are isolated from a patient and exposed to culture medium containing the retrovirus particles. Cells that have been used in the clinic include T-lymphocytes (ADA deficiency, TIL (tumor infiltrating lymphocytes)), bone marrow cells (ADA deficiency, Gauchers disease, gene marking studies), hepatocytes (for LDL-receptor deficiency) and tumor cells (e.g., melanoma). As cell division is needed for integration of retroviral DNA into the host cell, growth factors are usually added to the medium to stimulate division of the target cells and hence increasing gene transfer efficiency.

Retroviruses have been used in clinical gene marking protocols and gene therapy protocols (Anderson, 1992). Unlike gene therapy studies, gene marking studies have no therapeutic intent, but aim at demonstrating that an exogenous gene (e.g., easily detectable, non-human gene) can be safely transferred to a patient and at determining how long this gene is detectable in the patient's target cells. Most of the marking protocols address additional specific questions.

The first gene therapy protocol was for Adenosine Deaminase deficiency, a lethal inherited disorder leading to severe combined immunodeficiency. ADA patients can be cured by transplantation of bone marrow from a normal donor or by administration of the ADA protein. This indicates, that if sufficient bone marrow cells of a patient can be provided with a normal version of the ADA gene, cure of the disorder should be obtained.

The ADA gene therapy protocol was initiated in 1990. A 4 year old girl suffering from ADA deficiency received an intravenous infusion of her own gene-corrected T lymphocytes. Because T-lymphocytes have a limited lifespan, she received infusion at 1 to 2 months intervals. A second patient began treatment in 1991. Evaluation of the clinical results was difficult because the patients were treated with ADA enzyme also after gene therapy. Results suggest that this therapy was clinically useful, as both patients have shown improvement in their clinical condition after gene therapy was begun as well as in a battery of *in vitro* and *in vivo* immune function studies. Because of limited lifespan of mature T-cells (150–200 days), therapeutic correction of progenitors or stem cells present in the bone marrow would circumvent the frequent treatments required for gene therapy of T-lymphocytes. Based on encouraging data in rhesus monkeys, three ADA patients (two from France and one from the UK) have been treated in the Netherlands. No treatment-related toxicity was observed. Gene transfer to bone marrow stem cells could be demonstrated but remained low.

In addition, a number of cancer vaccination protocols have used retroviral vectors. Vaccination is most commonly attempted by surgically removing tumor cells from the patient, growing them *ex vivo* in tissue culture and inserting genes that stimulate inflammation and/or immunity. Vaccination with cells that produce cytokines has been shown to result in systemic immunity in mice, which leads to destruction of the tumor cells *in vivo*. Several gene therapy trials in humans have been approved, involving *ex vivo* retrovirus-mediated transfer of the IL-2, TNF-α or GM-CSF genes into melanoma, colorectal, renal cell carcinoma, neuroblastoma or breast cancer cells. Other protocols use insertion of the gene encoding IL-2 or IL-4 into autologous fibroblasts, which are then mixed with irradiated tumor cells from the patient and re-injected.

In vivo gene transfer using retroviral vectors for suicide genes has been applied to the treatment of brain tumors. In this protocol, retrovirus producing cells instead of retrovirus particles (which are relatively instable) were injected into growing brain tumors (Culver and Blaese, 1994). The retroviruses produced by these cells harbor the HSV-tk gene. Since retrovirus-mediated gene transfer is limited to dividing cells, the HSV-tk gene is expected to integrate only into the proliferating tumor cells and not into normal brain tissue (which is mostly non-dividing tissue). Patients received intravenous infusions of GCV. There was no evidence for toxicity related to the gene transfer and some patients showed a response of the tumor.

In general, *ex vivo* gene therapy is promising, although retroviral gene transfer efficiencies are still limiting. As retrovirus vectors need cell division for stable gene expression, terminally differentiated cells and other non-dividing cells will not be transduced by such vectors. In particular gene therapy of human hematopoietic stem cells is hampered by low transduction efficiencies. This is most probably caused by a combination of lack of stem cell cycling, low expression of an appropriate retroviral receptor and loss of stem cells during *ex vivo* culture.

Adenovirus Vectors

ADENOVIRUS LIFE CYCLE

Adenoviruses are non-enveloped DNA viruses, the genome of which is a linear, double stranded DNA molecule of about 36 kb. The virion has an icosahedral symmetry and a diameter of 88 nm. There are 49 distinct serotypes of adenoviruses (see for review on human adenoviruses: Horwitz, 1990). Adenoviruses used for the construction of recombinants are all belonging to subgroup C, which includes serotypes 1, 2, 5 and 6. In humans, those viruses are associated with mild respiratory disease only. The structure of the adenovirus genome is described on the basis of the adenovirus genes expressed following infection of human cells (Figure 7.7a). Several regions can be distinguished on the adenoviral genome (see Figure 7.7a), which are called Early (E) and Late (L), according to whether transcription of these regions takes place prior or after onset of DNA replication. The extremity of the viral genome has a short sequence, the inverted terminal repeat (ITR), which is necessary for viral replication. Sequences required for replication and encapsidation (ψ) of the virus have been mapped in a region of approximately 400 bp downstream of the left ITR.

Unlike retrovirus replication, where virions are released into the culture medium without affecting the viability of the cells, adenovirus replication causes lysis of the cells. The adenovirus lytic cycle is biphasic, comprising an early (E) phase which precedes viral DNA replication, and a late (L) phase, starting 6–8 hours later.

Following adhesion and receptor-mediated uptake of adenovirus into the cell, the adenovirus particle enters the endosomes that fuse with primary lysosomes. The low pH in the endosomes probably induces a conformational change of the surface of the virion, that leads to disruption of the endosomes. The adenovirus DNA is released and transported to the nucleus. The adenovirus DNA is not integrated into the host cell chromosomal DNA but remains episomal (extra-chromosomal). In the nucleus, the 'immediate early' E1 genes are first expressed, which trans-activate other early adenovirus genes (E2, E4) that shutdown host-cell protein synthesis and are involved in replication of the adenoviral DNA. After onset of DNA replication, the late genes L2-L5 are switched on. They encode structural adenovirus proteins, that in turn form virion particles in the nucleus of the cell, into which the adenoviral DNA becomes entrapped. Depending on the serotype, approxi-

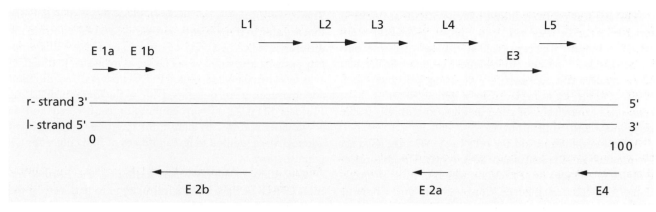

Figure 7.7a. Map of the adenovirus genome (courtesy of IntroGene). The 36 kb double stranded adenovirus DNA molecule is usually divided into 100 map units (mu). The early (E) and late (L) regions are indicated on the map. Note that both DNA strands contain protein coding regions.

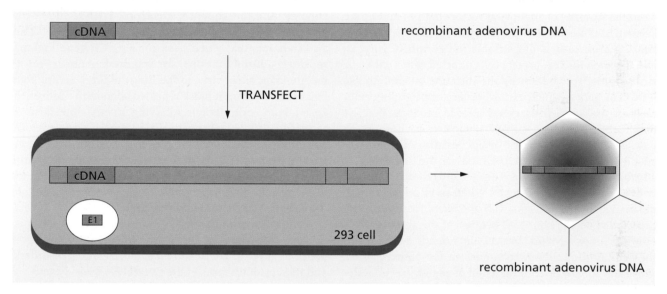

Figure 7.7b. Recombinant adenovirus (courtesy of IntroGene). All replication defective recombinant adenoviruses that are nowadays available contain a deletion of 'immediate early' E1 sequences. As E1 sequences are pivotal for activation of other adenovirus genes, E1 deletion mutants are not able to replicate unless E1 proteins are provided by the cell in which the adenovirus is propagated. The cell line most widely used at this moment is the 293 cell line, a human embryonic kidney cell transfected with the E1 sequences of adenovirus. Replication of recombinant adenovirus is similar to wild-type virus and virions of recombinant virus and wild-type virus are identical. The deletion of E1 sequences from adenovirus DNA gives also room for cloning recombinant genes to be used in gene therapy protocols.

mately 10,000 progeny adenovirus particles can be generated in a single cell.

RECOMBINANT ADENOVIRUSES

Gene-transfer vectors derived from adenoviruses (adenoviral vectors) have a number of features that make them particularly useful for gene transfer (Stratford-Perricaudet and Perricaudet, 1991): a) the biology of the adenoviruses is characterized in detail, b) the adenovirus is not associated with severe human pathology, c) the virus is extremely efficient in introducing its DNA into the host cell, d) the virus can infect a wide variety of cells and has a broad host-range, e) the virus can be produced in large quantities with relative ease, and f) replication defective recombinant adenoviruses, which lack the E1 region, can be propagated *in vitro* in human cell lines that harbor the E1 sequences in the genome and g) unlike retroviruses, adenoviruses are able to transduce terminally differentiated cells.

Vectors derived from human adenoviruses are deleted for at least the E1 region. E1 proteins are pivotal for replication, as they are first expressed after adenovirus infection and are needed to activate other adenovirus genes. So deletion of E1 renders the adenovirus replication defective. Such vectors, where E1 is replaced by a gene-of-interest, have been used extensively for gene therapy experiments in the pre-clinical and clinical phase.

Human embryonic kidney cells (293 cells) are used for the production of recombinant adenovirus. The genome of those cells includes the E1 region, which permits propagation of E1 deleted adenovirus. Consequently, an adenovirus deleted for the E1 region can be grown in 293 cells (Figure 7.7b). Adenoviruses can be purified and concentrated by cesium chloride density centrifugation and stored frozen until use. Titers of purified adenovirus up to 10^{11}–10^{12} infectious particles/mL are routinely obtained.

In the majority of adenoviral vectors both E1 and E3 are deleted. E1 is deleted to make the virus replication defective and E3, because it is dispensable for growth *in vitro*. E3 encodes proteins that protect cells infected with a wild-type virus against recognition by the immune system. Unlike retrovirus genes, which can expressed in packaging cells, most of the adenovirus genes encode products that are toxic to cells. Therefore, current adenovirus packaging cells only express the E1 genes of adenovirus. All the other adenovirus genes are maintained in the recombinant adenoviral vectors, which are deleted only for the E1 region and the E3 region (Figure 7.7b). When an E1 deleted recombinant adenovirus infects a cell, the adenovirus genes are expected to be not expressed because of the absence of E1. However, it was found that certain somatic cells support the activation of adenovirus genes in the absence of E1. This leads to (low level) production of adenovirus proteins, rendering the involved cell immunogenic. As a consequence, inflammations occur and the cells that are provided with the recombinant genes are wiped out by the immune system. A lot of research is being conducted to improve adenovirus technology by deleting more adenovirus genes from the recombinant virus and developing packaging systems that are able to complement genes deleted from the recombinant.

Adenovirus DNA does not integrate into the host cell genome and is therefore gradually lost after cell division. Life-long treatment of genetic disorders thus requires repeated virus administrations. *In vivo* administered recombinant adenovirus elicits a humoral immune response, that inhibits subsequent adenovirus-mediated gene deliveries. Adenoviruses seem therefore particularly useful for therapies that demand a single *in vivo* gene delivery and transient gene expression, such as gene therapy of cancer.

APPLICATION OF ADENOVIRAL VECTORS

The vast majority of somatic cells in adults is non-dividing.

Therefore, *in vivo* gene therapy should exploit strategies that are able to transduce non-dividing and even terminally differentiated cells. So far, adenoviruses do have this property and in addition, have been shown to be able to transfect cells *in vivo* in the intact organ. In first instance, recombinant adenoviruses were developed for gene therapy of Cystic Fibrosis (CF). As airway epithelium is involved and as adenovirus is tropic by nature for the lungs, recombinant adenoviruses seemed to be candidates of first choice for CF gene therapy.

Recombinant adenoviruses harboring the normal human CF cDNA have been administered to patients. In the beginning, they were added dropwise to the nasal epithelium. In patients treated in this way the defect in chloride transport was corrected, without appearance of toxic side effects. The correction lasted less than three weeks, because adenovirus DNA does not integrate into the host cell genome. As a consequence, adenovirus DNA is diluted out and eventually lost after division of transduced cells. This also indicates that when used for e.g., CF gene therapy, repeated administrations are required. Application of recombinant adenovirus to the lungs induces an antibody response, that might block repeated adenovirus deliveries. In addition, one patient receiving a moderate dose of recombinant adenovirus in the lungs showed transient toxic side effects, which were most likely caused by the administered adenovirus. This means that, in potential, adenovirus is a very powerful gene delivery system, but transient expression and immune responses against adenovirus might limit its use for treatment of genetic disorders.

Recombinant adenovirus is currently explored for muscle gene therapy (Duchenne Muscular Dystrophy), liver gene therapy (e.g., for treatment of blood clotting disorders) and therapy of diseases of the Central Nervous System.

A very promising area for adenoviral vector systems is gene therapy of cancer. Gene therapy of cancer aims at destruction of tumor cells, thereby demanding only transient expression of therapeutic genes. Adenovirus has proven to be very efficient in delivering genes *in vivo* to tumors. Clinical studies using adenovirus mediated delivery of cytokine genes, p53 tumor suppressor genes or suicide genes are in progress.

To summarize, both *in vivo* and *in vitro* gene delivery by means of recombinant adenovirus is very efficient. This is accompanied by relative ease of production and purification. The major limitation of its use for treatment of genetic disorders is the immune reponse (antibodies, cellular immune reponse against adenovirus infected cells) that is elicited after *in vivo* delivery. To avoid these limitations, recombinant adenoviruses that are further attenuated have to be constructed, and 'second generation vectors' have been produced, that partially circumvent these problems. Adenovirus seems to be particularly useful for treatment of cancer, where efficient *in vivo* gene delivery and high levels of expression of the therapeutic gene are salient characteristics. If it would be possible to combine adenovirus gene transfer with targeting to tumor cells, an extremely powerful system for the treatment of cancers would be generated.

Adeno-associated Virus Vectors

REPLICATION OF WILD-TYPE AAV

Adeno-associated viruses (AAV) are human members of the parvovirus family. They are icosahedrally shaped viruses that lack an envelope. The virus particles are very heat-stable and resistant to a variety of chemicals such as chloroform and alcohol. Their genome is a single stranded DNA molecule of approximately 5 kb. So far, wild-type AAV has not been associated with human disease. AAV is a dependo-virus. This means that the wild-type virus can not replicate on its own; it needs another virus, in this case adeno- or herpes virus, for efficient replication. In the absence of helper virus, AAV establishes a latent infection in which its genome becomes integrated into the cellular chromosomal DNA. In human target cells, wild-type AAV integrates preferentially into a discrete region (19q13.3-qter) of chromosome 19. The AAV genome contains two large open reading frames. The left half of the genome encodes so-called *rep* proteins, that are responsible for AAV DNA-replication during a lytic infection. The right half encodes the virus structural (*cap*) proteins that form the capsid of the virus (Figure 7.8a). The protein coding region is flanked by inverted terminal repeats (TR) of 145 bp. each, which appear to contain all the *cis*-acting sequences required for virus replication and encapsidation.

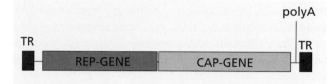

Figure 7.8a. Map of the adeno-associated virus genome (courtesy of IntroGene). The positions of terminal repeats (TR) and the REP and CAP genes are indicated.

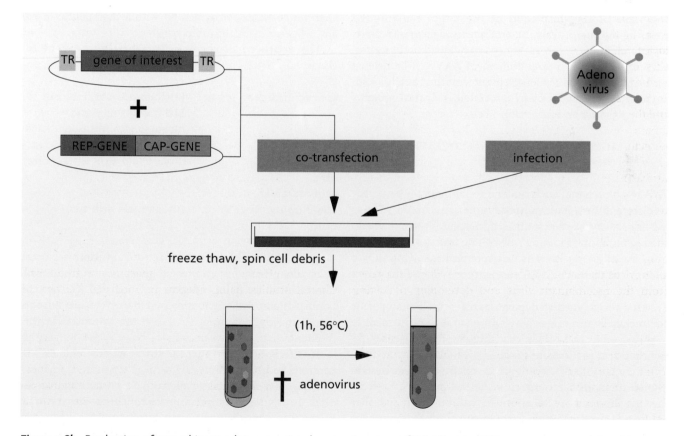

Figure 7.8b. Production of recombinant adeno-associated vector (courtesy of IntroGene). DNA constructs containing the therapeutic gene in between TR sequences are cotransfected into a cell together with constructs harboring the AAV genes. After infection with adenovirus, recombinant AAV is made from the construct containing the therapeutic gene because it contains TR sequences which are sufficient for replication and packaging of DNA into virions. Also the adenovirus replicates, so a mixture of recombinant AAV and adenovirus is generated. Unlike adenovirus, AAV particles are stable at 56°C; so after heating at this temperature only viable AAV particles remain.

Recombinant Adeno-associated Virus

In an AAV-vector, the entire protein-coding domain (±4.5 kb) can be replaced by the gene(s) of interest (for review see Einerhand and Valerio, 1995; Flotte and Carter, 1995). The ITRs are the only *cis*-acting elements required for all steps of the AAV life cycle, including replication of viral DNA, chromosomal integration, and packaging of the viral genome. Such vectors are packaged into virions by supplying the AAV-proteins *in trans*. This is achieved by transfecting the vector plasmid and the packaging plasmid into adenovirus infected cells. As a result, a mixture of recombinant AAV and wild-type adenoviruses is generated (Figure 7.8b). Due to the stability of the AAV-virion, the adenovirus contamination can be cleared from the virus-preparation by heat inactivation (1 hr. 56°C).

In the absence of helper virus AAV will stably integrate into the host cell genome and remain latent. AAV-vectors do integrate with high efficiency into the host chromosomal DNA. However, thus far they do not share the integration site specificity of wild-type AAV. Site specific integration would be of great importance since it reduces the risks of transformation of the target cell through insertional mutagenesis. In contrast to adenoviral vectors, where the majority of viral genes are retained in the vector, the entire protein coding domain of AAV can be deleted and replaced by the sequences of interest thus totally avoiding any immunity problem associated with viral proteins upon transduction of the target cell.

Application of Adeno-associated Viral Vectors

AAV-vector technology is under development for a number of different therapeutic purposes and target tissues. The as yet most developed system is perhaps AAV-vector mediated gene transfer to lung cells. Gene transfer and expression for at least 3 months was reported following *in vivo* delivery of the AAV-CFTR vector to one lobe of the rabbit lung.

AAV-vector mediated gene transfer to hematopoietic stem cells is also under development for the treatment of ß-thalassemia and sickle cell anemia. Both diseases severely affect erythrocyte function: ß-thalassemic erythrocytes contain insufficient ß-globin chains whereas mutant ß-globin chains are made in sickle cell anemia. Both inherited diseases are recessive in nature which indicates that one functional intact copy of the adult ß-globin gene is sufficient to correct the defect. Expression vectors carrying the human ß-globin gene with its promoter and local enhancer elements can direct erythroid specific globin RNA expression.

The results obtained with AAV-vectors thus far indicate that AAV-vector mediated gene transfer into hemopoietic stem cells might become a valuable tool in gene therapy protocols. Compared to retroviral and adenoviral vector technology, however, AAV-vector technology is still in its infancy. Although gene transfer into hemopoietic progenitor cells has been demonstrated using several functional assays, it still needs to be evaluated whether the vectors are indeed stably integrated into the host cell genome of primitive hemopoietic cells and whether infection frequency is sufficient to elicit a therapeutic response.

Clinical Studies

The first approved experiment in human gene therapy began in 1990, with the aim of treating adenosine deaminase deficiency, a rare immunodeficiency disorder (see above). Since that time, there has been substantial growth in the field of gene therapy, especially in the field of cancer gene therapy. By June 1995 a total of 112 clinical studies had been approved in the US Recombinant DNA Advisory Committee (RAC), of which 87 with a therapeutic intent and 25 gene marking protocols (Marshall, 1995).

The approved protocols with therapeutic intent include:

genetic disorders	21	(including Cystic Fibrosis, LDLR deficiency and hematological disorders such as ADA deficiency, Gaucher's disease and Fanconi anemia)
HIV	9	
cardiovascular	1	
autoimmune disease	1	(rheumatoid arthritis)
cancer	55	

In 82 of these trials, murine retroviral vectors are used, in 15 adenovirus and 12 involve liposomes, 2 groups will inject naked DNA (cf. Chapter 12), one will use particle bombardment and one is approved to use AAV. In Europe, approximately 20 protocols have been approved at this moment.

It is to be expected that the list of clinical studies will continue to grow rapidly.

Altogether, over 1000 patients have been treated so far (end of 1995), and the preliminary conclusions that can be drawn from these studies are that gene transfer to humans is possible, although the expression levels are still low in most cases, and that it is safe. Obviously, there is need for improvement of stable gene delivery for both in *ex vivo* and *in vivo* purposes.

Pharmaceutical Production and Regulation

In general, products that have the potential to be used in humans have to be tested for effectivity in an appropriate animal model before being introduced into the clinic. If this is not possible e.g., because an animal model does not exist, rigorous safety testing in rodents and large animals such as monkeys has to be performed. When proven to be safe in animal studies, clinical studies may be initiated after approval from the authorities. The objectives of the clinical studies are to assess toxicity and biological efficacy of the gene therapy product. When *in vivo* gene transfer is used, dose-related toxicity is assessed in dose escalation studies.

A fundamental prerequisite of gene therapy is that of safety, both for the patient and his environment. In addition, scientific and ethical questions are raised. All these issues have to be carefully reviewed when gene transfer experiments to humans are considered. The agents to be used in clinical studies have to be produced under strict adherence to Good Laboratory Practice (GLP) and Good Manufacturing Practice (GMP) principles. Control over both biological sources (e.g., packaging cell lines) and end products (e.g., batches of recombinant virus) is mandatory. Such a safety program must ensure that the biopharmaceuticals are not contaminated with adventitious agents such as microbial or viral contaminants and toxins (Ostrove, 1994). Most European countries have committees that must approve the clinical protocol, the production, safety testing program and ethics when gene transfer to humans is considered.

In the United States, proposals for experiments involving the transfer of recombinant DNA into humans require approval from the local Institutional Biosafety Committee and by the local Institutional Review Board. Then the proposal will be considered by the RAC (Recombinant DNA Advisory Committee of the National Institutes of Health (NIH) and the FDA (Food and Drug Administration). The RAC deals with ethical and social concerns, scientific evaluation and public discussion. The FDA is the relevant authority with respect to safety of these biological products.

Concluding Remarks

Although in the last decade gene therapy has evolved from 'possible in theory' to clinical testing in humans, we are still at the beginning of the gene therapy era.

Despite encouraging results obtained so far in clinical studies, a number of scientific questions have to be addressed to make gene therapy come to age. A few of the specific questions have already been addressed when discussing the different gene transfer systems. In general, retroviruses are used in *ex vivo* gene transfer protocols, where they are able to stably transduce the target cell population. The frequency of transduction depends on the cell type. *In vivo* gene transfer uses either liposome mediated gene transfer or recombinant adenovirus. Recombinant adenovirus is particularly effective. However, liposomes and adenoviruses do not or minimally integrate the transferred DNA into host cell chromosomes. This requires repeated administration protocols. Stable integration and efficient *in vivo* gene transfer has been reported for recombinant AAV. When the encouraging results that have been obtained in animals can be extended to humans, AAV seems to be a good candidate for future *in vivo* gene therapy for genetic disorders. AAV might be used in *ex vivo* protocols as well. Unlike retroviruses, AAV is able to infect non-dividing target cells. The main drawback of AAV is that large scale production is difficult and poorly reproducible. Non-viral gene transfer vectors need a lot of research to increase efficiencies of gene delivery. As already stated before, addition of (e.g., fusogenic) proteins or peptides may improve gene delivery significantly. This approach will result in 'artificial viruses'. By adding viral components, gene transfer of non-viral vectors may become more efficient, with a reduced risk to encounter the drawbacks associated with viral vectors.

The growth of medical interest in gene therapy is accompanied by growing commercial interests, which propels research in this area. However, increased commercial interest shouldn't lead to unrealistic expectations with respect to applications of gene therapy. The medical potential looks enormous, but sound scientific research is needed to turn the modest clinical effects of current studies into real cures. ∎

Further Reading

- **Ascadi G, Massie B, Jani A.** (1995). Adenovirus-mediated gene transfer into striated muscles. *J Mol Med*, 73, 165–180
- **Crystal RG.** (1995). Transfer of genes to humans: early lessons and obstacles to success. *Science*, 270, 404–410
- **Crystal RG.** (1995). The gene as the drug. *Nature Medicine*, 1, 15–17

- **Mulligan RC.** (1993). The Basic Science of Gene Therapy. *Science*, 260, 926–932
- **Spooner RA, Deonarain MP, Epenetos AA.** (1995). DNA vaccination for cancer treatment. *Gene Ther*, 2, 173–180
- **Wilson JM.** (1993). Vehicles for gene therapy. *Nature*, 365, 691–692
- **Yu M, Poeschla E, Wong-Staal F.** (1994). Progress towards gene therapy for HIV infection. *Gene Ther*, 1, 13–26

References

- **Anderson WF.** (1992). Human Gene Therapy. *Science*, 256, 808–813
- **Culver KW, Blaese RM.** (1994). Gene therapy for cancer. *Trends Genet*, 10, 174–178
- **Einerhand MPW, Valerio D.** (1995). Viral vector systems for bone marrow gene therapy. In *Hematopoietic stem cells*, edited by D Levitt and R Mertelsmann. New York: Marcel Dekker, Inc
- **Flotte TR, Carter BJ.** (1995). Adeno-associated virus vectors for gene therapy. *Gene Ther*, 2, 357–362
- **Horwitz MS.** (1990). Adenoviridae and their replication. In *Virology*, edited by BN Fields and DM Knipe. New York: Raven Press, Ltd, pp. 1679–1740
- **Jolly D.** (1994). Viral vector systems for gene therapy. *Cancer Gene Ther*, 1, 51–64
- **Ledley FD.** (1995). Nonviral gene therapy: the promise of genes as pharmaceutical products. *Human Gene Ther*, 6, 1129–1144
- **Marshall E.** (1995). Gene therapy's growing pains. *Science*, 269, 1050–1055
- **Miller AD.** (1992). Human gene therapy comes of age. *Nature*, 357, 455–460
- **Moolten FL.** (1994). Drug sensitivity ("suicide") genes for selective cancer chemotherapy. *Cancer Gene Ther*, 1, 279–287
- **Ostrove JM.** (1994). Safety testing programs for gene therapy viral vectors. *Cancer Gene Ther*, 1, 125–131
- **Smith AE.** (1995). Viral vectors in gene therapy. *Ann Rev Microbiol*, 49, 807–838
- **Stratford-Perricaudet LD, Perricaudet M.** (1991). Gene transfer into animals: the promise of adenovirus. In *Human Gene Transfer*, edited by O Cohen-Adenauer and M Boiron. John Libbey Eurotext, pp. 51–61
- **Valerio D.** (1992). Retrovirus vectors for gene therapy procedures, pp. 211–246. In *Transgenic Animals*, edited by F Grosveld and G Kollias. London: Academic Press
- **Yang NS, Sun WH.** (1995). Gene gun and other non-viral approaches for cancer gene therapy. *Nature Med*, 1, 481–483

Self-Assessment Questions

Question 1: What is the approach for treatment of CF with gene therapy?

Question 2: What makes it possible to generate retrovirus packaging cell lines?

Question 3: Why are hematopoietic stem cells such an attractive target for cure of diseases in which blood cells are affected?

Question 4: What is the key determinant for successful stem cell gene therapy with retroviral vectors?

Question 5: In vivo liposome-mediated gene transfer was found to be relatively inefficient as compared to virus-mediated gene delivery until now. In order to improve non-virus mediated gene delivery, several components, often derived from viruses, have been added to liposome/DNA mixtures to improve their efficiency. Optimal non-viral gene delivery vehicles might look like 'artificial viruses' in the end: particles containing all the components that make virus mediated gene delivery efficient but not having the safety drawbacks associated with the use of recombinant viruses. Which steps might be subject to improvement of the efficacy of non-virus mediated gene delivery?

Question 6: The treatment of a certain inherited disorder in which a number of different organs are affected demands delivery of the therapeutic gene to a number of different locations in the body. It is impossible to deliver the genes to all affected organs separately. Therefore, delivery of the therapeutic gene by intravenous injection is considered. What are the possibilities for having the therapeutic gene expressed only in the affected tissues?

Question 7: For suicide gene therapy of malignant brain tumors, two different gene delivery procedures are being exploited yet: 1) introduction of retrovirus producing cells into the tumor; 2) injection of recombinant adenovirus into the tumor.

Question 7A: What is the basic mechanism of suicide gene therapy?

Question 7B: What is the 'bystander' effect?

Question 7C: What are the advantages and disadvantages of each of the two gene delivery systems mentioned above?

Answers

Answer 1: To introduce a normal version of the CFTR gene into airway epithelium by in vivo gene transfer procedures.

Answer 2: Deletion of the packaging signal Ψ from the retroviral RNA prevents packaging of such an RNA molecule into a virus particle. However, synthesis of retroviral proteins from RNA molecules with a Ψ deletion is still possible.

Answer 3: Stem cells maintain at least one kg of bone marrow and blood cells in human adults. Therefore, correction of stem cells would result in life-long correction of the disease. Unlike stem cells, peripheral blood cells have a limited life span. Gene therapy of peripheral blood cells will therefore result only in transient correction of the disease.

Answer 4: For retrovirus mediated gene delivery, cell division is a pre-requisite. Therefore, the stem cells should be cycling when retroviral transduction is performed.

Answer 5: They should pass physical barriers (e.g. mucous layer should be passed for transfection of lung cells).
They should bind to (target cell specific) receptors (more efficient internalization).

Endosome disruption should be induced to prevent lysis of the DNA because of low pH in the endosomes/lysosomes.
They should transport the DNA to the nucleus.

Answer 6:
1) Targeting to the cells or organs that were affected, e.g., antibody mediated delivery.
2) Expression of the therapeutic gene is under the control of a tissue or cell-specific promoter, resulting in expression only in particular cell types.

Answer 7A:
Tumor cells are provided with a gene which encodes an enzyme that is able to convert a pro-drug (e.g., ganciclovir) into a toxic compound.

Answer 7B:
The fact that not all tumor cells have to be provided with the suicide gene to accomplish eradication of the complete tumor.

Answer 7C:
Re retrovirus-producing cells
Advantages:
– They infect only dividing cells, thereby preferentially transducing tumor cells and not the surrounding normal brain cells.
Disadvantages:
– A strong immune response against the retrovirus producing cells is evoked, preventing efficient repeat deliveries.
– No efficient gene delivery occurs when a large fraction of the tumor is non-dividing.

Re advantages and disadvantages of the use of recombinant adenovirus:
Advantages:
– Efficient gene delivery to both dividing and non-dividing tumor cells.
– If gene transfer to cells of normal tissues occurs, the adenovirus DNA does not integrate into the host chromosome and expression of the therapeutic gene is transient in nature.
Disadvantages:
– Gene transfer to non-dividing normal (brain) cells is also possible.
– An immune response against adenovirus particles is evoked.

8 Hematopoietic Growth Factors

by: Jeanne Flynn and Allen W. Rosman

Introduction

Hematopoietic or blood cells are vital to human life; they transport oxygen, provide host immunity, and clot blood. What may not be as familiar is the intricate, multistep process that allows immature precursor cells in the bone marrow to mature and become functional blood cells. Ordinarily, this regulatory process replaces cells lost through daily physiologic activities. The process is also capable of mass producing millions of cells to fight infection or replace losses due to hemorrhaging. This remarkable ability to form blood cells is called hematopoiesis.

As early as the first decade of this century, scientists recognized the presence of circulating factors that regulate hematopoiesis. Unfortunately, further progress was delayed for the next half century until cell culture systems were developed that could sustain cell colonies *in vitro*. The growth and survival of early blood cells required the presence of specific factors, which led to the term colony-stimulating factor (CSF) (Clark and Kamen, 1987; Kouides and DiPersio, 1995). Hematopoietic growth factor is the preferred term because it is more precise than the one based on laboratory observations.

Efforts to purify the hematopoietic growth factors progressed slowly throughout the 1970s and early 1980s for several reasons. Blood and most other specimens contain only minute amounts of growth factors. The presence of many growth factors confounded the search for a single growth factor with specific activity. Progress was temporarily interrupted until it was possible to purify sufficient quantities to fully evaluate the new biologics. The introduction of recombinant DNA technology triggered a flurry of studies and a virtual information explosion (Metcalf, 1990). Since that time, more than 20 hematopoietic growth factors have been isolated (Summerhayes, 1995), and the number is increasing.

The purpose of this chapter is to review the chemistry, pharmacology, pharmaceutical concerns, and clinical and practice aspects of hematopoietic growth factors. In view of the number of growth factors, it is not surprising that thousands of papers have been published on this topic. To cover the topic without overwhelming the reader, comprehensive reviews were selected over original research papers. References were also selected because of recent publication date, prestige, and relevance to pharmacy.

Definitions

Concepts and terms to be used in this chapter will be defined here. Hematopoietic growth factors regulate both hematopoiesis and the functional activity of mature cells. The former includes proliferation (i.e., reproduction of similar cells), differentiation (i.e., specialization or the acquisition of functions that are different from that of the most primitive cell form [i.e., stem cell]), and maturation (i.e., developmental changes that lead to functionally active cells). In addition, hematopoietic growth factors mobilize progenitor cells to move from the bone marrow to the peripheral blood (Kouides and DiPersio, 1995).

There are eight major lineages or types of mature blood cells, all of which are derived from a small population of primitive stem cells in the bone marrow. The myeloid pathway gives rise to red blood cells (erythrocytes), platelets, monocytes and macrophages, and granulocytes (neutrophils, eosinophils, and basophils). The lymphoid pathway gives rise to lymphocytes (Clark and Kamen, 1987; Kouides and DiPersio, 1995).

The name of each hematopoietic growth factor is derived from its predominant target cell. The growth factors to be covered in this chapter are listed below:

Granulocyte–colony-stimulating factor (G-CSF)
Granulocyte-macrophage–colony-stimulating factor (GM-CSF)
Erythropoietin (EPO)
Macrophage–colony-stimulating factor (M-CSF)
Interleukin-3 (IL-3)
Granulocyte-macrophage–colony-stimulating factor/IL-3 fusion protein (PIXY-321)
Thrombopoietin (TPO)
Stem cell factor (SCF)

This chapter focuses on the three growth factors that are produced by recombinant DNA technology and marketed in Europe and the United States, rG-CSF, rGM-CSF, and rEPO. The lower case "r" distinguishes recombinant from endogenous hematopoietic growth factors. The amount of data on investigational products is variable; information on the five (i.e., rM-CSF, rIL-3, PIXY-321, rTPO, and rSCF) that have been tested in humans is summarized whenever possible. Although the authors are more familiar with growth factors developed by their company, every effort has been made to provide a comprehensive, fair-balanced review.

Chemical Description

Hematopoietic growth factors are glycoproteins, which can be distinguished by their amino acid sequence and glycosylation (carbohydrate linkages). Hematopoietic growth factors have cysteine-cysteine disulfide bridges that dictate their three-dimensional configuration, which is necessary

for biologic activity. Most hematopoietic growth factors are single-chain polypeptides weighing approximately 14 to 21 kD. The carbohydrate content varies depending on the growth factor and production method, which in turn affects the molecular weight but not necessarily the biologic activity. Each hematopoietic growth factor is encoded by a unique gene, which can be obtained from different sources or cell lines, and expressed in different biologic systems (e.g., bacteria or yeast) to produce recombinant growth factors (Metcalf, 1990).

Chemical Properties of G-CSF and GM-CSF

The chemical properties of the myeloid hematopoietic growth factors, G-CSF and GM-CSF, have been characterized (Table 8.1). Two recombinant products of endogenous

	G-CSF			GM-CSF	
Endogenous growth factors					
Chromosomal location	17			5	
Animo acids	174 (and 177)*			127	
Glycosylation	O-glycosylation			N- and O-glycosylation	
Molecular weight (kD) †	18.6 (≈ 20)			14.7 (≈ 18-30)	
Recombinant human growth factors					
Proper name	Filgrastim	Lenograstim	Nartograstim	Molgramostim	Sargramostim
Company	Amgen/Kirin/ Roche/Dompé/ Esteve/Sankyo	Chugai/Rhône-Poulenc/Amrad/ Almirall	Kyowa	Schering/ Sandoz	Immunex
Animo acids	175 (N-terminal methionine)	174	174 (changes at 1st, 3rd, 4th, 5th and 17th amino acid)	128	127 (change at 23rd amino acid)
Glycosylation	no	O-glycosylation	no	no	N-glycosylation
Gene source	bladder carcinoma cell line (5637)	squamous carcinoma cell line (CHU-2)	?	human monocyte cell line (U937)	mouse T-lymphoma cell line (ATCC-CRL-8080)
Expression system	E. coli	Chinese hamster ovary	E. coli	E. coli	yeast

Table 8.1. Chemistry of selected hematopoietic growth factors (Lieschke and Burgess, 1992; Metcalf, 1990). * Native G-CSF exists in two forms; type a (177 amino acids) and is less active than type b (174 amino acids). † Molecular weight varies with the extent of glycosylation and is expressed for both core protein and glycosylated protein (in parentheses).

G-CSF, Filgrastim and Lenograstim and one of GM-CSF, Molgramostim are available in Europe. Filgrastim and the second recombinant GM-CSF, Sargramostim, are marketed in the United States. Filgrastim and Lenograstim are available in China and Japan. Less information is available on Nartograstim, a type of rG-CSF marketed in Japan, and on Regramostim, an early type of rGM-CSF that is no longer being evaluated by Sandoz.

The identification of two myeloid hematopoietic growth factors and various recombinant products of each invites comparison. The genes for endogenous G-CSF and GM-CSF are located on different chromosomes, 17 and 5, respectively. Interestingly, the gene for GM-CSF is located on the same chromosomal band as those for M-CSF and IL-3, but each hematopoietic growth factor is encoded by a unique gene. The implications of clustering are unknown (Clark and Kamen, 1987; Metcalf, 1990).

Genes provide the blueprint for producing large quantities of hematopoietic growth factors through recombinant DNA technology. The usual gene source is a tumor cell line because of its yield. After cloning, the gene is usually expressed in bacteria (*Escherichia coli*), mammalian cells (Chinese hamster ovary), or yeast (*Saccharomyces cerevisiae*), where large quantities of the glycoprotein can be produced (Metcalf, 1990). Of course, the entire production process requires multiple steps, which are described in Chapter 3.

The resultant recombinant hematopoietic growth factors closely resemble endogenous proteins except for slight modifications in amino acid sequence, extent of glycosylation, or both, which are determined by the production method. For example, Filgrastim differs from endogenous G-CSF in only two respects. Filgrastim has a terminal N-methionine that is absent from endogenous G-CSF. In addition, Filgrastim is not glycosylated because the bacterial expression system lacks glycosylation capability (Lieschke and Burgess, 1992). Crystallography studies reveal that these modifications are physically remote from the biologically active sites (Figure 8.1).

These minor differences between recombinant products and endogenous glycoproteins do not appear to translate to differences in biologic activity. The clinical consequences of different patterns of glycosylation are unknown and will be revisited in the appropriate section (Lieschke and Burgess, 1992; Metcalf, 1990).

Chemical Properties of Erythropoietin (EPO)

The gene that encodes EPO is located on chromosome 7. The mature polypeptide has 165 amino acids, two disulfide bonds, and three *N*- and one *O*-linked carbohydrate chains. Unlike G-CSF and GM-CSF, EPO requires glycosylation for its biologic activity. EPO is heavily glycosylated, which increases the molecular weight from 18.4 kD for the

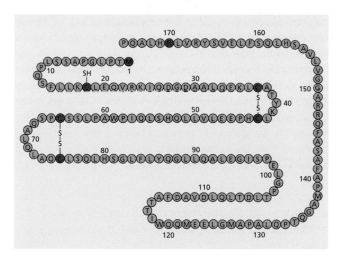

Figure 8.1a. Primary structure of Filgrastim (recombinant G-CSF).

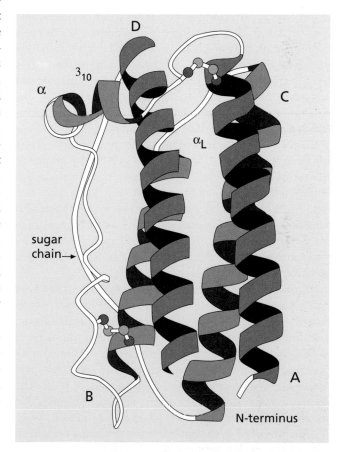

Figure 8.1b. Secondary structure of Filgrastim (recombinant G-CSF). Filgrastim is a 175-amino acid polypeptide. Its four anti-parallel α helices (A, B, C and D) and short 3-to-10 type helix (3_{10}) form a helical bundle. The two biologically active sites (α and $α_L$) are remote from modifications at the N terminus of the A helix and the sugar chain attached to loop C-D. *Note:* Filgrastim is not glycosylated; the sugar chain is included to illustrate its location in endogenous G-CSF.

unglycosylated molecule to approximately 34 kD. There are two recombinant EPO products; both are expressed in Chinese hamster ovary cells. In the United States, the proper name for recombinant erythropoietin alpha is Epoetin alpha, while the International nonproprietary name is Epoetinum alpha. Epoetin alpha is also available in Japan and China. The second recombinant erythropoietin is epoetin beta and is available in Europe and Japan. Both recombinant products have the same primary amino acid sequence and almost identical glycosylation (Abels, 1990, Veys et al., 1992).

Chemical Properties of Other Hematopoietic Growth Factors

M-CSF was the first hematopoietic growth factor to be purified and was isolated from human urine in 1975. As previously indicated, the gene for M-CSF is located on chromosome 5. In contrast with most other hematopoietic growth factors that are single polypeptides, M-CSF is a complex dimer. The molecular weight is 14 to 21 kD for each polypeptide or 28 to 42 kD for the dimer. M-CSF is heavily glycosylated, resulting in a final molecular weight of 70 to 90 kD (Metcalf, 1990). Recombinant M-CSF can be expressed in Chinese hamster ovary or African green monkey kidney cells (Clark and Kamen, 1987).

IL-3 was the fourth hematopoietic growth factor to be isolated after M-CSF, GM-CSF, and G-CSF. Also known as multi-CSF, IL-3 is encoded by a gene on chromosome 5. Differences in production methods and expression systems yield minor differences in the 133- or 134-amino acid sequence, glycosylation, and molecular weight (range, 14 to 26 kD). For example, rIL-3 is heavily glycosylated when expressed in yeast but is not glycosylated when expressed in bacteria (De Vries et al., 1993).

Immunex Corporation, Seattle, Washington, USA, is now concentrating on the fusion protein, PIXY-321, which consists of rGM-CSF and rIL-3 coupled by a flexible amino acid linker sequence that allows the binding domains to fold into their native conformation. Like its individual components, PIXY-321 has minor changes to its amino acid sequence, is glycosylated, and is expressed in yeast. The complete molecule has 271 amino acids and a molecular weight of approximately 35 kD (Dorr and Von Hoff, 1994).

The other two hematopoietic growth factors remain in early stages of development, so their chemical properties have not yet been thoroughly characterized. Initial attempts to purify thrombopoietin from body fluids or conventional cell lines failed because of the complex nature of the starting material and difficulties associated with in vivo assays. The search was hampered by the discovery of some platelet effects in other hematopoietic growth factors. Throughout the 1980s, scientists questioned the existence of this elusive glycoprotein. Finally, in 1994, three different strategies were used to obtain complementary DNA from pigs (Genentech Inc., San Francisco, California, USA) or dogs (Amgen Inc., Thousand Oaks, California, USA), mice (ZymoGenetics, a subsidiary of Novo Nordisk AS, Denmark), and rats (Kirin Brewery Company, Japan) or sheep (Kuter et al., 1994). Except for species-specific differences, each group described similar molecules. The gene for thrombopoietin is located on chromosome 3. Depending on the source, the mature polypeptide has 305 to 355 amino acids, which may undergo cleavage to a smaller polypeptide that retains biological activity. A wide range of molecular weights (18 to 70 kD) have been reported (Kaushansky, 1995).

The gene for SCF is located on chromosome 4. There are two forms of SCF, SCF-1 (248 amino acids) and SCF-2 (220 amino acids). SCF-1 can be cleaved to a soluble form (164 or 165 amino acids; 26 kD), which exists as a noncovalently associated dimer (53 kD). Both endogenous and recombinant SCF are heavily glycosylated, with O- and N-linked sugars (Galli et al., 1994).

A more recently cloned hematopoietic growth factor is flt3 (also known as flk-2) ligand, a protein structurally similar to SCF and its receptor. Sequence analysis of human flt3 ligand cDNA indicates that the protein has an N-terminal peptide of 26 amino acids, a 156 amino acid extracellular domain, a 23 amino acid transmembrane domain, and a 30-amino acid cytoplasmic domain. The protein is glycosylated and human recombinant soluble flt3 ligand has been produced in yeast.

Both SCF and flt3 ligand stimulate the proliferation and colony formation of human hematopoietic stem/progenitor cells (Lyman et al., 1994).

Pharmacology

Hematopoietic growth factors act by binding to specific cell surface receptors. The resultant complex sends a signal to the cell to express genes, which in turn induce cellular proliferation, differentiation, or activation. A hematopoietic growth factor may also act indirectly if the cell expresses a gene that causes the production of a different hematopoietic growth factor or another cytokine, which in turn binds to and stimulates a different cell (Figure 8.2). This indirect activity has made it difficult to delineate the pharmacologic activity of individual hematopoietic growth factors and accounts for some of the differences between in vitro and in vivo results. Cell culture studies can be designed to exclude indirect effects, but animal and clinical studies generally reflect the full scope of direct and indirect effects.

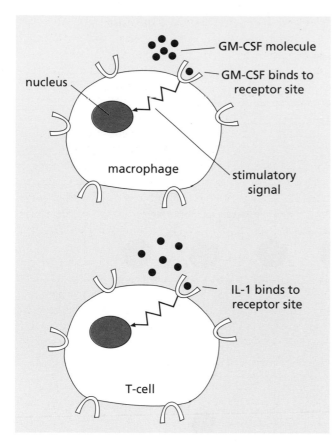

Figure 8.2. An example of a protein which acts both directly and indirectly on a cell is shown in this figure with GM-CSF binding to the receptor on a macrophage. GM-CSF may stimulate the macrophage to proliferate and differentiate. In addition, GM-CSF may induce the macrophage to produce and secrete a number of cytokines, including G-CSF, IL-1, and tumor necrosis factor. These cytokines then leave the macrophage and bind to cells with specific receptors for them, such as neutrophils, T-cells and fibroblasts, respectively. Thus, indirect acting CSFs may initiate a cytokine cascade.

In Vitro Activity

The hierarchy for hematopoiesis involves many steps and pathways. By definition, the pluripotent stem cell is the progenitor or precursor for all hematopoietic cells. The stem cell has the potential to replicate itself (i.e., self-renewal) or differentiate to more mature forms. Upon maturation, it loses its capacity for self-renewal and becomes highly specialized. Pluripotent refers to the stem cell's ability to differentiate along different pathways to give rise to myeloid cells (i.e., erythrocytes, platelets, monocytes and macrophages, and granulocytes [neutrophils, eosinophils, and basophils]) and lymphoid (i.e., B and T lymphocytes) cells.

The complex interactions among these progenitor cells were determined by evaluating the effects of adding hematopoietic growth factors to *in vitro* cell cultures containing immature progenitor cells from the bone marrow. Figure 8.3 illustrates key concepts such as synergy among hematopoietic growth factors. For example, sequential administration of rIL-3 followed by rGM-CSF expands myeloid cells (Kouides and DiPersio, 1995). Although the exact mechanism is unknown, the overlapping actions of different hematopoietic growth factors may constitute a control system (Metcalf, 1990).

This model also illustrates the concept of lineage specificity. Multilineage growth factors (e.g., GM-CSF, IL-3, and SCF) affect multiple cell lineages and tend to act on early progenitor cells before they become committed to one lineage. Lineage-specific growth factors (e.g., G-CSF, M-CSF, EPO, and presumably thrombopoietin) predominantly affect one cell type and act later in the hematopoietic cascade. For example, GM-CSF affects early and intermediate progenitor cells that give rise to erythrocytes, platelets, macrophages, neutrophils, and eosinophils. In contrast, G-CSF primarily acts at a later stage of differentiation in the pathway that gives rise to neutrophils (Clark and Kamen, 1987), although more recent models predict a slightly broader range of activity for some lineage-specific growth factors (Groopman *et al.*, 1989; Kouides and DiPersio, 1995; Vose and Armitage, 1995).

In addition to their effects on progenitor cells, hematopoietic growth factors bind to and regulate the functional activity of mature cells (Table 8.2). Again, multilineage growth factors (e.g., GM-CSF and IL-3) affect more than one cell lineage, whereas lineage-specific growth factors (e.g., G-CSF, M-CSF, and EPO) predominantly affect one cell type (Mertelsmann, 1991). This phenomenon is concentration dependent. The GM-CSF concentrations that regulate monocytes and granulocytes (5 to 20 pg/mL) are lower than those for eosinophils and platelets (20 to 2000 pg/mL) (Metcalf, 1990). See Table 8.3 for endogenous serum levels of these growth factors as measured in normal patient donors.

The last syllable of the proper names for the recombinant products of G-CSF and GM-CSF is based on their ability to <u>stim</u>ulate hematopoietic cells. The two recombinant G-CSF products, Fil<u>grast</u>im and Leno<u>grast</u>im, stimulate granulocytes, while the two recombinant GM-CSF products, Mol<u>gram</u>ostim and Sar<u>gram</u>ostim, stimulate both <u>granulo</u>cytes and <u>mono</u>cytes. The first syllable of <u>Sar</u>gramostim appears to be based on its expression system, *Saccharomyces*, but the derivation of the other hematopoietic growth factors is not as readily apparent.

Two hematopoietic growth factors are not listed in Table 8.2 because of the lack of definitive information. Thrombopoietin acts on mature megakaryocytes and platelets (Kaushansky, 1995, Debili *et al.*, 1997). On the other

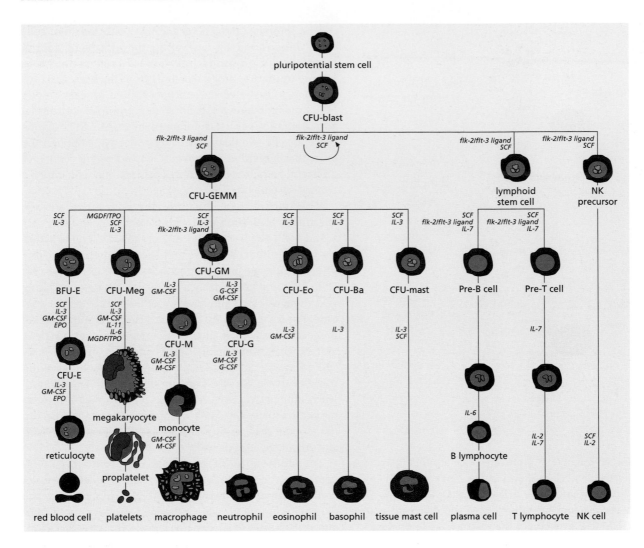

Figure 8.3. Hematopoietic cascade showing the pathways that give rise to mature blood cells and sites of action of hematopoietic growth factors (Clark and Kamen, 1987; Kaushansky, 1995; Vose and Armitage, 1995). Bas = basophil; BFU-E = burst-forming unit-erythroid; CFU = colony-forming unit; Eo = eosinophil; GEMM = granulocyte-erythrocyte-monocyte-megakaryocyte; Meg = megakaryocyte. For other abbreviations: see text.

Cell type	Multilineage		Lineage specific		
	GM-CSF	IL-3	G-CSF	M-CSF	EPO
Neutrophils	+	+	+		
Monocytes	+	+		+	
Basophils		+			
Eosinophils	+	+			
Erythrocytes		+			+
Platelets	+				

Table 8.2. In vitro effects of hematopoietic growth factors on mature hematopoietic cells (Mertelsmann, 1991).

Hematopoietic growth factor (normal range in serum)	Cellular source	Stimuli for release
G-CSF (9-51 pg/mL)	monocytes	lipopolysaccharide induction of monocytes
	fibroblasts	cytokine activation of fibroblasts and
	endothelial cells	endothelial cells
	bone marrow stromal cells	
GM-CSF (0.4-2 pg/mL)	T cells	antigen-mediated T cell activation
	monocytes	lipopolysaccharide induction of monocytes
	fibroblasts	cytokine activation of fibroblasts and
	endothelial cells	endothelial cells
EPO (3-7 mIU/mL)	kidney (>90%)	hypoxia (e.g. anemia)
	liver	
M-CSF (250-1700 pg/mL)	monocytes	T cell-mediated induction of monocytes
	fibroblasts	
	endothelial cells	
IL-3 (0.5-8 pg/mL)	T cells (primary source)	antigen-mediated T cell activation
	mast cells	
Thrombopoietin (20-300 pg/mL)	kidney	Constitutively expressed, not upregelated; levels determined through catabolism by platelets and megakaryocytes
	liver	
SCF (1200-1900 pg/mL)	fibroblasts	unknown

Table 8.3. Cellular sources, endogenous levels and stimuli for release of hematopoietic growth factors in humans (Groopman *et al.*, 1989; Kouides and DiPersio, 1995; Kuter *et al.*, 1994; Lok *et al.*, 1994; Nichol *et al.*, 1995, R&D Systems, 1997).

hand, the multilineage growth factor, SCF, does not appear to regulate the activity of mature blood cells; but it may interact with mast cells, melanocytes, and primitive sex cells (Galli *et al.*, 1994).

Studies by independent investigators provide insight regarding the types of *in vitro* actions that hematopoietic growth factors exert on mature cells such as neutrophils (Table 8.4). Both rG-CSF and rGM-CSF promote the destruction of foreign substances by enhancing phagocytosis, antibody-dependent cell-mediated cytotoxicity, and superoxide production. Recombinant G-CSF also primes neutrophils for enhanced release of arachidonic acid products in response to other stimuli (Dale *et al.*, 1995). Recombinant GM-CSF enhances neutrophil margination

and adhesion to the endothelium. The two growth factors appear to exert opposing effects on chemotaxis or neutrophil migration; rG-CSF enhances it, whereas rGM-CSF inhibits it (Clark and Kamen, 1987; Robinson and Quesenberry, 1990).

In Vivo Activity

The *in vivo* effects of hematopoietic growth factors can be assessed by measuring endogenous levels under different conditions or by administering the growth factors to animals or humans. Although the results are often consistent with those predicted by *in vitro* studies, there are some differences.

	rG-CSF	rGM-CSF
Phagocytosis	↑	↑
Antibody-dependent killing	↑	↑
Arachidonic acid product release	↑	
Superoxide production	↑	↑
Margination and adhesion to endothelium		↑
Chemotaxis or migration	↑	↓

Table 8.4. *In vitro* effects of rG-CSF and rGM-CSF on neutrophils (Clark and Kamen, 1987; Robinson and Quesenberry, 1990).

Cell lineage	rG-CSF	rGM-CSF
Neutrophil	↑ production and function	↑ production and function
Monocyte/ Macrophage	no effect	↑ production and function
Eosinophil	no effect	↑ production
Platelet	no effect	no consistent effect

Table 8.5. Hematologic effects of short courses of rG-CSF and rGM-CSF in phase I studies of patients with advanced cancer (Lieschke and Burgess, 1992).

CELLULAR SOURCES AND STIMULI FOR RELEASE

T lymphocytes, monocytes or macrophages, fibroblasts, and endothelial cells are the major cellular sources of most hematopoietic growth factors except for EPO (Table 8.3). EPO is initially produced in the liver, but the kidney becomes the primary source soon after birth (Groopman *et al.*, 1989; Kouides and DiPersio, 1995).

Many inflammatory stimuli are capable of promoting the cellular release of hematopoietic growth factors (see Table 8.3). Antigens, lectins, and interleukin-1 (IL-1) can signal T lymphocytes to produce GM-CSF and IL-3. Lipopolysaccharides such as endotoxin can induce monocytes and macrophages to release G-CSF and GM-CSF. Monocytes can produce M-CSF after stimulation by the products of activated T lymphocytes (e.g., γ-interferon, IL-3, and GM-CSF) or after exposure to tumor necrosis factor α (TNF α). Two cytokines, (IL-1 and TNF α), produced by activated monocytes can trigger the release of G-CSF and GM-CSF by fibroblasts and endothelial cells. The ability of hematopoietic growth factors to promote the release of more growth factors accounts for their indirect effects. In addition, these findings suggest that hematopoietic growth factors play a major role in host response to infection or antigen challenge and may also play a limited role in maintaining normal hematopoiesis (Groopman *et al.*, 1989).

PHYSIOLOGIC ROLE OF G-CSF AND GM-CSF

Animal and clinical studies provide further insight into the physiologic role of hematopoietic growth factors. G-CSF, but not GM-CSF, is usually detectable in the blood and increases during infection (Cebon *et al.*, 1994). Mice that lack endogenous G-CSF have chronic neutropenia and impaired neutrophil mobilization (Lieschke *et al.*, 1994). The collective results of these *in vivo* studies, together with *in vitro* observations, suggest that the two myeloid growth factors have complementary roles. G-CSF may help maintain neutrophil production during steady-state conditions and increase production during acute situations such as infection (Cebon *et al.*, 1994; Dale, 1994; Lieschke *et al.*, 1994; Rapoport *et al.*, 1992). GM-CSF may be a locally active growth factor that remains at the site of infection to retain and activate neutrophils (Rapoport *et al.*, 1992).

The results of phase I studies illustrate the *in vivo* actions of rG-CSF and rGM-CSF in patients with advanced cancer (Table 8.5). Both growth factors cause a transient leukopenia that is followed by a dose-dependent increase in the number of circulating mature and immature neutrophils (Lieschke and Burgess, 1992). The neutrophil response appears 1 to 2 days after rG-CSF (Lord *et al.*, 1989) and 4.5 to 6.5 days after rGM-CSF (Lord *et al.*, 1992), is sustained during continued administration, and disappears after stopping the growth factor administration (Lieschke and Burgess, 1992). Both growth factors enhance the *in vitro* function of neutrophils obtained from treated patients. Recombinant GM-CSF, but not rG-CSF, also increases the number of circulating monocytes and eosinophils, and *in vitro* monocyte cytotoxicity and cytokine production. In contrast with *in vitro* studies, rGM-CSF does not increase platelet production; in fact, there was a transient decrease in some phase I studies. These changes in the blood are accompanied by increases in bone marrow cellularity and ratio of myeloid to erythroid progenitor cells, but there is no change in the total number of progenitor cells (Lieschke and Burgess, 1992).

PHYSIOLOGIC ROLE OF EPO

EPO maintains a normal red blood cell count by causing committed erythroid progenitor cells to proliferate and differentiate into normoblasts. EPO also shifts marrow reticulocytes into circulation. EPO is ordinarily present in plasma in low, but detectable, quantities. Unlike some other hematopoietic growth factors, EPO release is not mediated by inflammatory stimuli. Hypoxia, such as the lack of oxygen caused by anemia, prompts the kidney to increase its production of EPO up to a hundredfold or more; however, patients with chronic renal failure are unable to produce EPO (Abels, 1990; Erslev, 1991).

PHYSIOLOGIC ROLE OF OTHER HEMATOPOIETIC GROWTH FACTORS

The *in vivo* and physiologic roles of the remaining hematopoietic growth factors are not as well defined. M-CSF is detectable in human serum (Groopman *et al.*, 1989), so it is tempting to speculate that it contributes to the survival and activation of monocytes and macrophages. However, its exact role remains an enigma (Clark and Kamen, 1987).

The physiologic role of IL-3 is elusive. Like GM-CSF, circulating IL-3 is not ordinarily detectable in blood. IL-3 levels increase after chemotherapy, which corresponds with platelet recovery (De Vries *et al.*, 1993). Recombinant IL-3 causes a multilineage increase in blood cell counts. In nonhuman primates exposed to total body irradiation, platelet recovery was quicker with rIL-3; neutrophil recovery was faster with rGM-CSF. Compared with rGM-CSF, the hematopoietic activity of rIL-3 is modest in magnitude, delayed in onset, and sustained. These findings, together with *in vitro* evidence of synergy, are the basis for combining rIL-3 and rGM-CSF (PIXY-321). In the nonhuman primate study, PIXY-321 accelerated neutrophil and platelet recovery more quickly than rGM-CSF (Vadhan-Raj, 1994).

Extensive *in vivo* evidence indicates that the physiologic role of thrombopoietin may be to stimulate the proliferation and differentiation of megakaryocyte progenitor cells. Thrombopoietin appears to be essential and sufficient for the full maturation of megakaryocytes. It appears to enhance platelet recovery after cancer chemotherapy or radiotherapy (Kuter, 1997, Kaushansky, 1995).

Preliminary *in vivo* experience indicates that SCF may help maintain normal hematopoiesis. It is not yet known whether the SCF acts on the stem cell per se because the most primitive progenitor cell has not yet been isolated. SCF can expand the number of other progenitor cells, presumably as a result of synergistic interactions with other hematopoietic growth factors. In humans with advanced cancer, this effect was predominantly observed among circulating hematopoietic progenitor cells; there was limited effect in the bone marrow. Other cell types are also affected. SCF enhances the development of mast cell or tissue basophils; SCF also enhances the release of mast cell mediators such as histamine (Galli *et al.*, 1994).

Pharmaceutical Concerns

Pharmaceutical concerns include the status and source, storage and stability, pharmacokinetics, and pharmacodynamics of hematopoietic growth factors. Unless otherwise indicated, the information in this section is taken from the package inserts.

Status and Source of Hematopoietic Growth Factors

Three hematopoietic growth factors are commercially available, rG-CSF (Filgrastim, Lenograstim, and Nartograstim), rGM-CSF (Molgramostim and Sargramostim), and rEPO (Epoetin or Epoetinum alpha and Epoetin beta) (Table 8.6). Recombinant EPO, launched in 1989, was the first to be approved by governmental regulatory agencies. Filgrastim, Lenograstim, and Sargramostim followed in 1991. Molgramostim was introduced in 1992. It is possible for a hematopoietic growth factor to be developed by one company, manufactured by another, and distributed by a third. These arrangements are dynamic, complex, and differ from country to country. Appropriate resources should be checked to determine the licensing and distribution agreements in a particular country.

The status of the investigational hematopoietic growth factors is even more dynamic and difficult to summarize. This topic was introduced in the section on chemical properties and will be revisited in the next section on clinical and practice aspects.

Storage and Stability

Commercially available hematopoietic growth factors should be stored under refrigeration (Table 8.7). Three recombinant products, Filgrastim, Sargramostim and Epoetin alpha, are available in ready-to-use solutions; the others (and Sargramostim) are supplied as lyophilized powders that must be reconstituted before use. After reconstitution or dilution for intravenous use, Filgrastim and Lenograstim are stable for up to 24 hours at room temperature (Neupogen® package insert, 1996; Granocyte package insert, 1993); Molgramostim and Sargramostim should be refrigerated (Leucomax package insert, 1992; Leukine package insert, 1996). Depending on the final concentration of intravenous solutions containing Filgrastim, Sargramostim, or Epoetin alpha, human serum albumin should be added to prevent adsorption to the plastic materials.

Pharmacokinetics

The pharmacokinetic profiles of selected available hematopoietic growth factors (Table 8.8) should not be compared

	Proper name	Trade name	Country	Company
rG-CSF	Filgrastim	Neupogen®	Europe, USA, Canada Australia, rest of world	Amgen, Roche
		Granulokine®	Italy	Dompé
			Spain	Esteve-Pensa
		Gran®	Japan, Taiwan, Korea, China	Kirin, Sankyo
	Lenograstim	Granocyte®	Europe	Rhône-Poulenc
		Euprotin®	Australia	Amrad
			Spain	Almirall
		Neutrogin®	Japan, China	Chugai
rG-CSF analog	Nartograstim	Neu-up®	Japan	Kyowa
rGM-CSF	Molgramostim	Leucomax®	Europe, Canada	Schering, Sandoz
	Sargramostim	Leukine®	USA	Immunex
			Canada	Wyeth-Ayerst Canada
rEPO	Epoetin alfa	Epogen®	USA	Amgen
		Procrit®	USA	Ortho
		Espo®	Japan	Kirin, Sankyo
			China	Kirin
		Eprex®	Europe, Australia, Canada	Ortho and its affiliates
	Epoetinum alfa	Eprex®	Europe	Ortho and its affiliates
	Epoetin beta	Epogin®	Japan	Chugai
		Recormon®	Europe	Boehringer Mannheim

Table 8.6. Status of commercially available hematopoietic growth factors as of October, 1995.

directly because of clinically relevant differences in study design, doses, regimens, administration routes, and study populations. For example, patients with advanced cancer typically receive many cancer chemotherapeutic agents, antibiotics, and other therapeutic interventions that may directly alter the disposition of hematopoietic growth factors or affect the organs that metabolize and eliminate these growth factors. Patients undergoing bone marrow transplantation are typically exposed to an even wider variety of therapeutic interventions.

In regards to rG-CSF, Filgrastim and Lenograstim exhibit first-order kinetics and yield increasing concentrations with increasing doses. Both are rapidly absorbed after subcutaneous administration, achieving peak concentra-

	Proper name	Storage temperature (centigrade)	Diluent for intravenous Use	Stability after dilution for IV use or reconstitution	Comments
rG-CSF	Filgrastim	+2° to +8°	5% dextrose	1 week (most of Europe) or 24 hours (USA, UK) at room temperature	final concentration must be > 5 μg/mL (USA), > 2 μg/mL (Europe); add HSA if < 15 μg/mL
	Lenograstim	+2° to +8°	normal saline	24 hours at +2° to + 8°	final concentration must be ≥ 2.5 μg/mL
rGM-CSF	Molgramostim	+2° to +8°	normal saline or 5% dextrose	24 hours at +2° to + 8°	final concentration must be > 7 μg/mL. Protect from light
	Sargramostim	+2° to +8°	normal saline	6 hours at +2° to + 8°	add HSA if final concentration < 10 μg/mL
rEPO	Epoetin alfa	+2° to +8°	normal saline	use immediately	may be admixed in syringe with 0.9% sodium chloride with benzyl alcohol 0.9% (bacteriostatic saline) at a 1:1 ratio using aseptic technique

Table 8.7. Stability and storage conditions of selected commercially available hematopoietic growth factors (as stated in respective package inserts). (HSA = human serum albumin; IV = intravenous; [a]: data on file, Amgen Inc., Thousand Oaks, California, USA.)

		C_{max} (dose)	$t_{1/2\beta}$ (h)	Comments
rG-CSF	Filgrastim	4-49 ng/mL (3.45-11.5 μg/kg s.c.)	3.5 (s.c. or i.v.)	first-order kinetics
		384 ng/mL (11.5 μg/kg i.v. over 30 min)		$t_{1/2\beta}$ independent of route
	Lenograstim	0.09-0.48 μg/L (10-40 μg s.c.)[a]	3-4 (s.c.)	profile dose and time dependent
			1-1.5 (i.v.)	
rGM-CSF	Molgramostim	0.35-3.9 μg/L (125 μg/m^2 s.c.)[b]	2-3 (s.c.)	
		22.5 μg/L (250 μg/m^2 i.v. over 2h)[b]	1-2 (i.v.)	
	Sargramostim	22,000-23,000 pg/mL (at end of 250 μg/m^2 i.v. over 120 min)	2 (i.v.)	
		350-3900 pg/mL (125 μg/m^2 q 12 h)		
rEPO	Epoetin alfa	104-288 mUnits/mL (100-300 s.c.)[c]	≈ 20 (s.c.)[c]	first-order kinetics
			4-13 (i.v., CRF)	

Table 8.8. Pharmacokinetic profiles of selected commercially available hematopoietic growth factors (as stated in respective package inserts, unless otherwise indicated).
C_{max} = peak concentration; $t_{1/2\beta}$ = β elimination half-life; h = hours; s.c. = subcutaneous; i.v. = intravenous; q = every; CRF chronic renal failure; [a]Sekino *et al.*, 1989; [b]Cebon *et al.*, 1990; Shadduck *et al.*, 1990; [c]Markham and Bryson, 1995.

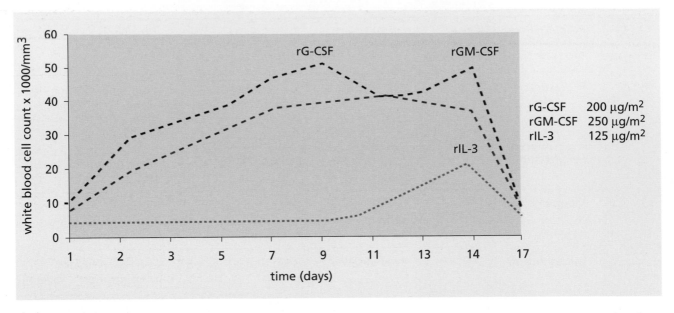

Figure 8.4. Effect of hematopoietic growth factors on white blood cell count in patients with advanced cancer (reproduced from Mertelsmann, 1991; with permission). Recombinant G-CSF (200 μg/m²), rGM-CSF (250 μg/m²), and rIL-3 (125 μg/m²) were administered by subcutaneous injection for approximately 14 days.

tions in 2 to 8 hours (Granocyte package insert, 1993; Neupogen® package insert, 1996; Sekino *et al.*, 1989). The elimination half-life of Filgrastim is approximately 3.5 hours in both normal volunteers and cancer patients, and after both intravenous and subcutaneous administration (Neupogen® package insert, 1996). The elimination half-life of Lenograstim is 3 to 4 hours after subcutaneous administration and 1 to 1.5 hours after intravenous administration (Granocyte® package insert, 1993).

Of the two recombinant GM-CSF products, the package inserts provide more comprehensive pharmacokinetic data on Sargramostim than for Molgramostim. In patients with advanced cancer, Sargramostim is rapidly absorbed after subcutaneous administration, achieving peak concentrations in 2 hours. After intravenous infusion over 2 hours, serum concentrations initially decline rapidly ($t_{1/2\alpha}$ = 12 to 17 minutes) followed by a more gradual decline ($t_{1/2\beta}$ = 2 hours) (Leukine package insert, 1996). The elimination half-life of Molgramostim is 2 to 3 hours after subcutaneous administration and 1 to 2 hours after intravenous administration (Leucomax package insert, 1992).

Recombinant EPO follows first-order kinetics. Peak serum concentrations occur 5 to 24 hours after subcutaneous administration and are lower than after intravenous administration. The elimination half-life of intravenously administered rEPO is 4 to 13 hours in patients with chronic renal failure and approximately 20% shorter in normal volunteers. The elimination half-life is longer after subcutaneous administration, resulting in more sustained plasma concentrations (Epogen® package insert, 1995; Erslev, 1991; Markham and Bryson, 1995).

Minimal pharmacokinetic information is available on the investigational hematopoietic growth factors. The disposition of rIL-3 has been described as rapid and possibly complex in patients with bone marrow failure. Peak concentrations of rIL-3 occur 2 to 4 hours after subcutaneous administration; the elimination half-life is 0.3 hours after intravenous administration and 3.5 hours after subcutaneous administration. In monkeys, PIXY-321 achieves peak concentrations 4 hours after subcutaneous injection; the elimination half-life is 2 to 7 hours after subcutaneous administration and 0.3 to 1 hours after intravenous administration (Dorr and Von Hoff, 1994).

Pharmacodynamics

The concept of pharmacodynamics was introduced in the previous section on the physiologic role of hematopoietic growth factors and will be revisited in the next section. This section provides additional details and emphasizes the onset of hematologic response.

Although there are no comparative studies, a series of phase I/II studies performed by the same group of investigators provide insight (Figure 8.4). In patients with advanced cancer not receiving chemotherapy, a hematopoietic growth factor was administered by subcutaneous injection and continued for approximately 2 weeks. Recombinant G-CSF induced a rapid increase in neutrophil counts, which

	Proper name	Indication	Dose[a]	Route	How supplied
rG-CSF	Filgrastim	chemotherapy-induced neutropenia	5 μg/kg/day, starting 24 h after last chemotherapy	s.c. bolus or over 24 h, or i.v. over 15-30 min (USA), 30 min (Europe) or 24 h.	ready-to-use solution in 300-μg (1 mL) and 480-μg (1.6 mL) vials
		bone marrow transplantation	10 μg/kg/day, starting 24 h after BMT	s.c. over 24 h, or i.v. over 4 or 24 h (30 min in Germany)	
		PBPC transplantation (Europe only)	10 μg/kg/day for 6 days before apheresis, followed by 5 μg/kg/day post chemotherapy	s.c. bolus or over 24 h (s.c. bolus only for post chemo)	
		(USA, Australia, Canada)	10 μg/kg/day for at least 4 days before apheresis and continued until the last pheresis	s.c. bolus or over 24 h	
		(Canada, Australia)	5 μg/kg/day post chemotherapy	s.c. bolus or as an i.v. infusion (Canada)	
		severe chronic neutropenia (Australia)	5 μg/kg/day (idiopathic or cyclic SCN) 6 μg/kg twice daily (congenital SCN) 12 μg/kg/daily (congenital SCN)	s.c. bolus	
		AIDS	1 μg/kg/day, titrate to maximum of 5 μg/kg/day to ANC of 2000/mm³		
	Lenograstim (Europe only)	chemotherapy-induced neutropenia	150 μg/m²/day, starting 24 h after last chemotherapy for ≤ 28 days	s.c.	lyophilized powder in 134- and 263-μg vials
		bone marrow transplantation	150 μg/m²/day, starting 24 h after BMT	i.v. over 30 min	

Table 8.9a. Established uses and dosing regimens for selected hematopoietic growth factors that are commercially available in Europe and the United States (as stated in respective package inserts). BMT = bone marrow transplantation; h = hour; i.v. = intravenous; PBPC = peripheral blood progenitor cell; s.c. = subcutaneous; SCN = severe chronic neutropenia; [a]Dose adjustments may be required for maintenance therapy, especially for severe chronic neutropenia and anemia.

was evident on day 2 and gradually increased through day 10. Thereafter, the neutrophil count declined gradually despite continued therapy and quickly returned to baseline after stopping therapy. Recombinant GM-CSF gradually expanded white blood cell counts throughout the treatment period; this finding was attributable to increases in neutrophils and bands, predominantly, and less striking increases in eosinophils and monocytes. Recombinant IL-3 had a much slower onset of action that was not evident before day 10. Recombinant IL-3 not only promoted the expansion of

	Proper name	Indication	Dose[a]	Route	How supplied
rGM-CSF	Molgramostim (Europe only)	chemotherapy-induced neutropenia	5-10 µg/kg/day, starting 24 h after last chemotherapy for 7-10 days	s.c.	lyophilized powder in 150-, 300-, and 700-µg vials
		bone marrow transplantation	10 µg/kg/day, starting 24 h after BMT for ≤ 30 days	i.v. over 4-6 h	
		AIDS	5 µg/kg/day (titrate after fifth day)	s.c.	
	Sagramostim (USA, Canada)	bone marrow transplantation (autologous only)	250 µg/m²/day, starting 2-4 h after BMT for 21 days	i.v. over 2 h	lyophilized powder in 250- and 500-µg vials
		bone marrow transplantation failure of engraftment delay	250 µg/m²/day for 14 days		
		chemotherapy-induced neutropenia (AML only)	250 µg/m²/day, titrate to bone marrow response, see PI	i.v. over 4 h	

Table 8.9b. For legends see Table 8.9a.

all types of white blood cells but also increased the numbers of reticulocytes and platelets (Mertelsmann, 1991).

These pharmacodynamic observations are consistent with *in vitro* predictions. Multilineage hematopoietic growth factors like rIL-3 have broad effects that occur early in the hematopoietic cascade and therefore take longer to become clinically apparent. In contrast, the lineage-specific growth factors act later in the cascade and appear to have a more rapid onset of action (Mertelsmann, 1991).

In patients with anemia due to chronic renal failure, rEPO (three times weekly) increases reticulocyte counts within 10 days, which is followed by increases in the red blood cell count, hemoglobin, and hematocrit within 2 to 6 weeks (Epogen package insert, 1995).

Clinical and Practice Aspects

Hematopoietic growth factors have been and continue to be evaluated in many clinical disorders involving different types of blood cells. This section focuses on established uses (Table 8.9) and introduces investigational uses.

Uses can become established through many mechanisms. In the United States, at least one randomized, pivotal study must be conducted before the Food and Drug Administration will consider a new indication for a bio-

logic. This official process can take many years, so biologics may be used for indications before they receive official governmental approval. These uses may be considered established if they appear in major medical textbooks or other respected resources. For example, the clinical practice guidelines recently adopted by the American Society of Clinical Oncology (1994), and recently updated (1996), are based on a meticulous literature review, extensive data collection, established scale to weigh the evidence, and general consensus by 25 renowned investigators. These guidelines and other eminent reviews will be cited in this section.

The term investigational uses also has different meanings and, for the purpose of this section, will refer to two types of ongoing studies. Commercially available hematopoietic growth factors are being evaluated for purposes that have not yet been established, which will be addressed in the section on future uses. Growth factors that are not yet commercially available will be addressed in the section on investigational hematopoietic growth factors.

Established Uses

Neutrophil disorders are a logical therapeutic target for the myeloid hematopoietic growth factors. The disorder may be qualitative or quantitative. Abnormal neutrophil function may occur because of defective adhesion, movement,

	Proper name	Indication	Dose[a]	Route	How supplied
rEPO	Epoetin alfa	anemia of chronic renal failure	50-100 units/kg three times weekly (titrate according to individual response)	i.v. or s.c.	ready-to-use solution in 1000- to 10,000-unit (single dose) and 10.000-unit (multi-dose) vials, and 500- to 10,000-unit prefilled syringes
	(Australia)		50 units/kg three times weekly (titrate according to individual response with maximum of 200)		
		anemia of zidovudine-treated AIDS	100 units/kg three times weekly (titrate after 8 weeks)	s.c.	
		anemia of cancer chemotherapy	150 units/kg three times weekly (titrate after 8 weeks)		
		reduction of allogeneic blood transfusion in surgery patients	300 units/kg/day for 10 days prior to, on the day of, and for 4 days after surgery		
	Epoetinum alfa	anemia of chronic renal failure	50-100 units/kg three times weekly (titrate according to individual response)	i.v. or s.c.	
		anemia of zidovudine-treated AIDS	??	??	
		anemia of cancer chemotherapy	150 units/kg three times weekly (titrate after 4 weeks)	s.c.	
		reduction of alloge-neic blood transfusion in surgery patients	??	??	

Table 8.9c. For legends see Table 8.9a.

or phagocytosis and killing. Insufficient numbers of neutrophils or neutropenia may occur because of accelerated destruction, maldistribution, or decreased production. In either case, patients generally have impaired host immunity and an increased risk of bacterial infection. Recombinant G-CSF is indicated for neutropenia associated with myelosuppressive cancer chemotherapy, bone marrow transplantation, and severe chronic neutropenia; rG-CSF is also indicated to mobilize peripheral blood progenitor cells (PBPC) for PBPC transplantation, and for reversal of clinically significant neutropenia and subsequent maintenance of adequate neutrophil counts in patients with HIV infection during treatment with antiviral and/or other myelosuppressive medications. Recombinant GM-CSF is indicated for neutropenia associated with myelosuppressive cancer chemotherapy, bone marrow transplantation, and antiviral therapy for AIDS-related cytomegalovirus; rGM-CSF is also indicated for failed bone marrow transplantation or delayed engraftment, and for use in mobilization and following transplantation of autologous peripheral blood progenitor cells. Recombinant EPO is indicated to treat anemia associated with chronic renal failure, zidovudine in HIV-infected patients, and chemotherapy. Recombinant EPO is also indicated to reduce allogeneic blood transfu-

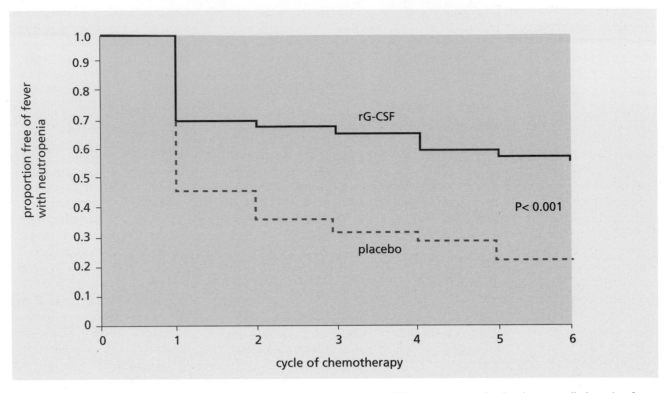

Figure 8.5. Effect of Filgrastim (rG-CSF) on febrile neutropenia in a double-blind, randomized, placebo-controlled study of 194 evaluable patients. Reprinted by permission of *The New England Journal of Medicine.* Crawford *et al.* (1991). Reduction by granulocyte colony-stimulating factor of fever and neutropenia induced by chemotherapy in patients with small-cell lung cancer. *New England Journal of Medicine,* 325, 164–170, Massachusetts Medical Society.

sions and hasten erythroid recovery in surgery patients. (Ortho Biologics Inc., data on file 1996). A representative pivotal study for each established use has been selected to illustrate the benefit of hematopoietic growth factors in patients with hematologic disorders. This section will also comment on the status of other hematopoietic growth factors for each established use.

CHEMOTHERAPY-INDUCED NEUTROPENIA

Neutropenia and infection are common dose-limiting effects of cancer chemotherapy. The risk of infection is directly related to the depth and duration of neutropenia. The severity of neutropenia depends on the intensity of the cancer chemotherapy regimen, as well as host- and disease-related factors. Fever may be the only manifestation of infection because underlying immunosuppression often obscures the classic signs and symptoms. Therefore, it is standard practice to administer broad-spectrum antibiotic therapy and even hospitalize patients who present with febrile neutropenia. Furthermore, clinicians may delay the start of subsequent cycles until neutrophil recovery, decrease the dose of cancer chemotherapy, or both. While this

practice may be deemed necessary to prevent infectious complications, it may also compromise otherwise effective cancer chemotherapy.

Filgrastim is indicated to decrease the incidence of infection, as manifested by febrile neutropenia, in patients with nonmyeloid malignancies receiving myelosuppressive cancer chemotherapy that is associated with a significant incidence of severe neutropenia and fever (Neupogen® package insert, 1996). In a double-blind, placebo-controlled study of 210 patients with small cell lung cancer, patients received standard-dose chemotherapy (cyclophosphamide 1 g/m² and doxorubicin 50 mg/m² on day 1, and etoposide 120 mg/m² on days 1 through 3) every 21 days. Filgrastim 4 to 8 μg/kg by daily subcutaneous injection was initiated 1 day after completing chemotherapy and continued for 2 weeks or until the absolute neutrophil count was >10,000/mm³. Compared with placebo, Filgrastim decreased the incidence of febrile neutropenia by 50%. The benefit was evident after the first cycle and persisted throughout six cycles of myelosuppressive chemotherapy (Figure 8.5). Filgrastim also reduced the duration of documented infections, antibiotic use, and hospitalization by approximately 50% (Crawford *et al.,* 1991).

Lenograstim (Granocyte® package insert, 1993) and Molgramostim (Leucomax® package insert, 1992) are also indicated to decrease the duration of neutropenia and risk of infection, respectively, associated with myelosuppressive cancer chemotherapy. Sargramostim was approved in the third quarter of 1995, but the indication is limited to the neutropenia associated with induction chemotherapy for acute myelogenous leukemia (see below).

The American Society of Clinical Oncology (1994) concluded that rGM-CSF is less consistently beneficial than rG-CSF in studies of patients at risk for chemotherapy-induced neutropenia. Molgramostim facilitated neutrophil recovery, decreased the incidence of febrile neutropenia, and reduced hospitalization in a randomized study of patients with non-Hodgkin's lymphoma; however, the benefit was limited to 72% of patients who tolerated Molgramostim 400 μg/day. Molgramostim improved some, but not all, endpoints in other randomized studies. Although Sargramostim had similar benefits in uncontrolled studies (Lieschke and Burgess, 1992), these results were not confirmed in a randomized double-blind placebo-controlled study (Jones et al., 1996). In this trial, 142 patients with stage II and III breast cancer were randomized to receive either placebo or Sargramostim 250 μg/m²/day on days 3 through 15 following each of 4 cycles of CAF chemotherapy (cyclophosphamide 750 mg/m², fluorouracil 600mg/m², doxorubicin 60mg/m² all administered IV on day 1). While the duration of severe neutropenia was significantly less with Sargramostim than with placebo (2.8 days versus 6.8 days, p < 0.001) there was no significant difference in the incidence of hospitalizations between the two arms. Sargramostim has, however, demonstrated benefit as an adjunct to chemotherapy in patients with acute myelogenous leukemia as described below (Rowe et al., 1995).

Hematopoietic growth factors are being tested in patients with acute myelogenous leukemia because induction therapy causes profound, prolonged neutropenia that is associated with substantial infection-related mortality. Randomized studies yielded disparate results. Sargramostim was the only recombinant growth factor to improve survival. Sargramostim 250 μg/m²/day shortened the duration of neutropenia, reduced serious infections, and improved survival (Rowe et al., 1995). Filgrastim has been the only growth factor associated with a reduction in the median duration of hospitalization, and fewer days of parenteral antibiotics. Filgrastim 5 μg/kg/day reduced the duration of neutropenia, median days of hospitalization, and days of parenteral antibiotics (Heil et al., 1995). A separate study of Filgrastim at 400 μg/m²/day demonstrated a reduction in the duration of neutropenia, but no effect on hospitalization (Godwin et al., 1995). Neither study demonstrated any effect of Filgrastim on median overall survival. Lenograstim 5 μg/kg/day and Molgramostim 5 μg/kg/day short-ened the duration of neutropenia, but they did not prevent infections or improve survival (Dombret et al., 1995; Stone et al., 1995).

Differences in study design may contribute to these discrepancies in the AML studies. The most obvious was the use of different recombinant GM-CSF products. Although the source of recombinant GM-CSF has not yet been shown to have efficacy implications, it appears to affect tolerability. Sargramostim was well tolerated (Rowe et al., 1995), but one third of the patients stopped Molgramostim because of toxicity. However, limiting the analysis to the subset who tolerated Molgramostim did not translate to survival benefits (Stone et al., 1995). These findings underscore the importance of carefully evaluating each hematopoietic growth factor on its own merits and not generalizing among different recombinant product or different growth factors.

These six studies have additional clinical implications. In the past, leukemia was considered to be a contraindication because of in vitro evidence showing that rGM-CSF promotes the proliferation of leukemic blast cells. None of these myeloid growth factors had an adverse effect on the complete remission rate or relapse rate in patients with acute myelogenous leukemia (Dombret et al., 1995; Heil et al., 1995; Godwin et al., 1995; Rowe et al., 1995; Stone et al., 1995), so these findings may trigger more studies to investigate their role in patients with myeloid malignancies.

BONE MARROW TRANSPLANTATION

Bone marrow transplantation enables the use of very high doses of chemotherapy, with or without radiotherapy, to eliminate malignant cells from patients with refractory tumors. The procedure involves administering ablative cancer chemotherapy and infusing bone marrow progenitor cells that were harvested from the patient (autologous transplantation) or another donor (allogeneic transplantation). Before the bone marrow recovers, the neutrophil count usually plunges to zero. Most patients experience profound pancytopenia and require multiple transfusions. Allogeneic is more complicated than autologous transplantation because donor white blood cells may recognize host antigens as foreign and attack host tissues. Graft-versus-host disease can be life-threatening and is manifested by epithelial damage to the skin, liver, and gastrointestinal tract. Consequently, these recipients receive immunosuppressive therapy, which further increases the risk of infection. Regardless of the source of the bone marrow, the procedure may necessitate prolonged hospitalization, which increases the cost of treatment.

Sargramostim is indicated to accelerate myeloid recovery following autologous bone marrow transplantation in patients with non-Hodgkin's lymphoma, acute lymphoblastic leukemia, or Hodgkin's disease. It is also indicated in patients undergoing allogeneic transplantation from human leukocyte antigen (HLA) matched related donors (Leukine package insert, 1996). In a double-blind, randomized, placebo-controlled study, 128 patients underwent autologous bone marrow transplantation for lymphoid cancer. Sargramostim 250 µg/m²/day by intravenous infusion over 2 hours was started within 4 hours of marrow infusion and continued for 21 days. Sargramostim shortened the duration of neutropenia by 7 days, antibiotic therapy by 3 days, and hospitalization by 6 days (Nemunaitis et al., 1991). Similarly, in a double-blind, randomized, placebo-controlled study, 109 patients underwent allogeneic bone marrow transplantation. Compared to placebo, Sargramostim significantly improved the time to neutrophil engraftment, duration of hospitalization, and the number of patients with bacteremia. Its use also reduced the overall incidence of infection (Leukine package insert, 1996).

The other recombinant GM-CSF product, Molgramostim (Leucomax® package insert, 1992), and a recombinant G-CSF product, Filgrastim (Neupogen® package insert, 1996), are indicated to reduce the duration of neutropenia and its sequelae following bone marrow transplantation for nonmyeloid malignancies. These two hematopoietic growth factors are not restricted to autologous bone marrow transplantation. Both Molgramostim and Filgrastim accelerated neutrophil recovery in randomized studies. Filgrastim also reduced the number of febrile days, and consistently shortened the duration of hospitalization (Stahel et al., 1994). Filgrastim reduced the duration of parenteral nutrition; investigators hypothesized that this may have been due to its beneficial effects on mucositis. Importantly, neither hematopoietic growth factor increased the risk of graft-versus-host disease, graft rejection, or relapse in patients undergoing allogeneic bone marrow transplantation (American Society of Clinical Oncology, 1994).

If engraftment is delayed or does not occur after bone marrow transplantation, the risk of infection and even death is considerable. Sargramostim's indication for failed autologous or allogeneic bone marrow transplantation or delayed engraftment is based on a historically controlled study of 243 patients. Patients were eligible if they had profound neutropenia 28 days after transplantation or infection plus profound neutropenia on day 21, or if they lost the marrow graft after transient engraftment. Sargramostim almost tripled survival, which is noteworthy because survival is the most definitive endpoint for a clinical study. The benefit was greatest among patients who had autologous (versus allogeneic) bone marrow transplantation, no total body irradiation, nonleukemic malignancy, and fewer impaired organs. The Sargramostim dosage is 250 µg/m² by intravenous infusion over 2 hours for 14 days. If response is not adequate after a 7-day interruption, this dosage may be

repeated. If the response is not adequate after a second 7-day interruption, Sargramostim 500 µg/m² may be given for 14 days. Further dose escalation is unlikely to be beneficial (Leukine package insert, 1996).

Peripheral Blood Progenitor Cell Transplantation

Progenitor cells found in the blood can be collected and concentrated for reinfusion after myelosuppressive cancer chemotherapy. PBPC transplantation is attractive because it is less invasive or technologically complex than bone marrow transplantation. PBPC transplantation can be performed in the outpatient setting without anesthetizing the donor, causes less morbidity and mortality, costs less, circumvents donor problems, and is therefore suitable for a larger number of patients.

Hematopoietic growth factors expand the population of circulating hematopoietic progenitor cells and may be used to facilitate peripheral collection, which in turn can be used to supplement and/or replace autologous bone marrow transplantation. The optimal scheduling is unknown and is the subject of intense research. Hematopoietic growth factors can be combined with cancer chemotherapy to enhance the mobilizing effect of the latter, used alone to induce de novo mobilization, or administered after transfusion. In fact, hematopoietic growth factors can even be added to cultures containing hematopoietic progenitor cells to expand them ex vivo. These approaches are being investigated using commercially available hematopoietic growth factors alone, and in combination with each other and investigational growth factors.

In the U.S., Filgrastim is indicated to mobilize PBPCs for collection by leukapheresis in patients undergoing myelosuppressive or myeloablative therapy followed by transplantation. In Europe, Filgrastim is indicated to mobilize PBPCs in patients undergoing myelosuppressive or myeloablative therapy followed by autologous PBPC transplantation with or without bone marrow transplantation (Neupogen package insert, 1996). Seventeen patients with nonmyeloid malignancies received Filgrastim 12 µg/kg/day by continuous subcutaneous infusion for 6 days. The number of granulocyte-macrophage progenitor cells (CFU-GM) in peripheral blood increased 58-fold. Progenitor cells were collected by three leukapheresis procedures and reinfused after high-dose chemotherapy to augment autologous bone-marrow rescue and post-transplant Filgrastim therapy. The time to platelet recovery was shorter in patients who received Filgrastim-mobilized PBPCs compared with controls (Sheridan et al., 1992). A more recent trial in 72 lymphoma patients compared the effects of Filgrastim-mobilized PBPC or autologous bone marrow reinfused after high-dose chemotherapy in a prospective randomized trial. In this study, Filgrastim-mobilized PBPC significantly reduced the number of platelet transfusions, the time to platelet and neutrophil recovery, and led to an earlier hospital discharge as compared to those patients receiving autologous marrow (Schmitz et al., 1996).

Sargramostim is indicated to mobilize PBPCs in patients undergoing myelosuppressive or myeloablative therapy followed by autologous PBPC transplantation. It is also indicated to further accelerate myeloid recovery following peripheral blood progenitor cell transplantation (Leukine package insert, 1996). Retrospective reviews of data from patients with cancer undergoing PBPC collections were conducted. These studies demonstrated that PBPCs from patients treated with Sargramostim 250 µg/m²/day had significantly more CFU-GMs than those collected without mobilization. After transplantation, mobilized patients had shorter times to myeloid engraftment, platelet transfusion independence, and duration of hospitalization compared to non-mobilized patients (Leukine package insert, 1996).

SEVERE CHRONIC NEUTROPENIA

Severe chronic neutropenia may be present from birth (congenital), periodic (cyclic), or of unknown etiology (idiopathic). The condition is manifested by decreased neutrophil counts, recurrent fever, chronic oropharyngeal inflammation, and severe infection. Filgrastim is indicated to reduce the incidence and duration of these sequelae (Neupogen package insert, 1996). In a phase III study, 123 patients were randomized to receive Filgrastim immediately or after a 4-month observation period. Filgrastim was given by subcutaneous injection at doses of 3.45 µg/kg/day for idiopathic neutropenia, 5.75 µg/kg/day for cyclic neutropenia, and 11.50 µg/kg twice daily for congenital neutropenia. The dose was adjusted to maintain the median monthly absolute neutrophil count between 1500 and 10,000/mm³. Hematologic responses were evident within a few days. Ninety percent of patients achieved complete responses, which were associated with improved bone marrow morphology and a lower incidence and duration of infection-related events (Dale et al., 1993).

AIDS

Neutropenia is a common complication of HIV infection, secondary infections, and antiviral drugs used in the treatment of HIV or secondary infection. For example, ganciclovir is a highly effective drug for the treatment and prevention of cytomegalovirus retinitis, the most common cause of AIDS-related blindness. However, therapy must be interrupted in up to half of the patients because of drug-induced neutropenia (Hardy, 1991).

Filgrastim has recently received approval in Australia in patients with HIV infection, for reversal of clinically significant neutropenia and subsequent maintenance of adequate neutrophil counts during treatment with antiviral and/or other myelosuppressive medications. In a study of 200 patients with HIV disease and neutropenia, Filgrastim reversed neutropenia in 96% of patients with a median time to reversal of 2 days, and at a median dose of 1 µg/kg/day (range 0.5–10) (Amgen, data on file 1996). Ganciclovir, zidovudine, co-trimoxazole and pyrimethamine were the medications most frequently considered to be causing neutropenia and 83% of patients received one or more of these on study. During the study, 84% of patients were able to increase or maintain dosing of these four medications or add them to their therapy (Amgen, data on file 1997). Various additional dosing regimens of Filgrastim have been used alone or in combination with rEPO to reverse the dose-limiting hematologic toxicity of ganciclovir or zidovudine (Frampton et al., 1994). For example, Filgrastim permitted higher doses of ganciclovir and improved the outcome of AIDS-related cytomegalovirus retinitis in a retrospective study of 28 patients (Morgan and Strickland, 1993).

Molgramostim is indicated as adjuvant therapy for patients with AIDS-related cytomegalovirus retinitis to maintain the recommended dosage of ganciclovir (Leucomax package insert, 1992). Fifty-three patients with AIDS and cytomegalovirus retinitis were randomized to receive ganciclovir with or without Molgramostim 1 to 8 µg/kg/day by subcutaneous injection to maintain absolute neutrophil counts between 2500 and 5000/mm³. Molgramostim reduced the risk of neutropenia and interruptions in ganciclovir therapy, which resulted in a trend toward delayed progression of retinitis (Hardy et al., 1994). Results of preliminary studies confirmed that this regimen did not alter the pharmacokinetic disposition of ganciclovir or promote HIV proliferation (Hardy, 1991).

ANEMIA

Anemia is characterized by a decrease in hemoglobin or red blood cells. Like other hematopoietic cells, red blood cells originate in the bone marrow and undergo a series of steps that are regulated by hematopoietic growth factors. It takes about a week for the progenitor cell to differentiate and mature in the bone marrow, and to incorporate the hemoglobin and iron that allow it to carry oxygen. When the cell becomes a reticulocyte, it is released into the blood where maturation continues. Over the next few days, the cell must lose its nucleus and shrink slightly before it becomes a mature red blood cell.

There are many types of anemia. Anemia is often a sign of an underlying disease such as chronic renal failure, which may decrease production of red blood cells. Or, anemia can be a complication of treatment such as antiviral therapy for AIDS or cancer chemotherapy, which may

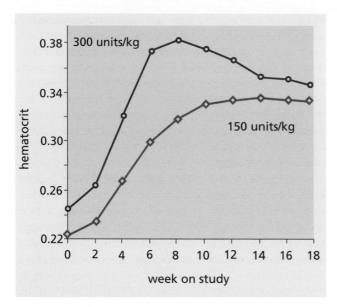

Figure 8.6. Effect of Epoetin alfa on mean hematocrit in 236 evaluable patients with anemia and end-stage renal disease. Epoetin alfa 150 or 300 Units/kg was given three times weekly by intravenous bolus (reproduced from Eschbach *et al.*, 1989; with permission).

increase destruction. Although the signs and symptoms vary depending on the etiology, they usually include pale or yellow skin, weakness and fatigue, shortness of breath, dizziness or lightheadedness, edema, enlarged spleen, and cardiovascular complications such as tachycardia or cardiac decompensation.

The kidney is the primary source of endogenous EPO, so is not surprising that patients without kidneys or with diseased kidneys produce suboptimal EPO levels. Epoetin alpha is indicated for the treatment of anemia associated with chronic renal failure, including patients on dialysis (Epogen package insert, 1995). In a phase III study of 333 patients with anemia and end-stage renal disease, Epoetin alpha increased the hematocrit and eliminated the need for red blood cell transfusions in virtually all patients. The response was dose dependent, evident within 2 weeks, and maximal at 6 to 10 weeks (Figure 8.6). Most patients experienced improved quality of life, which was manifested by improved sense of well being and increased energy levels (Eschbach *et al.*, 1989). Epoetin alpha was equally effective in studies of patients with chronic renal disease who did not require hemodialysis (Erslev, 1991). The recommended starting doses of Epoetin alpha in patients with chronic renal failure is 50–100 Units/kg three times weekly, administered either as an intravenous or subcutaneous injection. In patients on hemodialysis, Epoetin alpha is usually administered as an IV bolus three times weekly

into the venous line at the end of the dialysis procedure. In patients with chronic renal failure not on dialysis, Epoetin alpha is usually given either as an intravenous or subcutaneous injection (Epogen® package insert, 1995).

In Europe, the starting dosage for Epoetinum alpha is 50 Units/kg three times weekly for adult and pediatric hemodialysis patients and predialysis adults, and two times weekly for peritoneal dialysis adults (Eprex® package insert, 1994). Children weighing less than 30 kg may require higher maintenance doses than heavier children or adults. The package inserts (Epogen® 1995 and Eprex® 1994) contain more detailed recommendations on monitoring and dosage adjustments.

Zidovudine, an antiviral drug frequently prescribed for the treatment of AIDS, causes bone marrow suppression. Depending on baseline laboratory values, anemia occurs in up to one third of these patients. Epoetin alpha is indicated to elevate or maintain red blood cell level and decrease the need for transfusions in these patients (Procrit® package insert, 1995). In a double-blind, randomized, placebo-controlled study of 63 zidovudine-treated patients with AIDS, Epoetin alpha 100 Units/kg three times weekly by intravenous bolus increased hematocrit and reduced red blood cell transfusions during the second and third months of treatment. The benefit was apparent only if baseline EPO levels were ≤500 mUnits/mL but not if levels were >500 mUnits/mL (Fischl *et al.*, 1990).

These findings have dosing implications for zidovudine-treated patients. Epoetin alpha should be initiated at a dosage of 100 Units/kg three times weekly by subcutaneous or intravenous injection for 8 weeks. If the response is not satisfactory, the dosage may be increased by 50- to 100-Units/kg increments three times weekly at 4- to 8-week intervals. Dosages beyond 300 Units/kg three times weekly are unlikely to provide additional benefit (Procrit® package insert, 1995).

Myelosuppression is a well known complication of cancer chemotherapy. The risk of anemia depends on the agent, dose, duration, concomitant therapy, and patient factors. Cisplatin, a widely prescribed agent that is notorious for causing anemia, decreases the hemoglobin by at least 2 g/dL in 25% to 30% of patients. Epoetin alpha is indicated to decrease the need for transfusions in patients who will receive at least 2 months of concomitant chemotherapy for nonmyeloid malignancies (Procrit® package insert, 1995). In Europe, the regimen must contain cisplatin (Eprex® package insert, 1994). In a double-blind, randomized, placebo-controlled study of patients with chemotherapy-induced anemia, Epoetin alpha 150 Units/kg three times weekly was administered subcutaneously for 12 weeks. Patients were stratified according to whether they received cisplatin (n = 125) or not (n=153). Epoetin alpha increased the hematocrit and reduced the need for red blood cell transfusions in both groups. The benefit became statistically significant during the second and third months, and was maintained during an open-label extension for a total treatment period of 6 months. Epoetin alpha also improved the overall quality of life, energy level, and ability to carry out daily activities (Henry and Abels, 1994).

For patients receiving cancer chemotherapy, the recommended starting dosage of Epoetin alpha is 150 Units/kg subcutaneously three times weekly. If the response is not satisfactory, the dosage may be increased up to 300 Units/kg three times weekly. Higher dosages are unlikely to provide additional benefit (Procrit® package insert, 1993). The package insert provides additional details on laboratory monitoring and dosage adjustments (Eprex® package insert, 1994).

Epoetin alpha has recently been approved to treat patients with a hemoglobin of >10 to ≤13 g/dL who are undergoing major, elective noncardiac, nonvascular surgery. It is indicated to reduce allogeneic blood transfusions and hasten erythroid recovery in these patients. If the individual meets these criteria, Epoetin alpha 300 Units/kg/day subcutaneously for 10 days before surgery, on the day of surgery, and for 4 days after surgery should be administered. In addition, oral iron supplementation (e.g., elemental iron 200 mg/day) should be started as soon as possible and continued throughout Epoetin alpha therapy. In a placebo-controlled, double-blind trial of 316 patients scheduled for surgery, patients treated with Epoetin alpha 300 Units/kg/day administered as outlined above, had significantly fewer allogeneic transfusions than those treated with placebo (Ortho Biologics, Inc., 1996).

Future Uses

Many clinical studies are under way to evaluate the role of commercially available hematopoietic growth factors in the treatment of additional disease- and treatment-related cytopenias, infectious diseases, and other applications.

DISEASE-RELATED CYTOPENIA

Myelodysplastic syndrome was one of the first targets in early studies of myeloid hematopoietic growth factors. This condition is characterized by refractory cytopenia and abnormal cellular morphology and function. It has been difficult to confirm the potential benefits (e.g., decreased rates of infection or transfusion) or to evaluate the potential disadvantages (e.g., increased risk of malignant transformation) of rG-CSF and rGM-CSF because of the lack of information on the natural history of this disease and the inherent limitations of uncontrolled studies (Lieschke and Burgess, 1992). Although anemia is a common presenting sign, rEPO does not consistently reduce the need for red blood cell transfusions (Markham and Bryson, 1995).

Hematopoietic growth factors are being evaluated in many types of anemia. Aplastic anemia is a logical target because of the deficiency of hematopoietic progenitor cells. Recombinant G-CSF and rGM-CSF are beneficial in patients with mild to moderate disease but not in patients with severe hypoplasia (Lieschke and Burgess, 1992). Combination therapy with multilineage hematopoietic growth factors that act on early progenitor cells may be more effective. Patients with chronic inflammatory, infectious, or neoplastic processes may develop anemia of chronic disease. Recombinant EPO improved hematocrit or hemoglobin levels in small studies of patients with rheumatoid arthritis or juvenile arthritis. Premature infants often become anemic in part because of repeated blood sampling. Although high-dose rEPO reduced transfusion requirements in several double-blind, placebo-controlled studies of premature infants, rEPO had a slower onset of action and was more costly than transfusions. The preliminary results of small studies suggest that rEPO, especially in combination with hydroxyurea, may be beneficial in patients with sickle cell anemia (Markham and Bryson, 1995).

TREATMENT-RELATED CYTOPENIA, TRANSPLANTATION, AND TRANSFUSION

There is interest in expanding the role of hematopoietic growth factors for chemotherapy-induced cytopenias. Dose-intensive chemotherapy refers to the use of higher doses or a more frequent schedule compared with standard therapy. Both rG-CSF and rGM-CSF facilitate this goal (American Society of Clinical Oncology, 1994).

Radiation therapy is frequently added to chemotherapy to improve the therapeutic outcome. The American Society of Clinical Oncology (1994 and 1996) recommends against the use of hematopoietic growth factors in this setting. Although clinical trial experience is limited, available evidence suggests that myeloid growth factors are not beneficial and may increase the risk of thrombocytopenia when they are co-administered with radiation therapy. The expert panel hypothesized that growth factors may mobilize progenitor cells into the peripheral blood, rendering them vulnerable to the lethal effects of radiation (American Society of Clinical Oncology, 1994).

INFECTIOUS DISEASES

Infectious diseases are logical targets for myeloid hematopoietic growth factors because the therapeutic outcome of most infections is directly related to the supply and function of the host's phagocytic cells. The response to infection in an otherwise healthy host probably involves increased production of G-CSF, GM-CSF, M-CSF, IL-3 and other myeloid growth factors (Dale, 1994), which in turn regulate the proliferation, differentiation, and maturation

	Investigational use	Adjunct therapy
rM-CSF	refractory fungal infections	
rIL-3	chemotherapy-induced neutropenia and thrombocytopenia	± GM-CSF
	autologous bone marrow transplantation	± G-CSF or GM-CSF
	before (to mobilize) or after PBPC transplantation	G-CSF or GM-CSF
	ex vivo expansion of megakaryocytes and neutrophil progenitors	G-CSF, IL-6 and SCF
PIXY-321	chemotherapy-induced neutropenia and thrombocytopenia	
	autologous bone marrow transplantation	
	failed bone marrow transplantation	
	ex vivo or *in vivo* hematopoietic cell expansion	
PEG-rHuMGDF	chemotherapy-induced thrombocytopenia	
rSCF	chemotherapy-induced neutropenia and thrombocytopenia	
	ex vivo or *in vivo* hematopoietic cell expansion	G-CSF ± IL-3 and IL-6

Table 8.10. Status of clinical trials of investigational hematopoietic growth factors (Dorr and Von Hoff, 1994; Proceedings of meetings[a]; Vose and Armitage, 1995).
PEG-rHuMGDF = recombinant human megakaryocyte growth and development factor derivatized with poly(ethylene glycol) (cf. Chapter 5) (Amgen Inc., Thousand Oaks, California, USA); PBPC = peripheral blood progenitor cell; [a]American Society of Hematology, 1994; American Society of Clinical Oncology, 1995.

of these immature hematopoietic cells. The neutrophil is the first line of phagocytic defense, appearing at the site of infection within minutes of injury; macrophages are recruited several hours later. In addition, hematopoietic growth factors help fight infection by regulating the functional activity of mature neutrophils. For example, both G-CSF and GM-CSF enhance phagocytosis and antibody-dependent killing (see Table 8.3).

Extensive research programs have been started to evaluate rG-CSF and rGM-CSF in community-acquired pneumonia, as surgical prophylaxis, and in other nonneutropenic infections. The promising results of animal studies triggered a series of clinical studies that should provide insight in the near future. One small study of rM-CSF has been published; one fourth of the patients experienced resolution of refractory fungal infections during therapy with rM-CSF 100 to 2000 µg/m²/day (Nemunaitis *et al.*, 1993). More studies are needed to determine the role of hematopoietic growth factors as antimicrobial agents and in patients with fungal infections (Kouides and DiPersio, 1995; Vose and Armitage, 1995).

The role of therapeutically administered rG-CSF and rGM-CSF in patients with pre-existing neutropenia is controversial, except in severe chronic neutropenia. In a double-blind, placebo-controlled study, rG-CSF reduced the duration of neutropenia and febrile neutropenia, but it did not reduce the duration of fever, antibiotic use, or hospitalization (Maher *et al.*, 1994). These and similar findings have led to the conclusion that, although hematopoietic growth factors do not appear to be beneficial in the afebrile patient, they may be useful in selected subsets of febrile patients, such as those with protracted neutropenia, or evidence of tissue infection, such as pneumonia (American Society of Clinical Oncology, 1994).

Investigational Hematopoietic Growth Factors

A sample of potential indications for investigational hematopoietic growth factors was compiled from recent reviews and meetings (Table 8.10). Unfortunately, this type of list rapidly becomes obsolete as old ideas are abandoned and new studies are initiated. This list also demonstrates the impact of available hematopoietic growth factors on on-going studies. Because of the success of rG-CSF and rGM-CSF, thrombocytopenia has replaced neutropenia as the dose-limiting toxicity for some cancer chemotherapy regimens. Consequently, there is tremendous interest in hematopoietic growth factors that may expand platelets, such as thrombopoietin or other growth factors that exert broad effects earlier in the hematopoietic cascade. Many of these investigational agents are being tested in combination with each other or with rG-CSF or rGM-CSF (Vose and Armitage, 1995).

It is impossible to predict which investigational hemato-poietic growth factor will reach the market next. Recombinant M-CSF has been under clinical evaluation nearly as long as rG-CSF and rGM-CSF, which may have implications for the likelihood of marketing. Recombinant IL-3 was the next to enter clinical studies. Of the newer hematopoietic growth factors, PIXY-321 has been the most extensively evaluated. Recombinant SCF is also undergoing active investigation. As previously indicated, several companies are developing recombinant TPO and other Mpl related ligands. Amgen Inc. (Thousand Oaks, California, USA) started testing mega-karyocyte growth and development factor (PEG-rHuMGDF), a pegylated, truncated Mpl ligand related to TPO, in hu-mans in May 1995 and recently the first results of human trials were published (O'Malley et al., 1996; Basser et al., 1996a; Fanucchi et al., 1997). Genentech Inc. (San Fran-cisco, California, USA) has also begun clinical trials.

Toxicities

Many hematopoietic growth factors, especially multipotential factors that act on early progenitor cells, are associated with constitutional symptoms such as fever, chills, rash, myalgia, injection-site irritation, and edema. The safety of individual hematopoietic growth factors depends on their receptor sites and effects of secondary cytokine release (Vose and Armitage, 1995).

It is difficult to determine the relative toxicity of hemato-poietic growth factors because of the lack of comparative studies and confounding effects of different reporting methods and different cancer chemotherapy regimens. For example, patients who undergo bone marrow transplanta-tion experience toxicity that may obscure hematopoietic growth factor-related adverse effects. Formulations with different levels of glycosylation may also play a role. Therefore, this section will focus on the most common adverse effects and those that occurred more frequently in treated than control patients, summarize any comparative studies, and list toxicities described in the package inserts. Table 8.11 shows the relative frequency of events compared with placebo in two ways: statistically significant increases and 5% or greater increases in the frequency of adverse events.

RECOMBINANT G-CSF AND GM-CSF

The most common adverse effect associated with Filgrastim and Lenograstim is mild-to-moderate bone pain, which occurs in 15% to 39% of patients receiving Filgrastim 5 µg/kg/day, compared with 0% to 21% of control patients. Lenograstim is also associated with injection-site reaction. Loss of appetite, fever, and headache are mentioned in the Japanese package insert for Lenograstim, but published information does not indicate whether the frequency is higher compared with controls. Other adverse events are infrequent (American Society of Clinical Oncology, 1994).

A long list of adverse effects has been attributed to the two rGM-CSF products (see Table 8.11) in part because of the use of high doses in early, uncontrolled trials. For example, much has been written about the capillary-leak syndrome because of its potential severity. This complica-tion is manifested by fluid retention, pleural and/or peri-cardial effusions, peripheral edema, and hypoproteinemia. Fortunately, capillary-leak syndrome is rare and occurs at high doses (>15 µg/kg). Currently recommended doses of Sargramostim were not associated with this syndrome and did not even increase the incidence of most adverse events in a placebo-controlled study of bone marrow transplant recipients (Nemunaitis et al., 1991). Recombinant GM-CSF may also induce a first-dose reaction characterized by flushing, tachycardia, hypotension, musculoskeletal pain, dyspnea, nausea and vomiting, and leg spasms. This com-plication is much more common with Molgramostim and with intravenous administration (American Society of Clinical Oncology, 1994).

The results of noncomparative studies suggest differ-ences among hematopoietic growth factors and their recom-binant products, but comparative studies are needed to confirm these perceptions. Fever is thought to be more common with rGM-CSF, but the clinical relevance is un-known (American Society of Clinical Oncology, 1994). Glycosylation may be a factor and may prevent some ad-verse effects associated with rGM-CSF. The results of in-dependent studies (Rowe et al., 1995; Stone et al., 1995) suggest that glycosylated Sargramostim or Regramostim may be less likely to cause adverse effects than non-glycosylated Molgramostim (American Society of Clinical Oncology, 1994). Antibody formation has been reported with rGM-CSF but not rG-CSF. Differences in glycosylation may contribute to the higher incidence for Sargramostim (3.6%) compared with Molgramostim (1%) (Leucomax® package insert, 1992; Leukine® package insert, 1996), but the clinical significance of neutralizing antibodies is un-known (American Society of Clinical Oncology, 1994).

		Most frequent	Less frequent or rare
rG-CSF	Filgrastim	bone pain * nausea† (BMT patients only)	allergic-type reactions
	Lenograstim	bone pain * injection-site reaction *	
rGM-CSF	Molgramostim	fever nausea dyspnea diarrhea rash rigors injection-site reaction vomiting fatigue anorexia musculoskeletal pain asthenia	anaphylaxis bronchospasm cardiac failure capillary-leak syndrome cerebrovascular disorders confusion convulsions hypotension cardiac rhythm abnormalities intracranial hypertension pleural or pericardial effusion pericarditis pulmonary edema syncope
	Sagramostim	fever asthenia * headache bone pain chills myalgia malaise *	dyspnea peripheral edema rash * diarrhea * pleural or pericardial effusions capillary leak syndrome
rEPO	Epoetin alfa	hypertension * (CRF patients only) headache * arthralgia * diarrhea† clotted access * fever * cough respiratory congestion * dyspnea rash * edema† (cancer patients only)	nausea and vomiting

Table 8.11. Adverse effects listed in package inserts.
*More frequent in treated than control patients (i.e., occurring at a rate of $\geq 5\%$ of study patients compared with controls).
†Significantly more frequent in treated than control patients ($P < 0.05$).

EPOETIN ALPHA

Epoetin alpha is generally well tolerated. Many adverse effects are indistinguishable from those of underlying diseases such as chronic renal failure, AIDS, or cancer. The distribution of adverse effects is related to the underlying condition. For example, hypertension occurs in approximately one third of patients with chronic renal failure but not in those with nonrenal anemia. Acute hypertension occasionally leads to encephalopathy or seizures; the mechanism is unknown. In contrast, fever is limited to patients with AIDS or cancer and may reflect investigator sensitivity. Compared with placebo, rEPO lowered the incidence of nausea in patients with cancer and increased it only slightly in those with other conditions (Epogen® package insert, 1994; Eprex® package insert, 1994; Procrit® package insert, 1996).

INVESTIGATIONAL HEMATOPOIETIC GROWTH FACTORS

Comprehensive toxicity profiles are not yet available for the investigational hematopoietic growth factors. The dose-limiting toxicity of rM-CSF is thrombocytopenia (Vose and Armitage, 1995), which explains the waning research enthusiasm in this hematopoietic growth factor. Fever is the major adverse effect of rIL-3; others are headache and stiff neck, which may be caused by cytokine release (e.g., histamine). Facial flushing, mild local edema, injection site erythema, and bone pain are less common (Dorr and Von Hoff, 1994). As a fusion protein, PIXY-321 is expected to exhibit the toxicity of its individual components, rIL-3 and rGM-CSF. The most common adverse effect is erythema at the subcutaneous injection site; others are low-grade fever, chills, fatigue, headache and myalgia, and mild gastrointestinal symptoms (Dorr and Von Hoff, 1994; Vadhan-Raj, 1994). The toxicities of thrombopoietin are not yet known. The most common adverse effect of rSCF is local reaction at the subcutaneous injection site (Glaspy et al., 1994). Some rSCF-related adverse effects are attributable to its effects on mast cells and histamine release (Galli et al., 1994). A recombinant Mpl ligand, PEG-rHuMGDF, appears to be well tolerated in early clinical trials (Basser et al., 1996a; Basser et al., 1996b; Fanucchi et al., 1997).

Concluding Remarks

The field of hematopoietic growth factors is dynamic. New growth factors are being discovered. The indications for commercially available growth factors are expanding. Clinical experience is leading to more convenient administration methods. This information explosion provides an opportunity for pharmacists to contribute to the care of patients who are candidates for hematopoietic growth factor therapy. Health-care professionals should become familiar with similarities and differences in the chemistry, pharmacology, pharmaceutical concerns, and clinical and practice aspects of hematopoietic growth factors. Health-care professionals should be especially sensitive to differences in production methods and pharmacology that have the potential to translate to clinically relevant differences in effectiveness and safety. This review provides a brief introduction to commercially available and investigational hematopoietic growth factors. Appropriate resources should always be used for more current or detailed information. ■

References

- Abels R. (1990). Review of the hematologic effects of erythropoietin. *Seminars in Nephrology*, 10 (suppl 1), 1–10
- American Society of Clinical Oncology. (1994). American Society of Clinical Oncology recommendations for the use of hematopoietic colony-stimulating factors: evidence-based, clinical practice guidelines. *Journal of Clinical Oncology*, 12, 2471–2508
- American Society of Clinical Oncology. (1996). American Society of Clinical Oncology recommendations for the use of hematopoietic colony-stimulating factors: evidence-based, clinical practice guidelines. *Journal of Clinical Oncology*, 14, 1957–1960
- Basser RL, Rasko JEJ, Clarke K, Cebon J, Green MD, Hussein S, et al. (1996a). Thrombopoietic effects of pegylated recombinant human megakaryocyte growth and development factor (PEG-rHuMGDF) in patients with advanced cancer. *The Lancet*, 348, 1279–1281
- Basser R, Rasko J, Clarke K, Green M, Cebon J, Grigg A, et al. (1996b). Pegylated megakaryocyte growth and development factor (PEG-rHuMGDF) enhances the mobilization of peripheral blood progenitor cells (PBPC) by chemotherapy and Filgrastim. *Proceedings of the 38th Annual Meeting of the American Society of Hematology*, December 6–10, 2554.
- Cebon JS, Bury RW, Lieschke GJ, Morstyn G. (1990). The effects of dose and route of administration on the pharmacokinetics of granulocyte-macrophage colony-stimulating factor. *European Journal of Cancer*, 26, 1064–1069
- Cebon J, Layton JE, Maher D, Morstyn G. (1994). Endogenous haemopoietic growth factors in neutropenia and infection. *British Journal of Haematology*, 86, 265–274
- Clark SC, Kamen R. (1987). The human hematopoietic colony-stimulating factors. *Science*, 236, 1229–1237
- Crawford J, Ozer H, Stoller R, Johnson D, Lyman G, Tabbara I, et al. (1991). Reduction by granulocyte colony-stimulating factor of fever and neutropenia induced by chemotherapy in patients with small-cell lung cancer. *New England Journal of Medicine*, 325, 164–170
- Dale DC. (1994). Potential role of colony-stimulating factors in the prevention and treatment of infectious diseases. *Clinical Infectious Diseases*, 18 (suppl 2), S180–S188
- Dale DC, Bonilla MA, Davis MW, Nakanishi AM, Hammond WP, Kurtzberg J, et al. (1993). A randomized controlled phase III trial of recombinant human granulocyte colony-stimulating factor (filgrastim) for treatment of severe chronic neutropenia. *Blood*, 81, 2496–2502

- **Debili N, Cramer E, Wendling F, Vainchenker W.** (1997). *In vitro* effects of Mpl ligand on human hemopoietic progenitor cells. In *Thrombopoiesis and Thrombopoietins*, edited by DJ Kuter, P Hunt, W Sheridan, D Zucker-Franklin, 1st ed. Totowa, New Jersey, USA: Humana Press Inc, pp. 217–237
- **De Vries EGE, van Gameren MM, Willemse PHB.** (1993). Recombinant human interleukin 3 in clinical oncology. *Stem Cells*, 11, 72–80
- **Dombret H, Chastang C, Fenaux P, Reiffers J, Bordessoule D, Bouabdallah R, et al.** (1995). A controlled study of recombinant human granulocyte colony-stimulating factor in elderly patients after treatment for acute myelogenous leukemia. *New England Journal of Medicine*, 332, 1678–1683
- **Dorr RT, Von Hoff DD.** (1994). *Cancer Chemotherapy Handbook*, 2nd ed. Norwalk, Connecticut, USA: Appleton & Lange
- **Epogen® (epoetin alpha)** package insert. Thousand Oaks, California, USA: Amgen Inc, 1995
- **EPREX® (epoetinum alpha)** package insert. Bassersdorf, Switzerland: The R.W. Johnson Pharmaceutical Research Institute, 1994
- **Erslev AJ.** (1991). Erythropoietin. *New England Journal of Medicine*, 324, 1339–1344
- **Eschbach JW, Abdulhadi MH, Browne JK, Delano BG, Downing MR, Egrie JC, et al.** (1989). Recombinant human erythropoietin in anemic patients with end-stage renal disease. Results of a phase III multicenter trial. *Annals of Internal Medicine*, 111, 992–1000
- **Fanucchi M, Glaspy J, Crawford J, Garst J, Figlin R, Sheridan W, et al.** (1997). Effects of polyethylene glycol-conjugated recombinant human megakaryocyte growth and development factor on platelet counts after chemotherapy for lung cancer. *New England Journal of Medicine*, 336, 404–409
- **Fischl M, Galpin JE, Levine JD, Groopman JE, Henry DH, Kennedy P, et al.** (1990). Recombinant human erythropoietin for patients with AIDS treated with zidovudine. *New England Journal of Medicine*, 322, 1488–1493
- **Frampton JE, Lee CR, Faulds D.** (1994). Filgrastim. A review of its pharmacological properties and therapeutic efficacy in neutropenia. *Drugs*, 48, 731–760
- **Galli SJ, Zsebo KM, Geissler EN.** (1994). The kit ligand, stem cell factor. *Advances in Immunology*, 55, 1–96
- **Glaspy J, McNiece I, LeMaistre F, Menchaca D, Briddell R, Lill M, et al.** (1994). Effects of stem cell factor (rhSCF) and filgrastim (rhG-CSF) on mobilization of peripheral blood progenitor cells (PBPC) and on hematologic recovery posttransplant: early results from a phase I/II study. *Proceedings of the 30th Annual Meeting of the American Society of Clinical Oncology*, May 14–17, 1994
- **Godwin JE, Kopecky KJ, Head DR, Hynes HE, Balcerzak SP, Appelbaum FR.** (1995). A double blind placebo controlled trial of G-CSF in elderly patients with previously untreated acute myeloid leukemia. A Southwest Oncology Group Study. *Proceedings of the 37th Annual Meeting of the American Society of Hematology*, December 1–5, 1723
- **Granocyte® (lenograstim)** package insert. Antony, France: Chugai-Rhône-Poulenc, 1993
- **Groopman JE, Molina J-M, Scadden DT.** (1989). Hematopoietic growth factors. Biology and clinical applications. *New England Journal of Medicine*, 321, 1449–1459
- **Hardy WD.** (1991). Combined ganciclovir and recombinant human granulocyte-macrophage colony-stimulating factor in the treatment of cytomegalovirus retinitis in AIDS patients. *Journal of Acquired Immune Deficiency Syndrome*, 4 (suppl 1), S22–S28
- **Hardy D, Spector S, Polsky B, Crumpacker C, van der Horst C, Holland G, et al.** (1994). Combination of ganciclovir and granulocyte-macrophage colony-stimulating factor in the treatment of cytomegalovirus retinitis in AIDS patients. The ACTG 073 Team. *European Journal of Clinical Microbiology and Infectious Diseases*, 13 (suppl 2), S34–S40
- **Heil G, Hoelzer D, Sanz MA, Lechner K, Liu Yin J, Papa G, et al.** (1995). Results of a randomised, double-blind placebo controlled phase III study of Filgrastim in remission induction and early consolidation therapy for adults with de-novo acute myeloid leukaemia. *Proceedings of the 37th Annual Meeting of the American Society of Hematology*, December 1–5, 1053
- **Henry DH, Abels RI.** (1994). Recombinant human erythropoietin in the treatment of cancer and chemotherapy-induced anemia: results of double-blind and open-label follow-up studies. *Seminars in Oncology*, 21 (suppl 3), 21–28
- **Jones SE, Schottstaedt W, Duncan LA, Kirby RL, Good RH, Mennel RG, et al.** (1996). Randomized double-blind prospective trial to evaluate the effects of sargramostim versus placebo in a moderate-dose fluorouracil, doxorubicin, and cyclophosphamide adjuvant chemotherapy program for stage II and III breast cancer. *Journal of Clinical Oncology*, 14, 2976–2983
- **Kaushansky K.** (1995). Thrombopoietin: the primary regulator of platelet production. *Blood*, 86, 419–431
- **Kouides PA, DiPersio JF.** (1995). The hematopoietic growth factors. In *Cancer Treatment*, edited by CM Haskell, 4th ed. Philadelphia, Pennsylvania, USA: WB. Saunders Company, pp. 69–77
- **Kuter DJ, Beeler DL, Rosenberg RD.** (1994). The purification of megapoietin: a physiological regulator of megakaryocyte growth and platelet production. *Proceedings of the National Academy of Sciences of the United States of America*, 91, 11104–11108
- **Kuter DJ.** (1997). The regulation of platelet production *in vivo*. In *Thrombopoiesis and Thrombopoietins*, edited by DJ Kuter, P Hunt, W Sheridan, D Zucker-Franklin, 1st ed. Totowa, New Jersey, USA: Humana Press Inc, pp. 377–397
- **Leucomax® (molgramostim)** package insert. Suffolk, United Kingdom: Sandoz Pharmaceuticals, Surrey and Schering-Plough Ltd, 1992
- **Leukine® (sargramostim)** package insert. Seattle, Washington, USA: Immunex Corporation, 1996
- **Lieschke GJ, Burgess AW.** (1992). Granulocyte colony-stimulating factor and granulocyte–macrophage colony-stimulating factor. *New England Journal of Medicine*, 327, 28–35 and 99–106

- Lieschke GJ, Grail D, Hodgson G, Metcalf D, Stanley E, Cheers C, *et al.* (1994). Mice lacking granulocyte colony-stimulating factor have chronic neutropenia, granulocyte and macrophage progenitor cell deficiency, and impaired neutrophil mobilization. *Blood*, 84, 1737–1746
- Lok S, Kaushansky K, Holly RD, Kuijper JL, Lofton-Day CE, Oort PJ, *et al.* (1994). Cloning and expression of murine thrombopoietin cDNA and stimulation of platelet production *in vivo*. *Nature*, 369, 565–568
- Lord BI, Bronchud MH, Owens S, Chang J, Howell A, Souza L, *et al.* (1989). The kinetics of human granulopoiesis following treatment with granulocyte colony-stimulating factor *in vivo*. *Proceedings of the National Academy of Sciences of the United States of America*, 86, 9499–9503
- Lord BI, Gurney H, Chang J, Thatcher N, Crowther D, Dexter TM. (1992). Haemopoietic cell kinetics in humans treated with rGM-CSF. *International Journal of Cancer*, 50, 26–31
- Lyman SD, James L, Johnson L, Brasel K, De Vries P, Escobar S, *et al.* Cloning of the human homologue of the murine flt3 ligand: a growth factor for early hematopoietic progenitor cells. *Blood*, 83, 2795–2801
- O'Malley CJ, Rasko JE.J, Basser RL, McGrath KM, Cebon J, Grigg AP, *et al.* (1996). Administration of pegylated recombinant human megakaryocyte growth and development factor to humans stimulates the production of functional platelets that show no evidence of *in vitro* activation. *Blood*, 88, 3288–3298
- Maher DW, Lieschke GJ, Green M, Bishop J, Stuart-Harris R, Wolf M, *et al.* (1994). Filgrastim in patients with chemotherapy-induced febrile neutropenia. A double-blind, placebo-controlled trial. *Annals of Internal Medicine*, 121, 492–501
- Markham A, Bryson HM. (1995). Epoetin alpha. A review of its pharmacodynamic and pharmacokinetic properties and therapeutic use in nonrenal applications. *Drugs*, 49, 232–254
- Mertelsmann R. (1991). Hematopoietins: biology, pathophysiology, and potential as therapeutic agents. *Annals of Oncology*, 2, 251–263
- Metcalf D. (1990). The colony stimulating factors. Discovery, development, and clinical applications. *Cancer*, 65, 2185–2195
- Morgan KM, Strickland SR. (1993). The use of granulocyte stimulating factor (GCSF) has improved the outcome in AIDS related CMV retinitis (abstract PO-B16-1666). IX International Conference on AIDS, Berlin, June 6–11, 1993
- Nemunaitis J, Shannon-Dorcy K, Appelbaum FR, Meyers J, Owens A, Day R, *et al.* (1993). Long-term follow-up of patients with invasive fungal disease who received adjunctive therapy with recombinant human macrophage colony-stimulating factor. *Blood*, 82, 1422–1427
- Nemunaitis J, Rabinowe SN, Singer JW, Bierman PJ, Vose JM, Freedman AS, *et al.* (1991). Recombinant granulocyte–macrophage colony-stimulating factor after autologous bone marrow transplantation for lymphoid cancer. *New England Journal of Medicine*, 324, 1773–1778
- Neupogen® (Filgrastim) package insert. Thousand Oaks, California, USA: Amgen, 1996
- Neupogen® (Filgrastim) package insert. Hertfordshire, England: Roche Products Limited, 1995
- Nichol JL, Hokom MM, Hornkohl A, Sheridan WP, Ohashi H, Kato T, *et al.* (1995). Megakaryocyte growth and development factor. Analyses of *in vitro* effects on human megakaryopoiesis and endogenous serum levels during chemotherapy-induced thrombocytopenia. *Journal of Clinical Investigation*, 95, 2973–2978
- Nichol JL. (1997). Serum levels of thrombopoietin in health and disease. In *Thrombopoiesis and Thrombopoietins*, edited by DJ Kuter, P Hunt, W Sheridan, D Zucker-Franklin, 1st ed. Totowa, New Jersey, USA: Humana Press Inc, pp. 359–375
- Ortho Biologics Inc. 1996, data on file
- Proceedings of the 31st Annual Meeting American Society of Clinical Oncology, May 20–23, 1995
- Proceedings of the 36th Annual Meeting of the American Society of Hematology, December 2–6, 1994
- Procrit® (epoetin alpha) package insert. Raritan, New Jersey, USA: Ortho Biotech Inc, 1996
- R & D Systems, Personal Communication, 1997
- Rapoport AP, Abboud CN, DiPersio JF. (1992). Granulocyte-macrophage colony-stimulating factor (GM-CSF) and granulocyte colony-stimulating factor (G-CSF): receptor biology, signal transduction, and neutrophil activation. *Blood Reviews*, 6, 43–57
- Robinson BE, Quesenberry PJ. (1990). Hematopoietic growth factors: overview and clinical applications, Part II. *The American Journal of the Medical Sciences*, 300, 237–244
- Rowe JM, Andersen JW, Mazza JJ, Bennett JM, Paietta E, Hayes FA, *et al.* (1995). A randomized placebo-controlled phase III study of granulocyte-macrophage colony-stimulating factor in adult patients (>55 to 70 years of age) with acute myelogenous leukemia: a study of the Eastern Cooperative Oncology Group (E1490). *Blood*, 86, 457–462
- Schmitz N, Linch DC, Dreger P, Goldstone AH, Boogaerts MA, Ferrant A, *et al.* (1996). Randomised trial of filgrastim-mobilised peripheral blood progenitor cell transplantation versus autologous bone-marrow transplantation in lymphoma patients. *The Lancet*, 347, 353–357
- Sekino H, Moriya K, Sugano T, Wakabayashi K, Okazaki A. (1989). Recombinant human G-CSF (rG-CSF). *Shinryo to Shinyaku*, 26, 32–104
- Shadduck RK, Waheed A, Evans C, Sulecki C, Rosenfeld CS. (1990). Serum and urinary levels of recombinant human granulocyte-macrophage colony-stimulating factor: assessment after intravenous infusion and subcutaneous injection. *Experimental Hematology*, 18, 601
- Sheridan WP, Begley CG, Juttner CA, Szer J, To LB, Maher D, *et al.* (1992). Effect of peripheral-blood progenitor cells mobilised by filgrastim (G-CSF) on platelet recovery after high-dose chemotherapy. *Lancet*, 339, 640–644

- **Stahel R, Jost L, Cerny T, Pichert G, Honegger H, Tobler A, *et al.** (1994). Randomized study of recombinant human granulocyte colony-stimulating factor after high-dose chemotherapy and autologous bone marrow transplantation for high-risk lymphoid malignancies. *Journal of Clinical Oncology*, 12, 1931–1938

- **Stone RM, Berg DT, George SL, Dodge RK, Paciucci PA, Schulman P, *et al.** (1995). Granulocyte-macrophage colony-stimulating factor after initial chemotherapy for elderly patients with primary acute myelogenous leukemia. *New England Journal of Medicine*, 332, 1671–1677

- **Summerhayes M.** (1995). Myeloid haematopoietic growth factors in clinical practice — a comparative review — Parts I and II. *European Hospital Pharmacy*, 1, 30–36 and 67–74

- **Vadhan-Raj S.** (1994). PIXY321 (GM-CSF/IL-3 fusion protein): biology and early clinical development. *Stem Cells*, 12, 253–261

- **Veys N, Vanholder, R, Lameire N.** (1992). Pain at the injection site of subcutaneously administered erythropoietin in maintenance hemodialysis patients: a comparison of two brands of erythropoietin. *American Journal of Nephrology*, 12, 68–72

- **Vose JM, Armitage JO.** (1995). Clinical applications of hematopoietic growth factors. *Journal of Clinical Oncology*, 13, 1023–1035

Self-Assessment Questions

Question 1:   What are hematopoietic growth factors?

Question 2:   What are the eight major lineages or types of mature blood cells, all of which are derived from a small population of primitive stem cells in the bone marrow?

Question 3:   Generally, chemically describe the hematopoietic growth factors.

Question 4:   How do hematopoietic growth factors function?

Question 5:   Define the difference between multilineage growth factors and lineage-specific growth factors.

Question 6:   What are the in vivo actions of rG-CSF and rGM-CSF in patients with advanced cancer.

Question 7:   What is the physiologic role of EPO?

Question 8:   What are the currently commercially available hematopoietic growth factors?

Question 9:   What are the indications for rG-CSF?

Question 10:   What are the indications for rGM-CSF?

Question 11:   What are the indications for rEPO?

Question 12:   Why might infectious diseases be logical targets for myeloid hematopoietic growth factors?

Answers

Answer 1:   They regulate both hematopoiesis and the functional activity of mature cells (including proliferation, differentiation, and maturation). In addition, hematopoietic growth factors mobilize progenitor cells to move from the bone marrow to the peripheral blood .

Answer 2:   The myeloid pathway gives rise to red blood cells (erythrocytes), platelets, monocytes and macrophages, and granulocytes (neutrophils, eosinophils, and basophils). The lymphoid pathway gives rise to lymphocytes.

Answer 3:   They are glycoproteins, which can be distinguished by their amino acid sequence and glycosylation (carbohydrate linkages). Hematopoietic growth factors have cysteine-cysteine disulfide bridges that dictate their three-dimensional configuration, which is necessary for biologic activity. Most hematopoietic growth factors are single-chain polypeptides weighing approximately 14 to 21 kD. The carbohydrate content varies depending on the growth factor and production method, which in turn affects the molecular weight but not necessarily the biologic activity.

Answer 4:   Hematopoietic growth factors act by binding to specific cell surface receptors. The resultant complex sends a signal to the cell to express genes, which in turn induce cellular proliferation, differentiation, or activation. A hematopoietic growth factor may also act indirectly if the cell expresses a gene that causes the production of a different hematopoietic growth factor or another cytokine, which in turn binds to and stimulates a different cell.

Answer 5:   Multilineage growth factors (e.g., GM-CSF, IL-3, and SCF) affect multiple cell lineages and tend to act on early progenitor cells before they become committed to one lineage. Lineage-specific growth factors (e.g., G-CSF, M-CSF, EPO, and presumably thrombopoietin) predominantly affect one cell type and act later in the hematopoietic cascade.

Answer 6:   Both growth factors cause a transient leukopenia that is followed by a dose-dependent increase in the number of circulating mature and immature neutrophils. Both growth factors enhance the *in vitro* function of neutrophils obtained from treated patients. Recombinant GM-CSF, but not rG-CSF, also increases the number of circulating monocytes and eosinophils, and *in vitro* monocyte cytotoxicity and cytokine production.

Answer 7: EPO maintains a normal red blood cell count by causing committed erythroid progenitor cells to proliferate and differentiate into normoblasts. EPO also shifts marrow reticulocytes into circulation.

Answer 8: Three hematopoietic growth factors are commercially available, rG-CSF (Filgrastim, Lenograstim, and Nartograstim), rGM-CSF (Molgramostim and Sargramostim), and rEPO (Epoetin or Epoetinum alpha, Epoetin beta).

Answer 9: Recombinant G-CSF is indicated for neutropenia associated with myelosuppressive cancer chemotherapy, bone marrow transplantation, and severe chronic neutropenia; rG-CSF is also indicated to mobilize peripheral blood progenitor cells (PBPC) for PBPC transplantation; rG-CSF is indicated for reversal of clinically significant neutropenia and subsequent mainte-nance or adequate neutrophil counts in patients with HIV infection during treatment with antiviral and/or other myelosuppressive medications.

Answer 10: Recombinant GM-CSF is indicated for neutropenia associated with myelosuppressive cancer chemotherapy, bone marrow transplantation, and antiviral therapy for AIDS-related cytomegalovirus; rGM-CSF is also indi-cated for failed bone marrow transplantation or delayed engraftment, and for use in mobilization and following transplantation of autologous peri-pheral blood progenitor cells.

Answer 11: Recombinant EPO is indicated to treat anemia associated with chronic renal failure, zidovudine in HIV-infected patients, and chemotherapy. Recombinant EPO is also indicated to reduce allogeneic blood transfusions and hasten erythroid recovery in surgery patients.

Answer 12: Because the therapeutic outcome of most infections is directly related to the supply and function of the host's phagocytic cells. The response to infection in an otherwise healthy host probably involves increased produc-tion of G-CSF, GM-CSF, M-CSF, IL-3 and other myeloid growth factors, which in turn regulate the proliferation, differentiation, and maturation of these immature hematopoietic cells.

9 Interleukins and Interferons

by: Joseph Tami

Cytokines

Cytokines can generally be defined as soluble mediators or glycoproteins that aid in the communication between cells, primarily cells of the immunological, hematological, and neurological systems. Interleukins and interferons are groups of naturally occurring glycoproteins which belong to the overall category of cytokines. There are at least 60 different types of cytokines.

During the 1970's researchers began identifying molecules other than antibodies which were produced by the cells of the immune system. These molecules were involved in the communication network of the immune system. The released cytokines bind to their target cells via specific receptors found on the cell surface. Many cytokines are produced during the effector phases of immunity or host defense.

Cytokines are not the same as hormones. Cytokines can be distinguished from hormones by various criteria. An individual cytokine can be secreted by a number of different types of cells while hormones are typically produced by just one or two very specialized cell types. Cytokines also can act on a variety of cell types. While cytokines are usually targeted to produce a local effect, hormones are targeted to affect cells at distant sites. The release of a cytokine is often a brief, self-limited event.

The soluble mediators classified as cytokines are made up of a wide array of glycoproteins including interleukins, interferons, colony stimulating factors (hematopoietic growth factors), chemokines, inflammatory cytokines, and anti-inflammatory factors. The classification of cytokines can be broken down into a number of sub-categories. For example, cytokines can be classified by their source. Lymphokines are produced by lymphocytes, primarily from T cells but also from B cells. Monokines are cytokines that are secreted from mononuclear cells.

Many of the cytokines are also grouped according to functional definitions. The term interleukin comes from inter-leukocyte, or a cytokine which communicates between white blood cells. The term interferon originally came from the ability of the cytokine to interfere with the viral infection of a cell.

A complete bibliography can be found at the conclusion of this Chapter.

The Interleukins

Terminology

Interleukins are often designated as IL-(number). The World Health Organization-International Union of Immunologic Societies (WHO-IUIS) gives official nomenclature status to the interleukins. At the present time, seventeen different interleukins have been described, although not all these have been given official nomenclature status. The IUIS recommendations for a molecule to be classified as an interleukin is based on four guidelines:

1. The molecule must be purified, molecularly cloned, and expressed. It should be distinct from any previously described interleukin or other molecule.
2. The molecule must be a natural product of a cell of the immune system.
3. The molecule should not be part of a family of compounds that have a major function outside the immune system.
4. The molecule cannot be more suitably described by a descriptive designation.

A general description of the naturally occurring interleukins follows in the sections below. In general, once a unique interleukin has been identified, the protein sequence is determined in an attempt to further identify the gene encoding the protein. After the genetic sequence has been determined, recombinant DNA techniques are used to produce large quantities of the interleukin. This allows for the production of adequate supplies for basic and clinical studies. While many of the interleukins are in clinical studies, only one of the interleukins is currently approved by the FDA and commercially available for clinical use in the United States. This product is aldesleukin (IL-2). Table 9.1 provides a list of interleukins that have been discovered to date.

Interleukin	M_W (kD)	Primary cell source	Primary activities	Commercial product
IL-1a/IL-1b	17	macrophages, NK cells, B cells	inflammation	
IL-2	15.5	T cells	activates T cells	Aldesleukin
IL-3	28	T cells	hematopoietic growth factor	
IL-4	20	T cells	B cell growth	
IL-5	50 - 60	T cells	eosinophil and cell growth	
IL-6	25	T cells and fibroblasts	inflammation	
IL-7	25	stromal cells	B and T cell growth	
IL-8	8	macrophages	chemoattractant for neutrophils	
IL-9	30 - 40	activated T cells	T cell and erythroid growth	
IL-10	18	B cells, T cells	B cell growth/inhibition of cytokine synthesis by T cells	
IL-11	23	bone marrow stromal cells	hematopoietic co-factor	
IL-12	70	macrophages, B cells	induction of cell-mediated immunity	
IL-13	10	T cells	B cell growth	
IL-14	-	-	-	
IL-15	14	epithelial cells	T cell and NK cell growth	
IL-16	17	CD8+ T cells	T cell chemoattractant	
IL-17	-	CD4+ T cells	fibroblast stimulation	

Table 9.1. Interleukins.

Overview of the Interleukins

INTERLEUKIN-1

Interleukin 1 (IL-1) has been described by a variety of different names: lymphocyte activating factor (LAF), endogenous pyrogen, T cell replacing factor II, and B cell differentiation factor, as well as several others. It can thus be deduced that IL-1 exhibits a large variety of activities.

Interleukin 1 represents at least two distinct polypeptides (IL-1 α and IL-1 β). The molecular weights of the polypeptides are approximately 17,000 Daltons. Differences in glycosylation are responsible for the wide variation of reported molecular weights. IL-1 α and IL-1 β are encoded by two distinct genes. IL-1 α and IL-1 β are synthe-

sized as propeptides of approximately 30 kD, and are then cleaved to produce products of 159 and 153 amino acids respectively.

Both forms of IL-1 exert their effects by binding to two distinct types of IL-1 receptors. The first is IL-1 receptor type I which belongs to the immunoglobulin superfamily of receptors. The second IL-1 receptor is denoted type II and also belongs to the immunoglobulin superfamily. The two different forms of the IL-1 receptors bind IL-1 α and IL-1 β with different affinities.

IL-1 has been associated with numerous activities. Some of these include:
1) Induction of the IL-2 receptor
2) Stimulation of pre-B cell differentiation
3) Augmentation of NK-cell cytotoxicity

4) Induction of adhesion molecules on endothelial cells
5) Induction of fever
6) Stimulation of thymocyte proliferation
7) Enhancement of collagen production
8) Stimulation of the release of other cytokines involved in hematopoiesis

Overall, it is believed that IL-1 is an important mediator of the body's response to infection, inflammation, and injury. IL-1 is released as part of the acute phase reaction of hepatocytes. The primary producers of IL-1 in the immune system are macrophages, B cells and neutrophils. Potential clinical uses of IL-1 include the use as a radio-protective agent due to its stimulatory effects on hematopoiesis, and its ability to accelerate wound healing.

A naturally occurring inhibitor of IL-1 has been cloned. This molecule is termed the IL-1 receptor antagonist, or IL-1 ra. While it has limited sequence similarity to either IL-1 α or IL-1 β, it does have the ability to bind to the IL-1 receptors. However, it does not have IL-1 activity, thus serving as a useful blocker of the receptor. A recombinant version of IL-1 ra was investigated for its potential use in sepsis, however, the clinical trials were inconclusive as to the efficacy of the product in this setting.

INTERLEUKIN-2

Interleukin 2 (IL-2) was originally described as T cell growth factor (TCGF). IL-2 is synthesized and secreted primarily by T cells. It has direct effects on a number of immunological cells. IL-2 can stimulate the growth, differentiation and activation of T cells, B cells, and NK cells. Aldesleukin, a recombinant form of interleukin 2, has been approved by the FDA for use in patients with renal cell carcinoma.

IL-2 produces its immunological effects by binding to the cellular IL-2 receptor (IL-2R). There are various affinity forms of the IL-2R. Three chains are believed to comprise the cellular high affinity IL-2 receptor — the α, β and γ chains. A circulating form (also known as the soluble form) of the IL-2R has also been found in human serum. This circulating receptor is capable of binding IL-2. The circulating form of the IL-2R is a truncated version of the α chain, having no cytoplasmic tail. High levels of the circulating IL-2R have been found in patients with a wide variety of disorders including HIV infection, cancer, solid organ transplant rejection, and arthritis. It is believed that the circulating form of the IL-2R binds released IL-2 prior to IL-2 binding to cells in an attempt to prevent overstimulation of the immune system. Several other cytokine and adhesion molecule receptors also have circulating forms. It is believed that this is one manner in which the immunological cascade maintains a checks and balance system.

INTERLEUKIN-3

Interleukin 3 (IL-3) is a hematopoietic growth factor. The principle effects of IL-3 are on early hematopoietic progenitors in which IL-3 induces hematopoiesis and cell differentiation. Administration of IL-3 produces an increase in erythrocytes, neutrophils, eosinophils, monocytes and platelets. IL-3 can act synergistically or additively with other hematopoietic growth factors. IL-3 is believed to act early on in the hematological cascade.

INTERLEUKIN-4

Interleukin 4 (IL-4) is primarily derived from T cells. Its principle site of action is the B cell. IL-4 stimulates B cell proliferation and activation. It induces IgE and IgG1 expression from B cells, as well as class II MHC expression. In addition to its effects on B cells, IL-4 induces the differentiation of eosinophils and activity of T cytotoxic cells.

INTERLEUKIN-5

Interleukin 5 (IL-5) represents the compounds originally known as T cell replacement factor (TRF), eosinophil differentiation factor (EDF) and B cell growth factor (BCGFII). The primary effect of human IL-5 is on the eosinophilic lineage. It stimulates eosinophil chemotaxis as well as eosinophil expansion. It also appears to have activity on basophils.

INTERLEUKIN-6

Interleukin 6 (IL-6) is produced by lymphoid and non-lymphoid cells. It exerts a multitude of effects on a wide variety of cells. It acts on T cells and B cells. IL-6 stimulates multilineage hematopoiesis, including the maturation of megakaryocytes. IL-6 was also formerly known as interferon b_2, for its weak antiviral activity.

INTERLEUKIN-7

Interleukin 7 (IL-7) acts primarily on pre-B cells to stimulate their differentiation. It can also stimulate the development of human T cells. Overall, it appears that IL-7 is important in B and T cell development.

INTERLEUKIN-8

Interleukin 8 (IL-8) is a member of a group of glycoproteins known as chemokines. Chemokines are a family of small, inducible, secreted, pro-inflammatory cytokines that act primarily as chemoattractants and activators of specific types of leukocytes. IL-8 is a potent chemoattractant for neutrophils. It also has a wide variety of pro-inflammatory effects including the stimulation of neutrophil degranulation and the enhancement of neutrophil adherence to endothelial cells.

INTERLEUKIN-9 THROUGH INTERLEUKIN-16

Much more information will be needed in regards to the effects of the other interleukins before we see these interleukins used on a routine basis clinically. IL-9 appears to have effects on red blood cells, IL-10 is unique in that it appears to have immunosuppressive type activities, IL-13 is similar to IL-4 in its multiple inhibitory effects on monocytes and macrophages, and IL-15 appears to be very similar to IL-2.

INTERLEUKIN-17

Human Interleukin 17 (IL-17) has been described. This novel cytokine is derived from helper T cells (CD4+). Its effects on cells includes the induction of IL-6 and IL-6 secretion from fibroblasts, induction of ICAM-1 surface expression on fibroblasts, and costimulation of T cell proliferation.

Commercially Available Interleukins

INTRODUCTION: INTERLEUKIN-2

Interleukin 2 (IL-2) was originally referred to as T cell growth factor. IL-2 has a variety of immunoregulatory properties. IL-2 is produced primarily by activated T cells. The release of IL-2 results in increased T cell proliferation and differentiation. IL-2 has the ability to induce activation of natural killer (NK) cells and lymphokine activated killer (LAK) cells. IL-2 can also stimulate the production and activity of B cells. Cells activated by IL-2 release a variety of other cytokines such as tumor necrosis factor, IL-1, γ interferon, and granulocyte-macrophage colony stimulating factor. Thus the activities attributed to IL-2 can be mediated by direct (T cell and NK cell stimulation) and indirect (release of secondary cytokines) mechanisms.

Activation of T cells by IL-2 occurs by the binding of the IL-2 molecule to a specific receptor (IL-2R) on the cell surface. The IL-2 receptor (IL-2R) is displayed on the surface of inactive T cells and B cells. The IL-2R consists of at least three different chains: α (p55), β (p75) and γ. The highest affinity receptor is comprised of all three chains. The IL-2R α chain is also referred to as T cell activating antigen (Tac). A circulating form of the IL-2 receptor (p40) has been described which is derived from the p55 α chain. The circulating or soluble form of the IL-2R is capable of binding IL-2. Therefore, the circulating form of the IL-2R

may provide a mechanism for the down regulation of IL-2 effects.

CHEMICAL DESCRIPTION OF IL-2

Recombinant human interleukin 2 (rIL-2), known generically as aldesleukin, is available as Proleukin®. The chemical name is des-alanyl-1, serine-125-human interleukin-2. It is produced by a recombinant process involving genetically engineered *Escherichia coli*. Aldesleukin is not glycosylated. The molecule has no N-terminal alanine and has serine substituted for a cysteine at position 125. The molecular weight of the protein is approximately 15,300 daltons. The manufacturing process involves the use of tetracycline during fermentation. However, the presence of the antibiotic is not detectable in the final product.

PHARMACOLOGY OF IL-2

Indication
The approved indication for aldesleukin is for the treatment of metastatic renal cell carcinoma, based on reports of objective remissions in some patients.

Mechanism of Action
The exact mechanism of action of the antineoplastic effects of aldesleukin is unknown, although the immunomodulatory properties of recombinant IL-2 are believed to be involved. The effects of aldesleukin on cellular immunity include lymphocytosis, eosinophilia and thrombocytopenia. Activation of T cells, NK cells and LAK cells are believed to play an important role in the immune-mediated destruction of tumor cells.

Biotransformation
Greater than 80% of aldesleukin distributed to the plasma, cleared from the circulation, and presented to the kidney is metabolized to amino acids by the cells lining the proximal convoluted tubules of the kidney.

Elimination
Elimination is primarily from the kidney by glomerular filtration and peritubular extraction.

PHARMACEUTICAL CONCERNS OF IL-2

Aldesleukin is provided in a 22 million IU vial containing 1.3 mg of drug. It is reconstituted by adding 1.2 mLs of sterile water for injection to the vial. The injection of the diluent should be aimed at the side of the vial to prevent foaming and destruction of the protein. The reconstituted concentration is 18 million IU per mL. Undiluted vials should be stored refrigerated at 2–8°C. As the vials contain no preservative, the solutions should be used within 48 hours.

Administration can be given by the subcutaneous or intravenous routes. For administration by the intravenous route, the reconstituted solution should be further diluted into 50 mLs of a 5% dextrose solution. Bacteriostatic water and 0.9% sodium chloride solutions should not be used for reconstitution because of aggregation.

The approved dosing regimen in metastatic renal cell carcinoma is considered high dose therapy. Intravenous infusion of 600,000 International Units (IU) per kg of body weight is given over 15 minutes. This is given every 8 hours for a total of fourteen doses. Following nine days of rest, the schedule is repeated for another fourteen doses, thereby fulfilling one course of a maximum of twenty-eight doses. Two cycles constitute a treatment course. Plastic bags are recommended for infusion, in-line filters are not recommended due to the potential for protein adsorption.

CLINICAL AND PRACTICE ASPECTS OF IL-2

The FDA-approved regimen for aldesleukin administration is a high dose regimen in which there a high likelihood for adverse effects to occur. The capillary leak syndrome often seen with this regimen results due to an increase in capillary permeability. Hypotension and reduced organ perfusion occur in this syndrome, manifested by a variety of clinical signs and toxicities. Dose modification in response to toxicity is accomplished by holding a dose or interrupting a dose. Permanent withdrawal of aldesleukin is required in some instances, such as sustained ventricular tachycardia, renal function impairment requiring dialysis for more than 72 hours, and toxic psychosis lasting more than 48 hours, among others. Because of the potential life threatening toxicities, it has been recommended (USP DI Advisory Panel) that one carefully considers the risk-benefit of aldesleukin therapy using the approved dosing regimen. This regimen causes frequent, often serious, and on occasion fatal toxicity.

Current investigation is examining the use of lower dose regimens of aldesleukin for the treatment of a variety of neoplastic diseases. The relative efficacy of these lower toxicity regimens will need to be carefully examined in comparison to the approved high dose regimen.

One of the unique aspects of treatment of neoplastic diseases with aldesleukin is that significant responses have been seen in some individuals after a single course of therapy. This is in contrast to the traditional antineoplastic agents in which it is typically not until after several courses that a significant response is seen.

Interferons

The name interferon was coined prior to the identification of the actual compounds. The name was given to a substance that interfered with viral replication. There are currently three classes of interferons (IFN): interferon α, interferon β, and interferon γ. Products in all three classes have been approved for use by the FDA, with the most recent being the approval of interferon β-1b for use in patients with relapsing-remitting multiple sclerosis. Recombinant DNA versions of all three interferon classes exist.

Interferon α is the designation given to a group of substances which are of similar molecular weight and function. Interferons are produced by a large number of assorted cells. Leukocytes are the primary source of IFN α, IFN β is primarily produced by fibroblasts, and IFN γ is produced by T lymphocytes. The antiviral actions of IFN are achieved through multiple mechanisms. The release of IFN by virally infected cells can prevent the infection of other cells. Interferon α has been approved for a wide variety of uses including use in patients with genital warts, AIDS related Kaposi's sarcoma, hepatitis B and C, hairy cell leukemia and malignant melanoma. Interferon γ was approved for use in individuals with chronic granulomatous disease, a defect in phagocytic cells. Several interferon products are commercially available (described below).

α Interferon

There are a variety of systemic forms of α interferon commercially available. These can be broken down into recombinant versions of a specific α interferon subtype and purified blends of natural human α interferon. The natural family of human α interferon consists of at least 14 different subtypes. The recombinant cloning of a single α interferon gene allows for the production of one of the specific subtypes. The recombinant commercial versions of the subtypes include interferon α-2a and interferon α-2b. The available purified mixture is interferon α-n3 which is manufactured from pooled units of human leukocytes that have been induced to release interferon by incomplete infection with the avian Sendai virus. Immunoaffinity chromatography with monoclonal antibodies is used to purify the released interferon. Another version of natural α interferons (interferon α-n1, lns) is not commercially available in the US. It is a mixture of natural α interferons, but in different proportions from that in human leukocyte interferon.

The different forms of interferon α are approved for a variety of different uses. The basic use of interferon α is the upregulation of the immune system, whether that be in the stimulation of immunological cells to fight cancer or to fight off viral infections such as hepatitis or genital warts. Accepted indications for the use of interferon α include use in hairy cell leukemia; intralesional treatment of condylomata acuminata (genital warts); active, chronic hepatitis C; AIDS-associated Kaposi's sarcoma; treatment (intravesically) of bladder carcinoma; cervical carcinoma therapy; renal cell carcinoma, chronic myelocytic leukemia; laryngeal papillomatosis; non-Hodgkin's lymphoma; malignant melanoma; multiple myeloma; and mycosis fungoides. The various forms of the interferon α are FDA approved for different indications. It should be noted that while the efficacy of all α interferons for the various indications appears to be similar, there may be differences in the relative efficacy of a specific form for a particular indication. Very few comparative clinical studies exist to provide within-study efficacy data between one form of α interferon and another in a specific indication.

CHEMICAL DESCRIPTION OF α INTERFERON PRODUCTS

Recombinant interferon α-2a (Roferon-A®) is a synthetic version of interferon consisting of a protein chain of 165 amino acids. It is produced by genetically engineered *Escherichia coli*. It is therefore a non-glycosylated protein. The molecule has a lysine group at position 23. The purification process includes affinity chromatography with the use of murine monoclonal antibodies specific for the interferon. The final product contains a single α interferon subtype.

Recombinant interferon α-2b (Intron A®) is a synthetic version of interferon α consisting of 165 amino acids. It is produced by genetically engineered *Escherichia coli*. It is therefore a non-glycosylated protein. It has an arginine group at position 23. The purification of the molecule is done by proprietary methods. The final product contains a single α interferon subtype.

Interferon α-n3 (Alferon-N®) is a highly purified mixture of up to 14 natural human α subtypes. It consists of protein chains of approximately 166 amino acids. Sendai virus is used to infect pooled human white blood cells to produce the different subtypes of interferon α. The manufacturing process includes purification via immunoaffinity chromatography with a murine monoclonal antibody, acidification at a pH of 2 for 5 days at 4 degrees C, and gel filtration chromatography.

Interferon α-n1 (Wellferon®) is not commercially available in the United States. It is a purified blend of natural human α interferons obtained from human lymphoblastoid cells following induction with Sendai virus.

PHARMACOLOGY

α interferons have antiviral, antiproliferative, and immunomodulatory activities. Some of these activities are due to indirect effects. Most of the activities of α interferon are incompletely understood. Alterations in synthesis of RNA, DNA and proteins can be demonstrated after exposure to α interferon. This is believed to be the mechanism of action for the antiproliferative and antiviral activities of the α interferons available.

Since these are proteins, they are, as yet, not delivered by the oral route due to destruction by the gastric acidity. Thus, the route for administration of the α interferons is typically intramuscular, subcutaneous, intralesional, or intravesicular.

Absorption
Absorption from intramuscular and subcutaneous injection sites is typically greater than 80%. Although intralesional injections (genital warts) result in plasma concentrations which are below detectable levels, systemic effects have been reported.

Time to Peak Concentration
Subcutaneous injections, as compared to intramuscular injections, may result in a more delayed time to peak for recombinant interferon α-2a after a single dose. Intramuscular injection peaks in 3.8 hours, while a subcutaneous injection peaks in 7.3 hours. For recombinant interferon α-2b after a single dose, the time to peak for intramuscular or subcutaneous injection ranges from 3 to 12 hours.

Biotransformation
α interferons are totally filtered through the renal glomeruli and undergo degradation during reabsorption in the renal tubules. Elimination occurs as only negligible amounts of unchanged α interferon reappear in the systemic circulation.

Onset of Action
In hepatitis the normalization of serum alanine aminotransferase (ALT) concentrations may occur as early as 2 weeks after the initiation of the interferon treatment.

Time to Peak Effect
The time to peak effect in condylomata acuminata occurs in 1–2 months after the initiation of treatment.

PHARMACEUTICAL CONCERNS OF α INTERFERONS

The strengths and dosages of the available interferon α products are expressed in terms of Units. The Units are determined by a comparison of the antiviral activity of the particular interferon manufactured lot with the activity of the international reference preparation of human leukocyte interferon, which is established by the World Health Organization (WHO).

Packaging and storage. As proteins, the various forms of α interferon should not be frozen. Storage should be between 2 and 8 degrees C. The solutions should not be shaken to prevent foaming and loss of protein.

Interferon alfa-2a injection* (Roferon-A)	Interferon alfa-2a** (Roferon-A)	Interferon alfa-2b** (Intron A)
3 mU/ml (1 mL vials)	18 mU vials (3 mls diluent)	3 mU vials (1 mL diluent)
6 mU/ml (3 mL vials, 18 mU vial)		5 mU vials
10 mU/ml (0.9 mL, for Kaposi's sarcoma)		10 mU vials (1 mL diluent for condylomata acuminata)
36 mU/ml (1 mL vials for Kaposi's sarcoma		25 mU vials (5 mLs diluent for 5 mU/ml)
		50 mU vials (1 mL diluent for Kaposi's sarcoma)
* Liquid for injection ** Prepared for injection by addition of diluent		(mU = million units)

Table 9.2. Recombinant interferon α dosage forms in the U.S.

CLINICAL AND PRACTICE ASPECTS OF α INTERFERONS

The doses for the different indications of the various different α interferon products can vary greatly. For example, the dose for maintenance dosing of interferon α-2a in hairy cell leukemia is 3 million Units three times weekly. This can be compared to dosing in maintenance treatment of AIDS-associated Kaposi's sarcoma in which interferon α-2a is dosed at 36 million Units (1 mL) three times per week.

A selection of different strengths and vial volumes is available for the different recombinant products (see Table 9.2). In order to accurately dose, the higher concentration products should not be used to administer the lower doses. For example, the 36 million Unit per mL concentration of interferon α-2a should not be used for a 3 million Unit dose for a patient with hairy cell leukemia.

The interferon α-n3 product (Alferon N®) is available in the U.S. as a 5 million U/mL vial with a single labeled indication for intralesional dosing in condylomata acuminata. Dosing is performed with a 30 gauge needle at the base of the wart using 250,000 Units two times a week for up to eight weeks.

It should be noted that the different recombinant products are dosed differently within the same disease. For example in AIDS-associated Kaposi's sarcoma, interferon α-2a (Roferon-A®) is recommended to be dosed via the intramuscular or subcutaneous route at 36 million U per day for ten to twelve weeks, or to slowly increase the dose by starting at 3 million U per day on Days 1 to 3, then 9 million U per day on Days 4 to 6, then 18 million U per day on Days 7 to 9, followed by 36 million U per day for the remainder of the ten to twelve week induction period. This slow increase can help with the flu-like syndrome that is most pronounced during the first week of treatment as is gradually reduced as a result of tachyphylaxis. In contrast, for the use of interferon α-2b (Intron A®) in AIDS-associated Kaposi's sarcoma it is recommended to dose on a square meter regimen, at 30 million U per square meter three times a week.

SIDE EFFECTS OF α INTERFERONS

Patients should be informed about some of the side effects of interferon α administration in order to maximize therapy. The flu-like syndrome consists of aching muscles, fevers and chills, headaches, joint pain, back pain, and generalized malaise. This syndrome occurs in a majority of patients within the first week of therapy. Within continued treatment, the patient develops a "tolerance" or tachyphylactic response to the interferon usually within 2 — 4 weeks after the start of therapy. The use of acetaminophen prior to dosing is also recommended, as well as continued dosing to treat subsequent fever and chills. If a patient is told to expect this reaction before the start of therapy it is more likely that the patient will continue dosing after the first week.

Other side or adverse effects from interferon α administration include blurred vision, a change in taste, cold sores, diarrhea, dizziness, dry mouth, loss of appetite, nausea or vomiting, skin rash, and tiredness which can become more prominent with continued dosing and may necessitate a reduction in dosage. It can also be recommended to administer a dose at bedtime to minimize the inconvenience of fatigue. The more common adverse effects which may require medical attention include anemia, cardiotoxicity such as supraventricular arrhythmia, leukopenia and thrombocytopenia. The incidence of peripheral neuropathy, altered thyroid status and hepatotoxicity is less frequent. Partial loss of hair also occurs, with prompt return of hair growth after withdrawal of interferon α dosing.

Patients will at times develop an antibody response to the administered interferons. Sometimes these antibodies can actually inhibit the activity of the interferon (the formation of neutralizing antibodies). If a patient develops neutralizing antibodies to a particular product, one can switch to another product. Cross-reactive antibodies may be produced to the recombinant products; it has been suggested that it is less likely that antibodies will be produced against the various different subtypes found in the pooled interferon α-n3 product. It should also be noted that the interferon subtypes contained with the α-n3 product are glycosylated proteins. The recombinant versions are non-glycosylated proteins, having been produced by *E. coli*. It is theoretically possible that the recombinant versions are more immunogenic because they lack the sugars bound to the protein. The immune system could produce neutralizing antibodies to sites on the recombinant proteins which were once covered by carbohydrates on the natural interferon.

A consensus type-one interferon has also been developed. This is a synthetic, non-naturally occurring interferon designed through the use of genetic engineering. Consensus interferon is an investigational agent for the treatment of hepatitis C.

β Interferon

Interferon β has been shown to possess both antiviral and immunoregulatory effects. By binding to specific cellular receptors, interferon β exerts its activity. The activities of β interferon are species specific, thus much of what is known about the effects of human β interferon come from in vitro studies using human cell lines.

Recombinant interferon β has shown activity in relapsing-remitting multiple sclerosis. While recombinant interferon β-1b (Betaseron®) was first to market, recombinant β-1a (Avonex®) has been recently approved (see below). The exact mechanism of this activity is unknown, however, it is presumed to be due to immunomodulatory activity. In a randomized, double-blind, placebo-controlled study recombinant interferon β-1b (Betaseron®) was shown to have significant effects on exacerbation rates. There was a 31% reduction in the annual exacerbation rate in patients receiving Betaseron® as compared to placebo at the 2-year analysis. In the third year of analysis alone the difference between treatment groups was 28%, with a p value of 0.065, poten-

tially due to a lower number of patients. Antibody formation to Betaseron® was demonstrated; 45% of patients were found to have serum neutralizing activity at one point or more of the time points tested. The relationship between clinical efficacy of the drug and formation of antibody formation are not known.

CHEMICAL DESCRIPTION OF β INTERFERON PRODUCT

Interferon β-1b is a purified, lyophilized, sterile protein commercially available as Betaseron®. Interferon β-1b is produced by genetically engineered *Escherichia coli*. The native gene was obtained from human fibroblasts and was altered in a way that substitutes serine for the cysteine residue found at position 17. Interferon β-1b consists of a protein with a molecular weight of 18,500 daltons, and is non-glycosylated.

PHARMACOLOGY OF β INTERFERON

Interferon β-1b is indicated for use in ambulatory patients with relapsing-remitting multiple sclerosis to reduce the frequency of clinical exacerbations. Relapsing-remitting multiple sclerosis is characterized by recurrent attacks of neurologic dysfunction followed by complete or incomplete recovery. Betaseron® has not been evaluated in chronic progressive multiple sclerosis.

PHARMACEUTICAL CONCERNS OF β INTERFERON

Each vial of Betaseron® contains 0.3 mg (9.6 million IU) of interferon β-1b. The specific activity of the interferon is approximately 32 million IU per mg interferon β-1b. It should be noted that a different analytical standard was used prior to 1993. This assigned a value of 54 million IU per 0.3 mg of interferon β-1b. This should be remembered when reviewing articles and research dated prior to 1993 and comparing them to current dosing regimens.

Reconstitution of lyophilized product in vials is accomplished by adding 1.2 mLs of the supplied diluent (0.54% sodium chloride solution). Vials should not be shaken. After reconstitution, vials contain 0.25 mg (8 million IU) per mL of solution. Administration is given by the subcutaneous route using a syringe with a 27 gauge needle. Vials are for single use only. Reconstituted product should be used within 3 hours.

CLINICAL AND PRACTICE ASPECTS OF β INTERFERON

The recommended dose of Betaseron® is 0.25 mg (8 million IU) injected subcutaneously every other day in patients with relapsing-remitting MS. At this dose, many of the patients will experience the flu-like symptoms seen with other interferons such as the α interferons. The median time to the first occurrence of flu-like symptoms was 3 days, although the median duration per patient was 10.4 days per year. Injection site reactions were common (85%) in patients receiving Betaseron®, including inflammation, pain, hypersensitivity, necrosis and non-specific reactions. The median time to the first occurrence of an injection site reaction was 7 days; patients with injection site reactions reported these events 183.7 days per year.

Laboratory tests to follow in these patients include hemoglobin, complete white blood cell count with differential, platelet counts, and blood chemistries with liver function tests. In the clinical trial, patients were monitored every 3 months. Mental status should also be observed as changes in mental status including confusion, depression, anxiety and depersonalization were observed in the study. One suicide and four attempted suicides were reported. Whether these mental status changes were induced by Betaseron® or by the underlying neurological disease is unclear.

At this point, long term efficacy of Betaseron® beyond 2 years is unknown. More information needs to be gathered as patients continue on long-term therapy.

In May of 1996, the FDA approved the use of Avonex, a recombinant human interferon β-1a product. It was approved for use in treating relapsing forms of multiple sclerosis. The approval was based upon the results obtained from a multi-center, placebo-controlled, double-blinded clinical trial. The study demonstrated that over two years the risk of significant progression of physical disability was reduced by 37% in people taking Avonex compared to those on placebo.

Recombinant interferon β-1a (Avonex®) is administered by intramuscular injection once weekly (30 mcg), in comparison to recombinant interferon β-1b (Betaseron®) which is administered subcutaneously every other day. Recombinant interferon β-1a (Avonex®) is provided as lyophilized powder, containing 33 mcg (6.6 million International Units) in a vial to be reconstituted with 1.1 mL of diluent. The solution should be held at 2–8°C, and should not be frozen.

γ Interferon

γ interferon has antiviral, antiproliferative and immunomodulatory activities. The antiviral properties of γ interferon are probably less than that exerted by α interferon. γ interferon has a much more potent effect on phagocytic cells than α or β interferon. γ interferon is naturally produced by T cells which have been stimulated by antigen. It is usually released from T cells in conjunction with the release of IL-2. Natural killer (NK) cells can also secrete γ interferon.

By binding to cell surface receptors, γ interferon induces the activation of resting macrophages and monocytes. The stimulation increases the phagocytic activity of these cells, which is important in fighting off pathogens. One of the methods of killing engulfed pathogens by these cells is the intracellular production of toxic oxygen metabolites. γ interferon enhances the production of these toxic oxygen metabolites.

Antibody dependent cellular cytotoxicity (ADCC) and NK cell activity is increased by γ interferon. Increased expression of major histocompatibility (MHC) antigens is induced by γ interferon. Monocytes increase cell surface expression of immunoglobulin Fc receptors after exposure to γ interferon. The efficiency of macrophage-mediated killing of intracellular parasites is also increased upon exposure to γ interferon. Thus, an overall immunostimulation of phagocytic cells occurs with the release of γ interferon.

Natural γ interferon is a 143 amino acid protein that demonstrates little sequence homology to either the α or β interferons. Two different molecular weight forms of γ interferon have been described (20 kD and 25 kD) which vary in molecular weight due to differences in glycosylation.

γ interferon has shown efficacy in the treatment of chronic granulomatous disease (CGD). CGD is an inherited disorder which is characterized by a deficiency in phagocytic oxidative metabolism. γ interferon increases the phagocytic function of granulocytes, such as neutrophils, and monocytes. After exposure to γ interferon these cells have an increased ability to produce superoxide anion, which helps to eliminate phagocytosed pathogens. Early clinical trials in patients with CGD demonstrated the enhancement by γ interferon of phagocytic cell function, including the elevation of superoxide levels and improved killing of *Staphylococcus Aureus*.

In a randomized placebo controlled trial in patients with CGD a recombinant version of γ interferon (Actimmune®) significantly decreased the incidence of serious infection (p = 0.0036). CGD patients receiving placebo had a significantly higher number of serious infections and longer length of hospitalizations. Placebo patients required three times as many inpatient hospitalization days as compared to those receiving Actimmune®.

CHEMICAL DESCRIPTION OF γ INTERFERON PRODUCT

One recombinant version of γ interferon (interferon γ-1b) is currently available. Actimmune® is a single-chain polypeptide that contains 140 amino acids. Interferon γ-1b is produced by genetically engineered Escherichia coli. Purification of the product is performed by column chromatography.

PHARMACOLOGY OF γ INTERFERON

The accepted indication for interferon γ-1b is for reducing the frequency and severity of serious infections associated with chronic granulomatous disease. It appears that this product is effective in all genetic types of CGD. In patients with CGD, γ interferon-1b is believed to increase the activities of phagocytic cells.

Absorption
The fraction of the dose absorbed is more than 89%. Absorption is slow.

Time to Peak Plasma Concentration
Time to peak for an intramuscular injection is 4 hours, while time to peak for a subcutaneous injection is 7 hours.

Peak Plasma Concentration
Via the subcutaneous route, the peak plasma concentration from a 100 mcg per m² of body surface dose is 0.6 nanograms per mL.

PHARMACEUTICAL CONCERNS OF γ INTERFERON

The drug is available as a sterile clear solution containing 100 mcg (3 million U) of interferon γ-1b in 0.5 mLs. The vials are single use vials. The vials should not be shaken or frozen. They should be stored in a refrigerator at 2–8°C.

Prior to use, the unentered vials should not be left at room temperature for longer than 12 total hours.

Administration of the drug is by the subcutaneous route. The recommended dosage of interferon γ-1b for the treatment of patients with CGD is 50 mcg/m² (1.5 mU/m²) in those whose body surface area is greater than 0.5 m². For those patients equal to or less than 0.5 m², the recommended dose is 1.5 mcg/kg/dose. Injections are given three times weekly, typically on Monday, Wednesday and Friday. Because the vials do not contain a preservative they should be used for single use only.

CLINICAL AND PRACTICE ASPECTS OF γ INTERFERON

As with the α interferons, the flu-like syndrome occurs in most patients receiving γ interferon-1b. Severity of the syndrome is dose related, while a decrease in the symptoms may occur with continued treatment. Acetaminophen can be given prior to dosing to reduce the fever, headaches and flu-like symptoms. Medical attention should be sought in patients developing leukopenia and less frequently, in those patients developing hypotension, neurotoxicity, and thrombocytopenia.

The optimum sites for subcutaneous injection have been described as the right and left deltoids and the anterior portion of the thighs. No development of neutralizing antibodies has been reported in patients receiving γ interferon-1b. ∎

References

- **Alderson MR, Tough Tw, Zieger SF, Grabstein KH.** (1991). Interleukin-7 induces cytokine secretion and tumoricidal activity by human peripheral blood monocytes. *J Exp Med*, 173, 923–30
- **Aldesleukin.** Systemic. USP DI. (1995).
- **Anonymous.** (1993). Interferon β-1b is effective in relapsing-remitting multiple sclerosis. I. Clinical results of a multicenter, randomized, double-blind, placebo-controlled trial. The IFNB Multiple Sclerosis Study Group. *Neurology*, 43, 655–61
- **Anonymous.** (1995). Interferon β-1b in the treatment of multiple sclerosis: final outcome of the randomized controlled trial. The IFNB Multiple Sclerosis Study Group and The University of British Columbia MS/MRI Analysis Group. *Neurology*, 45, 1277–85
- **Bazan JF, Schall TJ.** (1996). Interleukin-16 or not? Letter. *Nature*, 381, 29–30
- **Bolinger AM, Taeubel MA.** (1992). Recombinant interferon γ for treatment of chronic granulomatous disease and other disorders. *Clin Pharm*, 11, 834–50
- **Cetus, Inc,** Proleukin package insert. Emeryville, CA: April 1992
- **Dinarello CA, Mier JW.** (1986). Interleukins. *Ann Rev Med*, 37, 173–78
- **Dinarello CA.** (1985). An update on human interleukin-1: from molecular biology to clinical relevance. *J Clin Immunol*, 5, 287–297
- **Genentech, Inc,** Actimmune package insert. San Franciso, CA: 1990 December
- **Gordon MS, McCaskill-Stevens WJ, Battiato LA,** *et al.* (1996). A phase I trial of recombinant human interleukin-11 (neumega rhIL-11 growth factor) in women with breast cancer receiving chemotherapy. *Blood*, 87, 3615–24
- **Interferons, α.** Systemic. USP DI. (1995). Drug information for the health care professional
- **Interferon, β, Recombinant, Human.** USP DI. (1995) Drug information for the health care professional
- **Interferon, γ-1b, Recombinant.** Systemic. USP DI. (1995). Drug information for the health care professional

- **Interleukin-2,** Recombinant, Human. Systemic. USP DI. (1995). Drug information for the health care professional
- **Jacobs LD,** et al. (1996). Intramuscular interferon β-1a for disease progression in relapsing multiple sclerosis. The Multiple Sclerosis Collaborative Research Group (MSCRG). *Ann Neurol*, 39, 285–94
- **Jaffe HS, Sherwin SA.** (1991). Immunomodulators. In *Basic and clinical immunology*, edited by DP Stites, AI Terr. East Norwalk, Conn: Appleton and Lange
- **Kintzel PE, Calis KA.** (1991). Recombinant interleukin-2: a biological response modifier. *Clin Pharm*, 10: 110–28
- **Koeller J, Tami JA.** (1992). *Concepts in immunology and immunotherapeutics.* 2nd edition. Bethesda: ASHP
- **Leutwyler K.** (1995). An inside job. IL-12 attacks tumors on two fronts, but can it win the battle? *Sci Am*, 273, 24
- **Lublin FD, Whitaker JN, Eidelman BH, Miller AE, Arnason BG, Burks JS.** (1996). Management of patients receiving interferon β-1b for multiple sclerosis: a consensus conference. *Neurology*, 46, 12–8
- **Maciaszek JW, Parada NA, Cruikshank WW, Center DM, Kornfeld H, Viglianti GA.** (1997). IL-16 represses HIV-1 promoter activity. *J. Immunol*, 158: 5–8
- **Male D, Champion B, Cooke A, Owen M.** (1991). *Advanced immunology.* Philadelphia: JB Lippincott Co
- **McKenzie AN, Culpepper JA, de Waal Malefyt R,** et al. (1993). Interleukin 13, a T-cell-derived cytokine that regulates human monocyte and B-cell function. *Proc Natl Acad Sci USA*, 90, 3735–9
- **Minty A, Chalon P, Derocq JM,** et al. (1993). Interleukin-13 is a new human lymphokine regulating inflammatory and immune responses. *Nature*, 362, 248–50
- **Neilly LK, Goodin DS, Goodkin DE, Hauser SL.** (1996). Side effect profile of interferon β-1b in MS: results of an open label trial. *Neurology*, 46, 552–4
- **Patchen ML MacVitte TJ, Williams JL, Schwartz GN, Souza LM.** (1991). Administration of interleukin-6 stimulates multilineage hematopoiesis and accelerates recovery from radiation induced hematopoietic depression. *Blood*, 77, 472–80
- **Paty DW, Li DK.** Interferon β-1b is effective in relapsing-remitting multiple sclerosis. II. MRI analysis results of a multicenter, randomized, double-blind, placebo-controlled trial. UBC MS/MRI Study Group and the IFNB Multiple Sclerosis Study Group. *Neurology*, 43, 662–7
- **Platanias LC, Vogelzang NJ.** (1990). Interleukin-1: biology, pathophysiology, and clinical prospects. *Am J Med*, 89, 621–629
- **Roche Labs,** Roferon-A package insert. Nutley, NJ: 1990 November
- **Roitt IM, Brostoff J, Male DK.** (1989). *Immunology.* 2nd ed. St. Louis, Gower Medical Publishing
- **Rosenberg SA, Lotze MT, Muul LM, Chang AE,** et al. (1987). A progress report on the treatment of 157 patients with advanced cancer using lymphokine-activated killer cells and interleukin-2 or high-dose interleukin-2 alone. *N Eng J Med*, 316, 889–97
- **Rosenberg SA, Packard BS, Aebersold PM, Solomon D,** et al. (1989). Use of tumor-infiltrating lymphocytes and interleukin-2 in the immunotherapy of patients with metastatic melanoma. *N Eng J Med, 319,* 1676–1680
- **Sechler JM, Malech HL, White CJ, Gallin JI.** (1988). Recombinant human interferon-γ reconstitutes defective phagocyte function in patients with chronic granulomatous disease of childhood. *Proc Natl Acad Sci USA*, 85, 4874–8
- **Sher A, Fiorentino D, Caspar P, Pearce E, Mosmann T.** (1991). Production of IL-10 by CD4+ T lymphocytes correlates with down regulation of TH1 cytokine synthesis in helminth infection. *J Immunol*, 147, 2713–16
- **Sideras P, Noma T, Honjo T.** (1988). Structure and function of interleukin 4 and 5. *Immunol Rev*, 102, 198–212
- **Stern AS, Magram J, Presky DH.** (1996). Interleukin-12 an integral cytokine in the immune response. *Life Sci*, 58, 639–54
- **Stites DP, Terr AI.** (1991). *Basic and clinical immunology.* 7th ed. Norwalk, Connecticut: Appleton and Lange
- **Tami JA, Parr MD, Thompson JS.** (1986). The immune system. *Am J Hosp Pharm*, 43, 2483–93
- **Tepler I, Elias L, Smith JW 2nd,** et al. (1996). A randomized placebo-controlled trial of recombinant human interleukin-11 in cancer patients with severe thrombocytopenia due to chemotherapy. *Blood*, 87, 3607–14
- **Weber JS.** (1995) Clinical trials with IL-6. *Ann NY Acad Sci*, 762, 357–8
- **Weening RS, Leitz GJ, Seger RA.** (1995) Recombinant human interferon-γ in patients with chronic granulomatous disease — European follow up study. *Eur J Pediatr*, 154, 295–8
- **WHO-ISUI Nomenclature Subcommittee on Interleukin Designation.** (1992). Nomenclature for secreted regulatory proteins of the immune system (interleukins). *Blood*, 79, 1645–1646
- **Wong GC, Clark SC.** (1991). Multiple actions of IL-6 within a cytokine network. *Immunol Today*, 9, 137–143
- **Yao Z, Painter SL, Fanskow WC, Ulrich D, Macduff BM, Spriggs MK, Armitage RJ.** (1995). Human IL-17: A novel cytokine derived from T cells. *J Immunol*, 155, 5483–5486

Self-Assessment Questions

Question 1: *What are cytokines?*

Question 2: *How do cytokines differ from hormones?*

Question 3: *What is a lymphokine?*

Question 4: *How many interleukins are approved for therapy in the U.S.?*

Question 5: *What is the physiological role of IL-1?*

Question 6: *What is IL-2R?*

Question 7: *How is IL-10 unique from the other ILs?*

Question 8: *How should undiluted vials of aldesleukin be stored?*

Question 9: *Where are interferons produced?*

Question 10: *What are the accepted indications for interferon α?*

Question 11: *What are the available forms of interferon α?*

Question 12: *What is the approved indication(s) of interferon β?*

Answers

Answer 1: Cytokines can generally be defined as soluble mediators or glycoproteins that aid in the communication between cells, primarily cells of the immunological, hematological, and neurological systems.

Answer 2: Cytokines can be distinguished from hormones by various criteria. An individual cytokine can be secreted by a number of different types of cells, while hormones are typically produced by just one or two very specialized cell types. Cytokines also can act on a variety of cell types. While cytokines are usually targeted to produce a local effect, hormones are targeted to affect cells at distant sites.

Answer 3: Lymphokines are cytokines produced by lymphocytes, primarily from T cells but also from B cells.

Answer 4: Only one of the interleukins is currently approved by the FDA and commercially available for clinical use in the United States. This product is aldesleukin (IL-2).

Answer 5: IL-1 is an important mediator of the body's response to infection, inflammation, and injury.

Answer 6: IL-2 produces its immunological effects by binding to the cellular IL-2 receptor (IL-2R). There are various affinity forms of the IL-2R. The circulating form of the IL-2R is a truncated version of the α chain, having no cytoplasmic tail. High levels of the circulating IL-2R have been found in patients with a wide variety of disorders including HIV infection, cancer, solid organ transplant rejection, and arthritis. It is believed that the circulating form of the IL-2R binds released IL-2 prior to IL-2 binding to cells in an attempt to prevent overstimulation of the immune system. Several other cytokine and adhesion molecule receptors also have circulating forms. It is believed that this is one manner in which the immunological cascade maintains a checks and balance system.

Answer 7: IL-10 is unique in that it appears to have immunosuppressive type activities.

Answer 8: Stored refrigerated at 2–8°C.

Answer 9: Interferons are produced by a large number of assorted cells. Leukocytes are the primary source of IFN α, IFN β is primarily produced by fibroblasts, and IFN γ is produced by T lymphocytes.

Answer 10: Accepted indications for the use of interferon α include use in hairy cell leukemia; intralesional treatment of condylomata acuminata (genital warts); active, chronic hepatitis C; AIDS-associated Kaposi's sarcoma; treatment (intravesically) of bladder carcinoma; cervical carcinoma therapy; renal cell carcinoma, chronic myelocytic leukemia; laryngeal papillomatosis; non-Hodgkin's lymphoma; malignant melanoma; multiple myeloma; and mycosis fungoides.

Answer 11: Recombinant interferon α-2a (Roferon-A®), recombinant interferon α-2b (Intron A®), interferon α-n3 (Alferon-N®), and interferon α-n1 (Wellferon®).

Answer 12: Recombinant interferon β has shown activity in relapsing-remitting multiple sclerosis.

10 Insulin

by: John M. Beals and Paul M. Kovach

Introduction

Insulin was discovered by Banting and Best in 1921 (Bliss, 1982). Soon afterward, manufacturing processes were developed to extract the insulin from porcine and bovine pancreata. From 1921 to 1980, efforts were directed at increasing the purity of the insulin and providing different formulations for altering time-action for improved glucose control (Brange, 1987a; Brange, 1987b; Galloway, 1988). Purification was improved by optimizing extraction and processing conditions and by implementing chromatographic processes (size exclusion, ion exchange, and reversed phase (Kroeff et al., 1989)) to reduce the levels of both general protein impurities as well as insulin-related proteins such as proinsulin and insulin polymers. Formulation development focused on improving chemical stability by moving from acidic to neutral formulations and by modifying the time-action profile through the uses of various levels of zinc and protamine. The evolution of recombinant DNA technology led to the unlimited availability of human insulin, which has eliminated issues with sourcing constraints while providing the patient with a natural exogenous source of insulin. Combining the improved purification methodologies and recombinant DNA technology, manufacturers of insulin are now able to provide the purest human insulin ever made available, > 98%.

Chemical Description

Insulin, a 51-amino acid protein, is a hormone that is synthesized as a proinsulin precursor in the β-cell of the pancreas and is converted to insulin by enzymatic cleavage. The resulting insulin molecule is composed of two polypeptide chains that are connected by two inter-chain disulfide bonds (Figure 10.1) (Baker et al., 1988). The A-chain is composed of 21 amino acids and the B-chain is composed of 30 amino acids. The inter-chain disulfide linkages occur between A^7–B^7 and A^{20}–B^{19}, respectively. A third intra-chain disulfide bond is located in the A-chain, between residues A^6 and A^{11}.

Bovine and porcine insulin preparations also are commercially available. The amino acid sequence of porcine insulin differs from human insulin at the B^{30} position, where $Thr^{B30}{\rightarrow}Ala^{B30}$ (Figure 10.1). The amino acid sequence of bovine insulin differs from human insulin at three positions, $Thr^{A8}{\rightarrow}Ala^{A8}$, $Ile^{A10}{\rightarrow}Val^{A10}$, and $Thr^{B30}{\rightarrow}Ala^{B30}$.

The net charge on the insulin molecule results from the four glutamic acid residues, four tyrosine residues, two α-carboxyl groups, two α-amino groups, two histidine residues, a lysine, and an arginine residue. Insulin has a isoelectric point (pI) of 5.3 in the denatured state, but because of its ability to associate as non-covalent dimers, insulin can exhibit an apparent pI of 6.4, which is presumed to be due to a masked carboxylate ionization under native conditions (Kaarsholm et al., 1990). Thus, the insulin molecule has a net negative charge at neutral pH. This net negative charge-state of insulin has been used in formulation development, as will be discussed later.

In addition to the net charge on insulin, another important intrinsic property of insulin is its ability to readily associate into dimers and higher-order associated states (Figure 10.2) (Pekar and Frank, 1972). The driving force for dimerization appears to be the formation of favorable hydrophobic interactions at the C-terminus of the B-chain (Ciszak et al., 1995). Insulin can associate into discrete hexameric complexes in the presence of various divalent metal ions (at 0.33 g-atom/monomer) (Goldman et al., 1974). Physiologically, insulin is stored as a zinc-containing hexamer in the β-cells of the pancreas. As will be discussed later, the ability to form discrete hexamers in the presence of zinc has been used to develop therapeutically useful formulations of insulin.

Commercial insulin preparations also contain phenolic excipients (e.g., phenol, m-cresol) as antimicrobial agents. As represented in Figure 10.2, these phenolic species also bind to specific sites on the Zn-insulin hexamers, causing a conformational change that increases the chemical stability of insulin in commercial preparations (Brange et al., 1992a). X-ray crystallographic data have identified the location of six phenolic ligand binding sites on the insulin hexamer and the nature of the conformational change that the binding of these ligands induces (Derewenda et al., 1989). The phenolic ligands are stabilized in a binding pocket between monomers of adjacent dimers by hydrogen bonds with the carbonyl oxygen of Cys^{A6} and the amide

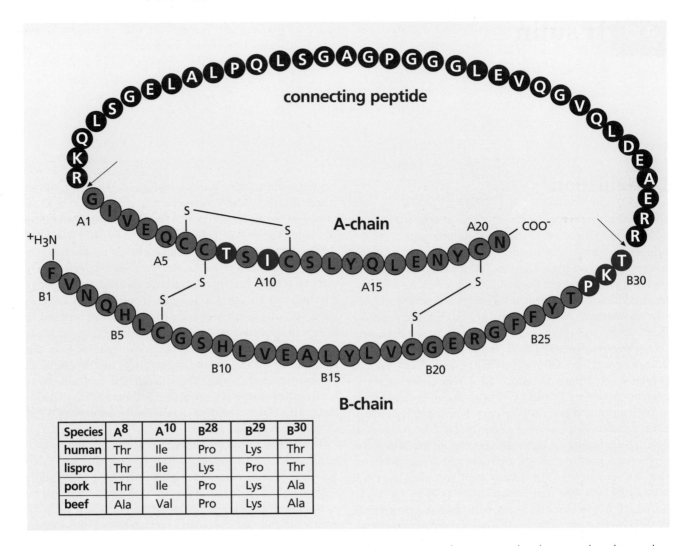

Species	A^8	A^{10}	B^{28}	B^{29}	B^{30}
human	Thr	Ile	Pro	Lys	Thr
lispro	Thr	Ile	Lys	Pro	Thr
pork	Thr	Ile	Pro	Lys	Ala
beef	Ala	Val	Pro	Lys	Ala

Figure 10.1. The primary structure of human proinsulin. The single-letter amino acid convention has been used to denote the amino acids (cf. Chapter 2). Insulin is represented by the brown/blue spheres. The connecting peptide that is excised by endopeptidase activity is represented by purple spheres. The blue spheres identify amino acids that are not conserved in other commercially available insulins. Note: sequence differences between species in the connecting peptide are not listed here.

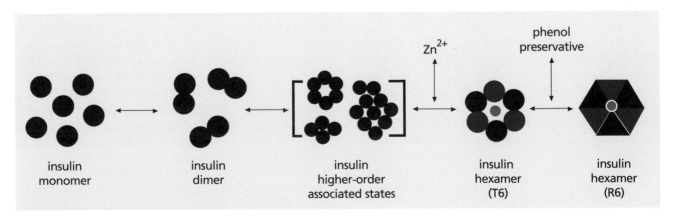

Figure 10.2. A schematic of the self-association of insulin. The hexamers are illustrated as a dimer of trimers. The monomers composing each trimer have been designated with either a blue or purple pattern. The small brown spheres represent zinc.

proton of Cys[AII] as well as numerous van der Waals contacts. The binding of these ligands stabilizes a conformational change that occurs at the N-terminus of the B-chain in each insulin monomer, shifting the conformational equilibrium of residues B1–B8 from an extended structure (T-state) to an α-helical structure (R-state), referred to as a T↔R transition (Brader et al., 1991).

In addition to the presence of zinc and phenolic preservatives, modern insulin formulations may contain an isotonicity agent (glycerol or NaCl) and/or a physiologic buffer (sodium phosphate). The former is used to minimize tissue damage and pain on injection. The latter is present to minimize pH drift in some pH-sensitive formulations.

Type [b]	Description	Appearance	Components	Action (hours) [a]		
				Onset	Peak	Duration
R [c]	Regular Soluble Insulin Injection	clear solution	metal: zinc (0.01-0.04 mg/100Units) buffer: none preservative: m-cresol isotonicity agent: glycerol	0.5	2-3	6-8
N	NPH Insulin Isophane Suspension	turbid or cloudy suspension	metal: zinc (0.01-0.04 mg/100Units) buffer: phosphate preservative: m-cresol and phenol isotonicity agent: glycerol modifying protein: protamine (0.32-0.44 mg/100Units)	1-2	6-12	18-24
L	Lente Insulin Zinc Suspension	turbid or cloudy suspension	metal: zinc (0.12-0.25 mg/100Units) buffer: acetate preservative: methylparaben isotonicity agent: glycerol modifying protein: none	1-3	6-12	18-24
U	Ultralente Extended Insulin Zinc Suspension	turbid or cloudy suspension	metal: zinc (0.12-0.25 mg/100Units) buffer: acetate preservative: methylparaben isotonicity agent: glycerol modifying protein: none	4-6	8-20	24-28
70/30 [d]	70% Insulin Isophane Suspension, 30% Regular Insulin Injection	turbid or cloudy suspension	metal: zinc (0.01-0.04 mg/100Units) buffer: phosphate preservative: m-cresol and phenol isotonicity agent: glycerol modifying protein: protamine (0.32-0.44 mg/100Units in NPH section)	0.5	2-12	14-24
50/50	50% Insulin Isophane Suspension, 50% Regular Insulin Injection	turbid or cloudy suspension	metal: zinc (0.01-0.04 mg/100Units) buffer: phosphate preservative: m-cresol and phenol isotonicity agent: glycerol modifying protein: protamine (0.32-0.44 mg/100Units in NPH section)	0.5	2-10	14-24

Table 10.1. A list of neutral human U100 insulin formulations. [a]The onset, peak and duration of insulin action depends on numerous factors, such as dose, injection site, presence of insulin antibodies, and physical activity. The action times listed below represent the generally accepted values in the medical community. [b]U.S. designation. [c]Another designation is S for soluble (Britain). Other soluble formulations have been designed for pump use and include Velosulin® and H-tronin®. [d]In Europe the ratio designation is inverted on the label, e.g., 30/70. In addition, other ratios are available in Europe and include 10/90, 20/80, and 40/60 (see text, "Clinical and Practice Aspects").

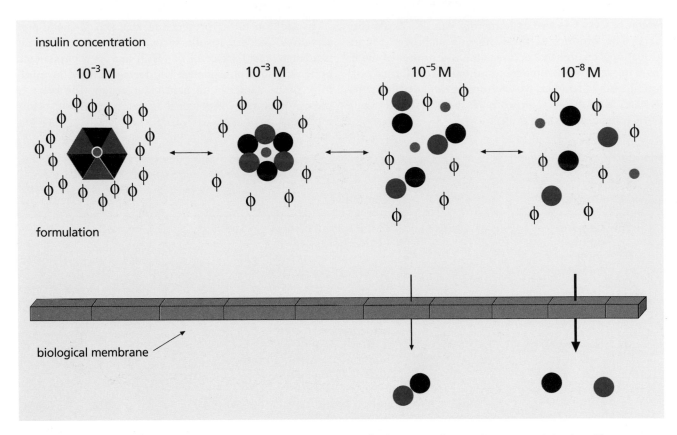

Figure 10.3. A schematic of the dissociation of a soluble human insulin hexamer after a subcutaneous injection. The hexamers are illustrated as a dimer of trimers. The monomers composing each trimer have been designated with either a blue or purple pattern. The small brown spheres represent zinc. Typically, soluble insulin has an onset time of 0.5 hour and peak action between 2–3 hours.

Pharmacology and Formulations

Regular and Rapid-acting Soluble Preparations

Initial soluble insulin formulations were formulated under acidic conditions and were chemically unstable. In these early formulations, considerable deamidation was identified at Asn[A21] and potency loss was observed during prolonged storage under acidic conditions. Efforts to improve the chemical stability of these soluble formulations led to the development of neutral, zinc-stabilized solutions.

The insulin in neutral, regular formulations is chemically stabilized by the addition of zinc (~0.4%) and phenolic preservatives. The zinc leads to the formation of discrete hexameric structures (containing 2 Zn atoms/hexamer) that can bind six molecules of phenolic preservatives, e.g., m-cresol (Figure 10.2). The binding of these excipients increases the stability of insulin by inducing the formation of a specific hexameric form (R_6), in which the B1 to B8 region of each monomer is in an α-helical conformation. This in turn decreases the availability of residues involved in deamidation and high molecular weight polymer formation (Brange et al., 1992a).

The pharmacodynamics of this soluble formulation is listed in Table 10.1. The neutral, regular formulations show peak insulin activity between 2 and 3 hours with a maximum duration of 6 to 8 hours. As with other formulations, the variations in time-action can be attributed to factors such as dose, site of injection, temperature, and patient's physical activity. Despite the soluble state of insulin in these formulations, a delay in action is still observed. This delay has been attributed to the time required for the hexamer to dissociate into the dimeric and/or monomeric substituents prior to adsorption through the biological membrane (Figure 10.3). This dissociation requires the diffusion of the preservative and insulin from the site of injection, effectively diluting the protein and shifting the equilibrium from hexamers to dimers and monomers (Brange et al., 1990).

Monomeric insulin analogs were designed to achieve a more natural response to post-prandial (after meal) glucose-level increases while providing convenience to the patient. The development of monomeric analogs of insulin

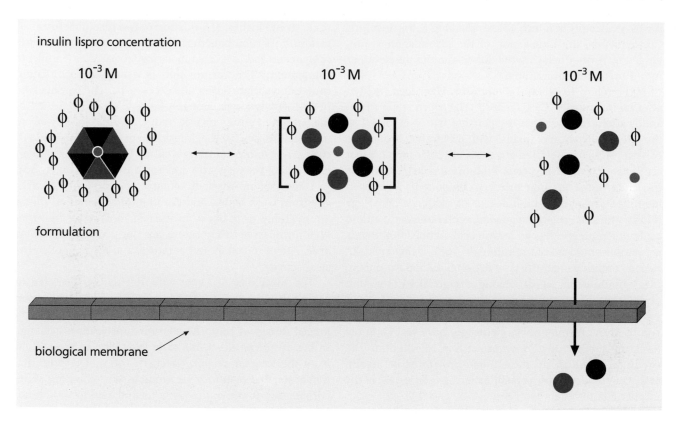

insulin lispro concentration

Figure 10.4. A hypothetical schematic of the dissociation of soluble insulin lispro hexamer after a subcutaneous injection. The hexamers are illustrated as a dimer of trimers. The monomers composing each trimer have been filled with blue or purple. The small brown spheres represent zinc. Insulin lispro typically has a 15 minute onset time and peak action by 1 hour.

for the treatment of insulin-dependent diabetes mellitus has focused on shifting the self-association properties of insulin to favor the monomeric species and consequently minimizing the delay in time-action (Brems *et al.*, 1992). One such monomeric analog, $Lys^{B28}Pro^{B29}$-human insulin (insulin lispro) has been developed and does have a more rapid time-action profile, with a peak activity of approximately 1 hour (Howey *et al.*, 1994). The sequence inversion at positions B28 and B29 yields an analog with reduced self-association behavior compared to human insulin. However, unlike some monomeric analogs, insulin lispro can be stabilized in a preservative-dependent hexameric complex that provides the necessary chemical and physical stability required by all insulin preparations. Despite the hexameric complexation of this analog, insulin lispro retains its rapid time-action. Based on the crystal structure of the insulin lispro hexameric complex, Frank and coworkers (Ciszak *et al.*, 1995) have hypothesized that the reduced dimerization properties of the analog coupled with the preservative dependence yield a hexameric complex that readily dissociates into monomers after rapid diffusion of the phenolic preservative into the subcutaneous tissue at the site of injection (Figure 10.4). Consequently, the substantial (10^5) dilution of the zinc insulin hexamers is not

necessary for the analog to dissociate from hexamers to monomers, which is required for adsorption.

In addition to the aforementioned rapid formulations, manufacturers have designed soluble formulations for use in external or implanted pumps. In most respects, these formulations are very similar to Regular insulin (i.e., hexameric association state, preservative, and zinc); however, buffer and/or surfactants may be included in these formulations to minimize the physical aggregation of insulin that can lead to clogging of the pump tubing. In early pump systems, gas-permeable tubing was used with the external pumps. Consequently, a buffer was added to the formulation in order to minimize pH changes due to dissolved carbon dioxide, that could lead to insulin precipitation. In addition, material advances have helped to minimize this problem.

Intermediate-acting Insulin Preparations

There are two widely used types of intermediate-acting insulin preparations: NPH and Lente: Both formulations achieve extended time-action by necessitating the dissolution of a precipitated and/or crystalline form of insulin. This dissolution is presumed to be the rate-limiting step in the bioavailability of intermediate- and long-acting insulins. Consequently, the time-action of the formulation is prolonged by further delaying the dissociation of the hexamer into dimers and monomers.

NPH refers to Neutral Protamine Hagedorn, named after its inventor H. C. Hagedorn (Hagedorn *et al.*, 1936), and is a neutral crystalline suspension that is prepared by the co-crystallization of insulin with protamine. Protamine consists of a closely related group of very basic proteins that are isolated from fish sperm. Protamine is heterogeneous in nature; however, four primary components have been identified and show a high degree of sequence homology (Hoffmann *et al.*, 1990). In general, protamine is ~30 amino acids in length and has an amino acid composition that is primarily composed of arginine, 65–70%. Using crystallization conditions identified by Krayenbühl and Rosenberg (Krayenbühl *et al.*, 1946), oblong tetragonal NPH insulin crystals with volumes between 1 and 20 μm^3 can be consistently prepared from protamine and insulin (Deckert, 1980). These formulations, by design, have very minimal levels of soluble insulin or protamine in solution. The condition at which no measurable protamine or insulin exists in solution after crystallization is referred to as the isophane point.

NPH has an onset of action from 1–2 hours, peak activity from 6–12 hours, and duration of activity from 18–24 hours (Table 10.1). As with other formulations, the variations in time-action are due to factors such as dose, site of injection, temperature, and patient's physical activity.

NPH can be readily mixed with Regular insulin either extemporaneously by the patient or as obtained from the manufacturer in a premixed formulation. Premixed insulin, e.g., 70/30 or 50/50 NPH/Regular, has been shown to provide the patient with improved dose accuracy and consequently improved glycemic control (Bell *et al.*, 1991). In these preparations, a portion of the soluble Regular insulin will reversibly adsorb to the surface of the NPH crystals through an electrostatically-mediated interaction under formulation conditions (Dodd *et al.*, 1995); however, this adsorption is reversible under physiological conditions and consequently has no clinical significance (Galloway *et al.*, 1982; Hamaguchi *et al.*, 1990; Davis *et al.*, 1991). Due in part to the reversibility of the adsorption process, NPH/Regular mixtures are uniquely stable and have a two-year shelf life.

Immunogenicity issues with protamine have been documented in a small percentage of diabetic patients (Kurtz *et al.*, 1983; Nell *et al.*, 1988). Individuals who show sensitivity to the protamine in NPH formulations are often switched to Lente or Ultralente preparations to control their basal glucose levels.

Lente insulin is a zinc insulin suspension that was designed for single daily injection (Hallas-Møller *et al.*, 1952). Lente insulin is a mixture of two insoluble forms of insulin, 70% rhombohedral zinc insulin crystals (Ultralente component) and 30% amorphous insulin particles (Semilente component). The formulation is a neutral formulation containing acetate buffer and excess zinc. The surplus zinc in the formulation presumably binds to weak metal sites on the insulin hexamer surface, reducing the solubility of the insulin, thus slowing the time-action of the insulin (Deckert, 1980). The volume of the crystalline Ultralente component is routinely between 200 and 1000 μm^3 (Deckert, 1980).

Lente has an onset of action of 1–3 hours, peak activity from 6–12 hours, and duration of action from 18–24 hours (Table 10.1). As with other formulations, the variations in observed time-action are due to factors such as dose, site of injection, temperature, and the patient's physical activity.

The mixability of Lente with Regular is restricted to extemporaneous mixtures that are used immediately upon preparation (Deckert, 1980; Galloway *et al.*, 1982). Prolonged storage of Lente/Regular mixtures leads to a change in the course of effect due to precipitation of the insulin from the Regular section (Deckert, 1980). The precipitation of Regular insulin is presumably due to binding of the surplus zinc found in the Lente formulation to weak binding sites on the soluble insulin hexamer.

Long-acting Insulin Formulations

Currently, the only long-acting insulin available is Ultralente. Ultralente is a crystalline insulin suspension. The crystals are identified as rhombohedral with a volume between 200 and 1000 μm^3 (Deckert, 1980). The formulation contains acetate buffer at neutral pH and a surplus of zinc.

Ultralente has an onset of action of 4–6 hours, peak activity between 8–20 hours, and duration of action from 24–28 hours (Table 10.1). As with other formulations, the variations in time-action are due to factors such as dose, site of injection, temperature, and the patient's physical activity. The mixability of Ultralente with Regular insulin is constrained to extemporaneous mixing with immediate use for the reasons described above for Lente.

Pharmaceutical Concerns

Chemical Stability of Insulin Formulations

Insulin has two primary routes of chemical degradation upon storage and use: hydrolytic transformation of amide to acid groups and formation of covalent dimers and higher order polymers. The rate of formation of these degradation products is influenced primarily by the pH, the storage temperature, and the components of the specific formulation. The purity of insulin formulations is typically assessed by high performance liquid chromatography using reversed-phase and size exclusion separation modes (USPC, 1995). In acidic solution, the main reaction is the transformation of asparagine (Asn) at the terminal 21 position of the A-chain to aspartic acid. This reaction is a relatively facile at low pH but is extremely slow at neutral pH (Brange et al., 1992b). This was the primary degradation route in early soluble (acidic) insulin formulations; however, the development of neutral solutions and suspensions has diminished the importance of this degradation route. Stability studies of neutral solutions indicate that the amount of A^{21} desamido insulin does not change upon storage. Thus the relatively small amounts of this bioactive material present in the formulation arise either from the source insulin or from pharmaceutical processing operations.

The deamidation of the Asn^3 of the B-chain is the primary degradation mechanism at neutral pH. The reaction proceeds through the formation of a cyclic imide that results in two products, aspartic acid (Asp) and iso-aspartic acid (iso-Asp) (Brennan et al., 1994). This reaction occurs relatively slowly in neutral solution (approximately 1/10 the rate of A^{21} desamido formation in acid solution) (Brange et al., 1992b). The relative amounts of these products are influenced by the flexibility of the B-chain, with approximate ratios of Asp:iso-Asp of 1:2 and 2:1 for solution and crystalline formulations, respectively. As noted earlier, the use of phenolic preservatives provides a stabilizing effect on the insulin hexamer that reduces the formation of the cyclic imide, as evidenced by reduced deamidation. The rate of formation also depends on temperature; typical rates of formation are approximately 2% per year at 5°C. Studies have shown these B^3 deamidated insulins to be essentially fully biopotent (Chance, 1995).

High molecular weight protein (HMWP) products form at both storage and room temperatures. Covalent dimers found between two insulin molecules are the primary condensation products in formulations. There is evidence that insulin-protamine heterodimers also form in NPH suspensions (Brange et al., 1992c). At higher temperatures, the probability of forming higher order insulin oligomers increases. The rate of formation of HMWP is less than that of hydrolytic reactions; typical rates are less than 0.5% per year for soluble neutral Regular insulin formulations. The rate of formation can be affected by the strength of the insulin formulation or by the addition of glycerol as an isotonicity agent. The latter increases the rate of HMWP formation presumably by introducing impurities such as glyceraldehyde. HMWP formation is believed to initiate in the stable hexamer form by N-terminal amino group reacting with the terminal A^{21} asparagine of a second insulin molecule.

Disulfide exchange leading to polymer formation is also possible at basic pH; however, the rate for these reactions is very slow under neutral pH formulation conditions. The quality of excipients such as glycerol is also critical because small amounts of aldehyde and other glycerol-related chemical impurities can accelerate the formation of HMWP. The biopotency of HMWP is significantly less (1/10 to 1/5 of insulin) than monomeric species (Chance, 1995).

Physical Stability of Insulin Formulations

The physical stability of insulin formulations is mediated by non-covalent aggregation of the insulin. The aggregation is typically driven by hydrophobic forces although electrostatics play a subtle but important role. Aggregation typically leads to a loss in potency of the formulation, and therefore should be avoided. Extreme aggregation may lead to the formation of fibrils of insulin. The physical stability of insulin formulations is readily assessed by visual observation for macroscopic characteristics as well as by instrumental methods such as light and differential phase contrast microscopy. Various particle sizing techniques also may be used to characterize microscopic phenomena.

In general, insulin solutions have good physical stability. Physical changes in soluble formulations may be manifested as color or clarity change or, in extreme situations, the formation of a precipitate. Insulin suspensions, such as NPH or Lente, are the most susceptible to changes in physical stability. These typically occur as a result of both elevated temperature and mechanical stress to the formulation. The increase in temperature favors hydrophobic interactions, whereas mechanical agitation serves to provide mixing and stress across interfacial boundaries. Nucleation of aggregation in suspensions can lead to conditions described as visible clumping of the suspension or "frosting" of the glass wall of the insulin vial by aggregates. In severe cases, resuspension may be nearly impossible because of caking of the suspension in the vial. Temperatures above normal ambient (>25°C) can accelerate the aggregation process, especially those at or above body temperature (37°C). Normal mechanical mixing of suspensions prior to administration is not deleterious to physical stability; however, vigorous shaking or mixing should be avoided. The necessity of rigorous resuspension may be the first sign of aggregation and should prompt a careful examination of the formulation to verify its suitability for use.

Clinical and Practice Aspects

Vial Presentations

Insulin is commonly available in 10-mL vials. In the United States, a strength of U–100 (100 U/mL) is the standard, whereas outside the U.S. both U–100 and U–40 (40 U/ mL) are commonly used. It is essential to obtain the proper strength and formulation of insulin in order to maintain glycemic control. In addition, species and brand/method of manufacture are important. Any change in insulin should be made cautiously and only under medical supervision (Galloway, 1988; Brackenridge, 1994) Common formulations, such as Regular, NPH, and Lente, are listed in Table 10.1. NPH/Regular mixtures, such as 70/30, are a popular choice for glycemic control. The ratio is defined as N/R 70/ 30 where 70% of a dose is available as NPH insulin and 30% as Regular insulin. Caution must be used in the nomenclature for NPH/Regular mixtures because it may vary depending on the country of sale and the governing pharmacopeial body. In the U.S., for example, the predominant species is listed first as in N/R 70/30, but in Europe the same formulation is described as R/N 30/70 (Soluble/ Isophane) where the base ("normal") ingredient is listed first. Currently an effort is being made to standardize worldwide to the European nomenclature. Mixtures available in the U.S. include 70/30 and 50/50 while Europe has R/N 10/90, 20/80, 30/70, 40/60, and 50/50.

Injectors

Insulin syringes should be purchased to match the strength of the insulin that is to be administered (e.g., for U–100 strength use 30– or 100–unit syringes designated for U–100). The gauge of needles available for insulin administration has been reduced to very fine gauges (28, 29, or 30 ga.) in order to minimize pain during injection. The use of a new needle for each dose maintains the sharp point of the needle and ensures a sterile needle for the injection.

In recent years the availability of insulin pen injectors has made dosing and compliance easier for the patient with diabetes. The first pen injector used a 1.5-mL cartridge of U–100 insulin. A needle was attached to the end of the pen, and the proper dose was selected and then injected by the patient. The cartridge was replaced when the contents were exhausted, typically three to seven days. More recently, larger 3.0-mL cartridges are becoming available in U–100 strength for Regular, NPH, and the range of N/R mixtures, for patients requiring larger doses. The advantages of the pen injectors are primarily better compliance for the patient through a variety of factors including more accurate and reproducible dose control, easier transport of the drug, more discrete dose administration, more timely dose administration, and greater convenience for the patient.

Storage

Insulin formulations should be stored in a cool place that avoids direct sunlight. Vials or cartridges that are not in active use should be stored under refrigerated (2–8°C)

conditions. Vials or cartridges in active use may be stored at ambient temperature. High temperatures, such as those found in non-air-conditioned vehicles in the summer, should be avoided. Insulin should not be frozen; if this occurs, the product should be disposed of immediately.

Usage

RESUSPENSION

Insulin suspensions (NPH, Premixtures, Lente, Ultralente) should be resuspended by gentle back-and-forth mixing and rolling of the vial between the palms to obtain a uniform, milky suspension. The homogeneity of suspensions is critical to obtaining an accurate dose. Any suspension that fails to a provide a homogeneous suspension should be discarded immediately. Pen injectors may be suspended in the same manner; however, the smaller size of the container and shape of the injector device may require slight modification of the resuspension method. A bead is added to cartridges to aid in the resuspension of NPH suspensions.

DOSING

Dose withdrawal should immediately follow the resuspension of any insulin suspension, especially Lente and Ultralente formulations because they settle relatively quickly. The patient should be instructed by their doctor or nurse educator in proper procedures for dose administration. Of particular importance are procedures for disinfecting the vial top and injection site. The patient is also advised to use a new needle and syringe for each injection. Reuse of these components, even after cleaning, may lead to contamination of the insulin formulation by microorganisms or by other materials, such as cleaning agents.

EXTEMPORANEOUS MIXING

As discussed above in the section on 'Intermediate-acting Insulin Preparations', Regular insulin can be mixed in the syringe with NPH, Lente, and Ultralente. However, only the Regular/NPH mixtures are stable enough to be stored for extended periods of time. The Lente/Regular and Ultralente/Regular formulations can be prepared but **must** be used immediately; otherwise, the time-action of the Regular component can be affected.

Acknowledgements

The authors would like to thank Bruce H. Frank, Ph.D., John H. Holcombe, M.D., and David J. Miner, Ph.D. for their critical review and commentary. ■

Further Reading

- Bliss M. (1982). *The Discovery of Insulin*. Toronto: McClelland and Stewart Limited
- Brange J. (1987). *Galenics of Insulin*. Berlin: Springer-Verlag
- Galloway JA, Potvin JH, Shuman CR. (1988). *Diabetes Mellitus*, 9th ed. Indianapolis, IN: Lilly Research Laboratories

References

- Baker EN, Blundell TL, Cutfield JF, Cutfield SM, Dodson EJ, Dodson GG, Hodgkin DMC, Hubbard RE, Isaacs NW, Reynolds CD, Sakabe K, Sakabe N, Vijayan NM. (1988). The structure of 2Zn pig insulin crystals at 1.5Å resolution. *Phil Trans R Soc Lond B*, 319, 369–456

- Bell DSH, Clements RS, Perentesis G, Roddam R, Wagenknecht L. (1991). Dosage accuracy of self-mixed vs premixed insulin. *Arch Intern Med.*, 151, 2265–2269

- Bliss M. (1982). Who discovered insulin. In *The Discovery of Insulin*. Toronto: McClelland and Stewart Limited, pp. 189–211

- Brackenridge B. (1994). Diabetes medicines: Insulin. In *Managing Your Diabetes*, edited by B Brackenridge. Indianapolis: Eli Lilly and Company, pp. 36–50

- Brader ML, Dunn MF. (1991). Insulin hexamers: New conformations and applications. *TIBS*, 16, 341–345

- Brange J. (1987a). Insulin Preparations. In *Galenics of Insulin*. Berlin: Springer-Verlag, pp. 17–39

- Brange J. (1987b). Production of bovine and porcine insulin. In *Galenics of Insulin*. Berlin: Springer-Verlag, pp. 1–5

- Brange J, Owens DR, Kang S, Vølund A. (1990). Monomeric insulins and their experimental and clinical applications. *Diabetes Care*, 13, 923–954

- Brange J, Langkjær L. (1992a). Chemical stability of insulin. 3. Influence of excipients, formulation, and pH. *Acta Pharm Nord*, 4, 149–158

- Brange J, Langkjær L, Havelund S, Vølund A. (1992b). Chemical stability of insulin. 1. Hydrolytic degradation during storage of pharmaceutical preparations. *Pharm Res*, 9, 715–726

- Brange J, Havelund S, Hougaard P. (1992c). Chemical stability of insulin. 2. Formation of higher molecular weight transformation products during storage of pharmaceutical preparations. *Pharm Res*, 9, 727–734

- Brems DN, Alter LA, Beckage MJ, Chance RE, DiMarchi RD, Green LK, Long HB, Pekar AH, Shields JE, Frank BH. (1992). Altering the association properties of insulin by amino acid replacement. *Prot Eng*, 6, 527–533

- Brennan TV, Clarke S. (1994). Deamidation and isoasparate formation in model synthetic peptides. In *Deamidation and Isoaspartate Formation in Peptides and Proteins*, edited by DW Aswad. Boca Raton: CRC Press, pp. 65–90

- Chance RE. (1995). Bioactivity data for insulin related substances. Personal Communication. Indianapolis, IN: Eli Lilly and Company

- Ciszak E, Beals JM, Baker JC, Carter ND, Frank BH, Smith GD. (1995). The role of the C-terminal B-chain residues in insulin assembly: The structure of hexameric $Lys^{B28}Pro^{B29}$-human insulin. *Structure*, 3, 615–622

- Davis SN, Thompson CJ, Brown MD, Home PD, Alberti KGMM. (1991). A comparison of the pharmacokinetics and metabolic effects of Human Regular and NPH mixtures. *Diabetes Res Clin Pract*, 13, 107–118

- Deckert T. (1980). Intermediate-acting insulin preparations: NPH and Lente. *Diabetes Care*, 3, 623–626

- Derewenda U, Derewenda Z, Dodson EJ, Dodson GG, Reynolds CD, Smith GD, Sparks C, Swenson D. (1989). Phenol stabilizes more helix in a new symmetrical zinc insulin hexamer. *Nature*, 338, 594–596

- Dodd SW, Havel HA, Kovach PM, Lakshminarayan C, Redmon MP, Sargeant CM, Sullivan GR, Beals JM. (1995). Reversible adsorption of soluble hexameric insulin onto the surface of insulin crystals cocrystallized with protamine: An electrostatic interaction. *Pharm Res*, 12, 60–68

- Galloway JA, Spradlin CT, Jackson RL, Otto DC, Bechtel LD. (1982). Mixtures of intermediate-acting insulin (NPH and Lente) with regular insulin: An update. In *Insulin Update: 1982*, edited by JS Skyler. Princeton: Exerpta Medica, pp. 111–119

- Galloway JA. (1988). Chemistry and clinical use of insulin. In *Diabetes Mellitus*, edited by JA Galloway JH. Potvin, CR Shuman, 9th ed. Indianapolis, IN: Lilly Research Laboratories, pp. 105–133

- Goldman J, Carpenter FH. (1974). Zinc binding, circular dichroism, and equilibrium sedimentation studies on insulin (bovine) and several of its derivatives. *Biochemistry*, 13, 4566–4574

- Hagedorn HC, Jensen BN, Krarup NB, Wodstrup I. (1936). Protamine Insulinate. *JAMA*, 106, 177–180

- Hallas-Møller K, Jersild M, Petersen K, Schlichtkrull J. (1952). Zinc insulin preparations for single daily injection. *JAMA*, 150, 1667–1671

- Hamaguchi T, Hashimoto Y, Miyata T, Kishikawa H, Yano T, Fukushima H and Shichiri M. (1990). Effect of mixing short and intermediate NPH insulin or Zn insulin suspension acting Human insulin on plasma free insulin levels and action profiles. *J Jpn Diabetes Soc*, 33, 223–229

- Hoffmann JA, Chance RE, Johnson MG. (1990). Purification and analysis of the major components of chum salmon protamine contained in insulin formulations using high-performance liquid chromatography. *Protein Expression and Purification*, 1, 127–133

- **Howey DC, Bowsher RR, Brunelle RL, Woodworth JR.** (1994). [Lys(B28),Pro(B29)]-human insulin: A rapidly-absorbed analogue of human insulin. *Diabetes*, 43, 396–402

- **Kaarsholm NC, Havelund S, Hougaard P.** (1990). Ionization behavior of native and mutant insulins: pK Perturbation of B13-Glu in aggregated species. *Arch Biochem Biophys*, 283, 496–502

- **Krayenbühl C, Rosenberg T.** (1946). Crystalline protamine insulin. *Rep Steno Hosp (Kbh)*, 1, 60–73

- **Kroeff EP, Owen RA, Campbell EL, Johnson RD, Marks HI.** (1989). Production scale purification of biosynthetic human insulin by reversed phase high performance liquid chromatography. *J Chromatography*, 461, 45–61

- **Kurtz AB, Gray RS, Markanday S, Nabarro JDN.** (1983). Circulating IgG antibody to protamine in patients treated with protamine-insulins. *Diabetologia*, 25, 322–324

- **Nell LJ, Thomas JW.** (1988). Frequency and specificity of protamine antibodies in diabetic and control subjects. *Diabetes*, 37, 172–176

- **Pekar AH, Frank BH.** (1972). Conformation of proinsulin. A comparison of insulin and proinsulin self-association at neutral pH. *Biochemistry*, 11, 4013–4016

- **USPC.** (1995). Official Monographs for USP 23. In *US Pharmacopeia*. Rockville: United States Pharmacopeia Convention, Inc, pp. 807–813

Self-Assessment Questions

Question 1: Which insulin formulations can be mixed and stored? Which insulin formulations must be extemporaneously mixed? Why?

Question 2: What are the primary chemical and physical stability issues with insulin formulations?

Answers

Answer 1: Mixtures of NPH/Regular can be prepared and have sufficient stability for long-term storage. NPH and Regular formulations can be mixed and stored because both formulations contain approximately the same level of zinc and consequently the soluble insulin will remain in solution after mixing. In addition, the adsorption of soluble insulin that occurs on the surface of NPH crystals is reversible under physiological conditions and therefore does not alter the bioavailability of the soluble insulin.

Mixtures of Lente/Regular and Ultralente/Regular must be prepared by extemporaneous mixing and be used immediately; otherwise, the time-action of Regular will be blunted. The time-action of Regular is blunted by the binding of surplus zinc, present in the Ultralente and Lente formulations, to sites on the surface of the soluble insulin hexamer, present in Regular formulations, causing the soluble insulin to precipitate. Consequently, the rapid absorption of the monomeric/dimeric insulin species arising from the dissociation of the soluble insulin hexamer is delayed due to the requirement of an additional dissolution step for the newly formed insoluble precipitate.

Answer 2: The two primary modes of chemical degradation are Asn^{B3} deamidation and HMWP formation. These routes of chemical degradation occur in all formulations; however, they are generally slower in suspension formulations. Physical instability is most often observed in insulin suspension formulations and pump formulations. In suspension formulations, non-covalent aggregation can occur resulting in the visible clumping of the crystalline and/or amorphous insulin. The soluble insulin in pump formulations has also been observed to form non-covalent aggregates that precipitate.

11 Growth Hormones

by: Melinda Marian

Introduction

Human growth hormone (hGH) is a protein hormone essential for normal growth and development in humans. hGH affects many aspects of human metabolism including lipolysis, the stimulation of protein synthesis and the inhibition of glucose metabolism. Human growth hormone was first isolated and identified in the late 1950's from extracts of pituitary glands obtained from cadavers or patients undergoing hypophysectomy. The first clinical use of these pituitary-extracted hGH's for stimulation of growth in hypopituitary children occurred in 1957 and 1958 (Raben, 1958). From 1958 to 1985 the primary material used for clinical studies was pituitary-derived growth hormone (pit-hGH). Human growth hormone was first cloned in 1979 (Goeddel *et al.*, 1979; Martial *et al.*, 1979). The first use in humans of recombinant human growth (rhGH) was reported in the literature in 1982 (Hintz *et al.*, 1982). The introduction of rhGH coincided with reports of a number of cases of Creutzfeldt-Jakob disease, a fatal degenerative neurological disorder, in patients receiving pituitary-derived hGH. Concern over possible contamination of the pituitary-derived hGH preparations by the prion responsible for Creutzfeldt-Jakob disease led to removal of pit-hGH products from the market in the US in 1985. The initial rhGH preparations were produced in bacteria (*E. coli*) and, unlike endogenous hGH, contained an N-terminal methionine group(met-rhGH). Natural sequence recombinant hGH products have subsequently been produced both in bacteria and mammalian cells.

hGH Structure and Isohormones

The major, circulating form of hGH is a non-glycosylated, 22 kD protein composed of 191 amino acid residues linked by disulfide bridges in two peptide loops. The three dimensional structure of hGH includes four antiparallel α-helical regions (Figure 11.1). Helix 4 and Helix 1 have been determined to contain the primary sites for binding to the growth hormone receptor (Wells *et al.*, 1993). Endogenous growth hormone is comprised of approximately 85% 22 kD monomer, 5–10% 20 kD monomer, and 5% a mixture of disulfide-linked dimers, oligomers and other modified forms (Baumann, 1991; Scanes and Campbell, 1995). The 20 kD monomer, dimers, oligomers and other modified forms occur as the result of different gene products, different splicing of hGH mRNA and posttranslational modifications. Glycosylated hGH forms less than 1% of pituitary hGH and appears to have biological effects comparable to non-glycosylated hGH.

There are two hGH genes in humans, the hGH-N gene and the hGH-V gene. The hGH-N gene is expressed in the pituitary gland and is responsible for the production of the "normal" 22 kD form of hGH. The hGH-V gene is expressed in the placenta and is responsible for the production of the "variant" form of hGH found in high levels in pregnant women during the third trimester.

Pharmacology

Growth Hormone Secretion and Regulation

Growth hormone is secreted from somatotrophs in the anterior pituitary. Multiple feedback loops are present in normal regulation of hGH secretion (Casanueva, 1992; Muller, 1987; Harvey, 1995) (Figure 11.2). Growth hormone release from the pituitary is regulated by a "short loop" of two coupled hypothalamic peptides — a stimulatory peptide, growth hormone releasing hormone (GHRH) and an inhibitory peptide, somatostatin. GHRH and somatostatin are, in turn, regulated by neuronal input to the hypothalamus. There is possibly also an "ultrashort loop" in which hGH release is feedback-regulated by growth hormone receptors present on the somatotrophs of the pituitary themselves. Growth hormone secretion is also regulated by a "long loop" of peripheral signals including, primarily, negative feedback via insulin-like growth factor (IGF-I). Growth hormone-induced peripheral IGF-I inhibits somatotroph release of hGH and stimulates somatostatin release.

Growth hormone secretion changes dramatically during human development with the highest production rates observed during gestation and puberty (Harvey and Daughaday, 1995; Brook *et al.*, 1992). Growth hormone production declines approximately 10–15% each decade from age 20 to 70. Endogenous hGH secretion also varies with sex, nutri-

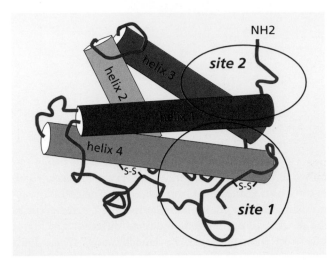

Figure 11.1. Schematic 3-D structure of hGH showing 4 antiparallel α-helices and receptor binding sites 1 and 2. Approximate positions of the two disulfide bridges (S-S) are also indicated. Modified from Wells *et al.*, 1993.

tional status, obesity, physical activity, and in a variety of disease states. Endogenous hGH is secreted in periodic bursts over a 24 hour period with great variability in burst frequency, amplitude and duration. There is little detectable hGH released from the pituitary between bursts. The highest endogenous hGH serum concentrations of 10–30 ng/mL usually occur at night when the secretory bursts are largest and most frequent.

Growth Hormone Biologic Actions

hGH has well-defined growth promoting and metabolic actions. hGH stimulates the growth of cartilage and bone directly, through hGH receptors in those tissues, and indirectly, via local increases in IGF-I (Isaksson *et al.*, 1987; Bouillon, 1991). Metabolic actions, which also may be directly controlled by hGH, include the elevation of circulating glucose levels (diabetogenic effect) and acute increases in circulating concentrations of free fatty acids (lipolytic effect). Other hGH anabolic and metabolic actions believed to be mediated through increases in local or systemic IGF-I concentrations include increases in net muscle protein synthesis (anabolic effect); modulation of reproduction in both males and females; maintenance, control and modulation of lymphocyte functions; increases in glomerular filtration rate and renal plasma flow rate (osmoregulation); influences on the release and metabolism of insulin, glucagon, and thyroid hormones (T3, T4); and possible direct effects on pituitary function and neural tissue development (Strobl and Thomas, 1994; Casanueva, 1992; Le Roith *et al.*, 1991).

hGH Receptor and Binding Proteins

The hGH receptor is a member of the hematopoietic cytokine receptor family. It has an extracellular domain consisting of 246 amino acids and a single transmembrane domain of 350 amino acids (Baumann, 1991; Bass *et al.*, 1991). The extracellular domain has at least six potential N-glycosylation sites and is usually extensively glycosylated. hGH receptors are found in most tissues in humans. However, the greatest concentration of receptors in humans and other mammals occurs in the liver.

As much as 40–45% of monomeric hGH circulating in plasma is bound to one of two binding proteins (GHBP) (Baumann, 1991; Harvey and Hull, 1995). Binding proteins decrease the clearance of hGH from the circulation (Baumann, 1979) and may also serve to dampen the biological effects of hGH by competing with cell receptors for circulating free hGH. The major form of GHBP in humans is a high affinity ($K_a = 10^{-9}$ to 10^{-8} M), low capacity form which preferentially binds the 22 kD form of hGH (Baumann *et al.*, 1986a; Herrington *et al.*, 1986). In humans, the high affinity GHBP is identical to the extracellular domain of the hGH receptor and arises by proteoloytic cleavage of liver hGH receptors (Harvey and Hull, 1995). Another low affinity ($K_a = 10^{-5}$M), high capacity GHBP is also present which binds the 20 kD form with equal or slightly greater affinity than the 22 kD form.

Molecular Endocrinology and Signal Transduction

X-ray crystallographic studies and functional studies of the extracellular domain of the hGH receptor suggest that two receptor molecules form a dimer with a single growth hormone molecule by sequentially binding to Site 1 on Helix 4 of hGH then to Site 2 on Helix 1 (Figure 11.3) (Wells *et al.*, 1993). Signal transduction may occur by activation/phosphorylation of JAK-2 tyrosine kinase followed by activation/phosphorylation of the extracellular signal-regulated kinase/mitogen-activated protein kinase (ERK/MAP) system (Figure 11.4) (Scanes, 1995). The details of subsequent signalling events have not been elucidated, however, hGH receptor activation results in rapid induction of the c-fos, c-myc and c-jun genes, possibly through activation of protein C kinase.

Dosing Schedules and Routes

The dosing levels and routes for exogenously administered growth hormone were first established for pit-hGH in growth hormone deficient (GHD) patients. This regimen, 0.05–0.1 mg/kg three times weekly by intramuscular (im) injection, was based on a number of factors including patient

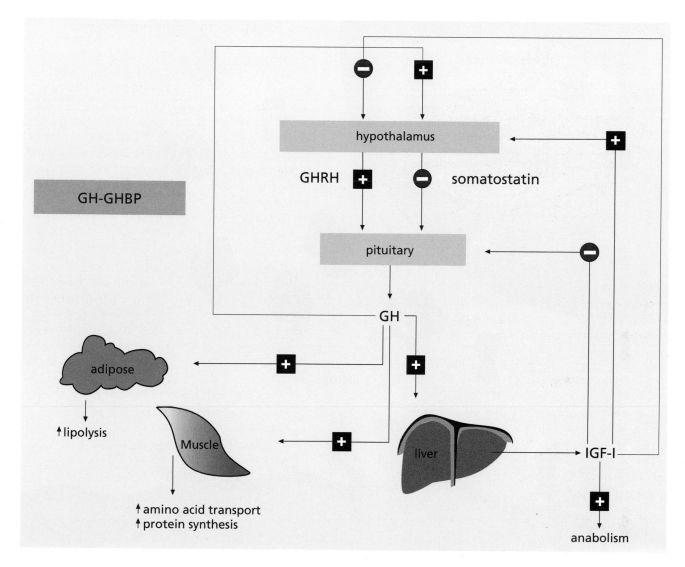

Figure 11.2. Schematic representation of hGH regulation and biologic actions in man. "Short loop" regulation of hGH secretion occurs between the hypothalamus and pituitary. "Long loop" of regulation of hGH secretion occurs through peripheral feedback signals, primarily from insulin-like growth factor I (IGF-I). hGH acts directly on muscle, bone and adipose tissue. Other anabolic actions are mediated through IGF-I.

compliance and availability of hGH derived from cadaver pituitaries. A re-evaluation of subcutaneous (sc) administration of hGH (Russo and Moore, 1982; Albertsson-Wikland *et al.*, 1986) found a very strong patient preference for the sc route. Furthermore, increased growth rates were observed with daily sc injections compared to the previous 2–3 times weekly im injection schedule (Takano *et al.*, 1988; Albertsson-Wikland *et al.*, 1986). The abdomen, deltoid muscle, and thigh are commonly used subcutaneous injection sites. Current dosing schedules are usually daily sc injections, often self-administered. Some studies (Jorgensen *et al.*, 1990; Christiansen *et al.*, 1983) suggest that evening injections, which emulate the normal evening increases in endogenous secretion, are better than morning injections.

Pharmacokinetics and Metabolism

The earliest pharmacokinetic studies were conducted with pituitary-derived hGH (pit-hGH). The pharmacokinetic profiles of pit-hGH, met-rhGH and rhGH have been compared (Takano *et al.*, 1983; Jorgenson *et al.*, 1987 and Wilton *et al.*, 1987) and shown to be very similar. The pharmacokinetics of hGH have been studied in normal, healthy children and adults and a variety of patient populations.

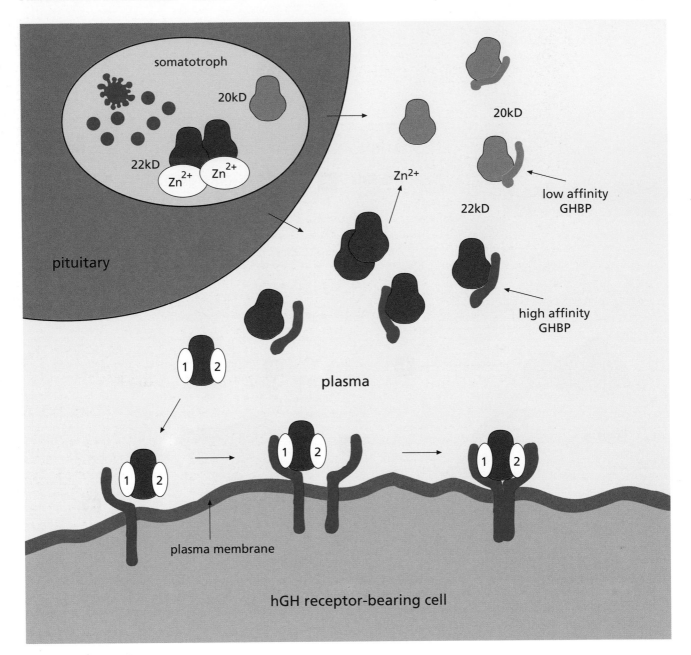

Figure 11.3. Growth hormone secreted isoforms, binding proteins and receptor interactions. Both 22kD and 20kD forms are secreted by the pituitary. Pituitary hGH is stored bound to zinc (Zn^{2+}) which is released upon secretion from the pituitary. Approximately 40% of secreted hGH is bound to either the low or high affinity GHBP in plasma. Receptor activation involves dimerization of two receptor molecules with one molecule of hGH. Modified from Wells *et al.*, 1993.

Table 11.1 summarizes clearance and terminal half-life values reported from studies in normal subjects and various patient populations. Pit-hGH, met-rhGH and rhGH are rapidly cleared following intravenous (iv) injection in normal subjects with terminal half lives ranging from 8 to 31 minutes. Distribution volumes usually approximate the plasma volume. hGH clearance in normal subjects ranges from 90–222 mL/hr/kg. The majority of the data indicate that the clearance of hGH in children and adults are similar. Comparative analyses of hGH clearance have not shown consistent differences on the basis of age, gender or hGH secretory status.

Human growth hormone is slowly, but relatively completely, absorbed after both intramuscular (im) and subcu-

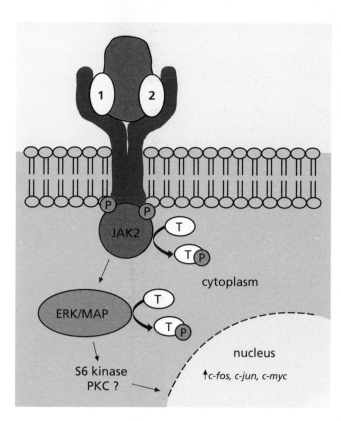

Figure 11.4. Molecule endocrinology and putative signal transduction pathway for hGH. JAK2 = Janus 2 tyrosine kinase; ERK = extracellular signal-regulated kinase; MAP = mitogen activated protein kinase; PKC = protein kinase C; T = target protein; P = phosphate.

taneous (sc) injection. Time to peak concentrations range from 3–4 hours following im bolus administration and 4–6 hours following sc bolus administration (Jorgensen, 1991). Subcutaneously administered rhGH is approximately 70–80% bioavailable (Wilton *et al.*, 1988). Elimination half-lives following extravascular administration (2–5 hr) are usually longer than the iv terminal half-lives indicating absorption rate-limited kinetics. Daily or thrice weekly dosing does not influence absorption or elimination (Kearns *et al.*, 1989). The extent of subcutaneous absorption appears to be independent of needle type, concentration of the injection solution or injection volume (Blok *et al.*, 1991; Laursen *et al.*, 1993).

The absorption and elimination in GHD patients are similar to published reports in healthy adults (Table 11.1). Changes in hGH pharmacokinetics due to the presence of diabetes, or diseases of the thyroid, liver and kidney have been investigated and results suggest disposition is not significantly altered compared with normal subjects except in severe liver or kidney dysfunction (Haffner *et al.*, 1994;

Owens *et al.*, 1973; Cameron *et al.*, 1972; Taylor *et al.*, 1969; Navalesi *et al.*, 1975; Refetoff and Sonksen, 1980). The reduction in clearance observed in severe liver (30%) or kidney dysfunction (40–75%) is consistent with the role of the liver and kidney as major organs of hGH elimination.

hGH is rapidly metabolized *in vivo*. Both the kidney and the liver have been shown to be important in the clearance of hGH in man (Bennett *et al.*, 1979; Cameron *et al.*, 1969; Carone *et al.*, 1979; Maack *et al.*, 1979; Owens *et al.*, 1973; Taylor *et al.*, 1969). The relative contribution of each organ has not been definitively determined in humans, but the preponderance of studies in laboratory animals, and isolated perfused organ systems, suggest a dominant role for the kidney at pharmacologic dose levels of hGH. Renal handling of hGH appears to involve filtration, re-absorption and intracellular catabolism (Maack *et al.*, 1979; Bennett *et al.*, 1979; Carone *et al.*, 1979). Little intact hGH (0.01% of serum concentrations) is normally excreted in human urine (Walker *et al.*, 1990; Sohmiya and Kato, 1992).

Protein Manufacture, Formulation and Stability

Commercially available hGH preparations are summarized in Table 11.2. All recombinant growth hormones except Serostim®/Saizen® are produced in *E. coli*. Met-rhGH is produced by direct cytoplasmic expression of the protein. Natural sequence rhGH is produced either by enzymatic cleavage of the methionine during the purification procedures or periplasmic secretion of rhGH into refractile bodies. The rhGH is then released from the refractile bodies by osmotic shock and the protein recovered and purified. rhGH synthesized in mammalian cells is transported across the endoplasmic reticulum and secreted directly into the culture medium from which it is recovered and purified.

Historically, the potency of hGH products has been expressed in International Units per mg (IU/mg). The initial standard, established in 1982 for pit-hGH preparations, was 2 IU/mg. The standard for rhGH products was 2.6 IU/mg until September 1994. The current WHO standard, established in September 1994, is 3.0 IU/mg. Dosages are usually expressed as IU/kg or IU/m² in Europe and Japan and as mg/kg in the US. However, the use of IU dosages may no longer be necessary due to the high level of purity and consistent potency of recombinant hGH products.

Most current formulations are lyophilized preparations which are reconstituted prior to injection. Lyophilized formulations usually include 5 or 10 mg of protein in a glycine and/or mannitol-containing phosphate buffer excipient. The materials are usually reconstituted with sterile water for injection for single use or with bacteriostatic water or

Population	CL (mL/hr/kg)[a]	Terminal $t_{1/2}$ (min)[a]	References
Normal adults	90-222	8-31	Haffner *et al.*, 1994 Rosenbaum and Gertner, 1989 Taylor *et al.*, 1969 Thompson *et al.*, 1972 Owens *et al.*, 1973 Navalesi *et al.*, 1975 Sohmiya and Kato, 1992 Henry *et al.*, 1987 Wilton *et al.*, 1988 Holl *et al.*, 1993 Parker *et al.*, 1962 Takano *et al.*, 1983
GHD children	125-245	8-13	Rosenbaum and Gertner, 1989 Albertsson-Wikland *et al.*, 1989
GHD adults	239	9-38	Hindmarsh *et al.*, 1989 Retetoff and Sonsken, 1970 Parker *et al.*, 1962 Hendricks *et al.*, 1985
CRI children	47-109	25-32	Haffner *et al.*, 1994
CRI adults	68-175	19-48	Haffner *et al.*, 1994 Owens *et al.*, 1973 Cameron *et al.*, 1972
Normal elderly	138	14	Sohmiya and Kato, 1992
Diabetes	87-175	22	Navalesi *et al.*, 1975 Taylor *et al.*, 1969 Owens *et al.*, 1973
Liver disease	86-124	29	Owens *et al.*, 1973 Cameron *et al.*, 1972
Acromegaly	46-190	33	Retetoff and Sonsken, 1980 Taylor *et al.*, 1969
Hyperthyroid	240	nr	Taylor *et al.*, 1969
Hypothyroid	122	nr	Taylor *et al.*, 1969
Thyrotoxicosis	201	16	Owens *et al.*, 1973
Myxedema	153	24	Owens *et al.*, 1973

Table 11.1. Intravenous pharmacokinetic parameters for hGH in various populations. [a]Values have been converted from units reported in the original publications for ease of comparison. Where specific activity of GH was not stated in the original publication, values of 2.6 IU/mg for rhGH and 2.0 IU/mg for pit-hGH were used. 70 kg/1.73 m² and 40 kg/1 m² were used as adult and child body weight/body surface values, respectively. Listed values are means or ranges of means. nr = not reported.

Growth hormone type	Source	Brand names	Supplier
Pituitary-derived human growth hormone (pit-hGH)	cadaver pituitaries	Crescormon® Nanormon®	KabiVitrum AB Novo Nordisk
Somatrem, methionyl human growth hormone (met-rhGH)	recombinant protein produced in bacteria (E. coli)	Somatonorm® Protropin®	KabiVitrum AB Genentech, Inc.
Somatropin, natural sequence human growth hormone (rhGH)	recombinant protein produced in bacteria (E. coli)	Genotropin® Norditropin® Nutropin® Humatrope® Bio-Tropin®	KabiVitrum AB Novo Nordisk Genentech, Inc. Eli Lilly & Co Bio-Technology General
	recombinant protein produced in mammalian cells (C127 mouse cell line-derived)	Serostim® Saizen®	Ares Serono

Table 11.2. Human growth hormone preparations.

bacteriostatic saline for multiple injection use. A liquid formulation of rhGH (Nutropin AQ®, Genentech, Inc.) has also been recently approved for use in the US which contains 10 mg of protein in citrate buffer containing polysorbate 20, phenol and sodium chloride. Product stability has been very good with shelf-lives of approximately 2 years at 2–8°C.

Clinical Usage

Early clinical use of hGH has been summarized by Frasier *et al.* (1983). Recent clinical usage has been reviewed by Jorgensen *et al.* (1991), Strobl and Thomas (1994), Kaplan (1993) and Harvey and Daughaday (1995). Investigations of clinical usages of hGH have focused, generally, in two major areas of hGH biologic action: 1) linear growth promotion and 2) modulation of metabolism. hGH has been approved for market in the US, Europe and Japan for treatment of growth hormone deficiency in children and chronic renal failure in children. hGH has also been approved for market in Europe and the US for treatment of Turner syndrome and, in several European countries and New Zealand, for treatment of growth hormone deficient adults. Indications for which hGH has been investigated as a possible therapeutic are summarized in Table 11.3 and detailed in the references contained within the reviews cited above. The following sections summarize observations from studies in the approved indications and selected indications under current investigation. Specific references for the investigated indications can be found in the cited review articles.

Growth Hormone Deficiency/Idiopathic Short Stature in Children

The major indication for therapeutic use of hGH is the long-term replacement treatment for children with classic growth hormone deficiency (GHD) in whom growth failure is due to a lack of adequate endogenous hGH secretion. Diagnosis of hGH deficiency is usually defined based on an inadequate response to two hGH provocation tests implying a functional deficiency in the production or secretion of hGH from the pituitary gland. Usual doses range from 0.08–0.35 mg/kg/week administered as daily subcutaneous injections. hGH treatment results in increased growth velocity and, at least in some populations, enhancement in final adult height. The growth response correlates positively with hGH dose and frequency of injections and negatively with chronological age at onset of treatment. hGH therapy in children is usually continued until growth has been completed, as evidenced by epiphyseal fusion. Partial GHD and idiopathic short stature (ISS) comprise a heterogeneous group of growth failure states due to impaired spontaneous hGH secretion, hGH resistance due to low levels of hGH receptors or possible other defects in either secreted hGH or hGH receptors. hGH treatment in these groups has resulted in acceleration of growth and improvement of final height.

Turner Syndrome

Turner syndrome is a disease of females caused by partial or total loss of one sex chromosome and is characterized by decreased intrauterine and postnatal growth, short final

Growth hormone biologic actions	Clinical indications
Promotion of linear growth	classic GHD partial GHD/Idiopathic short stature Turner syndrome Down's syndrome Prader-Willi syndrome Noonan's syndrome intrauterine growth retardation (IUGR) Silver-Russel syndrome thalassemia hypochondroplasia spina bifida myelomeningocele chronic renal insufficiency (CRI) growth impairment in chronic steroid therapy
Modulation of metabolism Stimulation of lipolysis Stimulation of protein synthesis	GHD in adults aging obesity weight training in athletes
Anabolism Stimulation of protein synthesis Improved nitrogen retention Prevention of starvation-induced hypoglycemia	catabolic states due to chronic disease, infections, surgery, trauma, burns, chronic obstructive pulmonary disease (COPD), short bowel syndrome (SBS), acquired immunodeficiency syndrome (AIDS)
Lipolysis Muscle anabolism	cardiovascular dysfunction
Stimulation of collagen formation	burns wound healing
Stimulation of bone formation	osteoporosis fractures
Stimulation of conversion of thyroxine (T4) to triiodothyronine (T3)	hypothyroidism
Osmoregulation Increased GFR, increased renal plasma flow	chronic renal disease
Maintenance of immune function	immune dysfunction
Enhancement of gonadotropin action	female and male infertility
Stimulation of lactation	lactational failure in women

Table 11.3. Growth hormone biologic actions and related clinical investigations.

adult height, incomplete development of the ovaries and secondary sexual characteristics, and other physical abnormalities. Although serum levels of hGH and IGF-I are not consistently low in this population, hGH treatment, alone or in combination with oxandrolone, significantly improves growth rate and final adult height in this patient group.

Chronic Renal Insufficiency (CRI)

Children with renal disease grow slowly, possibly related to defects in metabolism and/or defects in the IGF-I/hGH axis. Basal serum hGH concentrations and IGF-I responses to hGH stimulation are usually essentially normal. However, there are reported abnormalities in the IGF-binding protein levels in renal disease patients suggesting possible problems with GH/IGF-I action. Growth hormone therapy in children with chronic renal insufficiency has resulted in significant increases in height velocity. Increases were best during the first year of treatment for younger children with stable renal disease. Responses were less for children on dialysis or children post-transplant receiving corticosteroids.

Growth Hormone Deficient Adults and the Elderly

Early limitations in hGH supply severely limited treatment of adults with GHD. However, with rhGH abundantly available, replacement therapy for adults has received renewed clinical interest. Growth hormone has been used in three growth hormone deficient adult populations: a) adults with childhood onset GHD; b) adults with adult onset GHD usually due to pituitary tumors and subsequent hypophysectomy and c) elderly normal adults, 60 years of age or older. Adults with GHD show a predisposition to cardiovascular disease, have increased body fat and decreased lean muscle mass and strength. The elderly are considered growth hormone deficient due to the progressive decline in hGH secretion with ageing which results in substantial decreases in serum IGF-I levels. The elderly also show changes in body composition which are consistent with partial hGH deficiency (decreases in lean body mass and strength, increases in visceral fat, decreases in skin thickness and organ volumes).

Growth hormone treatment reduced body fat, increased lean body mass, increased exercise capacity and muscle strength in the elderly and adult GHD patients. Increases in bone density were observed in some bone types although treatment duration greater than 6 months may be necessary to see significant effects. hGH treatment consistently elevated both serum IGF-I and insulin levels. However, consistent reductions in serum cholesterol and/or LDL levels were not seen in all studies.

Clinical Malnutrition and Wasting Syndromes

The use of hGH therapy to ameliorate the catabolism seen in patients following surgery and/or infections have been investigated in a number of studies. Treatment with hGH alone improved nitrogen and phosphorous retention and increased body weight. Improvements in nitrogen balance were even greater with co-administration of GH and IGF-I. Growth hormone has also show benefit, when used with controlled diets, in increasing body weight and nitrogen retention in wasting associated with AIDS.

Other Indications

A number of studies have investigated the use of hGH in osteoporosis. Growth hormone was not successful in reducing the bone loss associated with osteoporosis, and use of this therapy must await further studies in which hGH is co-administered with inhibitors of bone reabsorption. Growth hormone use in various therapies for female infertility are the subject of a number of current studies. These studies have demonstrated that hGH may be useful for inducing hyperovulation for *in vitro* fertilization procedures and in increasing sensitivity to gonadotropin in ovulation stimulation. Studies on hGH effects in wound healing and burns have been modest with hGH showing significant effectiveness in mild injuries and in acceleration of healing in skin graft sites.

Safety Concerns

hGH has been widely used for many years and has been proven to be remarkably safe. Adverse events have been reported in a small number of children and include intracranial hypertension, glucose intolerance and the development of anti-hGH antibodies. The antibodies have not been positively correlated with a loss in efficacy. Additionally, leukemia has been reported in children receiving hGH therapy but a definite correlation with hGH treatment has not been established.

Growth hormone has caused significant, dose-limiting, fluid retention in adult populations resulting in increased body weight, swollen joints and arthralgias and carpal tunnel syndrome. Symptoms were usually transient and resolve upon reduction of hGH dosage or upon discontinuation of hGH treatment.

Concluding Remarks

The abundant supply of hGH, made possible by recombinant DNA technology, has allowed enormous advances to be made in understanding the basic structure, function and physiology of hGH over the past 10 years. As a result of those advances, recombinant hGH has been developed into a safe and efficacious therapy for growth failure in growth hormone deficiency, chronic renal insufficiency and Turner syndrome. Additional studies in other indications, notably hGH treatment in adults and the elderly, and catabolic wasting states hold promise for additional future uses for this versatile hormone. ∎

Further Reading

- **Baumann G.** (1991). Growth hormone heterogeneity: genes, isohormones, variants and binding proteins. *Endocr Rev*, 12, 424–449
- **Casanueva FF.** (1992). Physiology of growth hormone secretion and action. *Endocrinol Metab Clin N Am*, 21, 483–517
- **Harvey S, Scanes CG, Daughaday WH.** (1995). *Growth Hormone*, CRC Press, Inc, Boca Raton, Florida
- **Iranmanesh A, Veldhuis JD.** (1992). Clinical pathophysiology of the somatotropic (GH) axis in adults. *Endocrinol Metab Clin N Am*, 21, 783–816
- **Isaksson OG, Lindahl A, Nilsson A, Isgaard J.** (1987). Mechanism of the stimulatory effect of growth hormone on longitudinal bone growth. *Endocr Rev*, 8, 426–438
- **Johnson AJ, Blizzard RM.** (1990). Growth hormone treatment. In *Pediatric Endocrinology*, edited by F Lifshitz. New York: Marcel Dekker, Inc, pp. 61–75
- **Strobl JS, Thomas MJ.** (1994). Human growth hormone. *Pharm Rev*, 46, 1–34
- **Wells JA, Cunningham BC, Fuh G, Lowman HB, Bass SH, Mulkerrin MG, Ultsch M, DeVos AM.** (1993). The molecular basis for growth hormone-receptor interactions. *Recent Prog Horm Res*, 48, 253–275

References

- **Albertsson-Wikland K, Rosberg S, Libre E, Lundberg L-O, Groth T.** (1989). Growth hormone secretory rates in children as estimated by deconvolution analysis of 24-h plasma concentration profiles. *Am J Physiol (Endocrinol Metab 20)*, 257, E809–E814
- **Albertsson-Wikland K, Westphal O, Westgren U.** (1986). Daily subcutaneous administration of human growth hormone in growth hormone deficient children. *Acta Pediatr Scand*, 75, 89–97
- **Bass SH, Mulkerrin MG, Wells JA.** (1991). A systematic mutational analysis of hormone-binding determinants in the human growth hormone receptor, *Proc Natl Acad Sci USA*, 88, 4498–4502
- **Baumann G, Stolar MW, Buchanan TA.** (1986a) The metabolic clearance, distribution, and degradation of dimeric and monomeric growth hormone (GH): implications for the pattern of circulating GH forms. *Endocrinology*, 119, 1497–1501
- **Baumann G, Stolar MW, Amburn K, Barsano CP, De Vries BC.** (1986b) A specific growth hormone-binding protein in human plasma: initial characterization. *J Clin Endocrinol Metab*, 62, 134–141
- **Baumann G.** (1979). Metabolic clearance rates of isohormones of human growth hormone in man. *J Clin Endocrinol Metab*, 49, 495–499
- **Bennett HPJ, McMartin C.** (1979). Peptide hormones and their analogues: distribution, clearance from the circulation and inactivation *in vivo*. *Pharmacol Rev*, 30, 247–292
- **Beshyah SA, Anyaoku V, Niththyananthan R, Sharp P, Johnston DG.** (1991). The effect of subcutaneous injection site on absorption of human growth hormone: abdomen versus thigh. *Clin Endocrinol*, 35, 409–412
- **Blok GJ, Van der Veen EA, Susgaard S, Larsen F.** (1991). Influence of concentration and injection volume on the bioavailability of subcutaneous growth hormone: comparison of administration by ordinary syringe and by injection pen. *Pharmacol Toxicol*, 68, 355–359
- **Bouillon R.** (1991). Growth hormone and bone. *Horm Res*, 36 (suppl 1), 49–55
- **Brook CGD, Hindmarsh PC.** (1992). The somatotropic axis in puberty. *Endocrinol Metab Clin N Am*, 21, 767–782
- **Cameron DP, Burger HG, Catt KJ, Gordon E, Watts JMcK.** (1972). Metabolic clearance of human growth hormone in patients with hepatic and renal failure, and in the isolated perfused pig liver. *Metabolism*, 21, 895–904
- **Carone FA, Peterson DR, Oparil S, Pullman TN.** (1979). Renal tubular transport and catabolism of proteins and peptides. *Kidney Int*, 16, 271–278
- **Christiansen JS, Orskov H, Binder C, Kastrup KW.** (1983). Imitation of normal plasma growth hormone profile by subcutaneous administration of human growth hormone to growth hormone deficient children. *Acta Endocrinol*, 102, 6–10
- **Goeddel DV, Heyreker HL, Hozumi T, Arentzen R, Itakura K, Yansura DG, Ross MJ, Miozarri G, Crea R, Seeburg PH.** (1979). Direct expression in *Escherichia coli* of a DNA sequence coding for human growth hormone. *Nature*, 281, 544–548
- **Haffner D, Schaefer F, Girard J, Ritz E, Mehls O.** (1994). Metabolic clearance of recombinant human growth hormone in health and chronic renal failure. *J Clin Invest*, 93, 1163–71
- **Harvey S.** (1995). Growth hormone release: feedback regulation. In *Growth Hormone*, edited by S Harvey, CG Scanes, WH Daughaday. Boca Raton, Florida: CRC Press, Inc, 163–184

- **Harvey S, Daughaday WH.** (1995). Growth hormone action: clinical significance. In *Growth Hormone*, edited by S Harvey, CG Scanes, WH Daughaday. Boca Raton, Florida: CRC Press, Inc, 476–504

- **Harvey S, Hull K.** (1995). Growth hormone transport. In *Growth Hormone*, edited by S Harvey, CG Scanes, WH Daughaday. Boca Raton, Florida: CRC Press, Inc, 257–284

- **Hendricks CM, Eastman RC, Takeda S, Asakawa K, Gorden P.** (1985). Plasma clearance of intravenously administered pituitary human growth hormone: gel filtration studies of heterogeneous components. *J Clin Endocrinol Metab*, 60, 864–867

- **Herington AC, Ymer S, Stevenson J.** (1986). Identification and characterization of specific binding proteins for growth hormone in normal human sera. *J Clin Invest*, 77, 1817–1823

- **Hindmarsh PC, Matthews DR, Brain CE, Pringle PJ, DiSilvio L, Kurtz AB, Brook CGD.** (1989). The half-life of exogenous growth hormone after suppression of endogenous growth hormone secretion with somatostatin. *Clin Endocrinol*, 30, 443–450

- **Hintz RL, Rosenfeld RG, Wilson DM, Bennett A, Finno J, McClellan B, Swift R.** (1982). Biosynthetic methionyl human growth hormone is biologically active in adult man. *Lancet*, 1, 1276–1279

- **Holl RW, Schwarz U, Schauwecker P, Benz R, Veldhuis JD, Heinze E.** (1993). Diurnal variation in the elimination rate of human growth hormone (GH): the half-life of serum GH is prolonged in the evening, and affected by the source of the hormone, as well as by body size and serum estradiol. *J Clin Endocrinol Metab*, 77, 216–220

- **Jorgensen JOL.** (1991). Human growth hormone replacement therapy: pharmacological and clinical aspects. *Endocr Rev*, 12, 189–207

- **Jorgensen JOL, Moller N, Lauritzen T, Alberti KGMM, Orskov H, Christiansen JS.** (1990). Evening versus morning injections of growth hormone (gh) in gh-deficient patients: effects on 24-hour patterns of circulating hormones and metabolites. *J Clin Endocrinol Metab*, 70, 207–214

- **Jorgensen JOL, Flyvbjerg A, Dinesen J, Lund H, Alberti KGMM, Orskov H, Christiansen JS.** (1987). Serum profiles and sort-term metabolic effect of pituitary and authentic biosynthetic human growth hormone in man. *Acta Endocrinol*, 116, 381–386

- **Kaplan SL.** (1993). The newer uses of growth hormone in adults. *Adv Int Med*, 38, 287–301

- **Kearns GL, Kemp SF, Frindik JP.** (1991). Single and multiple dose pharmacokinetics of methionyl growth hormone in children with idiopathic growth hormone deficiency. *J Clin Endocrinol Metab*, 72, 1148–1156

- **Laursen T, Jorgensen JO.L, Susgaard S, Moller J, Christiansen JS.** (1993). Subcutaneous absorption kinetics of two highly concentrated preparations of recombinant human growth hormone. *Ann Pharmacother*, 27, 411–415

- **Le Roith D, Adamo M, Werner H, Roberts CT Jr.** (1991). Insulin-like growth factors and their receptors as growth regulators in normal physiology and pathologic states. *Trends Endocrinol Metab*, 2, 134–139

- **Maack T, Johnson V, Kau ST, Figueiredo J, Sigulem D.** (1979). Renal filtration, transport and metabolism of low-molecular weight proteins: a review. *Kidney Int*, 16, 251–270

- **Martial JA, Hallewell RA, Baxter JD.** (1979). Human growth hormone: complementary DNA cloning and expression in bacteria. *Science*, 205, 602–607

- **Muller EE.** (1987). Neural control of somatropin function. *Physiol Rev*, 67, 962–1031

- **Navalesi R, Pilo A, Vigneri R.** (1975). Growth hormone kinetics in diabetic patients. *Diabetes*, 24, 317–327

- **Owens D, Srivastava MC, Tompkins CV, Nabarro JDN, Sonksen PH.** (1973). Studies on the metabolic clearance rate, apparent distribution space and plasma half-disappearance time of unlabelled human growth hormone in normal subjects and in patients with liver disease, renal disease, thyroid disease and diabetes mellitus. *Europ J Clin Invest*, 3, 284–294

- **Parker ML, Utiger RD, Daughaday WH.** (1962). Studies on human growth hormone II. The physiological disposition and metabolic fate of human growth hormone in man. *J Clin Invest*, 41, 262–268

- **Raben MS.** (1958). Treatment of a pituitary dwarf with human growth hormone. *J Clin Endocrinol Metab*, 18, 901–903

- **Refetoff S, Sonksen PH.** (1970). Disappearance rate of endogenous and exogenous human growth hormone in man. *J Clin Endocr*, 30, 386–392

- **Rosenbaum M, Gertner JM.** (1989). Metabolic clearance rates of synthetic human growth hormone in children, adult women, and adult men. *J Clin Endocrinol Metab*, 69, 821–824

- **Russo L, Moore WV.** (1982). A comparison of subcutaneous and intramuscular administration of human growth hormone in the therapy of growth hormone deficiency. *J Clin Endocrinol Metab*, 55, 1003–1006

- **Scanes CG.** (1995). Growth hormone action: intracellular mechanisms. In *Growth Hormone*, edited by S Harvey, CG Scanes, WH Daughaday. Boca Raton, Florida: CRC Press, Inc, 337–346

- **Scanes CG, Campbell RM.** (1995). Growth hormone: chemistry. In *Growth Hormone*, edited by S Harvey, CG Scanes, WH Daughaday. Boca Raton, Florida: CRC Press, Inc, 1–24

- **Sohmiya M, Kato Y.** (1992). Renal clearance, metabolic clearance rate, and half-life of human growth hormone in young and aged subjects. *J Clin Endocrinol Metab*, 75, 1487–90

- **Takano K, Shizume K, Hibi I and Members of Committee for the Treatment of Pituitary Dwarfism in Japan.** (1988). A comparison of subcutaneous and intramuscular administration of human growth hormone (hgh) and increased growth rate by daily injection of hgh in gh deficient children. *Endocrinol Japon*, 35, 477–484

- **Takano K, Hizuka N, Shizume K, Asakawa K, Kogawa M.** (1983). Short-term study of biosynthesized hgh in man. *Endocrinol Japon*, 30, 79–84

- **Taylor AL, Finster JL, Mintz DH.** (1969). Metabolic clearance and production rates of human growth hormone. *J Clin Invest*, 48, 2349–2358

- **Thompson RG, Rodriguez A, Kowarski A and Blizzard RM.** (1972). Growth hormone: metabolic clearance rates, integrated concentrations, and production rates in normal adults and the effect of prednisone. *J Clin Invest*, 51, 3193–3199
- **Walker JM, Wood PJ, Williamson S, Betts PR, Evans AJ.** (1990). Urinary growth hormone excretion as a screening test for growth hormone deficiency. *Arch Dis Child*, 65, 89–92
- **Wilton P, Widlund L, Guilbaud O.** (1988). Pharmacokinetic profile of an iv and sc dose of recombinant human growth hormone. *Pediatr Res*, 23, 117
- **Wilton P, Widlund L, Guilbaud O.** (1987). Bioequivalence of genotropin and somatonorm. *Acta Paediatr Scand (Suppl)*, 337, 118–121

Self-Assessment Questions

Question 1: One molecule of hGH is required to sequentially bind to two receptor molecules for receptor activation. What consequences might the requirement for sequential dimerization have on observed dose-response relationships?

Question 2: Growth hormone is known or presumed to act directly upon which tissues?

Question 3: You are investigating the use of hGH as an adjunct therapy for malnutrition/wasting in a clinical population which also has severe liver disease. What effects would you expect the liver disease to have on the observed plasma levels of hGH after dosing and on possible efficacy (improvement in nitrogen retention, prevention of hypoglycemia, etc.)?

Answers

Answer 1: Sequential dimerization will potentially result in a "bell-shaped" dose response curve, i.e. response is stimulated at low concentrations and inhibited at high concentrations. The inhibition of responses at high concentrations is due to blocking of dimerization caused by the excess hGH saturating all the available receptors. Inhibition of *in-vitro* hGH binding is observed at high hGH (mM) concentrations. Reductions in biological responses (Total IGF-I increase and weight gain) have also been seen with increasing hGH doses in animal studies. However, inhibitory effects of high concentrations of hGH are not seen in treatment of human patients since hGH dose levels are maintained within normal physiological ranges and never approach inhibitory levels.

Answer 2: Growth hormone is known to act directly on both bone and cartilage and possibly also on muscle and adipose tissue. Growth hormone effects on other tissues appear to be mediated through the IGF-I axis or other effectors.

Answer 3: Severe liver disease may reduce the clearance of the exogenously administered hGH and observed plasma levels may be higher and persist longer compared to patients without liver disease (Table 11.1). However, the increased drug exposure may not result in increased anabolic effects. The desired anabolic effects require the production/release of IGF-I from the liver. Both IGF-I production and the number of hGH receptors may be reduced due to the liver disease. To understand the results (or lack of results) from the treatment, it is important to monitor effect parameters (i.e. IGF-I and possibly IGF-I binding protein levels, liver function enzymes, etc.) in addition to hGH levels.

12 Vaccines

by: Wim Jiskoot, Gideon F.A. Kersten and E. Coen Beuvery

Introduction

Vaccination aims to prevent infectious diseases. It can be considered as one of the most successful medical strategies in this century. The conventional vaccines routinely applied in man are very effective in preventing a number of infectious diseases. This is illustrated by the fact that mass vaccination has resulted in the worldwide eradication of smallpox in the 1970s. Moreover, diphtheria, pertussis, tetanus, poliomyelitis, measles, mumps, and rubella are under control in the developed countries as well as in an increasing number of developing countries because of the application of childhood vaccines.

In the rapidly evolving field of new vaccine technologies one can discern (1) the improvement of existing vaccines and (2) the development of vaccines for diseases against which there is no vaccine available yet. Modern biotechnology has an enormous impact on current vaccine development. The elucidation of the molecular structures of pathogens and the tremendous progress made in immunology during the past few decades have led to the identification of protective antigens. Together with technological advances, this has caused a move from empirical vaccine development to more rational approaches. A major goal of modern vaccine technology is to fulfil all requirements of the ideal vaccine as summarized in Figure 12.1, by expressing antigen epitopes (= the smallest molecular structures recognized by the immune system) and/or isolating those antigens that con-

fer an effective immune response, and eliminating structures that cause deleterious effects. Thus, 'cleaner', well-defined products can be obtained, resulting in improved safety and efficacy. In addition, modern methodologies may provide simpler production processes for selected vaccine components.

In the following section immunological principles that are important for vaccine design are summarized. Conventional vaccines, which are referred to as those products that are not a result of modern genetic or chemical engineering technologies, will be addressed in a separate section. Conventional and modern vaccines are listed in Table 12.1. Current strategies used in the development and manufacture of new vaccines are discussed in the section 'modern vaccine technologies'. It is not our intent to provide a comprehensive review of all possible vaccine options for all possible diseases. Rather, we will explain modern approaches to vaccine development and illustrate these approaches with representative examples. In the last two sections pharmaceutical aspects and regulatory and clinical aspects of vaccines are dealt with.

Immunological Principles

Introduction

After a natural infection the immune system in most cases launches an immunological response to the particular pathogen. After recovery from the disease, the immunological response indeed protects us from that disease, in the ideal case forever. This phenomenon is called immunity and is due to the presence of circulating antibodies, activated cytotoxic cells and memory cells (see below), the latter of which become active when the same type of antigenic material enters the body on a later occasion. Unlike the primary response after the first infection, the response after repeated infection is very fast and usually sufficiently strong to prevent reoccurrence of the disease.

The principle of vaccination is mimicking an infection in such a way that the natural specific defence mechanism of the host against the pathogen will be activated, but the host will remain free of the disease that normally results

---

The ideal vaccine

- is 100% efficient in all individuals of any age
- provides lifelong protection after single administration
- does not evoke an adverse reaction
- is stable under various conditions (temperature, light, transportation)
- is easy to administer, preferably orally
- is available in unlimited quantities
- is cheap

Figure 12.1. Characteristics of the (hypothetical) ideal vaccine.

Category	Technology	Live/non-living	Characteristics
Attenuated vaccines	conventional	live	bacteria or viruses attenuated in culture; empirically developed
Inactivated vaccines	conventional	non-living	heat-inactivated or chemically inactivated bacteria or viruses; empirically developed
Subunit vaccines	conventional	non-living	extracts of pathogens; combination of purified proteins with killed suspension; purified single components (proteins, polysaccharides); combination of purified components with adjuvant; purified components in a suitable presentation form; polysaccharide-protein conjugates
Genetically improved live vaccines	modern	live	genetically attenuated micro-organisms; live viral or bacterial vectors
Genetically improved subunit vaccines	modern	non-living	genetically detoxified proteins; proteins expressed in host cells; recombinant peptide vaccines
Anti-idiotype vaccines	modern	non-living	antigen-mimicking antibodies
Synthetic peptide-based vaccines	modern	non-living	linear or cyclic peptides; multiple antigen peptides; peptide-protein conjugates
Nucleic acid vaccines	modern	non-living	DNA or mRNA coding for antigen

Table 12.1. Categories of conventional vaccines and vaccines obtained by modern technologies.

from a natural infection. This is effectuated by administration of antigenic components that (1) consist of, (2) are derived from, or (3) are related to the pathogen. The success of vaccination relies on the induction of a long-lasting immunological memory. Vaccination is also referred to as active immunization, because the host's immune system is activated to respond to the 'infection' through humoral and cellular immune responses (see below), resulting in acquired immunity against the particular pathogen. The immune response is generally highly specific: it discriminates not only between pathogen species, but often also between different strains within one species (e.g., meningococci, poliovirus, influenza virus). Although this is sometimes a hurdle for vaccine developers, high specificity of the immune system allows an almost perfect balance between response to foreign antigens and tolerance with respect to self-antigens. Apart from active immunization, administration of specific antibodies can be utilized for short-lived immunological protection of the host. This is termed passive immunization (Figure 12.2).

Traditionally, active immunization has mainly served to prevent infectious diseases, whereas passive immunization has been applied for both prevention and therapy of infectious diseases. Owing to recent developments, new potential applications of vaccines for active immunization have emerged, such as the prevention of other diseases than infectious diseases (e.g., cancer) and of pregnancy. Furthermore, the use of vaccines in the treatment of chronic diseases, such as cancer and AIDS, is being explored; such vaccines are referred to as therapeutic vaccines. The difference between passive and active immunization for preventive and therapeutic applications is outlined in Figure 12.2. Since antibody preparations for passive immunization do not fall under the strict definition of a vaccine, they are not discussed here. Monoclonal antibodies for passive immunization will be addressed later in this book (Chapter 13).

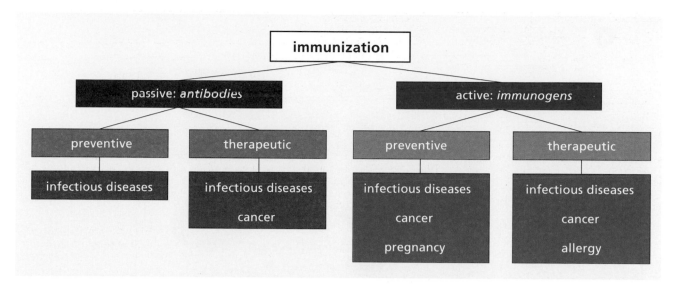

Figure 12.2. Scheme of active immunization (= vaccination) and passive immunization and examples of their fields of application.

Humoral and Cell-Mediated Immunity

Main stage players in the generation of an immune response are phagocytes (macrophages, dendritic cells, Langerhans cells) and lymphocytes (B- and T-cells). These cells communicate and stimulate each other via direct contact between surface bound receptors as well as via soluble lymphokines (interleukins and interferons). An extremely complicated network emerges from these interactions. Lymphocytes are classified by the presence or absence of certain receptors (CD molecules) and the secretion of lymphokines. It should be emphasized that cells can have different functions at different stages in the immune response (e.g., antigen presentation versus antibody produc-

tion; cytotoxicity versus help functions). Furthermore, a similar action of an effector mechanism may lead to different, sometimes even opposite results under different circumstances (e.g., at the start or at the end of a response).

Specific acquired immunity to infectious diseases can be divided into humoral and cell-mediated immunity (CMI) (see Figure 12.3 and Table 12.2). The humoral response results in antibody formation (but contains cell mediated events, see Figure 12.3, panel A); CMI results in the generation of cytotoxic cells (see Figure 12.3, panels B and C). The action of antibodies and of T-cells is dependent on accessory factors which are mentioned in Table 12.2. In general, after infection with a pathogen or a protective vaccine, both humoral and cellular responses are generated.

Immune response	Immune product	Accessory factors	Infectious agents
Humoral	IgG	complement, neutrophils	bacteria and viruses
	IgA	alternative complement pathway	micro-organisms causing respiratory and enteric infections
	IgM	complement, macrophages	(encapsulated) bacteria
	IgE	mast cells	parasites
Cell-mediated	CTL	cytolytic proteins	viruses and mycobacteria
	T_{DTH}	macrophages	viruses, mycobacteria, treponema (syphilis), fungi

Table 12.2. Immune products protecting against infectious diseases (adapted from Sell and Hsu, 1993).

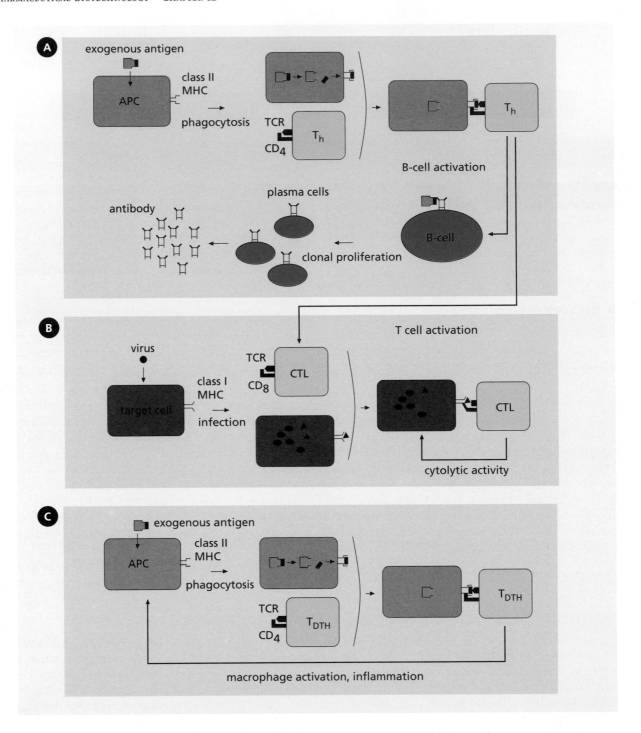

Figure 12.3. Schematic representation of antigen-dependent immune responses. (A) The humoral response. An antigen-presenting cell (APC) phagocytozes exogenous antigens (whole organisms or soluble antigens) and degrades them partially. Antigen fragments are presented via MHC class II to a (CD4 positive) T-helper cell (Th-cell). The Th-cell provides help (via lymphokines) to B-cells. They proliferate and the resultant plasma cells secrete soluble antibody. (B) The cytotoxic T-lymphocyte (CTL) response. Virally infected cells and tumor cells often express endogenous antigen fragments on their cell surface. The fragments plus the associated MHC class I molecules are recognized by CD8 positive CTLs. Upon binding, they destroy their target. Help is provided by Th-cells. (C) The delayed type hypersensitivity T-cell (T_{DTH}) response. In analogy to the humoral response, this is a class II restricted response. The T-cell becomes activated and secretes an array of (type 1) lymphokines, eventually resulting in macrophage activation and inflammatory reactions.

This indicates that both are needed for efficient protection. The balance between humoral and cellular responses, however, can differ widely between pathogens. This may have consequences for the design of a particular vaccine.

Antibodies are the typical representatives of humoral immunity. An antibody belongs to one of four different immunoglobulin classes (IgM, IgG, IgA or IgE). Upon immunization, the B-cells expressing specific antibodies on their cell surface are activated. The surface-bound antibodies recognize antigenic structures of the vaccine. These structures are called epitopes. Upon contact with the vaccine, and in close cooperation with T-helper cells (Th-cells), the B-cell becomes activated and massive clonal proliferation occurs. The proliferated B-cells are called plasma cells and excrete large amounts of soluble antibodies (Figure 12.3, panel A). Antibodies are able to prevent infection or disease by several mechanisms:

(1) Binding of antibody covers the antigen with Fc (constant fragment), the 'rear-end' of immunoglobulins. Phagocytic cells, like macrophages express surface receptors for Fc. This allows targeting of the opsonized (antibody-coated) antigen to these cells, followed by enhanced phagocytosis.

(2) Immune complexes (i.e. antibodies bound to target antigens) can activate complement, a system of proteins which then becomes cytolytic to bacteria, enveloped viruses or infected cells.

(3) Phagocytic cells may express receptors for complement factors associated with immune complexes. Binding of these activated complement factors enhances phagocytosis.

(4) Viruses can be neutralized by antibodies through binding at or near receptor binding sites on the virus surface. This may prevent binding to and entry into the host cell.

Antibodies are effective against certain but not all infectious microorganisms; they may have limited value when CMI is the major protective mechanism. CMI refers to induction of cytotoxic cells (see above). Of the cell types that are known to exhibit cytotoxicity, two are antigen-sensitized. Because of their specificity, they are of special importance with respect to vaccine design:

(1) Cytotoxic T-lymphocytes (CTLs) react with target cells and kill them by release of cytolytic proteins like perforin. Target cells express non-self antigens like viral proteins or tumor antigens, by which they are identified. CTL responses, as antibody responses, are highly specific.

(2) Delayed type hypersensitivity T-cells (T_{DTH}) can kill target cells as CTLs do, but also have helper (Th1-type, see below) functions that enable them to activate macrophages in an antigen-dependent fashion.

Activated macrophages, which can be activated as accessory factors in humoral as well as cellular immune responses (Table 12.2), engulf infected cells and foreign particulate material.

Besides plasma cells and cytotoxic cells, in many cases memory B- and T-cells develop. Memory B-cells do not produce soluble antibody, but on repeated antigen contact their response time is shorter compared to naive B-cells. Currently, it is not clear how immunization can result in immunity for tens of years. Induction of a long-lasting (preferably lifelong) memory is nevertheless one of the main objectives in vaccinology (see Figure 12.1).

The occurrence of different types of immune response to vaccines is the result of differences in antigen processing of the vaccine by antigen-presenting cells (APCs) and, as a result, in the activation of Th-cells (Figure 12.3). Major histocompatibility complex (MHC) molecules play an important role in the presentation of processed antigens to T-cells. Cells expose either MHC class I or II molecules on their surface. APCs carrying class II molecules process soluble, exogenous (extracellular) proteins or more complicated structures such as microorganisms (see Figure 12.3, panel A). After their endocytosis, the proteins are subject to limited proteolysis before they return as peptides to the surface of the APC in combination with the class II molecules for presentation to a T-cell receptor of CD4 positive Th-cells. The Th-cells provide type 2 help necessary for the effector function of B-cells. This type 2 help is characterized by the lymphokine pattern produced: interleukin 4, 5, 6, 10 and 13. These lymphokines trigger B-cells, which eventually results in the production of IgM and IgG antibodies.

Cells carrying MHC class I molecules process endogenous (intracellularly produced) antigens like viral and tumor antigens, and present them in combination with class I molecules on the cell surface (see Figure 12.3, panel B). The class I-antigen combination on the APC is recognized by the T-cell receptor of CD_8 positive CTLs. Th-cells provide help for the CTLs. For the induction of CMI (Figure 12.3, panels B and C), type 1 help is needed (production of IL-2 and 12, interferon-γ, and tumor necrosis factor). Th-cells are CD4 positive, regardless whether they have Th1 or Th2 functions. There is increasing evidence that the Th1/Th2 balance is an important immunological parameter since some diseases coincide with Th1 (autoimmunity) or Th2 (allergy) type responses.

Vaccine Design in Relation with the Immune Response

For the rational design of a new vaccine, understanding of the mechanisms of the protective immunity to the pathogen against which the vaccine is developed is crucial. For instance, to prevent tetanus a high blood titer of antibody against tetanus toxin is required; in mycobacterial diseases such as tuberculosis a macrophage-activating CMI is most effective; in case of an influenza virus infection CTLs probably play a significant role. The immune effector mechanisms triggered by a vaccine and, hence, the success of immunization not only depend on the nature of the protective components but also on their presentation form, the presence of adjuvants, and the route of administration (see below).

The response by B-cells is dependent upon the nature of the antigen and two types of antigens can be distinguished. (1) Thymus-independent antigens include certain linear antigens that are not readily degraded in the body and have a repeating determinant, such as bacterial polysaccharides. They are able to stimulate B-cells without the Th-cell involvement. Thymus-independent antigens do not induce immunological memory. (2) Thymus-dependent antigens provoke little or no antibody response in animals with few T-cells. Proteins are the typical representatives of thymus-dependent antigens. A prerequisite for thymus-dependency is that a physical linkage exists between the sites recognized by B-cells and those by Th-cells. When a thymus-independent antigen is coupled to a carrier protein containing Th-epitopes, it becomes thymus-dependent. As a result, these conjugates are able to induce memory.

When the vaccine is a protein, the epitopes can be continuous or discontinuous. Continuous epitopes involve linear peptide sequences (usually consisting of up to ten amino acid residues) of the protein (see Figure 12.7, panel A). Discontinuous epitopes comprise amino acid residues sometimes far apart in the primary sequence, which are brought together through the unique folding of the protein (see Figure 12.7, panel B). Antibody recognition of B-cell epitopes, whether continuous or discontinuous, is usually dependent on the conformation (= three-dimensional structure). T-cell epitopes, on the other hand, are continuous peptide sequences, the conformation of which does not seem to play a role in T-cell recognition.

Route of Administration

The immunological response to a vaccine is dependent on the route of administration. Most current vaccines are administered intramuscularly, with some exceptions such as live polio vaccine and live typhoid vaccine, which are administered orally. Parenteral immunization usually induces systemic immunity. However, local immunization may be preferred, because mucosal surfaces are the common entrance of many pathogens. The induction of a local humoral response of secretory IgA may prevent the attachment and entry into the host. For example, antibodies against cholera need to be in the gut lumen to inhibit

adherence to and colonization of the intestinal wall. Moreover, local (e.g., oral, intranasal, or intravaginal) immunization is attractive because it may induce not only mucosal immunity, but also systemic immunity. For example, orally administered Salmonella typhi not only invades the mucosal lining of the gut, but also infects cells of the phagocytic system throughout the body, thereby stimulating the production of both secretory and systemic antibodies, as well as CMI. Additional advantages of local immunization are the ease of administration and the avoidance of systemic side effects (Walker, 1994; Shalaby, 1995). Up to now, however, successful local immunization has only been achieved with a limited number of oral vaccines. The formulation of the antigens is probably crucial for the success of local immunization.

Conventional Vaccines

Classification

Conventional vaccines originate from viruses or bacteria and can be divided in live attenuated vaccines and non-living vaccines. In addition, three vaccine generations can be distinguished for non-living vaccines. The first generation vaccine consists of an inactivated suspension of the pathogenic microorganism. Little or no purification is applied. For the second generation of vaccines purification steps are applied, varying from the purification of a pathogenic microorganism (e.g., improved non-living polio vaccine) to the complete purification of the protective component (e.g., polysaccharide vaccines). The third generation vaccine is either a well-defined combination of protective components (e.g., pertussis vaccine) or the protective component with the desired immunological properties (e.g., polysaccharides conjugated with carrier proteins). An overview of the various groups of conventional vaccines and their generations is given in Table 12.3.

Live Attenuated Vaccines

Before the introduction of recombinant-DNA (rDNA) technology, a first step to improved live vaccines was the attenuation of virulent microorganisms by serial passage and selection of mutant strains with reduced virulence or toxicity. Examples are vaccine strains for oral polio vaccine, measles-rubella-mumps (MMR) combination vaccine, and tuberculosis vaccine consisting of bacille Calmette-Guérin (BCG). An alternative approach is chemical mutagenesis. For instance, by treating Salmonella typhi with nitrosoguanidine, a mutant strain lacking some enzymes that are responsible for the virulence was isolated (Germanier and Furer, 1975).

Type	Example	Marketed	Characteristics [a]
Live			
Viral	Adenovirus	yes	oral vaccine, USA military services only
	Poliovirus (Sabin)	yes	oral vaccine
	Hepatitis A virus	no	
	Measles virus	yes	
	Mumps virus	yes	
	Rubella virus	yes	whole organisms
	Varicella zoster virus	yes	
	Vaccinia virus	yes	
	Yellow fever virus	yes	
	Rotavirus	no	
	Influenza virus	no	
Bacterial	Bacille Calmette-Guérin	yes	whole organism
	Salmonella typhi	yes	whole organism, oral vaccine
Non-living (first generation products)			
Viral	Poliovirus (Salk)	yes	
	Influenza virus	yes	inactivated whole organisms
	Japanese B encephalitis virus	yes	
Bacterial	Bordetella pertussis	yes	
	Vibrio cholerae	yes	inactivated whole organisms
	Salmonella typhi	yes	
Non-living (second generation products)			
Viral	Poliovirus	yes	
	Rabies virus	yes	purified, inactivated whole organisms
	Hepatitis A virus	yes	
	Influenza virus	yes	subunit vaccine
	Hepatitis B virus	yes	plasma-derived hepatitis B surface antigen
Bacterial	Bordetella pertussis	yes	bacterial protein extract
	Haemophilus influenzae type b	yes	capsular polysaccharides
	Neisseria meningitidis	yes	capsular polysaccharides
	Streptococcus pneumoniae	yes	capsular polysaccharides
	Vibrio cholerae	yes	bacterial suspension + B subunit of cholera toxin
	Corynebacterium diphteriae	yes	diphteria toxoid
	Clostridium tetani	yes	tetanus toxoid
Non-living (third generation products)			
Viral	Measles virus	no	subunit vaccine, ISCOM formulation
Bacterial	Bordetella pertussis	yes	mixture of purified protein antigens
	Haemophilus influenzae type b	yes	polysaccharide-protein conjugates
	Neisseria meningitidis	no	polysaccharide-protein conjugates
	Streptococcus pneumoniae	no	polysaccharide-protein conjugates

Table 12.3. Conventional vaccines (source: Plotkin and Mortimer, 1994). [a]Unless mentioned otherwise, the vaccine is administered parenterally. ISCOMS: Table 12.6.

Live attenuated organisms have a number of advantages as vaccines over non-living vaccines. After administration, live vaccines may replicate in the host similar to their pathogenic counterparts. This confronts the host with a larger and more sustained dose of antigen, which means that few and low doses are required. In general, the vaccines give long-lasting immunity.

Live vaccines also have drawbacks. Live viral vaccines bear the risk that the nucleic acid is incorporated into the host's genome. Moreover, reversion to a virulent form may occur, although this is unlikely when the attenuated seed strain contains several mutations. For diseases such as viral hepatitis, AIDS and cancer, this drawback makes the use of conventional live vaccines virtually unthinkable. Furthermore, it is important to recognize that immunization of immunodeficient children with live organisms can lead to serious complications. For instance, a child with T-cell deficiency may become overwhelmed with BCG and die.

Non-Living Vaccines: Whole Organisms

An early approach for preparing vaccines was the inactivation of whole bacteria or viruses. A number of reagents (e.g., formaldehyde, glutaraldehyde) and heat are commonly used for inactivation. Examples of this first generation approach are pertussis, cholera, typhoid fever and inactivated polio vaccines. These non-living vaccines have the disadvantage that little or no CMI is induced. Moreover, they more frequently cause adverse effects as compared to live attenuated vaccines and second and third generation non-living vaccines.

Non-Living Vaccines: Subunit Vaccines

DIPHTHERIA AND TETANUS TOXOIDS

Some bacteria such as Corynebacterium diphtheriae and Clostridium tetani form toxins. Antibody-mediated immunity to the toxins is the main protection mechanism against infections with these bacteria. Both toxins are proteins. Around the beginning of this century, a combination of toxin and antibodies to diphtheria toxin was used as diphtheria vaccine. This vaccine was far from ideal and was replaced in the 1920s with formaldehyde-treated toxin. The chemically treated toxin is devoid of toxic properties and is called toxoid. The immunogenicity of this preparation was relatively low and was improved after adsorption of the toxoid to a suspension of aluminium salts. This combination of an antigen and an adjuvant is still used in existing combination vaccines. Similarly, tetanus toxoid vaccines have been developed. Diphtheria toxin has also been detoxified by chemical mutagenesis of Corynebacterium diphtheriae with nitrosoguanidine. These diphtheria toxoids are referred to as cross-reactive materials (e.g., CRM197).

ACELLULAR PERTUSSIS VACCINES

The relatively frequent occurrence of side effects of whole-cell pertussis vaccine was the main reason to develop subunit vaccines in the 1970s, which are referred to as acellular pertussis vaccines. These vaccines are prepared by either extraction of the bacterial suspension followed by purification steps, or purification of the cell-free culture supernatant. Their composition is variable; they all contain detoxified pertussis toxin. These second generation vaccines show relatively large lot-to-lot variations, as a result of their poorly controlled production processes.

The development of third generation acellular pertussis vaccines in the 1980s exemplifies how a better insight into factors that are important for pathogenesis and immunogenicity can lead to an improved vaccine. It was conceived that a subunit vaccine consisting of a limited number of purified immunogenic components and devoid of (toxic) lipopolysaccharide would significantly reduce undesired effects. Four protein antigens important for protection have been identified. However, as yet there exists no consensus about the optimal composition of an acellular pertussis vaccine. Candidate vaccines contain different amounts of two to four of these proteins.

POLYSACCHARIDE VACCINES

Bacterial capsular polysaccharides consist of pathogen-specific multiple repeating carbohydrate epitopes, which are isolated from cultures of the pathogenic species. Plain capsular polysaccharides (second generation vaccines) are thymus-independent antigens that are poorly immunogenic in infants and show poor immunological memory when applied in older children and adults. The immunogenicity of polysaccharides is highly increased when they are chemically coupled to carrier proteins containing Th-epitopes. This coupling makes them T-cell dependent, which is due to the participation of Th-cells that are activated during the response to the carrier. Examples of such third generation polysaccharide conjugate vaccines include Haemophilus influenzae type b polysaccharide vaccines that have recently been introduced in many national immunization programs. Four different conjugated polysaccharide structures are presently available, i.e. chemically linked to either tetanus toxoid, diphtheria toxoid, CRM197 (mutagenically detoxified diphtheria toxin, see above) or meningococcal outer membrane complexes. Apart from the carrier, the four structures vary in the size of the polysaccharide moiety, the nature of the spacer group, the polysaccharide-to-protein ratio, and the molecular size and aggregation state of the conjugates. As a result, they induce different

Vector	Antigens from	Advantages of vector	Disadvantages of vector
Viral			
Vaccinia	RSV, HIV, VSV, Rabies virus, HSV, Influenza virus, EBV, Plasmodium spp. (malaria)	widely used in man (safe) Large insertions possible (up to 41 kB)	sometimes causing side effects; Very immunogenic: repeated use difficult
Avipox viruses (canarypox, fowlpox)	Rabies virus, Measles virus	abortive replication in man low immunogenicity	
Poliovirus	Vibrio cholerae, Influenza virus, HIV, Chlamydia	widely used in man (safe) live/oral and inactivated/parenteral forms possible	small genome
Adenoviruses	RSV, HBV, EBV, HIV, CMV	oral route applicable	small genome
Herpes viruses (HSV, CMV, varicella virus)	EBV, HBV	large genome	
Bacterial			
Salmonella spp.	B. pertussis, HBV, Plasmodium spp., E. coli, Influenza virus, Streptococci, Vibrio cholerae, Shigella spp.	strong mucosal responses	
Mycobacteria (BCG)	Borrelia burgdorferi (lyme disease)	widely used in man (safe)	
E. coli	Bordetella pertussis, Shigella flexneri		

Table 12.4. Recombinant live vaccines. BCG = bacille Calmette-Guérin; CMV = cytomegalovirus; EBV = Epstein-Barr virus; HBV = hepatitis B virus; HIV = human immunodeficiency virus; HSV = herpes simplex virus; RSV = respiratory syncytial virus; VSV = vesicular stomatitis virus.

immunological responses. This illustrates that it is not only the nature of the antigen, but also its presentation form that determines the immunogenicity of a vaccine. Therefore, the determination of optimal conjugation procedures, the standardization of conjugation, as well as the separation of conjugates from free proteins and polysaccharides are of utmost importance.

Modern Vaccine Technologies

Genetically Improved Live Vaccines

Genetically Attenuated Microorganisms

The strategy of attenuation by genetic engineering of the live, intact pathogen has some potential drawbacks. The virulence and the life cycle of the pathogen have to be known in detail. It is also obvious that the protective antigens must be known: attenuation must not result in reduced immunogenicity. Last but not least, it has to be excluded that reversion of the attenuated micoorganism occurs during its production or its presence in the host. This means that subtle changes in the genome are not desirable. On top of that, live vaccines have the general drawbacks mentioned in the section about live conventionally attenuated vaccines. For these reasons, it is not surprising that homologous engineering is mainly restricted to pathogens that are used as starting materials for the production of subunit vaccines (see the section 'genetically improved subunit vaccines', below).

An example of an improved live vaccine obtained by homologous genetic engineering is an experimental, oral cholera vaccine. An effective cholera vaccine should induce a local, humoral response in order to prevent colonization of the small intestine. Initial trials with Vibrio cholerae cholera toxin (CT) mutants caused mild diarrhoea, which was thought to be caused by the expression of accessory toxins. A natural mutant was isolated that was negative for these toxins. Next, CT was detoxified by rDNA technology. The resulting vaccine strain, called CVD 103, is well tolerated by children (Suharyono *et al.*, 1992) and challenge experiments with adult volunteers showed protection (Tacket *et al.*, 1992).

LIVE VECTORS

A way to improve the safety or efficacy of vaccines is using live harmless (i.e. non-pathogenic or attenuated) viruses or bacteria as carriers for antigens from other pathogens.

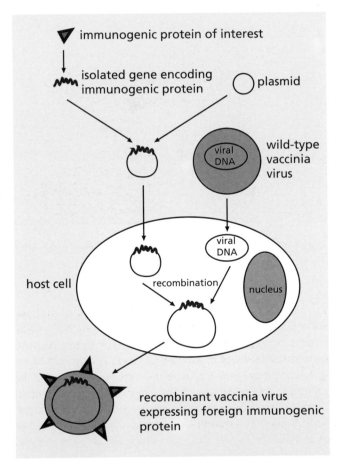

Figure 12.4. Construction of recombinant vaccinia virus as a vector of foreign protein antigens. The gene of interest encoding an immunogenic protein is inserted into a plasmid. The plasmid containing the protein gene and wild-type vaccinia virus are then simultaneously introduced into a host cell line to undergo recombination of viral and plasmid DNA, after which the foreign protein is expressed by the recombinant virus.

They are called vectors. Potentially useful vectors are listed in Table 12.4.

Most experience has been acquired with vaccinia virus by using the principle that is schematically shown in Figure 12.4. Advantages of vaccinia virus as vector include (1) its proven safety in humans as a smallpox vaccine, (2) the possibility for multiple immunogen expression, (3) the ease to produce, (4) its relative heat-resistance, and (5) its various possible administration routes. A multitude of live recombinant vaccinia vaccines with viral and tumor antigens have been constructed (Flexner and Moss, 1991), several of which are being tested in the clinic. It has been demonstrated that the products of genes coding for viral envelope proteins can be correctly processed and inserted into the plasma membrane of infected cells. Problems related with the side effects or immunogenicity of vaccinia may be circumvented by the use of attenuated strains or poxviruses with a non-human natural host.

Genetically Improved Subunit Vaccines

GENETICALLY DETOXIFIED PROTEINS

A biotechnological improvement of the acellular pertussis vaccine has been the switch from chemically to genetically inactivated pertussis toxin. The principle of both chemical and genetic inactivation is schematically illustrated in Figure 12.5. Chemical treatment with formaldehyde results in a cripple protein molecule with partial loss of conformational and antigenic properties (Figure 12.5, panel B). This reduces its immunogenicity, whereas potential reversal to a biologically active toxin is a major concern. Variations in the extent of detoxification can affect both the immunogenicity and the toxicity of the product. In contrast, genetic detoxification by site-directed mutagenesis warrants the reproducible production of a non-toxic mutant protein that is highly immunogenic because the integrity of immunogenic sites is fully retained (Figure 12.5, panel C). In the pertussis toxin example, codons for two amino acids were mutated in the cloned pertussis gene, which abolished the toxicity of the protein without changing its immunological properties. The altered gene was then substituted in Bordetella pertussis for the native gene (Nencioni *et al.*, 1990). Other candidates for genetic detoxification are diphtheria toxin, tetanus toxin, and cholera toxin. Alternatively, proteins can be detoxified by genetic deletion of active sites or subunits.

PROTEINS EXPRESSED IN HOST CELLS

To improve the yield, facilitate the production, and/or improve the safety of protein-based vaccines, protein antigens are sometimes expressed by host cells of the same (homologous) species or of different (heterologous) species that are safe to handle and/or allow high expression levels.

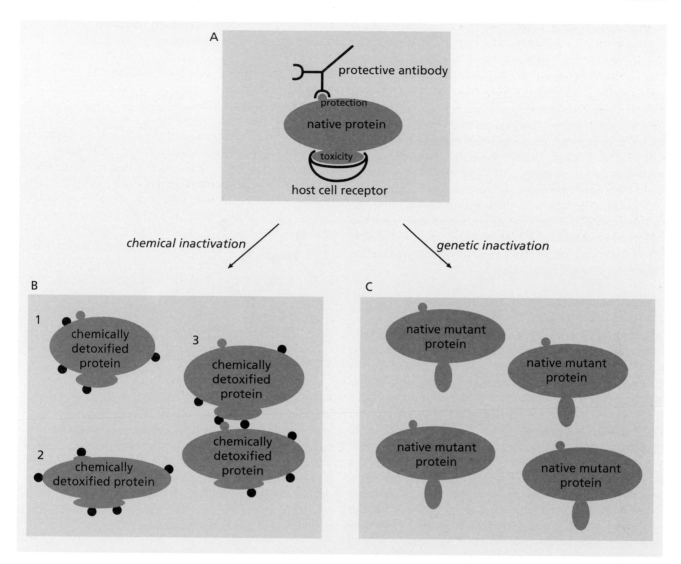

Figure 12.5. Schematic representation of chemical and genetic detoxification of immunogenic toxins. A hypothetical toxin contains an epitope recognized by protective antibodies and a site responsible for toxicity through interaction with a host cell receptor (panel A). Toxins can be chemically inactivated by treatment with (usually) formaldehyde, resulting in a heterogeneous population of chemically detoxified proteins that carry covalently bound formaldehyde residues on their surface (represented by black spheres in panel B). Chemically detoxified proteins preferably retain protective epitopes while the toxicity-related site is blocked (B1). However, part of the protein population may contain epitopes that are no longer recognized by protective antibodies (B2). Formaldehyde treatment may also lead to the formation of covalent multimers (B3) and slight perturbations of the three-dimensional protein structure (B2, B3). Apart from chemical inactivation, toxins can be genetically detoxified by selectively changing the amino acid sequence in the site responsible for toxicity without affecting the protective epitope, resulting in a homogeneous toxoid population (panel C).

Heterologous hosts used for the expression of immunogenic proteins include yeasts, bacteria, and mammalian cell lines. Hepatitis B surface antigen (HBsAg), which previously was obtained from plasma of infected individuals, has been expressed in baker's yeast (Saccharomyces cerevisae; Valenzuela *et al.*, 1982) and in mammalian cells (Chinese Hamster Ovary cells; Burnette *et al.*, 1985) by transforming the host cell with a plasmid containing the HBsAg-encoding gene. Both expression systems yield 22-nm HBsAg particles that are identical to those excreted by the native virus. Advantages are (1) safety, (2) consistent quality, and (3) high yields. The yeast-derived vaccine has become available worldwide and appears to be as safe and efficacious as the classical plasma-derived vaccine.

The experimental multivalent meningococcal vaccine is an example of the expression of multiple antigens in homologous host cells (Van der Ley *et al.*, 1995). The vaccine is prepared by extraction of vesicles from the meningococcal outer membrane. These vesicles serve as a natural carrier for immunogenic outer membrane proteins (OMPs), which are incorporated into the vesicle membrane. Each wild-type meningococcus strain expresses strain-specific OMPs. Taking a wild-type strain as starting point, mutant strains expressing OMPs specific for three strains have been made through transformation with plasmid constructs in E. coli and their recombination into the meningococcal chromosome. Outer membrane vesicles of two trivalent strains have been prepared and combined to a hexavalent vaccine, which is presently being evaluated in infants for its safety and efficacy.

RECOMBINANT PEPTIDE VACCINES

After identification of a protective epitope, it is possible to incorporate the corresponding peptide sequence into a carrier protein containing Th-epitopes through genetic fusion (Francis, 1991). The peptide-encoding DNA sequence is synthesized and inserted into the carrier protein gene. Such fusion proteins comprise HBsAg, hepatitis B core antigen, and β-galactosidase. An example of the recombinant peptide approach is a malaria vaccine based on a 16-fold repeat of the Asn-Ala-Asn-Pro sequence of a Plasmodium falciparum surface antigen. The gene encoding this peptide was fused with the HBsAg gene and the fusion product was expressed by yeast cells (Vreden *et al.*, 1991). Genetic fusion of peptides with proteins offers the possibility to produce protective epitopes of toxic antigens derived from pathogenic species as part of non-toxic proteins expressed by harmless species. Furthermore, a uniform product is obtained in comparison with the variability of chemical conjugates (see the section 'synthetic peptide-based vaccines', below).

Anti-Idiotype Antibody Vaccines

Antibodies can be elicited against any antigenic structure on almost any molecule, including antibodies themselves. The concept of anti-idiotype vaccines is eliciting antibodies against the antigen-binding site of protective antibodies (Figure 12.6). First, a monoclonal antibody (MAb-1) that recognizes a protective epitope of a particular immunogen is selected. Next, a monoclonal antibody (MAb-2) is generated against the idiotype, i.e. the three-dimensional structure of the antigen-binding site of MAb-1. Hence, MAb-2 immunologically mimics the protective epitope of the immunogen and may thus be used as a vaccine component. The original epitope is not necessarily of protein origin, which implies that immunological mimicry is not always present

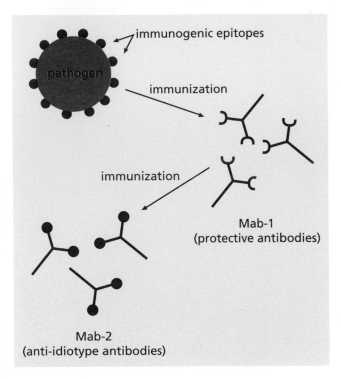

Figure 12.6. The anti-idiotype vaccine concept. Immunization of animals with a pathogen elicits antibodies against immunogenic epitopes on that pathogen. Antibodies are screened for protection and a protective monoclonal antibody (Mab-1) is selected. Subsequently, a different animal species is immunized with Mab-1. A selected monoclonal antibody (Mab-2) recognizing the antigen-binding site (the idiotype) of Mab-1 mimics the immunogenic epitope of the pathogen and can thus serve as vaccine component.

at the atomic level (Pan *et al.*, 1995). This makes the approach especially attractive for non-protein epitopes. For instance, anti-idiotype antibodies carrying the 'internal image' of carbohydrates that are difficult to produce and/or isolate in large quantities, or of immunogenic carbohydrate residues of toxic lipopolysaccharides or glycoproteins may serve as vaccine components. Large quantities of monoclonal antibodies are easy to produce using modern hybridoma technology. Experimental anti-idiotype vaccines that have been studied in animals include, amongst others, a Streptococcus pneumoniae vaccine based on phosphorylcholine-mimicking antibodies (McNamara *et al.*, 1984) and a vaccine consisting of anti-idiotype antibodies resembling lipopolysaccharide from Pseudomonas aeruginosa (Schreiber *et al.*, 1991). The clinical applicability of anti-idiotype antibodies, however, remains to be established. A drawback is that the major structural part of the anti-idiotype antibody molecule does not have any relationship with the structure of the original antigen and may give rise to unwanted

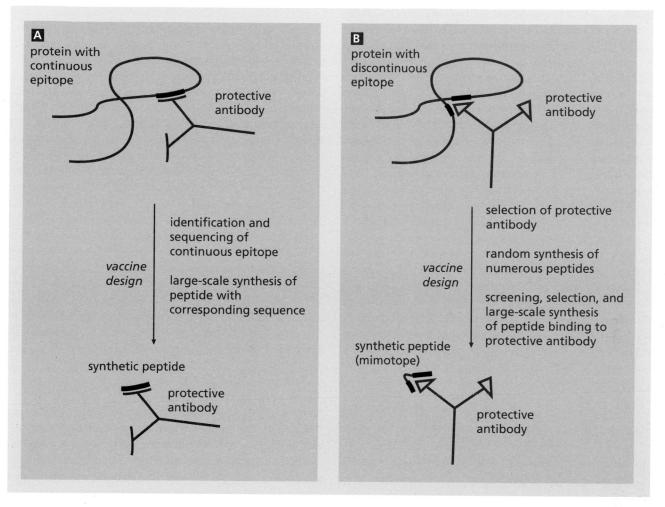

Figure 12.7. Two approaches for the design of synthetic peptide vaccines. Panel A: identification and sequencing of a continuous epitope on an immunogenic protein is followed by the synthesis of peptides with the amino acid sequence corresponding to that of the epitope. Panel B: synthesis of peptides mimicking discontinuous epitopes that are determined by the three-dimensional structure of the immunogenic protein; a peptide that strongly binds to a protective antibody recognizing the discontinuous epitope is selected. The peptide (mimotope) does not necessarily contain the exact amino acid sequence of the constituent fragments that form the epitope.

(immunological) reactions, unless human, humanized, and/or single-chain MAbs are used, as discussed later in Chapter 13.

Synthetic Peptide-Based Vaccines

Another form of molecular mimicry are synthetic peptides, which are vigorously being explored for immunization. Through recent improvements in solid-phase peptide synthesis, large quantities of oligopeptides that are capable of eliciting an immune response toward the native protein can be prepared nowadays. Primarily, peptide-based vaccines have been designed based on antibody recognition. Two approaches can be discerned, as outlined in Figure 12.7, depending on whether the epitope is continuous or discontinuous.

In the first approach (Figure 12.7, panel A) immunogenic epitopes are determined by DNA cloning and nucleotide sequencing of protein antigens, and serology studies. The small linear peptide sequence is chemically synthesized and can be used as a vaccine component. A limitation of this concept is that it is only applicable to continuous epitopes that are solely determined by the primary amino acid sequence and not by the conformation of the epitope. Many B-cell epitopes, however, are conformationally determined and/or discontinuous. For continuous conformational epitopes, synthetic peptides can be forced to adopt the proper conformation by cyclization (see below).

The second approach (Figure 12.7, panel B) is particularly useful for discontinuous epitopes. In this case, the optimal sequence of a synthetic peptide is not easy to determine a priori. With current technology, however, thousands of peptides can be rapidly synthesized at random and screened for optimal binding to protective antibodies (Geysen et al., 1986, 1987). The sequence of a selected peptide can, if necessary, be optimized for antibody binding by selectively substituting one or more amino acid residues. Such peptides approximating the native epitope (but not necessarily containing the exact (linear or non-linear) sequence of the epitope) are referred to as mimotopes. In theory, analogous with anti-idiotype antibodies, mimotopes may be useful as internal image not only of peptide epitopes but also of non-protein structures.

Similar to B-cell epitope peptides, T-cell epitope peptide vaccines can also be designed. T-cell epitopes usually have a continuous, non-conformational nature and are therefore relatively easy to mimic after their sequence has been identified, in analogy with the approach for continuous B-cell epitopes.

Synthetic peptide vaccines have the following advantages:

(1) they can be prepared in unlimited quantities using solid-phase technology;
(2) they are easily purified by HPLC methods;
(3) they do not contain infectious or toxic material.

The use of synthetic peptides as vaccine has two main complications regarding their immunogenicity. First, plain short peptide antigens are usually poorly immunogenic. This can be alleviated by (1) synthesizing them as multiple antigen peptides (MAPs; Tam, 1988) or (2) by coupling them to a carrier protein (Francis, 1991). MAPs consist of branched multimers with a small oligolysine core at the center. Apart from MAPs containing multiple copies of a single epitope, multivalent peptides consisting of different covalently linked epitopes can be constructed, including combinations of B-cell and T-cell epitopes. Examples of increased immunogenicity of synthetic MAPs are experimental malaria vaccines consisting of combined B-cell and T-cell epitopes (Tam et al., 1990) or a multimeric tetrapeptide with the sequence of a repetitive Plasmodium falciparum surface antigen epitope (Pessi et al., 1991). A convincing success of a synthetic peptide-carrier protein vaccine in vivo was reported by Langeveld et al. (1994). Peptides with the sequence of the amino-terminal region of protein VP2 of canine parvovirus were synthesized and chemically coupled to a protein (keyhole limpet hemocyanin). This vaccine induced full protection against virulent virus in dogs.

A second concern about synthetic peptide analogs is that they can adopt various conformations, which upon immunization may give rise to antibodies that recognize the peptide but not the native antigen. This is especially true for conformational epitopes. This problem may be overcome by the cyclization of peptides by using chemical linkers (usually oligopeptides). Thus, the conformation of the peptide is constrained to (hopefully) that of the native epitope. The nature of the peptide as well as the length and conformation of the cyclic construct determine the success of cyclization, as illustrated in Figure 12.8. One of the first examples of the successful induction of the proper conformation through cyclization has been reported by Muller et al. (1990). Antibodies raised to ovalbumin conjugates of cyclic peptide analogs of influenza virus hemagglutinin reacted with native hemagglutinin. The immunogenicity of the peptides was strongly dependent on the loop conformation and on the orientation of the peptide on the carrier protein. Recently, Hoogerhout et al. (1995) showed that the ring size and the cyclization chemistry are of crucial importance for the immunogenicity of cyclic peptide analogs (coupled to tetanus toxoid) of a meningococcal OMP epitope.

Nucleic Acid Vaccines

A revolutionary application of rDNA technology in vaccinology has been the recent introduction of nucleic acid vaccines (Davis and Whalen, 1995). In this approach plasmid DNA or messenger RNA encoding the desired antigen is directly administered into the vaccinee. The foreign protein is then expressed by the host cells and generates an immune response.

Plasmid DNA is produced by replication in E. coli or other bacterial cells and purification by established methods (e.g., density gradient centrifugation, ion-exchange chromatography). Only parenteral administration has proven to be effective in animals. Intramuscular injection seems to be the preferred administration route. The favorable properties of muscle cells for DNA expression are probably due to their relatively low turn-over rate, which prevents that plasmid DNA is rapidly dispersed in dividing cells. After intracellular uptake of the DNA, the encoded protein is expressed on the surface of host cells. After a single injection, the expression can last for more than one year.

Nucleic acid vaccines offer the safety of subunit vaccines and the advantages of live recombinant vaccines. Possible disadvantages of nucleic acid immunization concern acceptability issues. The main pros and cons of nucleic acid vaccines are listed in Table 12.5. An advantage of RNA over DNA is that it is not able to incorporate into host DNA. A drawback of RNA, however, is that it is less stable than DNA.

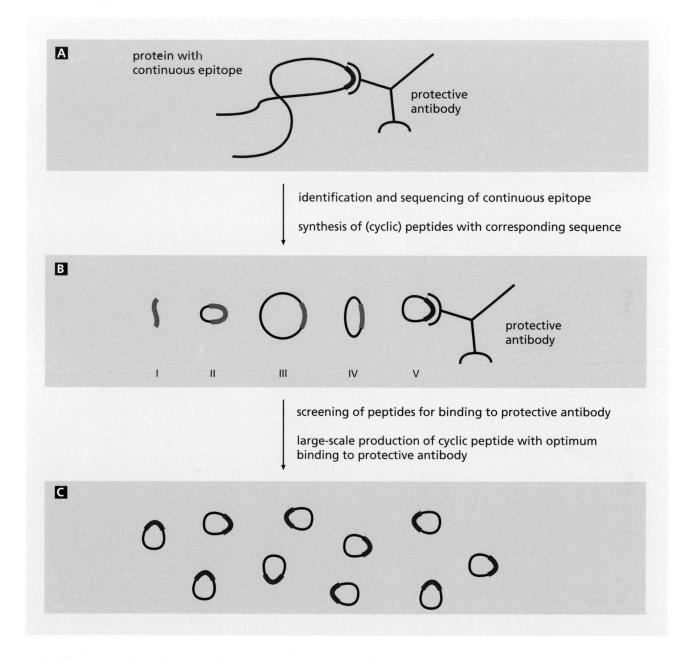

Figure 12.8. Design of synthetic peptide vaccines by cyclization of continuous, conformational epitopes. First, a continuous epitope that evokes protective antibodies is identified and sequenced (panel A). Next, peptides with the amino acid sequence corresponding to that of the epitope are synthesized (whether or not with a linker to form a loop structure and are screened for binding to protective antibody (panel B). In this example, immunization with peptides I-IV would induce non-protective antibodies to the misfolded epitope. Linear peptide I does not have the proper conformation corresponding to that on the native protein. Loops for cyclization in peptides II-IV are too short (II), too long (III) or improperly folded (IV), thereby inducing incorrect peptide conformations. Cyclic peptide V has the correct native conformation and is likely to induce protective antibody formation upon immunization. Therefore, cyclic peptide V is produced for vaccine purposes (panel C).

Advantages	Disadvantages
Low intrinsic immunogenicity of nucleic acids	effects of long-term expression unknown
Induction of long-term immune responses	formation of anti-nucleic acid antibodies possible
Induction of both humoral and cellular immune responses	possible integration of the vaccine DNA into the host genome
Possibility of constructing multiple epitope plasmids	concept restricted to peptide and protein antigens
Heat-stability	
Ease of large-scale production	

Table 12.5. Advantages and disadvantages of nucleic acid vaccines.

The concept is still in its infancy. In particular, the long-term safety of nucleic acid vaccines remains to be established. On the other hand, nucleic acids coding for a variety of antigens have shown to induce protective, long-lived humoral and cellular immune responses in various animal species. Examples are hepatitis B vaccine (Davis *et al.*, 1994), influenza vaccine (Webster *et al.*, 1994), and HIV vaccine (Coney *et al.*, 1994).

Pharmaceutical Aspects

Production

Except for synthetic peptides, vaccines are derived from microorganisms or from animal cells. For optimal expression of the required vaccine component(s), these microorganisms or animal cells can be genetically modified. Animal cells are used for the cultivation of viruses and for the production of some subunit vaccine components, and have the advantage that the vaccine components are released into the culture medium.

Three stages can be discerned in the manufacture of cell-derived vaccines: (1) cultivation, (2) downstream processing; and (3) formulation. In this section the first two stages will be presented briefly, whereas the formulation is addressed in the next section (cf. Chapters 3 and 4).

The development of the seed strain is a crucial part in the development of vaccines. The strain has to be characterized well in order to insure its genetic stability (e.g., with regard to the synthesis of the antigens) during cultivation. Next, the master and working seed lots are prepared. The development of the strain as well as the production and control of the seed lots have to be performed under 'good manufacturing practice' (GMP) conditions.

Bacteria and yeasts are relatively easily cultivated in bioreactors (cf. Chapter 3). The cultivation of animal cells is more complicated, because they are very sensitive to environmental factors like shear and oxygen concentration, and the composition of the culture media is complex. Both the seed culture, the medium composition, the cultivation conditions (such as pH, dissolved oxygen), and the criteria for harvesting should be well defined. The cultivation conditions have to be chosen in such a way that scaling up to production scale does not affect the quality of the vaccine component.

After cultivation, the vaccine component has to be separated from the bacteria, yeasts, or animal cells, and from other unwanted cell suspension components. The applied downstream processing procedures depend on several factors like the cell type, the localization (cellular or released) of the vaccine component, and the physico-chemical characteristics of the component. If the component is linked to a microorganism or a cell, the microorganisms or cells have to be collected; if the component is secreted, the cell-free culture liquid has to be collected. Filtration and centrifugation techniques are most commonly applied for the separation of cells and the cell-free culture liquid. For the release of cell-associated vaccine components, the cells have to be extracted or disrupted by physical, chemical or enzymatic methods, and the cellular mass has to be removed by filtration or centrifugation. Subsequently, the cell-free component will be processed in a series of purification steps (e.g., column chromatography, extraction with organic solvents, precipitation techniques), and an inactivation step, if necessary. After this stage the purified vaccine component (referred to as bulk product) is ready for formulation.

In modern vaccine production, consistency of production is a major issue. This means that lot-to-lot variations of bulk products should be minimal. This is realized by applying rigorous GMP rules, including control and validation of each production step, well-written standard operating procedures, collection of all relevant production data including results of the controls of intermediate and bulk products, and comparison of these data with those of previous lots. The implementation of automated production steps, in-process controls, and data analysis and collection is currently becoming common practice in production lines.

Formulation

ADDITIVES

Vaccine formulations may include buffer components, salts, preservatives, and stabilizers. These additives should not adversely affect vaccine components upon addition, storage, and application. Preservatives used include thimerosal, phenoxyethanol, phenol, and antibiotics. Stabilizers may be proteins or other (bio)polymers, carbohydrates, sugar alcohols or any other substances that can serve to prolong the vaccine shelf-life and/or to minimize deleterious effects of freeze-drying (cf. Chapter 4). Formaldehyde, which is used as inactivating agent of toxins and poliovirus, is often present in final products where it serves as a stabilizer of vaccine components. An alternative approach for vaccine stabilization is the encapsulation of vaccine components in biodegradable microspheres. This may prevent their degradation by low pH and lytic enzymes in the gastrointestinal tract upon oral administration (Morris *et al.*, 1994).

ADJUVANTS AND DELIVERY SYSTEMS

The success of immunization is not only dependent on the nature of the immunogenic components, but also on their presentation form. Therefore, the search for effective and acceptable adjuvants and delivery systems (Gupta *et al.*, 1993) is an important issue in modern vaccine development. Adjuvants are defined as any material that can increase the humoral and cellular response against an antigen. Colloidal aluminium salts (hydroxide, phosphate) are widely used in many classical vaccine formulations. Other adjuvants are in experimental testing or are sometimes used in veterinary vaccines. Delivery systems are injectable devices that allow multimeric presentation of antigens. They can also contain adjuvants. Table 12.6 shows a list of some well-known adjuvants and delivery systems.

Adjuvant	Characteristics
Aluminium salts	antigen adsorption is crucial
Lipid A and derivatives	fragment of lipopolysaccharide, a bacterial endotoxin
Muramyl peptides	active fragments of bacterial cell walls
Saponins	plant triterpene glycosides
NBP	synthetic amphiphiles
DDA	synthetic amphiphile
Cytokines	interleukins (1, 2, 3, 6, 12), interferon-γ, tumor necrosis factor
Cholera toxin, B subunit	mucosal adjuvant
Delivery system	Characteristics
Emulsions	both water-in-oil and oil-in-water emulsions are used; often contain amphiphilic adjuvants
Liposomes	phospholipid membrane vesicles; aqueous interior as well as lipid bilayer may contain antigens and/or adjuvants
ISCOMs	micellar lipid-saponin complex; not suitable for soluble antigens
Microspheres	biodegradable polymeric spheres, often poly(lactide-co-glycolide)

Table 12.6. Adjuvants and antigen delivery systems. DDA = dioctadecyldimethylammoniumbromide; ISCOM = immune stimulating complex; NBP = non-ionic block copolymers.

Unfortunately, the mode of action of adjuvants has not been fully unravelled yet. A better insight into adjuvant action would aid in the rational design of vaccine formulations. Mechanisms proposed for adjuvant action include:

(1) slow release of the antigen;
(2) attraction and stimulation of macrophages and lymphocytes;
(3) delivery of the antigen to regional lymph nodes.

COMBINATION VACCINES

Since oral immunization is not possible for most available vaccines (see the section 'route of administration', above), the strategy to mix individual vaccines in order to limit the number of injections has been common practice since many years. Traditional examples are diphtheria-tetanus-pertussis (DTP) vaccines and DTP with non-living (inactivated) polio vaccine (IPV) as a fourth component. Recently, a combination of DTP-IPV and Haemophilus influenzae type b vaccine has become available. Another example is measles-mumps-rubella (MMR) vaccine, alone or in combination with varicella vaccine.

Combining vaccine components may create pharmaceutical as well as immunological problems. For instance, formaldehyde-containing components may chemically react with other components; thimerosal (e.g., in DTP vaccine) is incompatible with IPV and can therefore not be added to combination vaccines containing the polio component. Components that are not compatible can be mixed prior to injection, if there is no short-term incompatibility. To this end, dual-chamber syringes have been developed, e.g., for DTP-IPV (Sawyer *et al.*, 1994).

From an immunological point of view, the immunization schedules of the individual components of combination vaccines should match. Even when this condition is fulfilled and the components are pharmaceutically compatible, the success of a combination vaccine is not warranted. Vaccine components in combination vaccines may exhibit a different behavior *in vivo* compared to separate administration of the components. For instance, enhancement (Paradiso *et al.*, 1993) as well as suppression (Gold *et al.*, 1994) of humoral immune responses have been reported as a result of field trials.

The use of live vectors such as vaccinia to express multiple antigens would technically facilitate the pharmaceutical formulation of combination vaccines. This may also hold true for nucleic acid vaccines, which can simply be mixed. Peptide or polysaccharide conjugate vaccine components can be combined after or perhaps during conjugation with a carrier protein.

Characterization

Second and third generation conventional vaccines and modern vaccines are well-defined products in terms of immunogenicity, structure, and purity. This means that the products can be characterized with a combination of appropriate biochemical, physico-chemical, and immunochemical techniques. Vaccines are considered as drugs and have to meet the same standards as other (biotechnological) pharmaceuticals. The use of modern analytical techniques for the design and release of new vaccines is currently gaining importance. These analytical techniques may eventually partly substitute for preclinical tests *in vivo*. During the development of the production process of a vaccine component, a combination of suitable assays can be defined. These assays can subsequently be applied during its routine production.

Column chromatographic (HPLC) and electrophoretic techniques like gel electrophoresis and capillary electrophoresis provide information about the purity, molecular weight, and electric charge of the vaccine component. For instance, formation of covalent bonds during the inactivation of toxins or viruses with formaldehyde is easily detected. Physico-chemical assays comprise mass spectrometry, nuclear magnetic resonance spectroscopy, and light spectroscopy, including circular dichroism and fluorescence spectroscopy. Information is obtained mainly about the molecular weight and the conformation of the vaccine component. Immunochemical assays, such as enzyme-linked immunoassays and radioimmunoassays, are powerful methods for the quantification of the vaccine component. By using well-defined monoclonal antibodies (preferably with the same specificity as those of protective human antibodies) information can be obtained about the conformation of the epitope to which the antibodies are directed. Moreover, the use of biosensors makes it possible to measure antigen-antibody interactions momentarily, allowing accurate determination of binding kinetics and affinity constants.

Storage

Depending on their specific characteristics, vaccines are stored in solution or in a freeze-dried formulation, usually at 2–8°C. The shelf-life depends on the physico-chemical characteristics of the vaccine formulation and on the storage conditions, and typically is in the order of several years.

Regulatory and Clinical Aspects

Vaccine manufacturers need a license to produce and to distribute a vaccine. This license is issued by the national control authority after inspection of the production facilities and review of the documentation of the production process as well as efficacy and safety data.

The quality requirements that conventional vaccines have to meet (e.g., sterility, absence of adventitious agents, antigen content, immunogenicity) have been formulated by the WHO. They have been published in the Technical Report Series issued by the WHO. Tests in order to assess whether vaccine lots and their intermediate products meet these requirements are performed in a quality control department that is independent of the production department. The vaccine lot is released for application in humans if both production data and those of the controls are in accordance with the specifications derived from the requirements.

The licensing of a vaccine is preceded by a premarketing stage. Field studies in man are crucial in this stage. First, all relevant information about the production and the control of the candidate vaccine has to be collected and described. This documentation and a detailed description of the proposed clinical study are submitted for permission to the responsible national authority. Local authorities (e.g., ethical committees) are linked to the clinical center in which the study is performed. Field studies are divided into phase I, II, and III trials. In phase I trials, the major side effects of a new vaccine are studied in a small number of healthy subjects. In phase II trials, the desired immune response and relative safety are investigated in a larger group of people. In phase III trials, the efficacy and safety of the vaccine are evaluated. After a successful completion of the clinical studies in which the efficacy and safety are assessed and documented in official reports, the stage of licensing the vaccine begins.

Most vaccines that are manufactured according to one of the strategies discussed in the section 'modern vaccine technologies' are still in the stage of clinical or preclinical testing. As yet, the only commercially available biotechnological vaccine is the yeast-derived hepatitis B vaccine, whereas the genetically improved acellular pertussis vaccine is in the process of being licensed. The slow introduction of modern vaccines on the market is partly due to the tremendous success of existing vaccines and to the fact that mass immunization of healthy children requires an almost reluctant attitude of regulatory authorities. Although classical whole-cell and chemically detoxified vaccines are pharmaceutically poorly defined and may exhibit fairly large lot-to-lot variations, they have proven their safety and efficacy in many national immunization programs throughout several decades. For instance, there is a great deal of reluctance to replace the classical whole-cell pertussis vaccine with the acellular pertussis vaccine. Also, the safety of recombinant live vaccinia as a vector for foreign antigens has yet to be determined, although extensive information about the safety of vaccinia as such is available. The uncertainties about the safety of nucleic acid vaccines (which have not been tested in the clinic up to now) make it unlikely that clinical trials will be initiated in healthy volunteers. Probably, target groups for the first field trials will be chronically, severely ill people such as cancer patients, for which the possibility of cure may outweigh a certain risk factor.

On the other hand, there are still many viral and parasitic diseases against which no effective vaccine exists. In addition, the growing resistance to the existing arsenal of antibiotics increases the need to develop vaccines against common bacterial infections. It is expected that novel vaccines against several of these diseases will become available, and in these cases several technologies described in this chapter have great promise. ∎

Further Reading

- **Davis HL, Whalen RG.** (1995). Genetic immunization. In *Molecular and Cell Biology of Human Genetic Therapeutics*, edited by G Dickson. London: Chapman & Hall, pp. 368–387
- **Dintzis RZ.** (1992). Rational design of conjugate vaccines. *Pediatr Res*, 32, 376–385
- **Plotkin SA, Mortimer EA.** (1994). *Vaccines*, second edition. Philadelphia, PA: WB Saunders Company
- **Roitt I.** (1994). *Essential Immunology*, eighth edition. London: Blackwell Scientific Publications
- **Roitt I, Brostoff J and Male D.** (1993). *Immunology*, third edition. St. Louis, MO: Mosby
- **Woodrow GC, Levine MM.** (1990). *New Generation Vaccines*. New York, NY: Marcel Dekker, Inc

References

- **Al-Shakhshir RH, Regnier FE, White JL, Hem SL.** (1995). Contribution of electrostatic and hydrophobic interactions to the adsorption of proteins by aluminium-containing adjuvants. *Vaccine*, 13, 41–44

- **Burnette WN, Samai B, Browne J and Ritter GA.** (1985). Properties and relative immunogenicity of various preparations of recombinant DNA-derived hepatitis B surface antigen. *Dev Biol Stand*, 59, 113–120

- **Coney L, Wang B, Ugen KE, Boyer J, McCallus D, Srikantin V, Agadjanyan M, Pachuk CJ, Herold K, Merva M, Gilbert L, Deng K, Moelling K, Newman M, Williams WV, Weiner DB.** (1994). Facilitated DNA inoculation induces anti-HIV-1 immunity *in vivo*. *Vaccine*, 12, 1545–1550

- **Davis HL, Michel M-L, Mancini M, Schleef M and Whalen RG.** (1994). Direct gene transfer in skeletal muscle: plasmid DNA-based immunization against the hepatitis B virus surface antigen. *Vaccine*, 12, 1503–1509

- **Davis HL, Whalen RG.** (1995), Genetic immunization. In *Molecular and Cell Biology of Human Genetic Therapeutics*, edited by G Dickson. London: Chapman & Hall, pp. 368–387

- **Flexner C and Moss B.** (1991). Vaccinia as a live vector carrying cloned foreign genes. In *New Generation Vaccines*, edited by GC Woodrow and MM Levine. New York: Marcel Dekker, Inc, pp. 189–206

- **Francis MJ.** (1991). Enhanced immunogenicity of recombinant and synthetic peptide vaccines. In *Vaccines: Recent Trends and Progress*, edited by G Gregoriadis, AC Allison and G Poste. New York, NY: Plenum Press, pp. 13–23

- **Germanier R and Furer E.** (1975). Isolation and characterization of gal E mutant Ty21a of Salmonella typhi: A candidate strain for a live oral typhoid vaccine. *J Infect Dis*, 114, 553–558

- **Geysen HM, Rodda SJ, Mason TJ.** (1986). A priori delineation of a peptide which mimics a discontinuous antigenic determinant. *Mol Immunol*, 23, 709–715

- **Geysen HM, Rodda SJ, Mason TJ, Tribbick G and Schoofs P.** (1987). Strategies for epitope analysis using peptide synthesis. *J Immunol Methods*, 102, 259–274

- **Gold R, Scheifele D, Barreto L, Wiltsey S, Bjornson G, Meekison W, Guasparini R and Medd L.** (1994). Safety and immunogenicity of Haemophilus influenzae vaccine (tetanus toxoid conjugate) administered concurrently or combined with diphtheria and tetanus toxoids, pertussis vaccine and inactivated poliomyelitis vaccine to healthy infants at two, four and six months of age. *Pediatr Infect Dis J*, 13, 348–355

- **Gupta RK, Relyveld EH, Lindblad EB, Bizzini B, Ben-Efraim S and Gupta CK.** (1993). Adjuvants — a balance between toxicity and adjuvanticity. *Vaccine*, 11, 293–306

- **Hoogerhout P, Donders EMLM, Van Gaans-van den Brink JAM, Kuipers B, Brugghe HF, Van Unen LMA, Timmermans HAM, Ten Hove GJ, De Jong APJM, Peeters CCAM, Wiertz EJHJ, Poolman JT.** (1995). Conjugates of synthetic cyclic peptides elicit bactericidal antibodies against a conformational epitope on a class 1 outer membrane protein of Neisseria meningitidis. *Infect Immun*, 63, 3473–3478

- **Langeveld JPM, Casal JI, Osterhaus ADME, Cortès E, De Swart R, Vela C, Dalsgaard K, Puijk WC, Schaaper WMM, Meloen RH.** (1994). First peptide vaccine providing protection against viral infection in the target animal: studies of canine parvovirus in dogs. *J Virol*, 68, 4506–4513

- **McNamara MK, Ward RE, Kohler H.** (1984). Monoclonal idiotope vaccine against Streptococcus pneumoniae infection. *Science*, 226, 1325–1326

- **Muller S, Plauè S, Samana JP, Valette M, Briand JP, Van Regenmortel MH.V.** (1990). Antigenic properties and protective capacity of a cyclic peptide corresponding to site A of influenza virus haemagglutinin. *Vaccine*, 8, 308–314

- **Nencioni L, Pizza M, Bugnoli M, De Magistris T, Di Tommaso A, Giovannoni F, Manetti R, Marsili I, Matteucci G, Nucci D, Olivieri R, Pileri P, Presentini R, Villa L, Kreeftenberg JG, Silvestri S, Tagliabue A and Rappuoli R.** (1990). Characterization of genetically inactivated pertussis toxin mutants: candidates for a new vaccine against whooping cough. *Infect Immun*, 58, 1308–1315

- **Pan Y, Yuhasz SC, Amzel LM.** (1995). Anti-idiotypic antibodies: biological function and structural studies. *FASEB J*, 9, 43–49

- **Paradiso PR, Hogerman DA, Madore DV, Keyserling H, King J, Reisinger KS, Blatter MM, Rothstein E, Bernstein HH, Pennridge Pediatric Associates and Hackell J.** (1993). Safety and immunogenicity of a combined diphtheria, tetanus, pertussis and Haemophilus influenzae type b vaccine in young infants. *Pediatrics*, 92, 827–832

- **Pessi A, Valmori D, Migliorini P, Tougne C, Bianchi E, Lambert P-H, Corradin G and Del Giudice G.** (1991). Lack of H-2 restriction of the Plasmodium falciparum (NANP) sequence as multiple antigen peptide. *Eur J Immunol*, 21, 2273–2276

- **Plotkin SA, Mortimer EA.** (1994). *Vaccines*, second edition. WB Saunders Company, Philadelphia, PA

- **Sawyer LA, McInnis J, Patel A, Horne AD, Albrecht P.** (1994). Deleterious effect of thimerosal on the potency of inactivated poliovirus vaccine. *Vaccine*, 12, 851–856

- **Schreiber JR, Nixon KL, Tosi MF, Pier GB, Patawaran MB.** (1991). Anti-idiotype-induced, lipopolysaccharide-specific antibody response to Pseudomonas aeroginosa. *J Immunol*, 146, 188–193

- **Sell S and Hsu, P-L.** (1993). Delayed hypersensitivity, immune deviation, antigen processing and T-cell subset selection in syphilis pathogenesis and vaccine design. *Immunol Today*, 14, 576–582

- **Shalaby WSW.** (1995). Development of oral vaccines to stimulate mucosal and systemic immunity: barriers and novel strategies. *Clin Immunol Immunopathol*, 74, 127–134

- **Suharyono, Simanjuntak C, Witham N, Punjabi N, Heppner DG, Losonsky G, Totosudirjo H, Rifai AR, Clemens J, Lim YL, Burr D, Wasserman SS, Kaper J, Sorenson K, Cryz S and Levine MM.** (1992). Safety and immunogenicity of single-dose live oral cholera vaccine CVD 103-HgR in 5–9-year-old Indonesian children. *Lancet*, 340, 689–694
- **Tacket CO, Losonsky G, Nataro JP, Cryz SJ, Edelman R, Kaper JB, Levine MM.** (1992). Onset and duration of protective immunity in challenged volunteers after vaccination with live oral cholera vaccine VCD 103-HgR. *J Infect Dis*, 166, 837–841
- **Tam JP.** (1988). Synthetic peptide vaccine design: synthesis and properties of a high-density multiple antigenic peptide system. *Proc Natl Acad Sci USA*, 85, 5409–5413
- **Tam JP, Clavijo P, Lu Y, Nussenzweig V, Nussenzweig R and Zavala R.** (1990). Incorporation of T and B epitopes of the circumsporozoite protein in a chemically defined vaccine against malaria. *J Exp Med*, 171, 299–306
- **Valenzuela P, Medina A, Rutter WJ, Ammerer G and Hall BD.** (1982). Synthesis and assembly of hepatitis B virus surface antigen particles in yeast. *Nature*, 298, 347–350
- **Van der Ley P, Van der Biezen J and Poolman JT.** (1995). Construction of Neisseria meningitidis strains carrying multiple chromosomal copies of porA gene for use in the production of a multivalent outer membrane vesicle vaccine. *Vaccine*, 13, 401–407
- **Vreden SGS, Verhave JP, Oettinger T, Sauerwein RW, Meuwissen JHE.** (1991). Phase I clinical trial of a recombinant malaria vaccine consisting of the circumsporozoite repeat region of Plasmodium falciparum coupled to hepatitis B surface antigen. *Am J Trop Med Hyg*, 45, 533–538
- **Walker RI.** (1994). New strategies for using mucosal vaccination to achieve more effective immunization. *Vaccine*, 12, 387–400
- **Webster RG, Fynan EF, Santoro JC, Robinson H.** (1994). Protection of ferrets against influenza challenge with a DNA vaccine to the haemagglutinin. *Vaccine*, 12, 1495–1498

Self-Assessment Questions

Question 1:   *What are the characteristics of the ideal vaccine? Which aspects should be addressed in the design of a vaccine in order to approach these characteristics?*

Question 2:   *How do antibodies neutralize antigens?*

Question 3:   *How do T-cells discriminate between exogenous (extracellular) and endogenous (intracellular) antigens? What is the eventual result of these differences in responsiveness?*

Question 4:   *Which categories of conventional vaccines exist and what are their characteristics?*

Question 5:   *Which technological approaches for modern vaccine development can be discerned? Mention at least one example of each category.*

Question 6:   *Mention two main problems related with the immunogenicity of peptide-based vaccines. How are these problems dealt with?*

Question 7:   *Mention at least three advantages and three disadvantages of nucleic acid vaccines. Give one advantage and one disadvantage of RNA vaccines over DNA vaccines.*

Question 8:   *Which stages are discerned in the manufacture of cell-derived vaccines?*

Question 9:   *Mention two or more examples of currently available combination vaccines. Which pharmaceutical and immunological conditions have to be fulfilled when formulating combination vaccines?*

Answers

Answer 1:   The characteristics of the ideal vaccine are listed in Figure 12.1. The first step in vaccine development is the identification of protective antigens. These antigens form the basis of the vaccine. Structures that cause deleterious effects should be eliminated. The antigens should be expressed by a safe expression system with high expression levels. The desired immunological effect as well as the route of administration are pivotal factors in the choice of a formulation form. The antigens may either be formulated as part of a live vaccine (either attenuated bacteria or viruses or live vectors), or isolated and formulated as a subunit vaccine, by using one of the modern strategies (including anti-idiotype, synthetic peptide, and nucleic acid vaccines) discussed in this chapter. An adjuvant is usually added to enhance the immune response. The immunogenicity of subunit vaccines can be improved by proper presentation forms, e.g., by incorporation of protein antigens into carrier systems such as liposomes or ISCOMs, or by chemical conjugation of peptide or polysaccharide antigens to carrier proteins. The physico-chemical stability of the vaccine components should also be addressed. The overall production process should be easy, consistent and cheap.

Answer 2:   Antibodies are able to neutralize antigens by at least four mechanisms:
(a) Fc mediated phagocytosis;
(b) complement activation resulting in cytolytic activity;
(c) complement mediated phagocytosis;
(d) competitive binding on sites that are crucial for the biological activity of the antigen.

Answer 3:   T-cells are able to distinguish exogenous from endogenous antigens by the type of self-antigen (MHC antigen) that is associated with processed antigen on the surface of the antigen-presenting cell. Processed antigen binds to MHC molecules, resulting in a cell surface located antigen/MHC complex. The complex is recognized by the T-cell receptor/CD4 or CD8 complex. A cell infected with a virus presents partially degraded viral antigen (i.e. endogenous antigen) complexed with class I MHC. The complex is recognized by CD8 positive T-cells, resulting in the induction of cytotoxic T-cells. Professional antigen-presenting cells like macrophages phagocytose exogenous antigen and present it in conjunction with class II MHC. CD4 positive T-cells bind to the MHC-antigen complex. Subsequent B-cell or macrophage activation leads to antibody or inflammatory responses, respectively.

Answer 4: Conventional vaccines consist of either live attenuated vaccines or non-living vaccines. For non-living vaccines we discern three generations. The first generation comprises suspensions of inactivated, pathogenic organisms. Second generation vaccines contain purified components, varying from whole organisms or extracts of organisms to purified single components. Third generation vaccines are either well-defined mixtures of purified components or protective components formulated in an immunogenic presentation form. Examples of these categories are given in Table 12.3.

Answer 5: Improved live vaccines are obtained by genetic engineering. The two main strategies are (a) genetic attenuation of organisms (e.g., oral cholera vaccine) and (b) use of live vectors expressing proteins from pathogenic species (e.g., live recombinant vaccinia vaccines carrying viral or tumor antigens).

Subunit vaccines can be improved by rDNA technology as follows: (a) genetic detoxification of proteins (e.g., genetically detoxified pertussis toxin), (b) expression of proteins in host cells (e.g., recombinant hepatitis B vaccine), and (c) genetic fusion of peptide epitopes with carrier proteins (e.g., experimental malaria vaccines based on epitopes genetically fused with hepatitis B surface antigen). Strategy (b) can be combined with (a) or (c).

Subunit vaccines also can be based on molecular mimicry according to two strategies: (a) anti-idiotype antibodies (e.g., experimental Pseudomonas and Streptococcus vaccines) and (b) synthetic peptides (e.g., experimental influenza vaccine).

Most recently, nucleic acids coding for pathogen-derived antigens have emerged as potential vaccine candidates. In particular, plasmid DNAs coding for viral antigens (e.g., hepatitis B, influenza, HIV) are being explored.

Answer 6: The first problem concerns the low immunogenicity of plain peptide vaccines. The immunogenicity can be improved by constructing multiple antigen peptides or by chemical coupling of peptides to carrier proteins. Alternatively, peptide epitopes can be incorporated into carrier proteins through genetic fusion of the peptide DNA with that of the carrier protein. The second problem of peptide antigens is that their conformation does not necessarily correspond to that of the epitope in the native protein, which may lead to poor immune responses or responses to irrelevant peptide conformations. Solutions to this problem are sought in constraining the conformation of the synthetic peptide by chemical cyclization methods.

Answer 7: The advantages and disadvantages of nucleic acid vaccines are listed in Table 12.5. An advantage of RNA is that there is no risk of incorporation into host DNA. On the other hand, RNA is less stable than DNA.

Answer 8: The three production stages are (a) cultivation of cells and/or virus, (b) purification of the desired components, and (c) formulation of the vaccine.

Answer 9: Examples of combination vaccines include diphtheria-tetanus-pertussis (polio) vaccines and measles-mumps-rubella(-varicella) vaccines. Prerequisites for combining vaccine components are:

(a) pharmaceutical compatibility of vaccine components and additives;
(b) compatibility of immunization schedules;
(c) no interference between immune responses to individual components.

13 Monoclonal Antibody-Based Pharmaceuticals

by: John R. Adair, Robert A. Zivin, Norberto A. Guzman and Khurshid Iqbal

Introduction

The recognition of a protective component (antibodies) in the serum of convalescent patients was made early in the development of preventive medicine (for review see Grundbacher, 1992). The use of these protective antibodies as crude immunoglobulin fractions to bind to antigens represented the first effective treatment of a number of infectious diseases (Imbach *et al.*, 1990). Sera have an established position in present medical practice (cf. Table 13.1).

Therapy with immunoglobulins is now into its second century of use. Today a large number of antibody-based products are being tested for efficacy in a variety of therapeutic and diagnostic models. The ability to produce monospecific (monoclonal) antibodies (MAbs) to immunologically distinct epitopes has been available since 1975 (Köhler and Milstein) (cf. Chapter 1). To date three monoclonal antibody products have been approved as therapeutics. The anti-CD3 antibody OKT3® has been approved for the prevention of rejection of kidney transplants since 1986 (cf. appendix A to this chapter). More recently have been approved ReoPro® for treatment of post coronary angioplasty complications (cf. appendix B to this chapter), and Panorex for treatment of colorectal cancers. Additionally, four *in vivo* diagnostics, Myoscint®, a cardiac imaging agent, and Oncoscint® CR/OV for detection, staging and follow-up of colorectal cancer (summarized in Adair and Bright, 1995), ProstaScint® for imaging prostate cancers and CeaScan® for recognizing the CEA antigen, present on many tumor types, are also approved and in use.

This chapter reviews progress in the design of antibody-based products for human use. See appendices 13A and 13B for additional pharmaceutical/clinical information on OKT3® and ReoPro®, respectively.

Disease	Biologic	Indication
Botulism	specific equine IgG	treatment
CMV infection	Hyperimmune human i.v. Ig	prophylaxis
Diphtheria	specific equine Ig	treatment
Ig deficiency	pooled human Ig	hepatitis A, measles
Ig deficiency, ITP Kawasaki disease	pooled human Ig	treatment
Hepatitis B	immune human Ig	hepatitis B
Rabies	immune human Ig	prophylaxis
Tetanus	immune human Ig	treatment
Vaccinia virus infection	immune human Ig	treatment
Varicella zoster infection	immune human Ig	prophylaxis

Table 13.1. US licensed products for passive immunization (adapted from Robbins *et al.*, 1995). CMV: cytomegalovirus; ITP: idiopathic thrombocytopenic purpura.

Antibody Structure

Antibodies are bifunctional molecules linking binding and effector elements (see below for a summary of the antibody structure). The binding site might be used in isolation as a simple blocking device, preventing the association of a ligand with its receptor. But, the binding site can also be used to target an associated effector element, either the natural Fc region itself, or conjugated heterologous proteins or drugs. Examples of bispecific antibodies and immunoconjugates are discussed in Chapter 4.

This summary is adapted from a review (Mountain and Adair, 1992). Immunoglobulin molecules consist of a number of protein chains which contain discrete structural domains, each of approximately 110 amino acids, capable of independent folding into their native structure of two stacked β sheets twisted into the 'immunoglobulin fold' and stabilized by disulphide bonds.

There are different isotypes of antibodies with isotype specific activities. An overview of the main human sets of antibody types and isotypes, their M_W and their main mechanism of action can be found in e.g., Roitt et al. (1996). Up until now, all monoclonal antibodies or antibody fragments approved in the U.S. for use in humans are of the IgG type. They are murine or mouse-human chimeric IgG (see below). Therefore, this chapter will focus on the IgG antibody structure and present approaches to modify it.

IgG antibodies (see Figure 13.1 for a schematic IgG structure) are 150 kD glycoproteins with a tetrameric structure consisting of two identical 50 kD glycosylated proteins (termed "heavy chains") and two identical 25 kD proteins, which are normally not glycosylated (termed "light chains") covalently linked by disulphide bridges.

Each light chain associates with and is covalently linked via a disulphide bridge to the N-terminal regions of one heavy chain and the C-terminal halves of the heavy chains associate with each other. The heavy chains are also covalently linked to each other via disulphide bridges in the so-called 'hinge' region. IgG molecules are therefore bilaterally symmetrical structures and adopt a Y or T shape. They have two binding sites for antigen per molecule.

Sequence information available for hundreds of antibodies of many different species reveals that the N-terminal domains of each chain are much more variable in sequence than the other domains. The N-terminal domains are therefore termed "variable domains" and the others "constant domains". Three non-contiguous regions within each of the variable domains (3 in the V_L and 3 in the V_H region) are particularly variable and are usually referred to as "hypervariable loops" or "complementarity determining regions" (CDR's). This sequence variation provides the diversity which enables antibodies to recognize and bind selectively to a very wide range of antigens.

Structural studies show that the six hypervariable sequences of a light chain-heavy chain pair are associated on the surface of the antibody as a set of loops. The loops form a large surface patch and, where structural information on the antibody-antigen complex is available, are shown to be in contact with antigen. The variable region residues which are not the CDR's or hypervariable loops together constitute the "framework" of the variable region and are arranged as anti-parallel β-stranded structures.

The constant regions tend to be conserved in sequence among antibodies of a given species, and also to a lesser extent between species. Light chains have a single constant domain for which there are two genes, Cκ and Cλ. IgGs have three constant domains on the heavy chains, C_H1, C_H2 and C_H3. Between the C_H1 and C_H2 domains of IgG is a short proline-rich peptide sequence termed the "hinge" which contains the cysteines that bridge the two heavy chains. These protein domains are encoded in the genome on separate exons separated by non-coding introns. Therefore, protein engineering of antibody genes is a relatively straightforward process.

IgGs also have a site in the C_H2 domain for the N-linked glycosylation, which can be required for structural integrity of the antibody and for some of its effector functions. Sequence motifs within the C_H2 and C_H3 domains (forming the F_c part) are responsible for the effector functions of MAbs, such as complement activation and binding to other cells of the immune system.

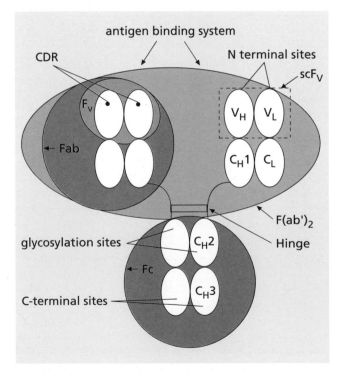

Figure 13.1. Schematic representation of the human IgG structure.

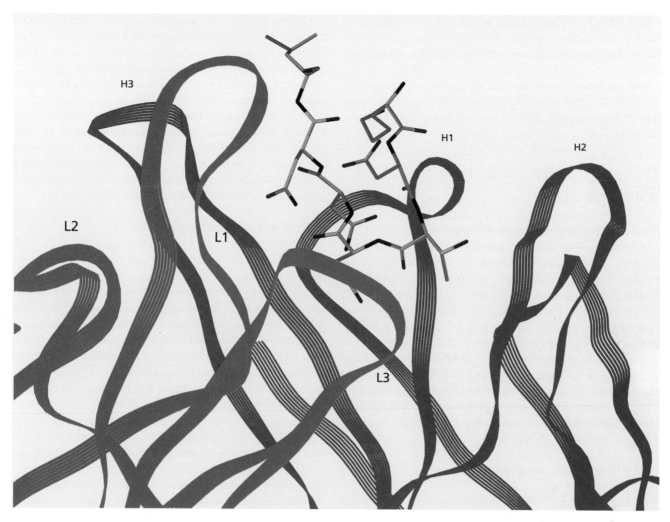

Figure 13.2. The Fab structure of the murine MAb M12 and the position of a bound antigen peptide. Structure determination at 2.6 Å resolution on the basis of X-ray crystallography analysis. The parts of the 6 CDR (L1, L2, L3 and H1, H2, H3) that interact with the antigen (peptide) are shown (Van den Elsen, 1996).

The modular structure of IgG allows the production of useful fragments of IgG: F(ab')$_2$ fragments and Fab' fragments (see Figure 13.1):

The F(ab')$_2$ fragment consists of the two light chains and the V_H, C_HI and hinge domains (together termed Fd') of the heavy chain. The F(ab')$_2$ fragment therefore has two binding sites for antigen, but does not retain the effector binding sites in the C terminal regions of the IgG.

The Fab fragment consists of a light chain and the V_H and C_HI domains (together termed Fd) of the heavy chain. The Fab fragment has a single antigen binding site.

The variable domains of the heavy and light chains (V_H and V_L) together comprise a fragment called the "F_V". This is the smallest fragment which retains the full antigen binding activity of the monovalent antibody.

Antibody fragments such as F(ab')$_2$, Fab, and in some cases F_V (see below) can be prepared by proteolysis of intact IgG. However, these methods are problematic, because they are expensive, they produce heterogeneous products, and the technology is not easily transferred from one antibody to another. These fragments can now be prepared in a defined manner by using molecular biology techniques. The design, construction and expression of genes which code for a desired section of the antibody is now a straightforward process (see the section on Assembly and Production).

F_V's have been produced, but in general they dissociate into V_H and V_L domains under physiological conditions and so they can not as such be used for *in vivo* applications. Several strategies for stabilization of F_V's have been attempted of which the production of single chain F_V's (scF$_V$) has proven the most successful one. The scF$_V$ has V_H and V_L domains linked by a short peptide linker and is expressed as a single polypeptide chain. It is possible to make scF$_V$ variants for most MAbs which retain the ability to bind to the original antigen, although obviously as monovalent binding species compared to the naturally divalent IgG.

All of these fragments can be routinely generated by recombinant and gene expression technologies and each has utility in various pharmaceutical and industrial applications.

Development of Antibody-Based Therapeutics

Granting the numerous potential opportunities for the use of MAbs and the different possibilities to produce them through advanced biotechnological techniques (see above), the question can be raised: why are there so few MAb based products for *in vivo* human use on the market? The main concerns include (1) developing MAbs of appropriate specificity and affinity, (2) engaging an appropriate effector mechanism, be it a natural immune effector mechanism or an exogenous entity such as drug, radioisotope, toxin cytokine or enzyme (cf. Chapter 4), (3) assembling the product so that suitable pharmacokinetics are obtained, (4) avoiding the generation of host immune responses to the administered MAb product and producing the material in a cost effective and safe formulation.

Antibody Binding Sites

The binding site for antigen on the antibody is a unique recognition surface which can bind with high affinity and selectivity to a specific antigen. A vast range of antibody binding sites are possible; they are the products of a process of modular, combinatorial construction. This construction process can be performed in quite different production systems. These sources include (1) murine or human hybridomas secreting murine and human monoclonal antibodies, respectively (cf. Chapter 1); (2) human B cells transformed by Epstein Barr virus; or (3) repertoires of antibody genes expressed on bacteriophage or bacterial display systems.

The phage display technology creates libraries with a large number of Fab or scF$_V$ molecules. The proper candidates that react with the antigen are selected and subsequently produced in E. coli.

A brief description of approaches using phage display technology is given below: human V$_H$ and V$_L$ can be isolated from B cell populations from 'naive', non-immunized individuals, or from immunized or convalescent individuals. Alternatively, they can be prepared *in vitro* from germline V, D, and J segment genes (encoding for the variable region of the heavy chains) by using PCR technology. The variable domain coding sequences are inserted into a filamentous bacteriophage genome, usually M13, so that after infection of E. coli the binding site is expressed on the outer surface of the 'phage as Fab or scF$_V$ fused with one of the 'phage coat proteins', usually the attachment protein, gpIII.

The phages are then purified and exposed to antigen. After an incubation period non-bound phages are washed away and bound phages are eluted from the antigen. These are then used to infect E. coli. Successive rounds of binding, elution and reinfection leads to the enrichment of one or a small number of binding sites from an initially mixed population of binders and non-binders. See Winter *et al.*, 1994, for a comprehensive review of phage display.

Antibody Humanization

Antibodies derived from non-human sources, or with non-human components usually require further modification so as to avoid immunological reactions when administered to patients. This "humanization" process is described below. Under special circumstances, the single dose usage of a murine MAb may not be an immediate problem. These may include immunocompromised patients or diagnostic situations (there are two licensed murine MAb diagnostic products (summarized in Adair and Bright, 1995). A recent survey by the Pharmaceutical Research and Manufacturers of America (cited in Genetic Engineering News 15: 14, 1995) identified 69 MAb products in clinical trials in the U.S.A., the majority of which are based on murine MAbs.

However, the repeated use of murine antibodies, and in some cases first generation recombinant antibodies which have murine variable regions attached to human constant regions (chimeric antibodies), is precluded because of the development of an immune response which leads to increased clearance and reduced half-life and may interfere with the function of the MAb (reviewed in Mountain and Adair, 1992).

Antibody "humanization", the transfer of the antigen binding specificity of a murine antibody to a human antibody, was developed to overcome this problem. Over 100 antibodies are known to have been humanized since the technique was first described in 1986. Of these, 20 have been or are now being entered into clinical studies. The most advanced of these antibodies are in Phase III studies (summarized in Adair and Bright, 1995).

The process of humanization involves the transfer of only those amino acids responsible for generating the correct binding site from a non-human antibody into a human antibody. This transfer may include some or all of the CDR regions, and may also require the transfer of some of the framework amino acids (cf. Figure 13.3).

The original description of the process involved simple substitution of the CDR regions from the murine antibody V region into a human V region (Jones *et al.*, 1986). Certain non-CDR alterations are also required to be made and this

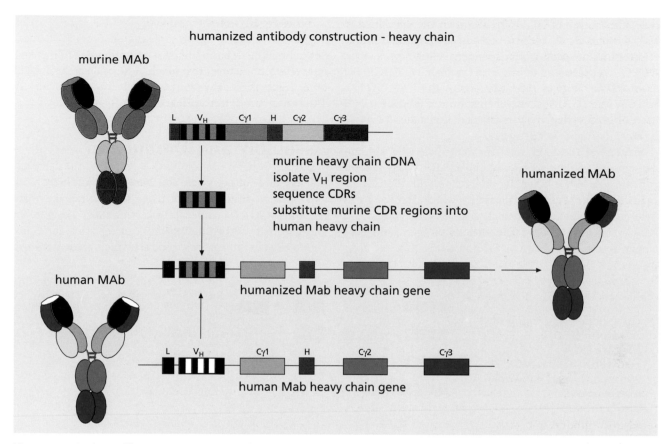

Figure 13.3. Outline of humanization strategy for murine MAb.

has led to a number of secondary procedures, each of which describes a method for the efficient generation of a humanized antibody. These secondary procedures have been recently reviewed (Adair, 1992; Mountain and Adair, 1992). Using these procedures it is now routinely possible to reconstitute the binding site specificity and affinity of a murine antibody within an otherwise human antibody. Where data is available from clinical trials it seems that any immune response to these antibodies is within the range seen for normal human antibodies. The antigen binding site (the idiotype) represents a unique structure and often anti-idiotypic antibodies are generated. This is a normal occurrence and is believed to be a part of the process of antibody regulation.

The Effector Element

In circumstances where the mode of action is to block the adsorption of the infectious agent to a cell, or to prevent cell-cell fusion mediated by viral proteins embedded in cell membranes, human isotypes such as IgG2 or IgG4, which have reduced ability to interact with cells of the immune system or complement, may be useful. Novel IgGs can be generated by site directed mutagenesis procedures with a modulated effector function of IgG (see for

example Duncan *et al.*, 1988; Alegre *et al.*, 1994). This allows the development of full length IgG, with the long half life profile of the IgG, while avoiding the interaction with other components of the immune system. Alternatively, where rapid (renal) clearance of antibody-antigen complex is desired, fragments only containing the antigen binding site may be sufficient. The pharmacokinetics of genetically engineered antibodies is becoming well understood and it is feasible to design antibody products with a particular biological half-life in mind.

However, many applications of antibody products use the binding site as a targeting element to bring an effector function to a particular location. The effector may be one or more of a number of elements including a recognition point for other components of the immune system (for example the Fc portion of IgG), cytokines, toxins, enzymes, radioisotopes or low molecular weight cytotoxic drugs. The various options have been recently reviewed (Adair and King, 1995) and are briefly summarized below:

The Fc as Effector

Most rodent MAbs are inefficient in recruiting human effector functions, although the mouse IgG2a and rat IgG2b isotypes are more efficient than other isotypes. In many cases the isotype of choice for a human therapeutic MAb will be human IgG1, because of the need to recruit immune effector functions (antibody dependent cellular cytotoxicity, ADCC; complement dependent cytotoxicity, CDC). For example, the human IgG1 versions of the CAMPATH-1, anti-Tac and L6 MAbs have been shown to mediate ADCC more effectively than the parent rodent antibodies (reviewed in Mountain and Adair, 1992).

In general, the ability of MAbs to mediate CDC strongly depends on antigen access and density. It is likely that the constitution of the hinge, its interaction with the C_{H1} domain and the segmental flexibility which results, partly determine efficiency in mediating CDC. Alterations to or removal of the carbohydrate portions of IgGs have been shown to diminish both ADCC and CDC.

Non-Ig Effectors

Several options for modification of antibodies to increase their effector function are under investigation at the present time. Some of those were described before in Chapter 4). The reader is referred to that section for more details.

Assembly and Production

The assembly of the genes for these novel antibody products is fairly straightforward using the polymerase chain reaction (PCR) (cf. Chapter 1) (Saiki *et al.*, 1985). The number and specificity of the binding sites can be varied, for example, to prepare a bispecific product which recognizes two

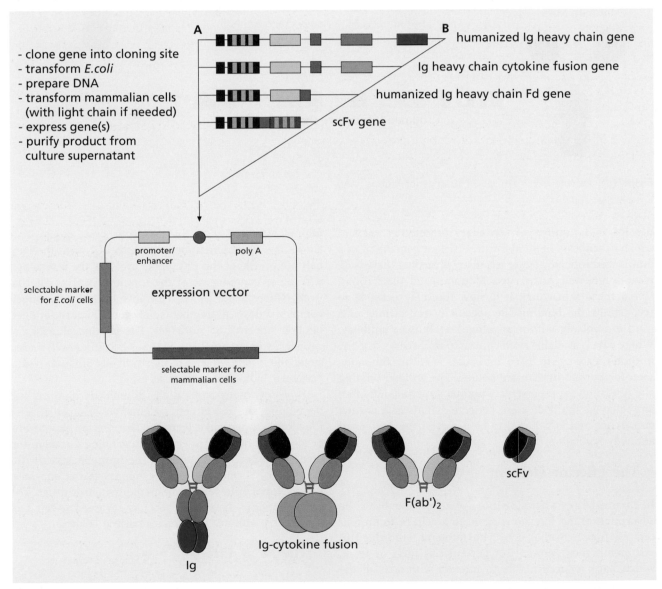

Figure 13.4. Scheme describing different steps necessary to produce human Abs *in vitro* by cloning and expression of Ab genes.

different target binding sites. The size of the overall product can be selected to accommodate pharmacokinetic considerations, for example, by using the minimal $_{sc}F_V$ binding site instead of Fab for attachment to the effector. The genes are then incorporated into a suitable expression vector for production. Figure 13.4. shows a scheme describing the different steps required to produce human Abs by cloning and expression of Ab genes *in vitro*.

In most situations where novel antibody products will be used, large scale production will be required. High level expression of antibodies in mammalian cell culture systems such as Chinese hamster ovary (CHO) or myeloma cells, and of antibody fragments in these mammalian systems, or in yeast or *E. coli* is now well understood and yields of kilogram quantities of purified antibody are feasible (reviewed in Bebbington, 1995; Mountain and Adair, 1992) (cf. Chapter 3).

Production of antibody based molecules from systems other than 'traditional' mammalian tissue culture and *E. coli*, such as transgenic animals, plants (Conrad and Fiedler, 1994), *Pichia* (Cregg *et al.*, 1993; Ridder *et al.*, 1995), *B. subtilus* (Wu *et al.*, 1993), baculovirus (Luckow, 1993) and filamentous fungi (Nyyssonen *et al.*, 1993) is increasing, although there is no sign that any products prepared from these systems have entered advanced stages of clinical testing. For the foreseeable future clinical material is likely to be derived from the traditional systems.

(Pre)Formulation of Monoclonal Antibody-Based Pharmaceuticals

Development and validation of quantitative assays are crucial at all stages of monoclonal antibody production, from unprocessed bulk lots of antibody in hybridoma medium or ascites fluid to purified antibody drug product in dosage form. The Federal Drug Administration (FDA) guidelines stipulate that certain quantitative assays should be validated, even at the Phase I investigational new drug (IND) stage, for specificity, linearity, precision, and accuracy (Little, 1995).

Traditionally, a number of instrumentations and methods have been applied and developed for the characterization of MAbs, including nephelometry, SDS-PAGE/densitometry (or imaging), HPLC, ELISA, UV/Vis spectrometry, and circular dichroism spectrometry. Capillary electrophoresis, an emerging analytical technique, has been successfully applied to the characterization of MAbs as well (Guzman *et al.*, 1997). The data obtained from these methods are used to obtain a comprehensive approach for characterization criteria of the MAbs (cf. Chapters 2 and 3). The chemical and physical changes that may occur during downstream processing of MAbs, ways to monitor these changes and strategies to avoid them, have been described in Chapters 2, 3 and 4.

Formulation aspects of proteins have been discussed in Chapter 4. Some of the marketed MAbs formulations are available in freeze dried form, some as an aqueous solution.

APPENDICES

This chapter on Monoclonal Antibodies does not provide detailed information on clinical aspects of MAbs. Information on clinical experience can be found in two appendices. Appendix A deals with therapeutic qualities of OKT3 and Appendix B describes the indications for the use of ReoPro. ∎

References

- **Adair JR.** (1992). Engineering antibodies for therapy. *Immunol. Rev.*, 130, 5–40
- **Adair JR, King DJ.** (1995). Reconstruction of monoclonal antibodies by genetic engineering. In *Monoclonal antibodies, The second generation*, edited by H Zola. Oxford UK: Bios Scientific Publishers Ltd, pp. 67–92
- **Adair JR, Bright SM.** (1995). Humanized antibodies — an update. *Exp. Opin. Invest. Drugs*, 4, 863–870
- **Alegre ML, Peterson LJ, Xu D, Sattar HA, Jeyarajah DR, Kowalkowski K, Thistlethwaite JR, Zivin RA, Jolliffe L, Bluestone JA.** (1994). A non-activating "humanized" anti-CD3 monoclonal antibody retains immunosuppressive properties *in vivo*. *Transplantation*, 57, 1537–1543
- **Bebbington CR.** (1995). Expression of antibody genes in mammalian cells. In *Monoclonal antibodies, The second generation*, edited by H Zola. Oxford UK: Bios Scientific Publishers Ltd, pp. 165–181
- **Conrad U, Fiedler U.** (1994). Expression of engineered antibodies in plant cells. *Plant Mol. Biol.*, 26, 1023–1030
- **Cregg JM, Vedvick TS, Raschke WC.** (1993). Recent advances in the expression of foreign genes in *Pichia pastoris*. *Bio/Technology*, 11, 905–910
- **Duncan AR, Woof JM, Partridge LJ, Burton DR, Winter G.** (1988). Localization of the binding site for the human high-affinity Fc receptor on IgG. *Nature*, 332, 563–564

- **Grundbacher FJ.** (1992). Behring's discovery of diphteria and tetanus antitoxins. *Immunology Today*, 13, 188–190
- **Guzman NA, Park SS, Schaufelberger DE, Hernandez L, Paez X, Rada P, Tomlinson AJ, Naylor S.** (1997). New approaches in clinical chemistry: On-line analyte concentration and microreaction capillary electrophoresis for the determination of drugs, metabolic intermediates, and biopolymers in biological fluids. *J. Chromatogr. B*, in press
- **Imbach P.** (1990). Immunotherapy with intravenous immunoglobulins. Academic Press
- **Jones PT, Dear PH, Foote J, Neuberger M, Winter G.** (1986). Replacing the complementarity-determining regions in a human antibody with those from a mouse. *Nature*, 321, 522–525
- **Little LA.** (1995). Validation of immunological and biological assays. *BioPharm*, 8, 36–42
- **Luckow VA.** (1993). Baculovirus systems for the expression of human gene products. *Curr. Opin. Biotechnol.*, 4, 654–572
- **Mountain A, Adair J.** (1992). Engineering antibodies for therapy. *Biotech. Gen. Eng. Rew.*, 10, 1–142
- **Nyssonen E, Penttila M, Harkki A, Saloheimo A, Knowles JKC, Keranen S.** (1993). Efficient production of antibody fragments by the filamentous fungus *Trichoderma reesei*. *Bio/Technology*, 11, 591–595
- **Ridder R, Schmitz R, Legay F, Gram H.** (1995). Generation of rabbit monoclonal antibody fragments from a combinatorial phage display library and their production in the yeast *Pichia pastori*. *Bio/Technology*, 13, 255–260
- **Robbins JB, Schneerson R, and Szu SC.** (1995). Perspective, Hypothesis, Serum IgG is sufficient to confer protection against infectious diseases by inactivating the inoculum. *Journal of Infectious Diseases*, 171, 1387–1398
- **Roitt I, Brostoff J, Male D.** (1996). Immunology, 4th edition. St. Louis: The C.V. Mosby Company
- **Saiki RK, Scharf S, Faloona F, Mullis KB, Horn GT, Erlich HA, Arnheim N.** (1985). Enzymatic amplification of β-globin genomic sequences and restriction site analysis for diagnosis of sickle anemia. *Science*, 230, 1350–1354
- **Van den Elsen J.** (1996). Antibody recognition of Neisseria meningitidis. Thesis, Utrecht University, The Netherlands
- **Winter G, Griffiths AD, Hawkins RE, Hoogenboom H.** (1994). Making antibodies by phage antibody display technology. *Ann. Rev. Immunol.*, 12, 433–455
- **Wu X-C, Ng S-C, Near RL, Wong S-M.** (1993). Efficient production of a functional single-chain antidigoxin antibody via an engineered *Bacillus subtilis* expression-secretion system. *Bio/Technology*, 11, 71–76

Self-Assessment Questions

Question 1: What is the difference between vaccines and sera?
Question 2: What are the domains one can recognize in a monoclonal antibody structure? What are the specific functions of the domains?
Question 3: Why should antibodies be 'humanized"?

Answers

Answer 1: Vaccination (the use of vaccines) is also referred to as active immunisation, because the host's immune system is activated resulting in acquired immunity against the particular pathogen (Chapter 12). The use of sera is also called passive immunization. Antibodies are being used to give the host short-lived immunological protection.

Answer 2: Figure 13.1 provides this information. The antigen binding sites are located at the N-terminal ends of the heavy and light chains. The effector functions (complement activation and binding sites for other cells of the immune system e.g., macrophages) can be found on the C_H2 an C_H3 domains.

Answer 3: Non-human antibodies induce immune responses against the host. Humanization of antibodies will reduce these adverse effects. However, idiotypic immune responses against the antigen binding site can not be avoided (cf. Chapter 12).

13A OKT3 Clinical Usage

by: David S. Ziska

Indications

Muromonab-CD3 (Orthoclone OKT3, also known as OKT3) is a mouse IgG2a product launched in the 1980's as a first generation therapeutic monoclonal antibody. In the United States, OKT3 is supplied in 5 mL ampoules containing 5 mg of antibody in solution. This product has received FDA approval for the treatment of acute rejection in renal transplant patients and steroid-resistant acute rejection in cardiac and hepatic transplant patients (Orthoclone OKT3 Package Insert, 1995). Non-FDA approved uses of OKT3 include: induction of immunosuppression for the prevention of acute rejection in solid organ transplantation (Debure et al., 1988; Millis et al., 1989; Welmar et al., 1989); ex vivo pretreatment of donor bone marrow to prevent acute graft-versus host disease (GvHD) in bone marrow transplantation (Prentice et al., 1982); and in vivo treatment of acute GvHD in bone marrow transplant patients (Gluckman et al., 1984).

Clinical Experience

Clinical uses of OKT3 in a variety of both approved and experimental applications are summarized in the review by Todd and Brogden 1989.

Renal Allograft Acute Rejection Prophylaxis

Effective induction and prophylaxis of acute rejection in renal transplant patients has been demonstrated with muromonab-CD3, although it is controversial whether this induction therapy is preferable to induction with cyclosporine. Several studies from the late 1980's demonstrated that OKT3 induction therapy (combined with azathioprine and corticosteroids) was more effective at preventing early acute rejection episodes than cyclosporine induction therapy (combined with azathioprine and corticosteroids) (Norman et al., 1988). More contemporary studies also uniformly demonstrate decreased rates of acute rejection in OKT3 versus cyclosporine based induction therapies, but the decision to choose one induction therapy over the other involves additional issues (Oplez, 1995).

Human Anti-Mouse Antibody (HAMA) production in patients induced with OKT3 is often cited as a reason to not use a monoclonal antibody (MAb) in induction therapy. HAMA can be produced to the isotypic region of the monoclonal antibody (constant region) or the idiotypic region (antigen binding region; cf. Chapter 12). Antibody generated to the isotypic region is usually less common than generation of anti-idiotypic antibody (Chatenoud et al., 1983). This is unfortunate, especially in induction therapy since anti-isotype antibody has little or no effect on immunosuppression and anti-idiotype antibody can prevent future use of OKT3 as acute rejection rescue therapy. Not having OKT3 available for rescue from corticosteroid resistant acute rejection is a significant concern since no other rescue therapy has proven to be more effective.

Another concern about using OKT3 as induction therapy is that rates of severe, life threatening infectious diseases increase (Portela et al., 1995). Most common of these life-threatening diseases is cytomegalovirus (CMV). CMV disease can severely injure the graft, cause leukopenia, and disseminate throughout the body if not treated promptly with effective antiviral therapy. Several expensive CMV prophylactic therapies have been developed, in part, because of OKT3's introduction as an immunosuppressant. When compared to cyclosporine induction regimens, OKT3 induction results in significantly higher rates of CMV disease.

In a study comparing the incidence of lymphoproliferative disorders (LPD) in patients treated with cyclosporine based immunosuppression versus those who had received OKT3, when receiving monoclonal antibody 11.4% of patients experienced LPD versus only 1.3% of those receiving cyclosporine (Walker et al., 1995).

Renal Allograft Acute Rejection Treatment

In the Ortho Multicenter Transplant Study Group trial in 1985 patients experiencing their first episode of acute rejection were randomized to treatment with OKT3 or conventional high-dose corticosteroids (Ortho Multicenter Transplant Study Group 1985). All patients participating in this study were 6 to 93 days post-transplantation and receiving low dose oral corticosteroids and azathioprine as maintenance immunosuppression. Both groups received a mean of 14 days of treatment for acute rejection. OKT3 reversed the first episode of acute rejection more frequently than did high dose corticosteroids, 94% vs. 75% reversal respectively. The one year graft survival rate was also significantly higher in OKT3 vs. high dose corticosteroid treated patients, 62% vs. 45%, respectively.

Reversal of steroid resistant rejections (rescue therapy) with OKT3 has been prospectively and retrospectively investigated. Goldstein *et al.* studied OKT3 as a rescue therapy and achieved a 70% rejection reversal rate in the 173 patients tested (Goldstein *et al.*, 1986). The patient population studied was receiving various combinations of cyclosporine, azathioprine, prednisone and antithymocyte globulin (a polyclonal antibody product) as maintenance immunosuppression.

Hirsch *et al.* studied OKT3 retrospectively as a rescue therapy. This study found that OKT3 was effective in reversing steroid resistant rejections. Interestingly, discontinuation of cyclosporine during OKT3 rescue increased rejection reversal to 67% when compared to only 50% reversal in patients continuing with cyclosporine during rescue therapy. Other investigators have demonstrated the opposite (Hricik *et al.*, 1987).

Other Applications

OKT3 has been tested in acute GvHD prophylaxis and treatment. In small trials of OKT3 vs. conventional therapies for prophylaxis and treatment of GvHD, MAb therapy seemed to be the superior therapy.

Safety

Safety issues are primarily a concern during the first two doses of OKT3 (Cosimi 1987). Within minutes of the first dose of monoclonal antibody being administered mature T lymphocytes are stimulated to produce cytokines. OKT3 induced T cell stimulated cytokine release is probably the primary mode of cytokine release. A less important source of possible cytokine release involves reticuloedothelial lysis of OKT3 opsonized T lymphocytes. This so called "cytokine release syndrome", results in flu-like symptoms and on rare occasions, may lead to life threatening pulmonary edema. Patients that are fluid overloaded by more than 3% of their post-dialysis body weight are at a greater risk for this cytokine-induced fluid collection in the lungs. Both the flu-like symptoms and pulmonary edema can, for the most part, be prevented through the use of prophylactic medications and diuretics or dialysis, respectively.

Concluding Remarks

Although monoclonal antibody therapy is very effective in both preventing and treating acute rejection in solid organ transplantation, this highly effective form of immunosuppression does not come without disadvantages. Anytime a transplant patient receives intensive immunosuppression (i.e. high dose corticosteroids, antithymocyte globulin, or OKT3) they are at an increased risk of experiencing infections and/or malignancies. Another drawback to using this highly effective agent to induce immunosuppression is that HAMA are sometimes formed. HAMA production reduces the efficacy of this product when it is later utilized as rescue therapy. New monoclonal antibodies are currently undergoing clinical trials that reduce the incidence of several of these problems. Through development of new products and vigilant prophylaxis and side effect monitoring of OKT3, these products can be utilized with relative safety as a highly effective weapon against acute rejection. ∎

Appendix 13A: References

- **Cosimi AB.** (1987). Clinical development of orthoclone OKT3. *Transplant Proc*, 19 (suppl 1), 7–16
- **Chatenoud L, Baudrihaye MF, et al.** (1983). Immunologic follow-up of renal allograft recipients treated prophylactically by OKT3 alone. *Transplant Proc*, 15, 643–5
- **Debure A, Chkoff N, Chatenoud L, Lacombe M, Campose H, et al.** (1988). One month prophylactic use of OKT3 in cadaver kidney transplant recipients. *Transplantation*, 45, 546–553
- **Gluckman E, Devergie A, Varin F, Rabian C, D Agay MF, et al.** (1984). Treatment of steroid resistant severe acute graft versus host. *Exper Haematol*, 2 (Suppl. 15), 66–67
- **Goldstein G, Fuccello AJ, Norman DJ, Shield CF, Colvin RB, et al.** (1986). OKT3 monoclonal antibody plasma levels during therapy and the subsequent development of host antibodies to OKT3. *Transplantation*, 42, 507–510
- **Hirsch RL, Layton PC, Barnes LA, Kremer AB, Goldsein G.** (1987). Orthoclone OKT3 treatment of acute renal allograft rejection in patients receiving maintenance cyclosporine therapy. *Transplant Proc*, 19 (Supl. 1), 32–36
- **Hricik DE, Zarconi H, Schulak JA.** (1989). Influence of low-dose cyclosporine on the outcome of treatment with OKT3 for acute renal allograft rejection. *Transplant Proc*, 47, 272–277

- **Millis JM, McDiarmid SV, Hiatt JR, Brems JJ, Colonna JO, *et al.*** (1989). Randomised prospective trial of OKT3 for early prophylaxis of rejection after liver transplantation. *Tranplantation*, 47, 82–88
- **Norman DJ, Shield CF, Barry J, Bennett WM, Henell K, *et al.*** (1988). Early use of OKT3 monoclonal antibody in renal transplantation to prevent rejection. *Am J Renal Dis*, 11, 107–110
- **Opelz, G.** (1995). Efficacy of rejection prophylaxis with OKT3 in renal transplantation. *Transplantation*, 60(11), 1220
- **Ortho Multicenter Transplant Study Group.** (1985). A randomized clinical trial of OKT3 monoclonal antibody for acute rejection of cadaveric renal transplants. *N Eng J Med*, 313, 337–342
- **Orthoclone OKT3 Sterile Solution.** (1995). Package Insert. Montvale, NJ: pp. 1762–1765
- **Portela D, Patel R, *et al.*** (1995). OKT3 treatment for allograft rejection is a risk factor for cytomegalovirus disease in liver transplantation. *J Infect Dis*, 171, 4, 1014–1018
- **Prentice HG, Blacklock HA, Janossy G, Bradstock KF, Skeggs D, *et al.*** (1982). Use of anti-T-cell monoclonal antibody OKT3 to prevent acute graft-versus-host disease in allogeneic bone-marrow transplantation for acute leukaemia. *Lancet*, 1, 700–703
- **Todd PA, Brogden RN.** (1989). Muromonab CD3, a review of its pharmacology and therapeutic potential. *Drugs*, 37, 871–899
- **Walker RC, Marshall WF, *et al.*** (1995). Pretransplantation assessment of the risk of lymphoproliferative disorder. *Clin Infect Dis*, 20, 5, 1346–1353
- **Welmar W, Essed CE, Balk AHMM, Simmons ML, Hendriks CFJ, *et al.*** (1989). OKT3 delays rejection crises after heart transplantation. *Transplant Proc*, 21, 2497–2498

13B The Pharmacodynamic Profile of Abciximab (ReoPro™)

by: Sven Warnaar and Robert Jordan

Introduction

Abciximab is the Fab fragment of the human/murine chimeric monoclonal antibody 7E3 (Knight *et al.*, 1995). Abciximab binds and blocks the platelet GPIIb/IIIa receptor. The parent molecule of abciximab is the murine 7E3 monoclonal antibody that was originally characterized by Coller and colleagues (Coller *et al.*, 1985). Abciximab is a potent inhibitor of platelet aggregation and prevents life-threatening thrombotic occlusion of coronary arteries (Coller, 1992) (cf. Figure 13B.1.). The potent anti-thrombotic efficacy of abciximab is due to its binding to platelet GPIIb/IIIa receptors and the prevention of platelet aggregate formation by natural adhesive molecules like fibrinogen that bind to these receptors. Abciximab is the first available agent in the new class of specific inhibitors of the binding of platelet GPIIb/IIIa receptors to its ligands (Coller, 1995; Topol and Plow, 1993).

Molecular Structure

Abciximab is produced from the human-murine chimeric monoclonal antibody, chimeric 7E3 IgG. Chimeric 7E3 IgG is a recombinant protein containing murine variable regions and human constant domains. The chimeric 7E3 IgG antibody is secreted into the culture medium by a hybridoma cell line into which the gene for chimeric 7E3 IgG has been inserted. Abciximab is produced by papain digestion of purified chimeric 7E3 IgG to yield the Fab fragments and the Fc domain (cf. Figure 13.1.). The 47.6 kD Fab fragment is purified by a series of steps involving viral inactivation and removal procedures, and column chromatography (cf. Chapter 3). The final abciximab product contains 439 amino acids and is constituted of approximately 50% murine sequences and 50% human sequences. Abciximab possesses no detectable carbohydrate groups and has an isoelectric point (pI) of approximately 8.3.

Mechanism of Action

Abciximab binds to the intact platelet GPIIb/IIIa protein, which is a member of the integrin family of adhesion

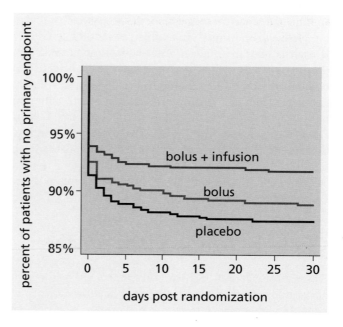

Figure 13B.1. Kaplan-Meier plot of the EPIC trial primary (30-day) endpoint (death, myocardial infarction, urgent intervention) event rates shown as the percentage of patients in each group who did not have a primary endpoint over the 30 day period. Event rates were accumulated at whole day intervals with events that occurred within 24 hours of randomization classified as day 0 events.

molecules and is the major platelet surface receptor for a variety of ligands involved in platelet aggregation (Plow and Ginsberg, 1989). Abciximab inhibits platelet aggregation by preventing the binding of fibrinogen, von Willebrand factor, and other adhesive molecules that bind to GPIIb/IIIa on activated platelets. The mechanism of action of abciximab is thought to involve steric hindrance and/or conformational effects within GPIIb/IIIa to block access of large adhesive molecules to the receptor. Binding of abciximab to platelet GPIIb/IIIa blocks the ability of platelets to aggregate in response to a wide variety of stimuli including collagen, adenosine diphosphate (ADP), thrombin, and others. The *in vivo* antithrombotic activity of abciximab in blocking platelet thrombus formation in coronary arteries is directly related to its binding to the platelet GPIIb/IIIa.

The results of *in vitro* platelet aggregation assays showed that c7E3 Fab inhibited GPIIb/IIIa-dependent platelet aggregation in a dose-dependent fashion (Jordan *et al.*, 1996). Both the rate and the final extent of platelet aggregation are correlated with the dosage. Subsequent *in vivo* studies of platelet aggregation in response to ADP in animal models confirmed this correlation and showed that the response was also directly related to the number of bound c7E3 Fab molecules per platelet.

The GPIIb/IIIa molecule is present only on platelets and the bone marrow megakaryocytes from which circulating platelets are formed. In addition to binding to GPIIb/IIIa, abciximab also binds to a related integrin, termed $\alpha_v\beta_3$ (Reverter *et al.*, 1996). The cross-reactivity of abciximab to both GPIIb/IIIa molecules and $\alpha_v\beta_3$ is due, at least in part, to the presence of the same β_3 subunit in both adhesion molecule receptors (in the integrin nomenclature, GPIIb/IIIa is designated $\alpha II\beta_3$). Studies are in progress to define the binding and pharmacological implications of abciximab binding to $\alpha_v\beta_3$ that may occur on activated and injured cells at a site of a balloon angioplasty injury within a diseased coronary artery.

Clinical Pharmacology Studies

Dose-response and clinical pharmacology studies of abciximab were conducted in normal healthy subjects, in patients with stable coronary artery disease who did not receive concomitant heparin therapy and in patients with coronary artery disease who were receiving concomitant heparin therapy (Weisman *et al.*, 1995; Weisman, 1996). Based on the preclinical data, human Phase I studies were designed to identify the bolus dose required to achieve at least 80% GPIIb/IIIa receptor blockade and to achieve complete or nearly-complete inhibition of platelet aggregation. Dose response studies with the earlier murine form of 7E3 Fab in patients with stable coronary disease indicated that a bolus of 0.25 to 0.30 mg/kg achieved >75% receptor blockade, prolongation of the bleeding time to >20 minutes and marked inhibition of ADP-induced platelet aggregation (Bhattacharya *et al.*, 1995). Subsequent dose response studies with abciximab (c7E3 Fab) confirmed that at doses of 0.25 mg/kg or higher, ≥ 80% GPIIb/IIIa receptor blockade was attained in most patients and was accompanied by prolongation of the bleeding time and a profound inhibition of platelet function as measured by *ex vivo* platelet aggregation induced by a variety of weak and strong platelet agonists (ADP, collagen, thrombin receptor activating peptide (TRAP), epinephrine, shear force).

The anti-platelet effects of single bolus doses of abciximab were not long lasting and *ex vivo* platelet aggregation and the bleeding time showed a significant degree of recovery within 6–12 hours. In an attempt to achieve a more sustained duration of platelet inhibition, dose regimens comprising a bolus dose followed by either a repeat bolus dose or a continuous infusion were tested. Repeat bolus dose regimens were not effective in providing sustained inhibition of platelet function and caused undesirable fluctuations in the degree of anti-platelet effect. On the other hand, patients who received a bolus dose of 0.25 mg/kg followed by a continuous infusion of 10 µg/min, exhibited high-grade inhibition of platelet aggregation that was maintained for the duration of the infusion period (Tcheng *et al.*, 1994). Lower infusion rates (5 µg/min) did not maintain sufficient receptor blockade. Numerous clinical pharmacology studies performed at the dose defined above, showed that abciximab inhibited *ex vivo* platelet aggregation. These results also confirmed that abciximab inhibits platelet aggregation induced by the known physiological pathways including a variety of weak and strong platelet agonists.

A large fraction of the clinical dose of abciximab becomes bound to platelets (Coller *et al.*, 1991). Following a bolus dose of 0.25 mg/kg, more than 60% or more of the abciximab can be found associated with platelet GPIIb/IIIa receptors as determined by the radiometric receptor blockade assay. This suggests that the platelet GPIIb/IIIa is the primary *in vivo* site for abciximab binding. Immunohistology studies on tissues obtained from non-human primates treated with abciximab do not indicate substantial binding of abciximab to normal cells or tissues except to platelets and megakaryocytes (Jordan *et al.*, 1996).

Key Clinical Efficacy Studies

Abciximab first gained approval for protection against ischemic complications that may accompany high-risk percutaneous transluminal coronary angioplasty (PTCA) procedures. This indication was established in a 2099-patient, randomized placebo controlled clinical trial (The EPIC Investigators, 1994). All patients in the EPIC trial also received standard antiplatelet (aspirin) and anticoagulant (heparin) therapy and other appropriate cardiovascular medications. A bolus plus 12-hour infusion of abciximab demonstrated a 35% reduction in the 30-day composite primary endpoint which consisted of a combination of death, or myocardial infarction or the need for urgent repeat revascularization. The bolus dose was a weight-adjusted injection of 0.25 mg of abciximab per kg of body weight and the infusion was non-weight-adjusted, 12-hour infusion at 10 µg/min. A group of patients receiving the same bolus dose without the accompanying 12-hour infusion did not demonstrate a statistically-significant benefit at 30 days. A Kaplan-Meier plot of the 30-day primary end point results is presented in Figure 13.B1. In the EPIC trial, there was an increased rate of bleeding episodes in patients who received abciximab plus the standard anticoagulant dose of heparin.

A subsequent 4800-patient Phase III clinical trial that included patients at lower risk for PTCA complications designated EPILOG, confirmed the 30-day benefit of abciximab seen in the EPIC trial. This trial was terminated ahead of schedule based on the highly significant efficacy seen at interim analysis (Ferguson, 1996). The 0.25 mg/kg bolus plus a weight-adjusted, 0.125 µg/kg/min 12-hour infusion dose resulted in a 65% decrease of ischemic complications at 30 days. Importantly, the use of a lower, 70 unit/kg weight-adjusted dose of heparin in EPILOG reduced bleeding rates in the abciximab-treatment group to the same level as in patients receiving heparin alone. The dramatic increase in efficacy in EPILOG compared to EPIC may be related to procedural factors and the lowered heparin dose that reduced bleeding side effects. In both the EPIC and EPILOG clinical trials, the abciximab bolus was given at the time of the PTCA procedure and the abciximab infusion was continued for 12 hours thereafter.

An alternative abciximab dose regimen was used in another large randomized, placebo-controlled Phase III clinical trial conducted in patients with severe unstable angina (CAPTURE trial). Unstable angina is caused by recurrent thrombotic ischemia within the coronary circulation. In the 1400 patient CAPTURE trial, abciximab-treated patients received a 0.25 mg/kg bolus approximately 24 hours before PTCA followed by a non-weight adjusted 10 µg/min abciximab infusion until approximately 1 hour following PTCA. This trial was also stopped ahead of schedule due to significant reduction of thrombotic ischemic complications due to PTCA (Ferguson, 1996). Thus, confirmation of 30-day anti-thrombotic benefit was gained in 3 large placebo-controlled trials in different patient groups. In the EPIC trial, long-term benefit against ischemic events was maintained at 6-months following the PTCA (Topol et al., 1994).

Pharmacokinetics and Pharmacodynamics

Abciximab is administered as an intravenous bolus injection of 0.25 mg/kg followed by a non-weight-adjusted continuous infusion of 10 µg/minute for 12 hrs. The effects of abciximab on platelet aggregation occur immediately after binding. This binding of abciximab to platelets and its presence in plasma is detectable soon after administration of the initial bolus injection. To investigate the in vivo pharmacokinetic profile of abciximab, quantitative methods for measuring both platelet-bound abciximab and free plasma abciximab were used.

Pharmacodynamics of Platelet-bound Abciximab

The primary method for measuring in vivo bound abciximab assesses the number of platelet GPIIb/IIIa molecules available for ex vivo binding by a radiolabeled form of abciximab. In this assay, ^{125}I labeled 7E3 IgG is incubated with platelet samples obtained from a patient at different times after abciximab administration (Coller, 1985). Measurements performed on samples obtained prior to abciximab treatment quantify the average total number of receptors per platelet. Later measurements reveal lower numbers of binding sites for ^{125}I 7E3 IgG that correspond with the blockade occurring in vivo from abciximab treatment. Following a dose of 0.25 mg abciximab per kg body weight, most patients exhibit greater than 80% blockade of the total number of GPIIb/IIIa receptors. Following cessation of the continuous infusion, there is a gradual recovery of unblocked receptors that results in the average degree of receptor blockade falling below 80% within several hours. Partial recovery of platelet function, as measured by ex vivo platelet aggregation, is evident when receptor blockade is less than 80%. The continued recovery of unblocked receptors occurs in a gradual, tapered manner. At one week following therapy, an average receptor blockade of approximately 10–20% is still evident in most patients.

A second method for detection of platelet-bound abciximab is a flow cytometric measurement of individual platelets. This method uses a fluorescent second antibody procedure to detect platelet-bound abciximab. The flow cytometric method differs from the radiometric receptor blockade technique in that it provides information about individual platelets whereas the radiometric method represents an average measurement on all platelets in the sample being tested. Flow cytometry provided important data on the distribution and pharmacodynamics of abciximab. Immediately after treatment with abciximab, all platelets in circulation are highly fluorescent indicating the presence of abciximab on all platelets. During therapy, the degree of fluorescence on circulating platelets gradually decreases in parallel with the gradually decreasing number of abciximab molecules on the platelet surface. Importantly, all circulating platelets continue to possess surface-bound abciximab even 2 weeks after administration when the level of fluorescence returns to near baseline levels. No evidence of a second peak of non-fluorescent platelets is seen at any point in the post-treatment period when abciximab is still detectable. Since new platelets are continually being synthesized in the bone marrow and then circulate for 7–10 days, the data suggest that new platelets also acquire abciximab. Thus, these results are consistent with a pharmacodynamic pattern in which abciximab slowly re-equilibrates among circulating platelets to yield a homogeneous, unimodal population of platelets with a gradually decreasing receptor blockade. The duration of attachment of abciximab on circulating platelets exceeds the period of several days of measurable inhibition of platelet aggregation, which is the desired pharmaco-dynamic effect.

Pharmacokinetics of Free Plasma Abciximab

Free plasma abciximab is quantified in platelet-poor plasma by an EIA method in which abciximab is captured and detected by antibodies that specifically bind to abciximab. Following a bolus dose of 0.25 mg/kg, a maximum plasma concentration of approximately 1 to 2 µg/mL is detected soon (< 20 minutes) after injection. The plasma concentration of abciximab rapidly declines thereafter, typically resulting in a concentration < 0.5 µg/mL and < 0.1 µg/mL at 1 hour and 12 hours, respectively. If an administration protocol of 0.25 mg/kg bolus plus 12-hour infusion of 10 µg/minute (or alternatively, a weight-adjusted 0.125 µg/kg-min infusion) is used, a different pattern is observed. Throughout the duration of the continuous abciximab infusion, detectable concentrations of abciximab are maintained at approximately 0.1 to 0.3 µg/mL. An abciximab concentration of 0.1 to 0.3 µg/mL is lower than the ~1 µg/mL IC50 for inhibition of *in vitro* platelet aggregation, but is sufficient to sustain the inhibition of platelet aggregation that resulted *in vivo* from the bolus injection. Following cessation of the infusion, the plasma abciximab concentration rapidly declines within 2 hours to < 0.1 µg/mL.

Partial reversal of the anti-platelet effect of abciximab occurs spontaneously within several hours after the termination of treatment. In more acute situations, the transfusion of donor platelets into an abciximab-treated patient results in an immediate, partial normalization of platelet function. Reversal occurs immediately because of the low concentration of free plasma abciximab that is insufficient to inhibit the function of the newly-transfused platelets.

There are no data from systematic studies involving re-administration of abciximab. Administration of abciximab may result in human anti-chimeric antibody (HACA) formation that can cause allergic or hypersensitivity reactions (including anaphylaxis), thrombocytopenia or diminished benefit upon re-administration of abciximab. In the Phase III EPIC trial, positive HACA responses occurred in 6.5% of the patients in the bolus plus infusion group. There was no evidence of excess hypersensitivity or allergic reactions related to initial abciximab treatment compared with placebo treatment in the EPIC trial.

Formulation and Dosage Information

The recommended dosage of abciximab is an intravenous bolus of 0.25 mg/kg administered 10–60 minutes before the start of PTCA, followed by a continuous infusion of 10 µg/min for 12 hours.

Abciximab (2 mg/mL) is supplied in 5 mL vials. Each vial contains 2 mg/mL of abciximab in a buffered solution (pH 7.2) of 0.01 M sodium phosphate, 0.15 M sodium chloride and 0.001% polysorbate 80 in Water for Injection. No preservatives are added. Vials should be stored at 2 to 8°C. Under correct storage conditions, abciximab has been shown to be stable for 3 years.

From the instructions for administration as per the 1996 package insert for abciximab the following is excerpted (also see Chapter 17):

1. Hypersensitivity reactions should be anticipated whenever protein solutions such as abciximab are administered. Epinephrine, dopamine, theophylline, antihistamines and corticosteroids should be available for immediate use. If symptoms of an allergic reaction or anaphylaxis appear, the infusion should be stopped and appropriate treatment given.
2. Withdraw the necessary amount of abciximab (2 mg/mL) for bolus injection through a sterile, non-pyrogenic low protein-binding 0.2 or 0.22 µm filter (Millipore SLGV025LS or equivalent) into a syringe. The bolus should be administered 10–60 minutes before the procedure.
3. Withdraw 4.5 mL of abciximab for the continuous infusion through a sterile, non-pyrogenic low protein-binding 0.2 or 0.22 µm filter (Millipore SLGV025LS or equivalent) into a syringe. Inject into 250 mL of sterile 0.9% saline or 5% dextrose and infuse at a rate of 17 mL/hour (10 µg/min) for 12 hours via a continuous infusion pump equipped with an in-line sterile, non-pyrogenic, low protein-binding 0.2 or 0.22 µm filter (Abbot #4524 or equivalent). Discard the unused portion at the end of the 12 hour infusion.
4. Abciximab should be administered in a separate intravenous line; no other medication should be added to the infusion solutions.
5. No incompatibilities have been observed with glass bottles or polyvinyl chloride bags and administration sets. ■

Appendix 13B: References

- **Bhattacharya S, Jordan R, Machin S, Senior R, Mackie I, Smith CR, Schaible TF, Weisman HF, Lahiri A.** (1995). Blockade of the human platelet GPIIb/IIIa receptor by a murine monoclonal antibody Fab fragment (7E3), Potent dose-dependent inhibition of platelet function. *Cardiovasc Drugs Ther*, 9, 665–675

- **Coller BS.** (1985). A new murine monoclonal antibody reports an activation-dependent change in the conformation and/or microenvironment of the platelet glycoprotein IIb/IIIa complex. *J Clin Invest*, 76, 101–108

- **Coller BS.** (1992). Platelets in cardiovascular thrombosis and thrombolysis. In *The Heart and Cardiovascular System*, edited by HA Fozzard, *et al*. New York: Raven, pp. 219–273

- **Coller BS.** (1995). Blockade of platelet GPIIb/IIIa receptors as an antithrombotic strategy. *Circulation*, 92, 2373–2380

- **Coller BS, Scudder LE, Beer J, Gold HK, Folts JD, Cavagnaro J, Jordan R, Wagner C, Iuliucci J, Knight D, Ghrayeb J, Smith C, Weisman HF, Berger H.** (1991). Monoclonal antibodies to platelet glycoprotein IIb/III as antithrombotic agents. *Ann NY Acad Sci*, 614, 193–213

- **Ferguson III, JJ.** (1996). EPILOG and CAPTURE trials halted because of positive interim results. *Circulation*, 93, 637

- **Jordan RE, Wagner CL, Mascelli MA, Treacy G, Nedelman MA, Woody JN, Weisman HF, Coller BS.** (1996). Preclinical development of c7E3 Fab; a mouse/human chimeric monoclonal antibody fragment that inhibits platelet function by blockade of GPIIb/IIIa receptors with observations on the immunogenicity of c7E3 Fab in humans. In *Adhesion Receptors as Therapeutic Targets*, edited by MA Horton. London: CRC, pp. 281–305

- **Knight DM, Wagner C, Jordan R, McAleer MF, DeRita R, Fass DN, Coller BS, Weisman HF, Ghrayeb J.** (1995). The immunogenicity of the 7E3 murine monoclonal Fab antibody fragment variable region is dramatically reduced in humans by substitution of human for murine constant regions. *Mol Immunol*, 32, 1271–1281

- **Plow EF, Ginsberg MH.** (1989). Cellular adhesion, GPIIb/IIIa as a prototypic adhesion receptor. *Prog Hemost Thromb*, 9, 117–156

- **Reverter JC, Beguin S, Kessels H, Kumar R, Hemker HC, Coller BS.** (1996). Inhibition of platelet-mediated, tissue factor-induced thrombin generation by the mouse/human chimeric 7E3 antibody. *J Clin Invest*, 98, 863–874

- **Tcheng JE, Ellis SG, George BS, Kereiakes DJ, Kleiman NS, Talley JD, Wang AL, Weisman HF, Califf RM, Topol EJ.** (1994). Pharmacodynamics of chimeric glycoprotein IIb/IIIa integrin antiplatelet antibody Fab 7E3 in high-risk coronary angioplasty. *Circulation*, 90, 1757–1764

- **The EPIC Investigators.** (1994). Use of a monoclonal antibody directed against the platelet glycoprotein IIb/IIIa receptor in high-risk coronary angioplasty. *NEJM*, 330, 956–961

- **Topol EJ, Califf RM, Weisman HF, Ellis SG, Tcheng JE, Worley S, Ivanhoe R, George BS, Fintel D, Weston M, Sigmon K, Anderson KM, Lee KL, Willerson JT.** (1994) on behalf of the EPIC investigators. Randomised trial of coronary intervention with antibody against platelet IIb/IIIa integrin for reduction of clinical restenosis, results at six months. *Lancet*, 343, 881–886

- **Topol EJ, Plow EF.** (1994). Clinical trials of platelet receptor inhibitors. *Thromb Haemost*, 70, 94–98

- **Weisman HF.** (1996). ReoPro clinical development, Future directions and therapeutic approaches. *J Invasive Cardiology*, 8, 51B-61B

- **Weisman HF, Schaible TF, Jordan RE, Cabot CF, Anderson KM.** (1995). Anti-platelet monoclonal antibodies for the prevention of arterial thrombosis, experience with ReoPro, a monoclonal antibody directed against the platelet GPIIb/IIIa receptor. *Therapeutic Monoclonals*, 23, 1052–1057

14 Recombinant Tissue-Type Plasminogen Activator and Factor VIII

by: Nishit B. Modi

Introduction

Coagulation and fibrinolysis normally exist in a mutually compensatory or balanced state. Endogenous regulatory mechanisms ensure that the process of hemostasis and blood coagulation at a site of injury and the subsequent fibrinolysis of the blood clot is normally localized and well controlled. This ensures a rapid and efficient hemostatic response at the site of injury while avoiding thrombogenic events at sites distant from the site of injury or the hemostatic response from persisting beyond its physiologic need. This chapter will focus on the therapeutic aspects of recombinant tissue-type plasminogen activator (rt-PA) and Factor VIII which are now available through recombinant technology.

Tissue-Type Plasminogen Activator

Introduction

Deposition of fibrin and platelets in the vasculature causes thromboembolic diseases which are responsible for considerable mortality and morbidity. Early thrombolytic therapy can decrease mortality and improve coronary artery patency in patients with an acute myocardial infarction (AMI) (Bates and Topol, 1989). During fibrinolysis, the inactive zymogen plasminogen is enzymatically converted to the active moiety, plasmin, by various physiologic plasminogen activators, such as tissue-type plasminogen activator and single-chain urokinase-type plasminogen activator (scu-PA). Plasmin subsequently digests the insoluble fibrin matrix of a thrombus to yield soluble fibrin degradation products (Figure 14.1). Tissue plasminogen activator (t-PA) exhibits fibrin-specific plasminogen activation (Hoylaerts *et al.*, 1982), with minimal systemic fibrinogenolysis. The relative absence of systemic fibrinogenolysis with t-PA means that there are fewer systemic side effects compared to other plasminogen activators. Furthermore, t-PA is not associated with the allergic and hypotensive effects reported for the non-endogenous plasminogen activators, streptokinase and acylated plasminogen-streptokinase activator complex (APSAC).

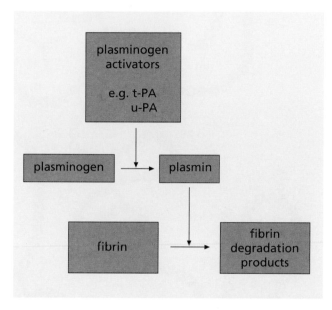

Figure 14.1. Schematic representation of the fibrinolytic pathway.

Structure

Native tissue-type plasminogen activator is a serine protease synthesized by vascular endothelial cells as a single chain polypeptide of 527 amino acids and has a molecular mass of 64 kD (Pennica *et al.*, 1983). Approximately 6–8% of the molecular mass consists of carbohydrate. A schematic primary structure of human t-PA is shown in Figure 14.2. There are seventeen disulfide bridges and four putative N-linked glycosylation sites recognized by the consensus sequence Asn-X-Ser/Thr at residues 117, 184, 218, and 448 (Pennica *et al.*, 1983). In addition, the presence of a fucose attached to Thr61 via an O-glycosidic linkage has been reported (Harris *et al.*, 1991). Two forms of t-PA that differ by the absence or presence of a carbohydrate moiety at Asp184 have been characterized (Bennett, 1983). Type I t-PA is glycosylated at asparagines 117, 184 and 448 whereas Type II t-PA lacks a glycosylation at asparagine 184. The asparagine at 218 is normally not occupied in either form of t-PA (Vehar *et al.*, 1984a). Asparagine 117 contains a high

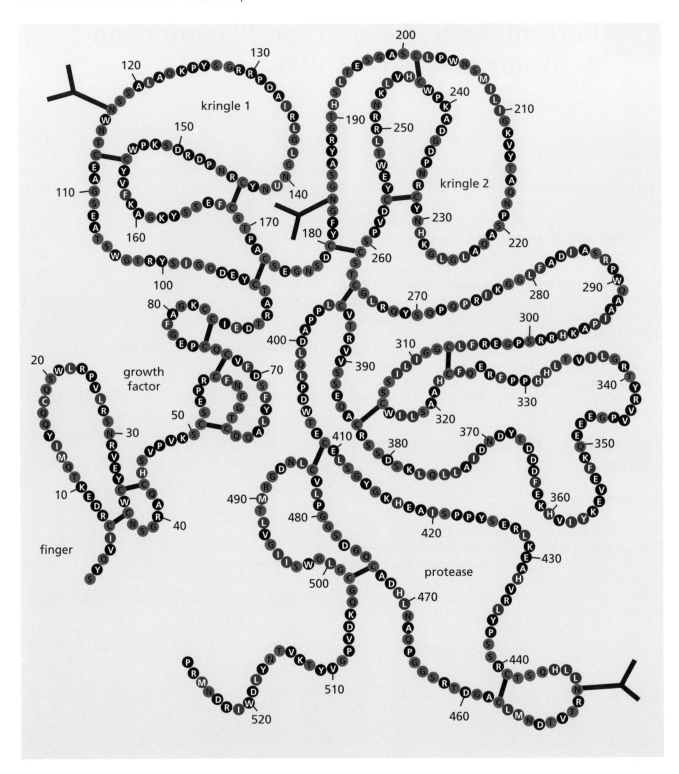

Figure 14.2. Primary structure of tissue-plasminogen activator.

mannose oligosaccharide whereas Asn184 and Asn448 are of the complex carbohydrate type (Spellman *et al.*, 1989). Complex N-linked glycan structures are ones containing a disaccharide Galβ(1,4)GlcNac and terminate in sialic acids while an oligomannose (high mannose) type glycan contains only mannose in the outer arms (see recommended reading for further details). Type II t-PA has a slightly higher specific activity *in vitro* compared with type I t-PA

(Einarsson *et al.*, 1985). During fibrinolysis, the single chain polypeptide is cleaved between Arg275 and Ile276 by plasmin to yield 2-chain t-PA. Two chain t-PA consists of a heavy chain (A-chain) derived from the amino terminus and a light chain (B-chain) linked by a single disulfide bridge between Cys264 and Cys395. The A-chain consists of the finger, growth factor and two kringle domains. The finger domain and the second kringle are responsible for t-PA binding to fibrin and for the activation of plasminogen. The function of the first kringle is not known. The B chain contains the serine protease domain consisting of the His-Asp-Ser triad that cleaves plasminogen (Pennica *et al.*, 1983).

Recombinant t-PA (rt-PA)

Recombinant t-PA (alteplase) is identical to endogenous human t-PA. Like melanoma-derived t-PA, rt-PA lacks a glycosylation at Asn218 and exists as two forms differing by the absence or presence of a carbohydrate at residue Asn184 (Vehar *et al.*, 1986). Initially, rt-PA was produced as a two-chain form in Chinese Hamster Ovary (CHO) cells using a roller bottle (RB) process. Most of the initial pharmacology and clinical studies were conducted using rt-PA derived from this process. Subsequently, a large scale suspension culture (SC) process that produced primarily (80%) single chain rt-PA was developed for commercialization. A pharmacokinetic comparison of rt-PA derived from the RB and SC processes showed that the SC-derived rt-PA was cleared from the circulation approximately 30% faster than RB-derived rt-PA (Data on file, Genentech, Inc.). However, when used at pharmacokinetically similar doses, both had similar pharmacodynamic and therapeutic properties.

Pharmacology

During fibrinolysis the inactive zymogen plasminogen is converted to the active enzyme plasmin by plasminogen activators. Plasmin then degrades the insoluble fibrin clot into soluble degradation products. Tissue plasminogen activator has a high affinity for fibrin and is a strong activator of plasminogen. Tissue plasminogen activator is a poor enzyme in the absence of fibrin, however, there is a > 600-fold enhancement in the activation of plasminogen by t-PA in the presence of fibrin (Hoylaerts *et al.*, 1982). Plasminogen activators are inhibited by the action of plasminogen activator inhibitors 1 and 2 (PAI-1 and PAI-2), which normally circulate at a concentration of 5–20 µg/L in the plasma (Collen and Lijnen, 1994). Mean t-PA antigen concentrations at rest in humans are approximately 5 µg/mL (Holvoet *et al.*, 1985) and can increase about 1.5–2-fold in venous occlusion (Holvoet *et al.*, 1987). Circulating plasmin is rapidly inactivated by α_2-antiplasmin whereas plasmin formed on the fibrin clot surface is only slowly inactivated. This allows for efficient plasminogen activation at the target site (the fibrin clot) with less systemic activation and fewer systemic side effects compared to other thrombolytic agents currently approved for the management of acute myocardial infarction. If the amount of plasmin produced is sufficient to deplete the available α_2-antiplasmin, a systemic fibrinolytic state, characterized by activation of plasminogen, depletion of α_2-antiplasmin, decreased fibrinogen levels and increased fibrinogen degradation products, can occur. This can subsequently lead to hemorrhagic complications. Decreases in plasma levels of fibrinogen (to 54–61% of baseline), plasminogen (to 54–70% of baseline), and α_2-antiplasmin (to 25–35% of baseline) have been reported following 100 mg rt-PA over 1.5–3 hours (Seifried *et al.*, 1989; Tanswell *et al.*, 1992). These effects had reverted to 70–88% of baseline levels by 24 hours after treatment.

DISPOSITION OF RT-PA

The pharmacokinetics of rt-PA have been studied in mice, rats, rabbits, dogs, primates, and humans. After intravenous administration, the plasma concentrations decline rapidly with an initial dominant half-life of less than 5 minutes in all species. The clearance ranges from 27 mL/min in rabbits (Hotchkiss *et al.*, 1988), 29 mL/min in monkeys (Baughman, 1987), and 0.62 L/min in humans (Tanswell *et al.*, 1989). Recombinant t-PA exhibits non-linear pharmacokinetics at high plasma concentrations (Tanswell *et al.*, 1990). The estimated Km and Vmax computed by simultaneously fitting multiple plasma concentration-time curves following several different doses were 12–15 µg/mL and 3.7 µg/mL/hr, respectively, with little species variation in these parameters. The pharmacokinetics are essentially linear in cases where the plasma concentration does not exceed 10–20% of Km (i.e. 1.5–3 µg/mL). A pharmacokinetic summary of rt-PA following intravenous administration in humans is presented in Table 14.1. There was no difference in the pharmacokinetics following the different regimens. Recombinant t-PA has an initial volume of distribution that approximates plasma volume, and shows a rapid plasma clearance. The initial half-life was less than 5 minutes.

The primary route of rt-PA clearance is via receptor-mediated mechanisms in the liver. Three liver cell types are responsible for the clearance of t-PA: parenchymal cells, endothelial cells, and Kupffer cells. Kupffer cells and endothelial cells mediate t-PA clearance via the mannose receptor (Otter *et al.*, 1992). Hepatocytes clear t-PA via a carbohydrate-independent, receptor-mediated mechanism. Recent data suggests that this carbohydrate-independent clearance is mediated via the low density lipoprotein receptor-related protein (LRP) (Bu *et al.*, 1993).

Reference	Administration regimen	Health status	Cmax (µg/mL)	CL (L/min)	V_1 (L)	V_{ss} (L)	$t_{1/2\alpha}$ (min)	$t_{1/2\beta}$ (min)
Tanswell et al, 1989	0.25 mg/kg/30 min	Healthy	0.96±0.18	0.64±0.05	4.6±0.3	8.1±0.8	4.4±0.2	39±2.6
	0.5 mg/kg/30 min	Healthy	1.8±0.25	0.60±0.09	4.3±0.8	8.0±0.9	4.4±0.4	40±3.1
Seifried et al, 1989[b]	100 mg/2.5 hr[c]	AMI	3.3±0.95	0.38±0.07	2.8±0.9	9.3±5.0	3.6±0.9	16±5.4
Tanswell et al, 1992	100 mg/1.5 hr[d]	AMI	4±1	0.57±0.1	3.4±1.5	8.4±5	3.4±1.4	72±68

Table 14.1. Clinical pharmacokinetic profile of rt-PA following intravenous administration in healthy volunteers and patients with acute myocardial infarction (AMI). All data reported are based on an immunoreactive assay.[a]
[a] Cmax = maximum rt-PA concentration; CL = plasma clearance; V_1 = initial volume of distribution; V_{ss} = Steady-state volume of distribution; t1/2 = half-life 3-compartment model was used. The β half-life corresponds to the second phase. [b] A 3-compartment model was used. The β half-life corresponds to the second phase. The terminal half-life was 3.7 ± 1.4 hr. [c] 10 mg bolus, 50 mg over 1 hr, then 30 mg in 1.5 hr. Note that the second infusion is of a shorter duration but at a similar rate to the standard dosage regimen. [d] 15 mg bolus, 50 mg over 0.5 hr, then 35 mg in 1 hr.

Several reports have shown a correlation between a change in hepatic blood flow and plasma concentration of thrombolytic agents in healthy volunteers. The therapeutic implications of pharmacokinetic and pharmacodynamic drug interactions with thrombolytic agents were recently reviewed (De Boer *et al.*, 1995). Clinical data correlating rt-PA plasma concentrations in patients with acute myocardial infarction and hepatic blood flow are currently lacking and it is unclear if dose adjustments of thrombolytics are therapeutically necessary in patients receiving drugs that might affect liver blood flow.

PHARMACEUTICAL CONSIDERATIONS

Recombinant human t-PA (Alteplase, Activase®, Genentech, Inc; Actilyse®, Boehringer Ingelheim) is supplied as a sterile, white to off-white lyophilized powder. Recombinant t-PA is practically insoluble in water and arginine is included in the formulation to increase the aqueous solubility. Phosphoric acid and/or sodium hydroxide may be used prior to lyophilization to adjust the pH. The sterile lyophilized powder should be stored at controlled room temperatures not to exceed 30°C, or refrigerated at 2–8°C and should be protected from excessive light.

The powder is reconstituted by adding the accompanying Sterile Water for Injection, USP to the vial resulting in a colorless to pale yellow transparent solution containing 1 mg/mL rt-PA, with a pH of 7.3 and osmolality of approximately 215 mOs/kg. Recombinant t-PA is stable in solution over a pH range of 5 to 7.5. Since the reconstituted solution does not contain any preservatives, it should be used within eight hours of preparation and should be refrigerated prior to use. The solution is incompatible with bacteriostatic water for injection. Other solutions such as Sterile Water

for Injection or preservative containing solutions should not be used for further dilution. The 1 mg/mL solution may be diluted further in an equal volume of 0.9% Sodium Chloride for Injection, USP or 5% Dextrose Injection, USP to yield a concentration of 0.5 mg/mL and is compatible with glass bottles or poly-vinyl chloride bags.

Clinical Application

Recombinant human t-PA is indicated for use in the management of acute myocardial infarction and acute massive pulmonary embolism in adults. Two dosage regimens have been studied in patients experiencing acute myocardial infarction (AMI). Initially, rt-PA was administered as a 100 mg dose over 3 hours with a reduction in dosage for patients weighing less than 65 kg. In this regimen, 10 mg was administered as a bolus with 50 mg being infused over 1 hour, then 40 mg was infused over the subsequent 2 hours. Infarct artery-related patency rates of 70 to 77% are achieved at 90 minutes with this 3-hour regimen (Verstraete *et al.*, 1985; Carney *et al.*, 1992). Patency grades of blood flow in the artery are defined by the Thrombolysis in Myocardial Infarction (TIMI) trial and are assessed angiographically with TIMI grade 0 representing no flow; grade 1, minimal flow; grade 2, sluggish flow; and grade 3 indicating complete or full, brisk flow. Recently, the efficacy of an accelerated rt-PA regimen compared to streptokinase was demonstrated in 41,000 AMI patients (The GUSTO Investigators, 1993a,b). In the accelerated regimen, a bolus dose of 15 mg is administered over 2 minutes, followed by an infusion of 50 mg over 30 minutes. A dose of 35 mg is infused over the subsequent 60 minutes. For patients weighing less than 67 kg, a weight adjusted regimen is recommended with a bolus of 15 mg, followed by

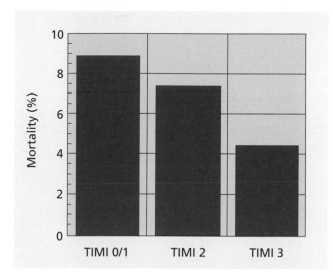

Figure 14.3. Correlation between TIMI flow and mortality demonstrating a decrease in mortality with improvement in TIMI flow.

0.75 mg/kg over 30 minutes, not to exceed 50 mg and then a rate of 0.5 mg/kg over 60 minutes, not to exceed 35 mg. The comparative efficacy of the two rt-PA regimens has not been evaluated. The GUSTO trial demonstrated a higher infarct-related artery patency rate (90-minute patency rate of 81%) and reduced mortality (an additional 10 lives saved per 10,000 patients treated) in the group treated with rt-PA with IV heparin compared to streptokinase with either subcutaneous or intravenous heparin (90-minute patency

of 54–60%) (The GUSTO Investigators, 1993b). The rt-tPA group had an approximate 1% rate of intracranial hemorrhage. The GUSTO trial also indicated a decline in 30-day mortality with improvement in TIMI flow regardless of treatment assignment (Figure 14.3).

CONTRAINDICATIONS

Since thrombolytic therapy increases the risk of bleeding, rt-PA is contraindicated in patients who have a history of cerebrovascular accidents, or have any kind of active internal bleeding, intracranial neoplasm, arteriovenous malformation, aneurism or have had recent intracranial or intraspinal surgery or trauma.

Second Generation Thrombolytic Agents

The rapid clearance of rt-PA from the circulation by the liver necessitates that it be administered as an intravenous infusion. Considerable preclinical and clinical research is currently underway to develop a rt-PA variant that is fibrin-specific and can be administered as an intravenous bolus injection. Several reviews (e.g. Higgins and Bennet, 1990) have outlined the progress of these efforts. Strategies that have been used to develop these rt-PA variants include domain deletions, glycosylation changes, or site directed amino acid substitutions (see Chapter 5). Several of these rt-PA variant have shown efficacy in animal models following bolus administration and are currently undergoing extensive clinical trials, hence, their availability is several years away.

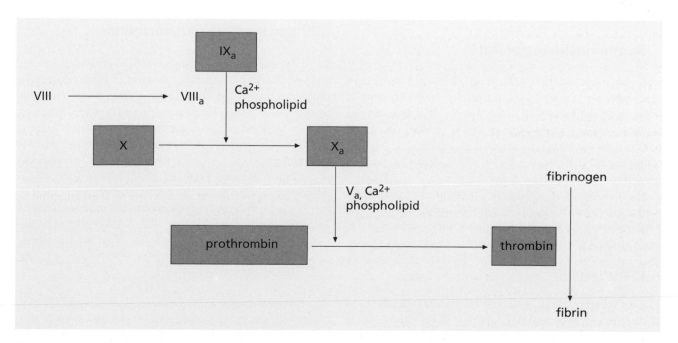

Figure 14.4. Simplified scheme showing the role of Factor VIII in the coagulation pathway.

Factor VIII

Factor VIII (antihemophilia factor) is a plasma protein that functions as a cofactor by increasing the Vmax in the activation of Factor X by Factor IXa in the presence of calcium ions and negatively charged phospholipid (Figure 14.4) (Jackson and Nemersen, 1980). The congenital absence of Factor VIII is characterized by a bleeding disorder termed Hemophilia A, an X-linked recessive disorder that afflicts approximately 1 in 10,000 males (Antonarakis et al., 1987). The introduction of Factor VIII concentrates derived from plasma increased the quality of life and the life expectancy of individuals with hemophilia A, however, reliance on plasma as a source for Factor VIII also exposed patients to alloantigens and transfusion-associated viral disease (Schwartz et al., 1990). Factor VIII derived from recombinant technology has the potential to eliminate many of the shortcomings of plasma derived antihemophilia factor and be available in an unlimited supply.

Factor VIII Structure

Factor VIII is synthesized as a single chain polypeptide of 2332 amino acids (Eaton et al., 1987). Shortly after synthesis, cleavage occurs and most plasma Factor VIII circulates as a 80 kD light chain associated with a series of about 210 kD heavy chains in a metal ion-dependent complex. There are 25 potential N-linked glycosylation sites and 22 cysteines (Vehar et al., 1984). The about 210 kD heavy chain is further proteolytically cleaved to a series of proteins of Mr 90–188 kD (Eaton et al., 1986). The 90–210 kD proteins form a complex with the light chain that is mediated by a metal ion (Eaton et al., 1986).

Recombinant Factor VIII

Recombinant Factor VIII from Baxter Healthcare (Recombinate®) is produced in a batch refeed culture process using transfected CHO cells whereas that from Bayer/ Miles Inc (Kogenate®) is produced in a continuous cell culture process using transfected Baby Hamster Kidney cells. A major difference between recombinant Factor VIII from Bayer/Miles and Baxter is the presence of a Galα1-> 3Gal carbohydrate moiety in the Baxter product (Hironaka et al., 1992). Recombinant factor VIII consists of multiple peptides including an 80 kD protein and various extensions of about 90 kD subunit protein (Schwartz et al., 1990).

Pharmacology

The concentration of Factor VIII in plasma is about 200 ng/mL (Hoyer, 1981). It is not known with certainty where Factor VIII is synthesized. There is evidence that several different tissues, including the spleen, liver, and kidney, may play a role. Factor VIII is normally covalently associated with a 50-fold excess of Von Willebrand factor. von Willebrand factor protects Factor VIII from proteolytic cleavage and allows concentration at sites of hemostasis. Circulating von Willebrand factor is bound by exposed subendothelium and activated platelets at sites of injury allowing localization of von Willebrand factor and Factor VIII.

Factor VIII circulates in blood as a large precursor polypeptide devoid of coagulant activity. Cleavage by thrombin at Arg372-Ser373, Arg740-Ser741, and Arg1689-Ser1690 results in procoagulant function (Vehar et al., 1984b). While cleavage at Arg740 is not essential for coagulant activity, cleavage at the other two sites is necessary. Although factor VIII is synthesized as a single chain polypeptide, shortly after synthesis, the single chain polypeptide is cleaved and most of the factor VIII in plasma exists as a 80 kD light chain and a series of heavy chains. The heavy and light chains circulate as a population of heterodimers that require a divalent cation to maintain their interaction and procoagulant potential.

DISPOSITION OF RECOMBINANT FACTOR VIII

Several studies have evaluated the clinical pharmacokinetics of recombinant factor VIII. The pharmacokinetic profile is summarized in Table 14.2. Following administration, the increase in Factor VIII concentration is dose proportional and the disposition is similar following a single and chronic dosing. The terminal half-life is 14–16 hours and the initial volume of distribution approximates plasma volume.

Pharmaceutical Considerations

Recombinant Factor VIII (Kogenate®, Bayer/Miles; Recombinate®, Baxter) is supplied as sterile, single dose vials containing 250 to 1000 IU of Factor VIII activity. The preparation is stabilized with human albumin and is lyophilized. The product contains no preservatives and should be stored at 2–8°C. The lyophilized powder may be stored at room temperature (up to 25°C) for up to 3 months without loss of biological activity. Freezing should be avoided as the diluent bottle may break. Factor VIII is reconstituted with the diluent provided. The reconstituted product must be administered intravenously by either direct syringe injection or drip infusion within 3 hours of reconstitution.

Clinical Application

Recombinant Factor VIII, antihemophilic factor, (Recombinate®, Kogenate®) is indicated for the treatment of classical hemophilia (hemophilia A), for the prevention and

Reference	Administration regimen	CL (mL/hr/kg)	V (mL/kg)	$t_{1/2}$ (hr)	MRT (hr)
Morfini et al, 1992	50 U/kg Recombinate	3.1±1.2	62±18[a]	14.5±4.3	NR[b]
Schwartz et al, 1990[c]	50 IU/kg Kogenate	2.5+0.8 2.6±0.9 2.2±0.7	51±13[d] 48±12 49±18	15.8±3.9 13.9±3.2 16.6±3.0	21.2±5.3 19.1±4.5 22.6±4.1
Harrison et al, 1991	50 U/kg Kogenate	2.4±0.7	51±13	16.5±3.5	22.2±4.9

Table 14.2. Clinical pharmacokinetic profile of recombinant factor VIII following intravenous administration in patients with hemophilia A. [a] V_{d-area}; [b] Not reported; [c] Data reported for Weeks 1, 13 and 25; [d] V_{ss}.

control of hemorrhagic episodes and in the perioperative management of patients with hemophilia A. Since recombinant antihemophilic factor is indicated in the treatment of bleeding disorders arising from a deficiency in factor VIII, it is essential that this deficiency be identified before administration of rAHF. Recombinant Factor VIII is also approved for the treatment of hemophilia A in certain patients with inhibitors to Factor VIII. Recombinant factor VIII is not indicated for the treatment of von Willebrand disease. Factor VIII replacement should be based on the minimal effective hemostatic concentration necessary for treatment, the volume of distribution and the elimination half-life.

Schwartz *et al.* (1990) investigated the pharmacokinetics, safety and efficacy of recombinant factor VIII in patients with hemophilia A. In this study, the mean residence time and elimination half-life of recombinant factor VIII were equal to or exceeded that for plasma derived factor VIII, whereas the clearance and steady-state volume of distribution for recombinant factor VIII were slightly smaller than that for plasma derived factor VIII. In the safety and efficacy portion of the study, the mean incremental recovery of factor VIII following 50 IU/kg of recombinant factor VIII given at weeks 1, 5, 9, 13, and 25 was 2.49–2.92% per IU administered per kilogram and was not statistically dependent on multiple dosing.

The incidence of formation of inhibitors to recombinant factor VIII in previously untreated patients is approximately 20% (Lusher *et al.*, 1993). This incidence rate is similar to that for plasma derived factor VIII, where approximately 10–15% of patients treated develop antibodies which neutralize factor VIII and result in resistance to treatment (McMillan *et al.*, 1988). A direct comparison of incidence rates is difficult since studies investigating the incidence of inhibitor development to recombinant factor VIII used previously untreated patients whereas those investigating plasma derived factor VIII were conducted in previously treated patients, a group that may be at lower risk for inhibitor development (Lusher *et al.*, 1993). The study by Lusher *et al.* (1993) showed that the risk of developing antibodies to recombinant factor VIII correlated with the severity of the disease and the intensity of exposure to factor VIII. Inhibitors were detected 1 to 15 months after the initial exposure with factor VIII. In several of the patients in whom inhibitors were detected, they disappeared completely or remained at a low level (≤ 10 Bethesda units) despite continued treatment with factor VIII.

CONTRAINDICATIONS

Since trace amounts of mouse or hamster protein may be present in recombinant Factor VIII as contaminants from the expressions system, caution should be exercised when administered to individuals with known hypersensitivity to plasma-derived antihemophilic factor or with hypersensitivity to biological preparations with trace amounts of murine or hamster proteins.

Concluding Remarks

This chapter has provided an overview of two hematologic products currently available throughout recombinant technology that have made a significant impact on patient care. Several other recombinant products that could have a further clinical benefit (e.g., second generation thrombolytics, Factor IX) are currently under investigation. ■

References

- **Antonarakis SE, Youssoufian H, Kazazian HH Jr.** (1987). Molecular genetics of hemophilia A in man (factor VIII deficiency). *Mol Biol Med*, 4, 81–94

- **Bates ER, Topol EJ.** (1989). Thrombolytic therapy for acute myocardial infarction. *Chest*, 95(Suppl 1), 257S–64S

- **Baughman RA.** (1987). Pharmacokinetics of tissue plasminogen activator. In *Tissue Plasminogen Activator in Thrombolytic Therapy*, edited by B Sobel, D Collen and E Grossbard. New York: Markel Dekker, pp. 41–53

- **Bennett WF.** (1983). Two forms of tissue-type plasminogen activator (tPA) differ at a single specific glycosylation site. *Thromb Haemostas*, 50, 106

- **Bu G, Maksymovitch EA, Schwartz AL.** (1993). Receptor-mediated endocytosis of tissue-type plasminogen activator by low density lipoprotein receptor-related protein on human hepatoma HepG2 cells. *J Biol Chem*, 268, 13002–13009

- **Carney RJ, Murphy GA, Brandt TR, *et al.*** (1992). Randomized angiographic trial of recombinant tissue-type plasminogen activator (alteplase) in myocardial infarction. *J Am Coll Cardiol*, 20, 17–23

- **Collen D, Stassen, J-M, Yasuda T, Refino C, Paoni N, Keyt B, Roskams T, Guerrero JL, Lijnen HR, Gold HK, Bennett WF.** (1994). Comparative thrombolytic properties of tissue-type plasminogen activator and of a plasmiogen activator inhibitor-1-resistant glycosylation variant, in a combined arterial and venous thrombosis model in the dog. *Thromb Haemostas*, 72, 98–104

- **Collen D and Lijnen HR.** (1994). Fibrinolysis and the control of hemostasis. In *The Molecular Basis of Blood Diseases WB*, edited by G Stamatoyannopoulos, AW Nienhuis, PW Majerus and H Varmus. Philadelphia: Saunders Company, pp. 725–752

- **De Boer A, Kluft C, Kroon JM, Kasper FJ, Shoemaker HC, Pruis J, Breimer DD, Soons PA, Emeis JJ, Cohen AF.** (1992). Liver blood flow as a major determinant of the clearance of recombinant human tissue-type plasminogen activator. *Thromb Haemostas*, 67, 83–87

- **De Boer A, Kluft C, Kasper FJ, Kroon JM, Schoemaker HC, Breimer DD. Soons PA, Cohen AF.** (1993). Interaction study between nifedipine and recombinant tissue-type plasminogen activator in healthy subjects. *Br J Clin Pharmac*, 36, 99–104

- **De Boer A, van Griensven JMT.** (1995). Drug interactions with thrombolytic agents. Current perspectives. *Clin Pharmacokinet*, 28, 315–326

- **Eaton D, Rodriguez H, Vehar GA.** (1986). Proteolytic processing of human factor VIII. Correlation of specific cleavages by thrombin, factor Xa, and activated protein C with activation and inactivation of factor VIII coagulant activity. *Biochemistry*, 25, 505–512

- **Eaton DL, Hass PE, Riddle L, Mather J, Wiebe M, Gregory T, Vehar GA.** (1987). Characterization of recombinant human Factor VIII. *J Biol Chem*, 262, 3285–3290

- **Einarsson M, Brandt J, Kaplan L.** (1985). Large-scale purification of human tissue-type plasminogen activator using monoclonal antibodies. *Biochim Biophys Acta*, 830, 1–10

- **Giles AR, Tinlin S, Hoogendoorn H, Fournel MA, Ng P, Pancham N.** (1988). *In vivo* characterization of recombinant Factor VIII in a canine model of hemophilia A (Factor VIII deficiency). *Blood*, 72, 335–339

- **The GUSTO Investigators.** (1993a). An international randomized trial comparing four thrombolytic strategies for acute myocardial infarction. *N Engl J Med*, 329, 673–682

- **The GUSTO angiographic investigators.** (1993b). The effects of tissue plasminogen activator, streptokinase, or both on coronary-artery patency, ventricular function, and survival after acute myocardial infarction. *N Engl J Med*, 329, 1615–1622

- **Harris RJ, Leonard CK, Guzzetta AW, Spellman MW.** (1991). Tissue plasminogen activator has an O-linked fucose attached to Threonine-61 in the epidermal growth factor domain. *Biochemistry*, 30, 2311–2314

- **Higgins DL, Bennett WF.** (1990). Tissue Plasminogen activator: The biochemistry and pharmacology of variants produced by mutagenesis. *Annu Rev Pharmacol Toxicol*, 30, 91–121

- **Hironaka T, Furukawa K, Esmon PC, Fournel MA, Sawada S, Kato M, Minaga T, Kobata A.** (1992). Comparative study of the sugar chains of factor VIII purified from human plasma and from the culture media of recombinant baby hamster kidney cells. *J Biol Chem*, 267, 8012–8020

- **Holvoet P, Cleemput H, Collen D.** (1985). Assay of human tissue-type plasminogen activator (t-PA) with an enzyme-linked immunosorbent assay (ELISA) based on three murine monoclonal antibodies to t-PA. *Thromb Haemostas*, 54, 684–687

- **Holvoet P, Boes J, Collen D.** (1987). Measurement of free, one-chain tissue-type plasminogen activator in human plasma with an enzyme-linked immunosorbent assay based on an active site-specific murine monoclonal antibody. *Blood*, 69, 284–289

- **Hotchkiss A, Refino CJ, Leonard CK, O'Connor JV, Crowley C, McCabe J, Tate K, Nakamura G, Powers D, Levinson. A, Mohler M, Spellman MW.** (1988). The influence of carbohydrate structure on the clearance of recombinant tissue-type plasminogen activator. *Thromb Haemostas*, 60, 255–261

- **Hoyer LW.** (1981). The Factor VIII complex: Structure and function. *Blood*, 58, 1–13

- **Hoylaerts M, Rijken DC, Lijnen HR, Collen D.** (1982). Kinetics of the activation of plasminogen by human tissue plasminogen activator: role of fibrin. *J Biol Chem*, 257, 2912–2919

- **Jackson CM, Nemersen Y.** (1980). Blood coagulation. *Ann Rev Biochem*, 49, 767–811

- **Lusher JM, Arkin S, Abildgaard CF, Schwartz RS, and the Kogenate previously untreated patient study group.** (1993). Recombinant Factor VIII for the treatment of previously untreated patients with hemophilia A. *N Eng J Med*, 328, 453–459

- **McMillan CW, Shapiro SS, Whitehurst D, Hoyer LW, Rao AV, Lazerson J.** (1988). The natural history of factor VIII:C inhibitors in patients with hemophilia A: a national cooperative study. II. Observations on the initial development of factor VIII:C inhibitor. *Blood*, 71, 344–348

- **Morfini M, Longo G, Messori A, Lee M, White G Mannucci P, and the Recombinate Study Group.** (1992). Pharmacokinetic properties of recombinant factor VIII compared with a monoclonally purified concentrate (Hemofil® M). *Thromb Haemostas*, 68, 433–435

- **Otter M, Kuiper J, Van Berkel TJC, Rijken DC.** (1992). Mechanisms of tissue-type plasminogen activator (tPA) clearance by the liver. *Annals NY Acad Sci*, 667, 431–442

- **Pennica D, Holmes WE, Kohr WJ, Harkins RN. Vehar GA, Ward CA, Bennett WF, Yelverton E, Seeburg PH, Heyneker HL, Goeddel DV, Collen D.** (1983). Cloning and expression of human tissue-type plasminogen activator cDNA in E. coli. *Science*, 301, 214–221

- **Schwartz RS, Abildgaard CF, Aledort LM, et al.** (1990). Human recombinant DNA-derived antihemophilic factor (Factor VIII) in the treatment of hemophilia A. *N Engl J Med*, 323, 1800–1805

- **Seifried E, Tanswell P, Ellbrück D, Haerer W, Schmidt A.** (1989). Pharmacokinetics and haemostatic status during consecutive infusions of recombinant tissue-type plasminogen activator in patients with acute myocardial infarction. *Thromb Haemostas*, 61, 497–501

- **Spellman MW, Basa LJ, Leonard CK, Chakel JV. O'Connor JV, Wilson S, Van Halbeek H.** (1989). Carbohydrate structures of human tissue plasminogen activator expressed in Chinese Hamster Ovary cells. *J Biol Chem*, 264, 14100–14111

- **Tanswell P, Seifried E, Su PCAF, Feuerer W, Rijken DC.** (1989). Pharmacokinetics and systemic effects of tissue-type plasminogen activator in normal subjects. *Clin Pharmacol Ther*, 46, 155–162

- **Tanswell P, Heinzel G, Greischel A, Krause J.** (1990). Nonlinear pharmacokinetics of tissue-type plasminogen activator in three animal species and isolated perfused rat liver. *J Pharmacol Exp Ther*, 255, 318–324

- **Tanswell P, Tebbe U, Neuhaus, K-L, Gläsle-Schwarz L, Wojcik J, Seifried E.** (1992). Pharmacokinetics and fibrin specificity of alteplase during accelerated infusions in acute myocardial infarction. *J Am Coll Cardiol*, 19, 1071–1075

- **Vehar GA, Kohr WJ, Bennett WF, Pennica D, Ward CA, Harkins RN, Collen D.** (1984a). Characterization studies on human melanoma cell tissue plasminogen activator. *Bio/Tech*, 2, 1051–1057

- **Vehar GA, Keyt B, Eaton D, Rodrigues H, O'Brien DP, Rotblat F, Oppermann H, Keck R, Wood WI, Harkins RN, Tuddenham EGD, Lawn RM, Capon DJ.** (1984b). Structure of human Factor VIII. *Nature*, 312, 337–342

- **Vehar GA, Spellman MW, Keyt BA, Ferguson CK, Keck RG, Chloupek RC, Harris R, Bennett WF, Builder SE, Hancock WS.** (1986). Characterization studies of human tissue-type plasminogen activator produced by recombinant DNA technology. *Cold Spring Harbor Symp Quant Biol*, 51, 551–562

- **Verstraete M, Bernard R, Bory M, et al.** (1985). Randomized trial of intravenous recombinant tissue-type plasminogen activator versus intravenous streptokinase in acute myocardial infarction. *Lancet*, 1, 842–7

Self-Assessment Questions

Question 1: *Several biopharmaceutical companies are developing second generation thrombolytic agents. What are the motivations for this ?*

Question 2: *Design a therapeutic regimen for a 30 kg patient with a laceration. Assume that the desired plasma concentration of factor VIII is 30 U/dL.*

Answers

Answer 1: While rt-PA has demonstrated an increase in the patency rate of the infarct-related artery and a decrease in the mortality, there are potentially several areas where further benefits can be made in the treatment of acute myocardial infarction :

(i) Due to the rapid hepatic clearance of rt-PA from the circulation, currently administration is via an intravenous infusion regimen to maintain therapeutic concentrations. Several of the second generation agents are claimed to have a longer half-life and slower plasma clearance allowing administration via a single or double bolus regimen (cf. Figure 5.18).

(ii) Although rt-PA results in fewer systemic side effects compared to other thrombolytic agents, there is an approximate 30–50% fall in systemic fibrinogen levels. A more fibrin specific second generation thrombolytic could result in a further reduction in systemic fibrinogenolysis and potentially a reduction in the incidence of intracranial hemorrhage.

Answer 2: Dose = 30 U/dL × 50 mL/kg (volume of distribution) × 30 kg = 450 IU.

15 Recombinant Human Deoxyribonuclease

by: Melinda Marian and Sharon Baughman

Introduction

Deoxyribonuclease I (DNase) is a human endonuclease, normally present in saliva, urine, pancreatic secretions and blood, which catalyzes the hydrolysis of extracellular DNA into oligonucleotides. Aerosolized recombinant human DNase (rhDNase) has been developed for inhalation to assist in the treatment of pulmonary disease in patients with cystic fibrosis (CF).

Cystic fibrosis (CF) is the most common autosomal recessive, lethal disease in Caucasians and is caused by mutations of a gene that regulates the synthesis of a chloride ion transfer protein (Riordan et al., 1989). Clinical manifestations of the disease include obstruction of the airways and pancreatic ducts. The abnormal ion transport has been implicated in the formation of the dehydrated, viscous mucus found in the airway secretions of CF patients. Retention of viscous purulent mucus in the airways contributes both to reduced pulmonary function and to exacerbations of infection (Boat et al., 1988; Collins, 1992). A cycle of pulmonary obstruction and infection leads to progressive lung destruction and eventual death before the age of thirty for most CF patients.

Two macromolecules which contribute to the physical properties of lung secretions are mucus glycoproteins and DNA. Experiments in the 1950's and 1960's revealed that DNA is present in very large concentrations (3–14 mg/mL) in infected, but not in uninfected lung secretions (Chernick and Barbero, 1950; Potter et al., 1960; Matthews et al., 1963). The high levels of extracellular DNA are released by degenerating neutrophils that accumulate in response to infection (Potter et al., 1969). The high concentrations of DNA make the secretions very viscous. The DNA-rich secretions also bind aminoglycoside antibiotics commonly used for treatment of pulmonary infections and may reduce their efficacy (Ramphal et al., 1988; Bataillon et al., 1992).

Early *in vitro* studies in which lung secretions were incubated for several hours with partially purified bovine pancreatic DNase I showed a large reduction in viscosity (Armstrong and White, 1950; Chernick et al., 1961). Based on these observations, bovine pancreatic DNase I (Dornavac or Pancreatic Dornase) was approved in the United States

for human use in 1958. Numerous uncontrolled clinical studies in patients with pneumonia and one study in patients with cystic fibrosis suggested that bovine pancreatic DNase I was effective in reducing the viscosity of lung secretions (Elmes and White, 1953; Salomon et al., 1954; Spier et al., 1961; Lieberman, 1968). However, severe adverse reactions did occasionally occur, perhaps as a consequence of allergic reactions to a foreign protein or "irritation" due to contaminating proteases, as up to 2% trypsin and chymotrypsin were present in the final product (Raskin, 1968; Lieberman, 1962). Both bovine DNase I products were eventually withdrawn from the market.

Recombinant human deoxyribonuclease I (rhDNase) was cloned, sequenced and expressed (Shak et al., 1990) to reevaluate the potential of DNase I as a therapeutic for cystic fibrosis. *In-vitro* incubation with catalytic concentrations of rhDNase reduced the viscoelasticity of purulent sputum from CF patients (Shak et al., 1990). The reduction in viscoelasticity was directly related to both rhDNase concentration and to reduction in the size of the DNA in the samples. Reduction of high molecular weight DNA into smaller fragments by treatment with aerosolized rhDNase was, therefore, proposed as a mechanism to reduce the mucus viscosity and improve mucus clearability from obstructed airways in patients. Improved clearance of the purulent mucus was hoped to improve pulmonary function and reduce recurrent exacerbations of respiratory symptoms requiring parenteral antibiotics.

Protein Chemistry and Structure

Recombinant human DNase I is a monomeric, 260-amino acid glycoprotein produced in Chinese hamster ovary (CHO) cells (Shak et al., 1990). The molecule has four cysteines and two potential N-linked glycosylation sites. The molecule has an approximate molecular weight from polyacrylamide gel electrophoresis (PAGE) of 37 kD. The predicted molecular mass from the amino acid sequence is 29.3 kD. The higher molecular weight and the broad band observed on PAGE gels is due to glycosylation. The primary amino acid structure (Figure 15.1) is identical to that of the native human enzyme purified from urine. The X-ray

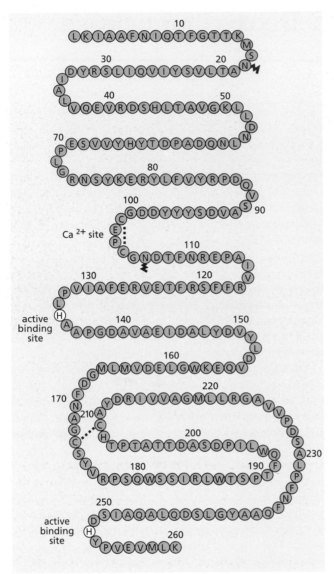

Figure 15.1. Primary amino acid sequence of rhDNase.

crystal structure of human pancreatic DNase I, which shares 78% identity with bovine DNase I, has recently been solved by molecular replacement and refined at 2.2 Å resolution (Wolf *et al.*, 1995). The structure of the human enzyme is essentially the same as that reported for bovine DNase I (Oefner and Suck, 1986). The two structures superimpose with an overall root mean square deviation for main chain atoms of 0.56 Å.

DNase I is an endonuclease that cleaves double-stranded DNA, or to a much lesser degree single-stranded DNA, into 5'-phosphate-terminated polynucleotides. Optimal DNase enzymatic activity depends upon the presence of calcium and magnesium ions. DNase is inactivated by heat, is specifically inhibited by actin or EDTA and shows optimal

activity at neutral (5.5–7.5) pH. The active binding site includes two histidine residues (residue 134 and 252).

Pharmacology

In Vitro Actions on Sputum

In vitro, rhDNase hydrolyzes the DNA in sputum of CF patients and reduces sputum viscoelasticity (Figure 15.2a, Shak *et al.*, 1990). Effects of rhDNase were initially examined using a "pourability" assay. Pourability was assessed qualitatively by inverting the tubes and observing the movement of sputum after a tap on the side of the tube. Catalytic amounts (50 µg/mL) greatly reduced the viscosity of the sputum, rapidly transforming it from a viscous gel to a flowing liquid. More than 50% of the sputum moved down the tube within 15 minutes of incubation and all the sputum moved freely down the tube within 30 minutes.

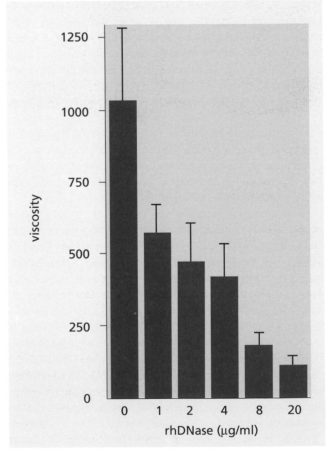

Figure 15.2a. *In vitro* reduction in viscosity in $10^3.kg.m^{-1}.s^{-1}$ of cystic fibrosis sputum by cone-plate viscometry. Cystic fibrosis sputum was incubated with various concentrations of rhDNase for 15 minutes at 37°C.

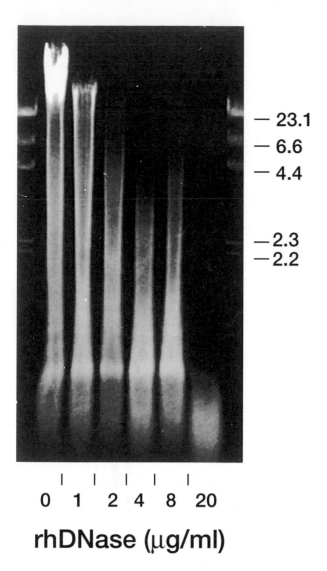

0 1 2 4 8 20

rhDNase (μg/ml)

Figure 15.2b. *In vitro* reduction in sputum DNA size as measured by agarose gel electrophoresis. Cystic fibrosis sputum was incubated with increasing concentrations (0–20 μg/mL) of rhDNase for 150 minutes at 37°C. Outside lanes are molecular weight standards for DNA in Kilodaltons.

The qualitative results of the pourability assay were confirmed by quantitative measurement of viscosity using a Brookfield Cone-Plate viscometer. The reduction of viscosity by rhDNase is rhDNase concentration-dependent (Figure 15.2a) and is associated with reduction in size of sputum DNA as measured by agarose gel electrophoresis (Figure 15.2b).

In vitro studies of CF mucus samples (Zahm *et al.*, 1995) treated with rhDNase have also demonstrated a dose-dependent improvement in cough transport and mucociliary transport of CF mucus using a frog palate model and a

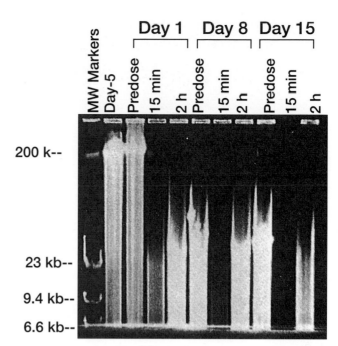

Figure 15.3. Sustained reduction in DNA length in sputum recovered from a CF patient treated with 2.5 mg rhDNase BID for up to 15 days. Samples analysed by pulsed field agarose field gel electrophoresis.

reduction in adhesiveness as measured by mucus contact angle. The improvements in mucus transport properties and adhesiveness were associated with a decrease in mucus viscosity and mucus surface tension and suggest rhDNase treatment may improve clearance of mucus from airways.

In Vivo Actions of rhDNase on Sputum

In vivo confirmation of the proposed mechanism of action for rhDNase has been obtained from direct characterization of apparent DNA size (Figure 15.3) and measurements of enzymatic and immunoreactive (ELISA) activity of rhDNase (Figure 15.4) in sputum from cystic fibrosis patients (Sinicropi *et al.*, 1994). Sputum samples were obtained at various times 1 to 6 hours postdose from adult cystic fibrosis patients after inhalation of 5 to 20 mg of rhDNase. rhDNase therapy produced a sustained reduction in DNA size in recovered sputum (Figure 15.3).

Inhalation of the therapeutic dose of rhDNase produced sputum levels of rhDNase which have been shown to be effective *in-vitro* (Figure 15.4) (Shak, 1995). The recovered rhDNase was also enzymatically active. Enzymatic activity was directly correlated with rhDNase concentrations in the sputum. Viscoelasticity was also reduced in the recovered sputum.

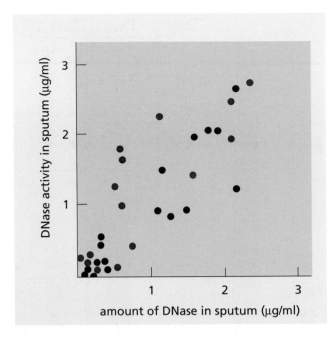

Figure 15.4. Immunoreactive concentrations and enzymatic activity of DNase in sputum following aerosol administration of either 10 mg (●) or 20 mg (●) rhDNase to patients with cystic fibrosis. Each data point is a separate sample measured in duplicate.

In addition, results from scintigraphic studies in rhDNase-treated patients suggested possible reductions in pulmonary obstruction and increased rates of mucociliary sputum clearance from the inner zone of the lung compared to controls (Laube *et al.*, 1993).

Pharmacokinetics and Metabolism

Non-clinical ADME data in rats and monkeys suggest minimal systemic absorption of rhDNase following aerosol inhalation of clinically-equivalent doses. rhDNase is cleared from the systemic circulation without any accumulation in tissues following acute exposure (Green, 1994). Additionally, non-clinical metabolism studies suggest that the low rhDNase concentrations present in serum following inhalation will be bound to binding proteins, and therefore inactive (Mohler *et al.*, 1993; Green 1994).

When 2.5 mg of rhDNase was administered by inhalation to 18 CF patients, mean sputum concentrations of 3 µg/mL DNase were measurable within 15 minutes. Mean sputum concentrations declined to an average of 0.6 µg/mL two hours following inhalation. Inhalation of up to 10 mg three times daily of rhDNase by 4 CF patients for 6 consecutive days did not result in significant elevation of serum concentrations of DNase above normal endogenous levels (Aiken *et al.*, 1992). After administration of up to

2.5 mg of rhDNase twice daily for 6 months to 321 CF patients, no accumulation of serum DNase was noted (assay limit of detection = approximately 0.5 ng DNase/mL serum).

Protein Manufacture and Formulation

Genentech's approved rhDNase product [Pulmozyme® (dornase alpha)] is a sterile, clear, colorless aqueous solution containing 1.0 mg/mL dornase alpha, 0.15 mg/mL calcium chloride dihydrate and 8.77 mg/mL sodium chloride. The solution contains no preservative and has a nominal pH of 6.3. Pulmozyme® is administered by inhalation of an aerosol mist produced by a compressed air-driven nebulizer system. Pulmozyme® is supplied as single-use ampoules which deliver 2.5 mL of solution to the nebulizer.

The choice of formulation components was determined by a need to provide 1–2 years stability and to meet additional requirements unique to aerosol delivery. In order to avoid adverse pulmonary reactions such as cough or bronchoconstriction, aerosols for local pulmonary delivery should be formulated as isotonic solutions with minimal or no buffer components and should maintain pH > 5.0. rhDNase has an additional requirement for calcium to be present for optimal enzymatic activity. Limiting formulation components raised concerns about pH control since protein stability and solubility can be highly pH-dependent. Fortunately, the protein itself provided sufficient buffering capacity at 1 mg/mL to maintain pH stability over the storage life of the product.

The droplet or particle size of an aerosol is also important in defining the site of deposition of the drug in the patient's airways (Gonda, 1990). A distribution of particle or droplet size of 1–6 µm was determined to be optimal for uniform deposition of rhDNase in the airways (Cipolla *et al.*, 1994). Jet nebulizers were used since they are the simplest method of producing aerosols in the desired respirable range. However, recirculation of protein solutions under high shear rates in the nebulizer bowl presented risks to the integrity of the protein molecule. rhDNase survived recirculation and high shear rates during the nebulization process with no apparent degradation in protein quality (Cippola *et al.*, 1994).

Clinical Usage

Indication and Clinical Dosage

rhDNase (Pulmozyme®) is currently approved for use in cystic fibrosis patients, in conjunction with standard thera-

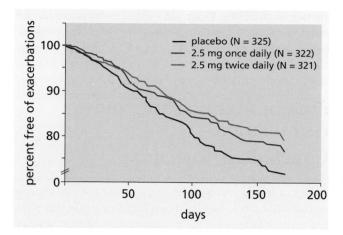

Figure 15.5. Proportion of patients free of exacerbations of respiratory symptoms requiring parenteral antibiotic therapy from a 24-week study. Reprinted by permission of *The New England Journal of Medicine* from HJ Fucus *et al.* Effect of aerosolized recombinant human DNase on exacerbations of respiratory symptoms and on pulmonary function in patients with cystic fibrosis, *N Engl J Med*, v 331, p. 637–642, copyright 1994, Massachusetts Medical Society.

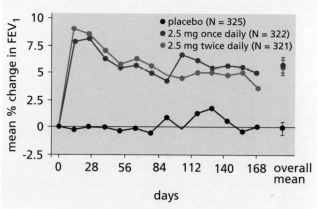

Figure 15.6. Mean percent change in FEV1 from baseline through a 24-week study. Reprinted by permission of *The New England Journal of Medicine* from HJ Fucus *et al.* Effect of aerosolized recombinant human DNase on exacerbations of respiratory symptoms and on pulmonary function in patients with cystic fibrosis, *N Engl J Med*, v 331, p. 637–642, copyright 1994, Massachusetts Medical Society.

pies, to reduce the frequency of respiratory infections requiring parenteral antibiotics and to improve pulmonary function. The recommended dose for use in most cystic fibrosis patients is one 2.5 mg dose inhaled daily using a tested, recommended nebulizer.

Clinical Experience

Clinical usage and therapeutic potential of rhDNase is summarized in reviews by Bryson and Sorkin, 1994; Fuchs *et al.*, 1994 and Shak, 1995.

CYSTIC FIBROSIS

rhDNase has been evaluated in a large, randomized, placebo-controlled trial of clinically stable CF patients, 5 years of age or older, with baseline forced vital capacity (FVC) greater than or equal to 40% of predicted (Fuchs *et al.*, 1994). All patients were receiving additional standard therapies for CF. Patients were treated with placebo, 2.5 mg of rhDNase once or twice a day for six months. When compared to placebo, both once daily and twice daily doses of rhDNase resulted in a 28–37% reduction in respiratory tract infections requiring use of parenteral antibiotics (Figure 15.5). Within 8 days of the start of treatment with rhDNase, mean forced expiratory volume in one second (FEV$_I$) increased 7.9% in patients treated once a day and 9.0% in those treated twice a day compared to the baseline values. The mean FEV$_I$ observed during long-term therapy

increased 5.8% from baseline at the 2.5 mg daily dose level and 5.6% from baseline at the 2.5 mg twice daily dose level (Figure 15.6). The risk of respiratory tract infection was reduced even in patients whose pulmonary function (FEV$_I$) was not improved. This finding is thought to result from improved clearance of mucus from the small airways in the lung which may have little effect on FEV$_I$ or FVC but may significantly reduce the risk of exacerbations of infection (Shak, 1995). The administration of rhDNase also lessened shortness of breath, increased the general perception of well-being and reduced the severity of other cystic fibrosis-related symptoms.

OTHER STUDIES

rhDNase did not produce a pulmonary function benefit in short-term usage in the most severely ill CF patients (FVC less than 40% of predicted) (Shah *et al.*, 1995). These patients with end-stage lung disease represent approximately 7% of the CF population. Many are being prepared for lung transplantation but die while still awaiting an organ due to the shortage of donors. Studies are in progress to assess the impact of chronic usage on pulmonary function and infection risk in this population. Additional clinical studies are ongoing to evaluate the usefulness of rhDNase therapy in CF patients under age 5 and to assess the possible impact of rhDNase therapy on slowing disease progression in CF patients with mild disease.

Clinical trials have indicated that rhDNase therapy can be continued or initiated during an acute respiratory exacerbation (Wilmott *et al.*, 1993). Short-term dose ranging studies demonstrated that doses in excess of 2.5 mg twice daily did not provide further improvement in FEV_1 (Hubbard *et al.*, 1992; Aiken *et al.*, 1992; Ramsey *et al.*, 1993). Patients who have received drug on a cyclical regimen (i.e. administration of rhDNase 10 mg twice daily for 14 days, followed by a 14-day washout period) showed rapid improvement in FEV_1 with the initiation of each cycle and a return to baseline with each rhDNase withdrawal.

Other agents for CF therapy, such as N-acetylcysteine, which acts on mucus glycoproteins, amiloride which blocks sodium absorption in airway epithelial cells, anti-*Pseudomonas* antibodies, anti-proteases, gelsolin, ibuprofen and gene therapy are under active investigation (Rosenstein, 1994). Further clinical studies will be necessary to determine whether use of these agents in combination with rhDNase and/or other standard CF therapies will result in significant improvements in the management of CF.

Clinical studies have also recently started which will evaluate rhDNase for treatment of lupus nephritis, a type of kidney damage resulting from systemic lupus erythematosus (SLE), an inflammatory connective tissue disease.

Safety Concerns

Administration of rhDNase has not been associated with an increase in major adverse events. Most adverse events were not more common with rhDNase than with placebo treatment and probably reflect complications related to the underlying lung disease. Most events associated with dosing were mild, transient in nature, and did not require alterations in dosing. Observed symptoms included hoarseness, pharyngitis, laryngitis, rash, chest pain, and conjunctivitis. Within all the studies a small percentage (average 2–4%) of patients treated with rhDNase developed serum antibodies to rhDNase. None of these patients developed anaphylaxis, and the clinical significance of serum antibodies to rhDNase in unknown.

Concluding Remarks

DNase, a human enzyme responsible for the digestion of extracellular DNA, has been developed as a safe and effective adjunctive agent in the treatment of pulmonary disease in cystic fibrosis patients. rhDNase reduced the viscoelasticity and improved the transport properties of viscous mucus both *in vitro* and *in vivo*. Inhalation of aerosols of rhDNase reduced the risk of infections requiring antibiotics, improved pulmonary function and improved the well-being of CF patients with mild to moderate disease. Continuing studies will assess the usefulness of rhDNase in early-stage CF pulmonary disease and other disease states.

Acknowledgments

This review benefited greatly from the contributions and comments of DNase project team members at Genentech, notably Steve Shak, Dominick Sinicropi, Steve Shire, Victoria Hale and John O'Connor. ∎

Further Reading

- **Boat TF.** (1988). Cystic fibrosis. In *Textbook of respiratory medicine 1*, edited by JF Murray and JA Nadel. Philadelphia: WB Saunders, pp. 1126–1152
- **Bryson HM, Sorkin EM.** (1994). Dornase alfa, a review of its pharmacological and therapeutic potential in cystic fibrosis. *Drugs*, 48 (6), 894–906
- **Collins FS.** (1992). Cystic fibrosis: molecular biology and therapeutic implications. *Science*, 256, 774–779
- **Fuchs HJ, Borowitz DS, Christiansen DH, Morris EM, Nash ML, Ramsey BW, Rosenstein BJ, Smith AL, Wohl MEW.** (1994). Effect of aerosolized recombinant human DNase on exacerbations of respiratory symptoms and on pulmonary function in patients with cystic fibrosis. *New Engl J Med*, 331, 637–642
- **Gonda I.** (1990). Aerosols for delivery of therapeutic and diagnostic agents to the respiratory tract. *Crit Rev Ther Drug Carrier Systems*, 6 (4), 273–313
- **Rosenstein BJ.** (1994). Cystic fibrosis in the year 2000. *Semin Respir Crit Care Med*, 15, 446–451
- **Shak S.** (1995). Aerosolized recombinant human DNase I for the treatment of cystic fibrosis. *Chest*, 107(suppl), 65s–70s
- **Shak S, Capon DJ, Helmiss R, Marsters SA, Baker CL.** (1990). Recombinant human DNase I reduces the viscosity of cystic fibrosis sputum. *Proc Natl Acad Sci USA*, 87, 9188–9192

References

- Aiken ML, Burke W, McDonald G, Shak S, Montgomery AB, Smith A. (1992). Recombinant human DNase inhalation in normal subjects and patients with cystic fibrosis. *J Am Med Assoc*, 267(14), 1947–1951
- Armstrong JB, White JC. (1950). Liquifaction of viscous purulent exudates by deoxyribonuclease. *Lancet*, 2, 739–742
- Bataillon V, Lhermitte M, Lafitte, JJ, Pommery J, Roussel P. (1992). The binding of amikacin to macromolecules from the sputum of patients suffering from respiratory diseases. *J Antimicrob Chemother*, 29, 499–508
- Chernick WS, Barbero GJ, Eichel HJ. (1961). *In-vitro* evaluation of effect of enzymes on tracheobronchial secretions from patients with cystic fibrosis. *Pediatrics*, 27, 589–596
- Chernick WS, Barbero GJ. (1959). Composition of tracheobronchial secretions in cystic fibrosis on the pancreas and bronchiectasis. *Pediatrics*, 24, 739–745
- Cipolla DC, Gonda I, Meserve KC, Weck S, Shire SJ. (1994). Formulation and aerosol delivery of recombinant deoxyribonucleic acid derived human deoxyribonuclease I. In *Formulation and Delivery of Protein and Peptides*, edited by JL Cleland and R Langer. Washington, DC: ACS Symposium Series 567, American Chemical Society, pp. 322–342
- Elmes PC, White JC. (1953). Deoxyribonuclease in the treatment of purulent bronchitis. *Thorax*, 8, 295–300
- Green JD. (1994). Pharmaco-toxicological expert report, Pulmozyme™, rhDNase, Genentech, Inc, *Human & Expt Tox*, 13, Suppl 1, S1–S42
- Hubbard RC, McElvaney NG, Birrer P, Shak S, Robinson WW, Jolley C, Wu M, Chernick MS, Crystal RG. (1992). A preliminary study of aerosolized recombinant human deoxyribonuclease I in the treatment of cystic fibrosis. *New Engl J Med*, 326, 812–815
- Laube BL, Auci RM, Shields DE, Christiansen D, Fuchs HJ, Rosenstein BJ. (1993). A randomized, placebo-controlled trial of the effect of recombinant human DNase I (rhDNase) on the deposition homogeneity and mucociliary clearance of radioaerosol in patients with cystic fibrosis. *Pediatr Pulmonol*, Suppl 9, 155–156
- Lieberman J. (1968). Dornase aerosol effect on sputum viscosity in cases of cystic fibrosis. *J Am Med Assoc*, 205, 312–313
- Lieberman J. (1962). Enzymatic dissolution of pulmonary secretions. *Am J Dis Child*, 104, 3342–348
- Matthews LW, Spector S, Lemm J, Potter JL. (1963). The over-all chemical composition of pulmonary secretions from patients with cystic fibrosis, bronchiecstatis and laryngectomy. *Am Rev Respir Dis*, 88, 119–204
- Mohler M, Cook J, Lewis D, Moore J, Sinicropi D, Championsmith A, Ferraiolo B, Mordenti J. (1993). Altered pharmacokinetics of recombinant human deoxyribonuclease in rats due to the presence of a binding protein. *Drug Met Disp*, 21, 71–75
- Oefner C, Suck D. (1986). Crystallographic refinement and structure of DNase I at 2 Å resolution. *J Mol Biol*, 192, 605–632
- Potter JL, Spector S, Matthews LW, Lemm J. (1969). Studies on pulmonary secretions. 3. The nucleic acids in whole pulmonary secretions from patients with cystic fibrosis bronchiectasis and laryngectomy. *Am Rev Resp Dis*, 99, 909–915
- Potter J, Matthews LW, Lemm J, Spector S. (1960). The composition of pulmonary secretions from patients with and without cystic fibrosis. *Am J Dis Child*, 100, 493–495
- Ramphal R, Lhermitte M, Filliat M, Roussel P. (1988). The binding of anti-pseudomonal antibiotics to macromolecules from cystic fibrosis sputum. *J Antimicrob Chemother*, 22, 483–490
- Ramsey BW, Astley SJ, Aitken ML, Burke W, Colin AA, Dorkin HL, Eisenberg JD, Gibson RL, Harwood IR, Schidow DV, Wilmott RW, Wohl ME, Meyerson LJ, Shak S, Fuchs H, Smith AL. (1993). Efficacy and safety of short-term administration of aerosolized recombinant human deoxyribonuclease in patients with cystic fibrosis. *Am Rev Respir Dis*, 148, 145–151
- Raskin P. (1968). Bronchospasm after inhalation of pancreatic Dornase. *Am Rev Respir Dis*, 98, 697–698
- Riordan JR, Rommens JM, Kerem B, Alon N, Rozmahel R, Grzelczak Z, Zielenski J, Lok S, Plavsic N, Chou J, Drumm ML, Iannuzzi MC, Collins FS, Tsui LC. (1989). Identification of the cystic fibrosis gene: genetic anaysis. *Science*, 245, 1073–1080
- Salomon A, Herchfus JA, Segal MS. (1954). Aerosols of pancreatic Dornase in bronchopulmonary disease. *Ann Allergy*, 12, 71–79
- Shah PL, Bush A, Canny GJ, Colin AA, Fuchs HJ, Geddes DM, Johnson CAC, Light MC, Scott SF, Tullis DE, DeVault A, Wohl ME, Hodson ME. (1995). Recombinant human DNase I in cystic fibrosis patients with severe pulmonary disease: a short-term, double-blind study followed by six months of open-label treatment. *Eur Respir J*, 8, 954–958
- Sinicropi DV, Williams M, Prince WS, Lofgren JA, Lucas M, DeVault A, Baughman S, Nash M, Fuchs H, Shak S, DNase Clinical Investigators. (1994). Sputum pharmacodynamics and pharmacokinetics of recombinant human DNase I in cystic fibrosis. *Am J Respir Crit Care Med*, 149, suppl 4, A671
- Spier R, Witebsky E, Paine JR. (1961). Aerosolized pancreatic Dornase and antibiotics in pulmonary infections. *J Am Med Assoc*, 178, 878–886
- Wilmott R, Amin RS, Collin A, et al. (1993). A phase II, double-blind. multicenter study of the safety and efficacy of aerosolised recombinant human DNase I (rhDNase) in hospitalized patients with CF experiencing acute pulmonary exacerbations. *Pediatr Pulmonol*, Suppl 9, 154
- Wolf E, Frenz J, Suck D. (1995). Structure of human pancreatic DNase I at 2.2 Å resolution. *Protein Eng*, 8 (Suppl), 79
- Zahm JM, de Bentzmann SG, Deneuville E, Perrot-Minnot C, Dabadie A, Pennaforte F, Roussey M, Shak S, Puchelle E. (1995). Dose-dependent *in vitro* effect of recombinant human DNase on rheological and transport properties of cystic fibrosis respiratory mucus. *Eur Respir J*, 8, 381–386

Self-Assessment Questions

Question 1: *Why would reduction in apparent size of DNA molecules in mucus improve pulmonary function and/or reduce the risk of infections?*

Question 2: *What factors must be considered when choosing formulation components for an aerosolized protein?*

Answers

Answer 1: Reduction in DNA size reduces viscoelasticity of mucus and improves clearability of the mucus from the airways. Clearance of the DNA-rich mucus from the airways may also improve the efficacy of antibiotics typically administered for chronic lung infections since the aminoglycoside antibiotics commonly used have been shown to bind to DNA.

Answer 2: The formulation should be isotonic, have minimal additives (buffer agents, surfactants, etc.) and maintain a pH >5.0. Stability of the protein and development of possible protein aggregates should be carefully monitored if using minimal buffering agents and surfactants.

16 Follicle-Stimulating Hormone (FSH)

by: Tom Sam and Willem de Boer

Introduction

About 15% of all couples experience infertility at some time during their reproductive lives. Increasingly, infertility can be treated by the use of assisted reproductive technologies, such as *in-vitro* fertilization (IVF), gamete intra-fallopian transfer (GIFT) and intracytoplasmic sperm injection (ICSI). Gonadotropin treatment to increase the number of oocytes is a common element of these programmes. A major cause for female infertility is chronic anovulation. Patients suffering from this condition are also treated with gonadotropins with the aim to achieve monofollicular development.

Gonadotropin preparations for infertility treatment are traditionally derived from postmenopausal urine. The urinary preparations contain Follicle-Stimulating Hormone (FSH), but are typically less than 5% pure and contain by nature also Luteinizing Hormone (LH) as contaminant. Recombinant DNA technology allowed the reproducible manufacture of FSH preparations of high purity and specific activity, and devoid of urinary contaminants. Recombinant FSH is produced using a Chinese Hamster Ovary (CHO) cell line, transfected with the genes encoding for the two human FSH subunits (Howles, 1996). The isolation procedures render a product of high purity (at least 97%), devoid of LH activity and very similar to natural FSH.

Currently, there are two clinically approved recombinant FSH-containing drug products on the market. These are Gonal-F®, manufactured by Ares-Serono, and Puregon®, manufactured by NV Organon. Regulatory authorities have issued two distinct International Non-proprietary Names for the two corresponding recombinant FSH drug substances, i.e. follitropin alpha (Gonal-F®) and follitropin beta (Puregon®). Thus, the two products should be considered as similar, but not identical preparations containing distinct active ingredients.

Biological Role

The primary function of the glycoprotein hormone FSH in the female is the regulation of follicle growth. FSH is produced and secreted by the anterior lobe of the pituitary, a gland at the base of the brain. Its target is the FSH receptor at the surface of the granulosa cells that surround the oocyte. FSH acts synergistically with oestrogens and LH to stimulate proliferation of these granulosa cells thereby leading to follicular growth. This explains why deficient endogenous production of FSH may cause infertility.

Chemical Description

Follicle-stimulating hormone belongs to a family of structurally related glycoproteins also including luteinizing hormone (LH), chorionic gonadotropin (CG) and thyroid-stimulating hormone (TSH). Each hormone is a dimeric protein consisting of two non-covalently associated glycoprotein subunits, denoted α and β. The α-subunit is identical for all these gonadotropins, and it is the β-subunit that provides each hormone with its specific biological function.

The glycoprotein subunits of FSH consist of two polypeptide backbones with carbohydrate side-chains attached to the two asparagine (Asn) amino acid residues on each subunit. The oligosaccharides are attached to Asn-52 and Asn-78 on the α-subunit (92 amino acids), and to Asn-7 and Asn-24 on the β-subunit (111 amino acids). The glycoprotein FSH has a molecular mass of approximately 35 kD. For the FSH preparation to be biologically active, the two subunits must be correctly assembled into their 3-dimensional dimeric protein structure and post-translationally modified (Figure 16.1).

Assembly and glycosylation are intracellular processes, taking place in the endoplasmatic reticulum and in the Golgi apparatus. This glycosylation process leads to the formation of a population of hormone isoforms differing in their carbohydrate side chain composition. The carbohydrate side chains of FSH are essential for its biological activity since they 1) influence FSH receptor binding, 2) play an important role in the signal transduction into the FSH target cell and 3) affect the plasma residence time of the hormone.

Recombinant FSH contains approximately 36% carbohydrate on a mass per mass basis. The carbohydrate side chains are composed of mannose, fucose, N-acetyl-

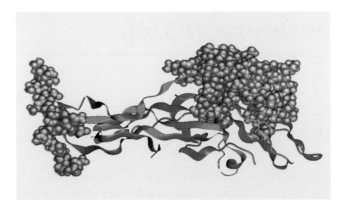

Figure 16.1. A 3-dimensional model of FSH. The ribbons represent the polypeptide backbones of the α-subunit (green ribbon) and the β-subunit (blue ribbon). The carbohydrate side chains (yellow and pink space filled globules) cover large areas of the surface of the polypeptide subunits. The sialic acid carbohydrates are depicted in pink.

glucosamine (GlcNAc), galactose and sialic acid. Structure analysis by ^{1}H-NMR spectroscopy on oligosaccharides enzymatically cleaved from follitropin beta, reveals minor differences with natural FSH. For instance, the bisecting GlcNAc residues are lacking in the recombinant molecule, simply because the FSH-producing CHO cells do not possess the enzymes to incorporate these residues. Furthermore, the carbohydrate side chains of recombinant FSH exclusively contain α2–3 linked sialic acid, whereas in the natural hormone α1–6 linked sialic acid occurs as well. All carbohydrate side chains identified in recombinant FSH are, however, moieties normally found in other natural human glycoproteins.

Production of Recombinant FSH

The genes coding for the human FSH α-subunit and β-subunit were inserted in cloning vectors (plasmids) to enable efficient transfer into recipient cells. These vectors also contained promoters that can direct transcription of foreign genes in recipient cells. CHO cells were selected as recipient cells since they are easily transfected with foreign DNA, and are capable of synthesizing glycoproteins. Furthermore they can be grown in cell cultures on a large scale. To construct an FSH-producing cell line NV Organon, the manufacturer of Puregon®, used one single vector containing the coding sequences for both subunit genes (Olijve, 1996). Ares Serono, the manufacturer of Gonal-F® used two separate vectors, one for each subunit gene (Howles, 1996). Following transfection, a genetically stable transformant producing biologically active recombinant FSH is isolated. For the CHO cell line used for the manufacture

of Puregon® it was shown that approximately 150–450 gene copies were present.

In order to establish a master cell bank (MCB) identical cell preparations of the selected clone are stored in individual vials and cryopreserved until needed. Subsequently a working cell bank (WCB) is established by expansion of cells derived from a single vial of the MCB and aliquots are put in vials and cryopreserved as well. Each time a production run is started, cells from one or more vials of the WCB are cultured.

Both recombinant FSH products are isolated from cell culture supernatant collected from a perfusion-type of bioreactor containing recombinant FSH-producing CHO cells grown on microcarriers. This is because CHO cells are anchorage-dependent cells, which implies that a proper surface must be provided for cell growth. The reactor is perfused with growth-promoting medium during a period that may continue up to 3 months (cf. Chapter 3).

The down-stream purification processes for the isolation of the two recombinant FSH products are different. For Puregon® a series of chromatographic steps including anion and cation exchange chromatography, hydrophobic chromatography and size-exclusion chromatography is used. Recombinant FSH in Gonal-F® is obtained by a similar process of five chromatographic steps, but also includes an immunoaffinity step using a murine FSH-specific monoclonal antibody. In both production processes, each purification step is rigorously controlled in order to ensure the batch-to-batch consistency of the purified product.

Isohormones

Structural Characteristics

As explained above, FSH exists in many distinct molecular forms (isohormones), with identical polypeptide backbones, but differing in oligosaccharide structure, in particular in the degree of terminal sialylation. These isohormones can be separated by chromatofocusing or isoelectric focusing on the basis of their different isoelectric points (pI), as has been demonstrated for follotropin beta (De Leeuw et al., Figure 16.2). The typical pattern for FSH indicates an isohormone distribution between pI values of 6 and 4. To obtain structural information at the subunit level, the two subunits were separated by RP-HPLC and treated to release the N-linked carbohydrate side chains. Fractions with low pI values (acidic fractions) displayed a high content of tri- and tetrasialo-oligosaccharides and a low content of neutral and monosialo oligosaccharides. For fractions with a high pI (basic fractions) value the reverse was found. The β-subunit carbohydrate side chains appeared to be more heavily sialylated and branched than the α-subunit carbohydrate side chains. The low pI value isohormones of follitropin

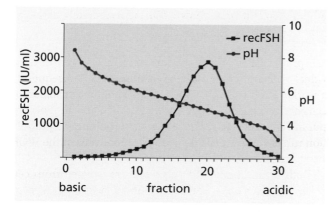

Figure 16.2. Isohormone profile of recombinant follicle stimulating hormone (follitropin beta) after preparative free flow focussing (De Leeuw *et al.*, 1996). The FSH concentration was determined by a two-site immunoassay that is capable of quantifying the various isohormones equally well.

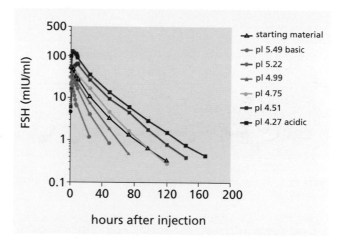

Figure 16.3. Kinetic behavior of FSH isoforms after a single intramuscular injection (20 IU/kg) in Beagle dogs.

beta have a high sialic acid/galactose ratio and are rich in tri- and tetra-antennary N-linked carbohydrate side chains as compared with the side chains of the high pI value isohormones.

Biological Properties of Recombinant FSH Isohormones

An FSH preparation can be characterised with four essentially different assays, each having its own specific merits. The immunoassay (1) determines FSH-specific structural features and provides a relative measure for the quantity of FSH. The receptor binding assay (2) provides information on the proper conformation for interaction with the FSH receptor. Receptor binding studies with calf testis membranes showed that FSH isoform activity in follitropin beta decreases when going from high to low pI isoforms. The *in-vitro* bioassay (3) measures the capability of FSH to transduce signals into target cells (the intrinsic bioactivity). The *in-vitro* bioactivity, assessed in the rat Sertoli cell bioassay, also decreases when going from high to low pI isoforms. The *in-vivo* bioassay (4) provides the overall bioactivity of an FSH preparation. It is determined by the number of molecules, the plasma residence time, the receptor binding activity and the signal transduction. Surprisingly, in contrast to the receptor binding and *in-vitro* bioassays, the *in-vivo* biological activity determined in rats shows an approximate 20-fold increase between isoforms with a pI value of 5.49 as compared to those with a pI of 4.27. These results indicate that the basic isohormones exhibit the highest receptor binding and signal transduction activity, whereas the acidic isohormones are the more active forms under *in-vivo* conditions.

Pharmacokinetic Behavior of Recombinant FSH Isohormones

The pharmacokinetic behaviour of follitropin beta and its isohormones was investigated in Beagle dogs, that were given an intramuscular bolus injection of a number of FSH isohormone fractions each with a specific pI value. With a decrease in pI value from 5.49 (basic) to 4.27 (acidic), the AUC increased and the clearance rate decreased, each more than ten-fold (Figure 16.3). A more than two-fold difference in elimination half-life between the most acidic and the most basic FSH isohormone fraction was calculated. The absorption rate of the two most acidic isoforms was higher than the absorption rates of all other isoforms. The AUC and the clearance rate for the follitropin beta preparation, being a mixture of all isohormone fractions, corresponded with the centre of the isohormone profile (Figure 16.3). In contrast, the elimination of the follitropin beta preparation occurred at a rate similar to that of the most acidic fractions, indicating that the elimination rate is largely determined by the removal of the most acidic isoforms from the plasma. Thus for follitropin beta isohormone fractions a clear correlation exists between pI value and pharmacokinetic behaviour. Increasing acidity leads to an increase in extent of absorption and elimination half life, but to a decrease in clearance rates.

Pharmaceutical Formulations

Protein drugs are generally lyophilized, because of their limited stability in aqueous solutions. Also the FSH preparations are freeze-dried. They are available in different strengths and presentation forms (see Table 16.1). Follitropin alpha

Market preparation	Freeze-dried presentation	Container	Strength
Gonal-F® (follitropin alpha) Ares-Sereno	powder powder	ampoule, vial ampoule, vial	75 IU 150 IU
Puregon® (follitropin beta) NV Organon	lyosphere cake lyosphere lyosphere	ampoule vial ampoule ampoule	50 IU 75 IU 100 IU 150 IU

Table 16.1. The presentation forms of recombinant FSH products.

is formulated with sucrose (bulking agent, lyoprotectant), sodium dihydrogen phosphate/disodium hydrogen phosphate, phosphoric acid and sodium hydroxide (for pH adjustment). Follitropin beta is formulated with sucrose, sodium citrate (stabilizer), polysorbate 20 (lyoprotectant and agent to prevent adsorption losses), and hydrochloride/sodium hydroxide (for pH adjustment).

Recombinant FSH preparations distinguish themselves by their high purity (at least 97%) e.g. from urinary FSH preparations, typically having a purity of less than 5%. Pure proteins are, however, relatively unstable and difficult to process. Due to their high affinity for glass and polymers substantial losses of activity through adsorption can be anticipated. The activity yields of conventionally freeze-dried recombinant FSH preparations may therefore be substantially lower than 100 percent. The newly developed lyosphere formulation and process, however, yielded a freeze-dried FSH product with significantly less activity loss (Skrabanja and Vromans, 1996). Lyospheres are frozen drops of aqueous solution, which are freeze-dried in bulk and subsequently put in ampoules. Compared to the traditional freeze-dried cake formulation, lyospheres have the advantage of high dose uniformity, less adsorption to the glass walls of the ampoule, instantaneous dissolution, and in case of FSH, improved stability.

The shelf-life of the recombinant FSH products is two years when stored in the containers in which they are supplied, at temperatures below 30°C, not frozen and protected from light.

Clinical Aspects

Both recombinant FSH products on the market have been approved for two indications. The first indication is anovulation (including polycystic ovarian disease) in women, who are unresponsive to clomiphene citrate. The second indication is controlled ovarian hyperstimulation to induce the development of multiple follicles in medically assisted reproduction programs such as IVF and embryo transfer.

In anovulatory infertility, FSH treatment aims for the development of a single follicle, whereas in IVF FSH treatment is aimed at multifollicular development. For the treatment of anovulatory patients it is recommended to start Puregon® treatment with 50 IU per day for 7 to 14 days and gradually increase dosing with steps of 50 IU in case no sufficient response is seen. This gradually dose-increasing schedule is followed in order to prevent multifollicular development and the induction of ovarian hyperstimulation syndrome (a serious condition of unwanted hyperstimulation).

The most commonly applied treatment regimen in IVF starts by suppressing endogenous gonadotropin levels by a GnRH (gonadotropin releasing hormone) agonist. It is recommended to start Puregon® treatment with 100–200 IU of recombinant FSH followed by maintenance doses of 50–350 IU. The availability of a surplus of collected oocytes allows replacement of 2–3 embryos. Similar treatment regimens are recommended for Gonal-F®.

Serum levels of FSH do not correlate with pharmacological responses such as production of oestradiol, inhibin response or follicular development. Moreover, there is a large variability found for the individual pharmacological response to a fixed dose of recombinant FSH. This emphasises the importance of a patient individualised dosing and treatment regimen when using recombinant FSH.

Follitropin beta has an elimination half life of approximately 40 h. Steady-state levels of follitropin beta are therefore reached after four daily doses. At that time, the concentrations of circulating immunoreactive FSH are about a factor of 1.5–2.5 higher than after a single dose. This increase is relevant in attaining therapeutically effective plasma concentrations of FSH. Follitropin beta can be administered via the intramuscular as well as via the subcutaneous route, because the absence of impurities results in an improved local tolerance. Bioavailability via both routes is approximately 77%. Injections of the highly pure follitropin beta preparations do not require medical personnel, but can be given by the patient herself or her partner. In a large number of patients treated with follitropin beta, no formation of antibodies against recombinant FSH or CHO-cell derived proteins was seen.

Differences with Urinary FSH Preparations

In IVF, follitropin beta treatment is more effective and efficient than treatment with urinary FSH, since more follicles, oocytes, embryos and pregnancies are obtained with a lower total dose of recombinant FSH in a shorter treatment period. Treatment of patients with anovulatory infertility with either follitropin beta or urinary FSH was equally effective, but follitropin beta treatment was more efficient (a lower total dose was needed in a shorter duration of treatment). ∎

Further Reading

- **Damm JBL.** (1995). Application of Glycobiology in the Biotechnological Production of Pharmaceuticals. *Pharm. Tech. Europe*, 9, 28–34

- **Groves MJ.** (1996). Pharmaceutical Biotechnology: Drugs for the Future. In *Innovations in drug delivery: impact on pharmacotherapy*, edited by AP Sam, JG Fokkens, 2nd Edition. The Netherlands: Anselmus Society, Houten, pp. 146–156

- **Sam AP, Metsers FAAJ.** (1997). Chemistry and Pharmacy Aspects of Applications for Marketing Authorisations for Peptide and Protein Medicines. In *Minutes 8th Intern. Pharm. Techn. Symp. "Recent Advances in Peptide and Protein Delivery"*, edited by AA Hincal. Paris: Editions de Santé

References

- **De Boer W, Mannaerts B.** (1990). Recombinant follicle stimulating hormone. II. Biochemical and biological characteristics. In *From clone to clinic, Developments in Biotherapy*, edited by DJA Crommelin, H Schellekens, Vol. 1. Dordrecht: Kluwer Academic Publishers, pp. 253–259

- **European Public Assessment Report Gonal-F (Follitropin alpha)**, CPMP/415/95, European Agency for the Evaluation of Medicinal Products

- **European Public Assessment Report Puregon (Follitropin beta)**, CPMP/003/96, European Agency for the Evaluation of Medicinal Products

- **Howles CM.** (1996). Genetic engineering of human FSH (Gonal-F®). *Human Reproduction Update*, 2, 172–191

- **De Leeuw R, Mulders J, Voortman G, Rombout F, Damm J, Kloosterboer L.** (1996). Structure-function relationship of recombinant follicle stimulating hormone (Puregon®). *Mol. Human Reproduction*, 2, 361–369

- **Olijve W, de Boer W, Mulders JWM, van Wezenbeek PMGF.** (1996). Molecular biology and biochemistry of human recombinant follicle stimulating hormone (Puregon®). *Mol. Human Reproduction*, 2, 371–382

- **Out HJ, Mannaerts BMJL, Driessen SGAJ, Coelingh Bennink HJT.** (1996). Recombinant follicle stimulating hormone (rFSH; Puregon®) in assisted reproduction: More oocytes, more pregnancies. Results from five comparative studies. *Human Reprod. Update*, 2, 162–171

- **Skrabanja A, Vromans H.** (1996). Lyospheres, a new pharmaceutical parenteral dosage form for proteins. *Orgyn*, 6, 34

Self-Assessment Questions

Question 1:   *What makes the formulation process of recombinant FSH difficult?*

Question 2:   *What makes the biological properties of glycoprotein hormone preparations so complex?*

Answers

Answer 1:   Recombinant FSH preparation are highly purified, not stabilised by the presence of other (contaminating) proteins. Urinary FSH preparations contain, for instance, more than 95% of proteins of largely undetermined origin. Recombinant protein formulations can be protected against the destabilising effect of the freeze-drying process and against the effect of adsorption losses by the addition of albumin or gelatin in their formulations. This is however not desirable, since it unnecessarily contaminates the highly purified protein, and may lead to immunological and/or local tolerance problems. This requires, therefore, optimisation of the formulation and the freeze-drying process (cf. Chapter 4).

Answer 2:   FSH is a glycoprotein existing of a large array of isohormones, differing in the composition of their four carbohydrate side chains. The fate of such an isohormone in an organism is a function of its intrinsic activity and its pharmacokinetics. It has been demonstrated that for recombinant FSH isohormone fractions, a clear correlation exists between their pI value and their receptor binding activity on one hand and their pharmacokinetic behaviour on the other. The relatively basic isoforms display high receptor binding and high intrinsic bioactivity with a short plasma residence time. Relatively acidic isohormones, that are more heavily sialylated, combine low receptor binding and low intrinsic bioactivity with a long plasma residence time. Increasing acidity of the isohormone leads to an increase in absorption rate and elimination half-life, and to a decrease in clearance rate. The longer blood residence times of the acidic isohormones counterbalance their relatively lower intrinsic activities.

17 Dispensing Biotechnology Products: Handling, Professional Education and Product Information

by: Gary H. Smith and Peggy Piascik

Introduction

Pharmacists have traditionally been responsible for the preparation and/or dispensing of pharmaceuticals. Up until now most products for parenteral use have been available in ready to use containers or required dilution with water or saline prior to use without any special handling requirements. In hospitals, pharmacists have been involved with the preparation and dispensing of parenteral products for individual patients for many years. Biotechnology products are proteins subject to denaturation and thus require special handling techniques. While (hospital) pharmacists are skilled in handling parenteral products, biotechnology products may provide additional challenges which will be explained in more detail in this chapter.

Pharmacist Reluctance

Practicing pharmacists may be reluctant to provide pharmaceutical care services to patients who require therapy with biotechnology drugs for a variety of reasons including (1) lack of knowledge about the tools of biotechnology; (2) lack of understanding of the therapeutic aspects of recombinant protein products; (3) unfamiliarity of the side effects and patient counseling information; (4) unfamiliarity with the storage, handling and reconstitution of proteins; and (5) difficulty of handling reimbursement issues.

Some pharmacists may incorrectly view these drugs as quite different from traditional drug products which are normally dispensed as familiar oral dosage forms. However, in most respects the services offered by pharmacists when dispensing biotechnology products are basically the same as those provided for traditional tablets, or injectable products. In addition, pharmacists have dispensed insulin and a variety of other proteins routinely for years. As more of these novel protein products come to market and the indications for existing agents are expanded for ambulatory patients, pharmacists will be increasingly required to deal with protein pharmaceuticals. While the first protein/peptide recombinant products were used primarily in hospital settings, many of those agents have become commonplace in ambulatory settings such as home health pharmacies and home infusion services. Even the traditional community pharmacy is now likely to be dispensing products like colony stimulating factors, growth hormone, and interferons to name a few.

Types of Information Needed by Pharmacists

What types of information do pharmacists require to be confident dispensers of biotech drugs? For pharmacists who have been out of school for more than five to ten years, a basic understanding of (or updated information regarding) the immune system, diseases related to immunosuppression and autoimmune mechanisms, and ways in which drugs may modify the immune system is essential. Several appropriate books which can provide a basic background in immunology are listed in Table 17.1. Additionally, practitioners may enroll in organized courses of continuing education programs which can provide up-to-date information in the area of immunology. Most current pharmacy students will be sufficiently trained in basic immunology as part of their professional curriculum.

Many pharmacists and pharmacy students upon hearing the word biotechnology imagine a discipline too technical or complicated to be understood by the typical practitioner. Pharmacists merely need to learn that biotechnology refers to a set of tools which has allowed great strides to be made in basic research, the understanding of disease and development of new therapeutic agents. All pharmacists should have a basic understanding of recombinant DNA technology and monoclonal antibody technology. It is not necessary that pharmacy practitioners know how to use these tools in the laboratory but rather how the use of these tools provides us with new products and a greater understanding of disease processes.

Pharmacists may also need to review or learn anew about protein chemistry and those characteristics that affect therapeutic activity, product storage and routes of administration of these drugs. Apart from this textbook, several publications, videotapes and continuing professional education programs from industry and academic institutions are available to pharmacists for learning about the technical aspects of product storage and handling. Pharmacists need to become familiar with the drug delivery

■ **Cellular and Molecular Immunology.**
Abbas AK, Lichtman AH, Pober JS.
Philadelphia: W.B. Saunders Company, 1994: 331
pp. *Softbound book providing basic
immunology concepts and clinical issues.*

■ **Immunology: a short course.** 2nd ed.
Benjamin E.
New York: Wiley-Liss, 1991: 459 pp.
*Softbound elementary text with review
questions for each chapter.*

■ **Concepts in Immunology and
Immunotherapeutics.** 2nd ed.
Koeller J, Tami J, eds. Bethesda, MD:
American Society of Hospital Pharmacists, 1992:
537 pp.
*Review of basic immunology including
therapeutic applications.*

■ **Medical Immunology for Students.**
Playfair JHL, Lydyard PM.
New York: Churchill Livingstone, 1995: 104 pp.
*Softbound, simple overview of basic
immunology, immunopathology and clinical
immunology.*

■ **Immunology: clinical, fundamental and
therapeutic aspects.**
Ram BP, Harris MC, Tyle, P, eds.
New York: VCH, 1990: 364 pp.
*Review of basic immunology, immunobiology,
clinical immunology and related drugs; a
scientific viewpoint.*

■ **Essential immunology.** 8th ed.
Roitt IM.
Oxford; Boston: Blackwell Scientific Publications,
1994: 448 pp.
Softbound basic immunology textbook.

Table 17.1. Selected texts to enhance immunology knowledge.

systems currently in use for biotech drugs as well as those which are likely to be used in the next few years (cf. Chapter 4).

Sources of Information for Pharmacists

Many pharmacists do not know where to obtain the information which will allow them to be good providers of products of biotechnology. This textbook provides much of the essential background information in one source.

Examples of practical resources which are available to pharmacists when learning about biotech drugs are listed in Table 17.2.

A number of continuing education programs and journal articles in the past have focused on biotechnology methods describing recombinant DNA technology and how monoclonal antibodies are made. Many manufacturer-sponsored programs are now on the market describing biotech products which are currently available and those likely to come to market in the near future. An excellent source of information on biotechnology in general and specific products in particular is the biotech drug industry. Manufacturers are prepared to help pharmacists in the most effective provision of products and services to patients, both hospital-based and ambulatory (Table 17.3). However, many pharmacists are unaware of these services and how to obtain them.

A variety of manufacturer-sponsored programs and services are available to both health professionals and patients. The information provided by manufacturers can help pharmacists confidently provide biotechnology products to their patients. The services provided generally fall into three categories: reimbursement information, customer/medical services and support, and educational materials.

The Pharmacist and Handling of Biotech Drugs

For biotech based pharmaceuticals, it is logical for the pharmacist to be responsible for their storage, preparation and dispensing as well as patient education. However it will require, in many cases, that additional education be obtained by the pharmacist in order to be prepared for this role. This is especially true for pharmacists who practice primarily in the ambulatory care setting since many of these products will be administered by the patient him or herself in the home. The hospital as well as the community pharmacy of the future will handle different kinds of materials than they do today. The future community pharmacy will stock pumps, patches, timed-release tablets, liposomes, implants, and vials of tailored monoclonal antibodies. With gene therapy and gene splicing on the horizon it is not inconceivable that the pharmacist may well be involved with related products. A list of currently available and future products is presented in Chapters 8–16 and 18 (Check, 1984; Koeller *et al.*, 1991; Stewart *et al.*, 1989).

This chapter will discuss the general principles that pharmacists will need to know about storage, handling, preparation, administration of biotech products and issues related to outpatient/home care. Specific examples will be discussed for illustrative purposes. Most available products can be found in Table 17.4, which lists the products along with specific handling requirements. For more current

The Pharmacists' Role with Biotechnology Products. Jim Koeller J, Fields S. Contemporary Pharmacy Issues, The Upjohn Company, 1991. *Discusses issues which must be addressed when evaluating or working with biotech drugs.* **Pharmaceutical Considerations in the Use of Biotechnology Agents.** Pharmacy Rounds, Developed by the School of Pharmacy, University of California at San Francisco, produced by American Medical Communications; accredited for continuing education through July 1, 1996; 1994. *Consists of a video program which describes appropriate reconstitution and administration of peptide products and individual monographs of most biotech drugs; a technical chart summarizing storage and handling considerations is included.*	**Biotech Rx: Opportunities in Therapy Management,** a program focusing on integrating biotechnology products into ambulatory care pharmacy practice: designed for practitioners in community pharmacy, outpatient clinics, and home infusion agencies; series consists of 3 executive reports and 4 learning modules; each module contains a workbook with hands on tools and forms; program is available from the American Pharmaceutical Association, 2215 Constitution Avenue NW, Washington DC 20037-2985, 1-800-237-APhA. approved for continuing education credit through October 1, 1996.
Executive Report Series 1. Perspective on Biotechnology: The Pharmacist's Role 2. Effective Patient Care: From Drug Therapy to Reimbursement 3. Biotechnology in Oncology: Focus on Cytokines	**Learning Modules** 1. Reimbursement for Biotechnology Products 2. Marketing Biotechnology Pharmacy Services to the Medical Community 3. Counseling Patients Taking Biotechnology Products 4. Negotiating Contracts Associated with Provision of Biotechnology Pharmacy Service

Table 17.2. Selected practical resources for information about biotechnology drugs.

information you may need to contact the manufacturer. A list of manufacturers and their telephone numbers can be found in Table 17.3.

Storage

Biotech products have special storage requirements which in most cases differ from the majority of products pharmacists normally dispense. The shelf life of these products is often considerably shorter than for traditional compounds. E.g., interferon α 2a (McEvoy, 1995; Roche, 1992) is only stable in a refrigerator in the ready-to-use solution for 12 months. Since most of these products need to be kept at refrigerated temperatures some facilities may need to increase cold storage space in order to accommodate the storage needs.

Temperature Requirements

Since biotech products are primarily proteins, they are subject to denaturation when exposed to extreme temperatures. In general, most biotech products are shipped by the manufacturer in gel ice containers and need to be stored at 2–8°C (Banga *et al.*, 1994). Once reconstituted, they should be kept stored under refrigeration until just prior to use. There are, of course, exceptions to this rule as exemplified by alteplase (tissue plasminogen activator). Alteplase is stable at room temperature for several years (Genentech, 1994). For individual product requirements for temperature requirements, the product brochure or the manufacturer should be contacted. Table 17.4 also lists temperature requirements for most of the available products. The variability between products with respect to temperature is exemplified by granulocyte-colony stimulating factor (G-CSF; filgrastim) (Amgen, 1992) and erythropoietin (Amgen, 1993) which are stable in ready-to-use form at room temperature for 24 hours and 14 days, respectively. Granulocyte macrophage-colony stimulating factor (GM-CSF; sargramostim) (Immunex, 1992) on the other hand is packaged as a lyophilized powder but still requires refrigeration and once reconstituted is stable at room temperature for 30 days or refrigerator for 2 years. Aldesleukin (interleukin-2) is stable for 48 hours at room temperature or up to 18 months in a refrigerator (Chiron, 1994). Betaseron

Manufacturer	Product	Professional services	Reimbursement hotline/ indigent patient programs
Amgen Inc.	Neupogen Epogen	1-800-77-AMGEN	1-800-272-9376[1]
Baxter Hyland	Recombinate	1-800-423-209	1-800-548-4448
Bayer	KoGENate	1-800-468-0894	1-800-998-9180
Berlex Lab.	Betaseron	1-800-888-4112	1-800-788-1467[2]
Chiron Therapeutic	Proleukin	1-800-244-7668	1-800-775-7533
Genentech Inc.	Activase Actimune Protropin Pulmozyme	1-800-821-8590	1-800-879-4747
Genzyme Corporation	Cerezyme	1-800-326-7002	1-800-326-7002
Immunex Corporation	Leukine	1-800-334-6273	1-800-321-4669
Lilly	Humatrope ReoPro	1-800-545-5979	1-800-545-6962
Ortho Biotech	Procrit	1-800-325-7504	1-800-553-3851
Roche	Roferon A	1-800-526-6367	1-800-526-6367
Schering	Intron A	1-800-521-7157	1-800-521-7157

1. In Washington, DC metropolitan area, phone 1-202-637-6698
2. Adverse reaction reporting   1-800-237-5392

Table 17.3. Toll-free assistance numbers for selected biopharmaceuticals in USA and Canada.

(interferon β-1b) must be stored in a refrigerator and should be used within three hours after reconstitution (Berlex, 1994). While most products require refrigeration to maintain stability due to denaturation by elevated temperatures, extreme cold such as freezing may be just as harmful to most products. The key is to avoid extremes in temperature be it heat or cold (Banga *et al.*, 1994).

Storage in Dosing and Administration Devices

Most biotech products may adhere to either plastic or glass containers such as syringes, polyvinyl chloride (PVC) intravenous bags, infusion equipment, and glass intravenous bottles. The effectiveness of the product may be reduced by three or four fold due to adherence. In order to decrease the amount of adherence, human serum albumin (HSA) is usually added to the solutions (cf. Chapter 4). The relative loss through adherence is usually concentration dependent, i.e., the more concentrated the final solution the less significant the adherence becomes. The amount of human serum albumin added varies with the product (Banga *et al.*, 1994; Koeller *et al.*, 1991). Those products requiring the addition of HSA include filgrastim, sargromostim, aldesleukin, erythropoietin and interferon α. In the case of filgrastim at a concentration of 5–15 mcg/mL the addition of 2 mg/mL of HSA to the final solution is required (Amgen, 1992). With sargramostim, 1 mg/mL of HSA is required for concentrations of <10 mcg/mL. (Immunex, 1992). For aldesleukin 0.1% HSA is required for all concentrations (Chiron, 1995). For erythropoietin 2.5 mg HSA is required per injection, and 1 mg/vial of HSA for interferon α.

Product Name	Storage	Stability		Reconstitution sol	Stability after reconstitution	
		RT	Ref		RT	Ref
Aldesleukin	2-8° C	48h	18m	SWFI	48 h	48 h
Alteplase	2-8°C	2 y	2 y	SWFI	8 h	8 h
Antihemophiliac Factor VIII	2-8° C	3 m	2 y	SWFI	3 h	DNF
Dornase Alpha	2-8° C	24 h	NA	-------	24 h	NA
Erythropoetin Alpha	2-8° C	14 d	2 y	NA	NA	NA
Filgrastim	2-8° C	24 h	2 y	NA	NA	NA
Interferon Alpha 2a	2-8° C 24h	RTU	RTU 12m; sol 24 h; powd 3m	dil	24 h	30 d
Interferon Alpha 2b	2-8° C	7 d	ex da	dil	48 h	30 d
Interferon Beta 1b	2-8° C	NA	ex da	dil	NA	3 h
Interferon Gamma 1b	2-8° C	12 h	ex da	NA	NA	NA
Sargromastim	2-8° C	30 d	2 y	SBWFI	30 d	30 d
Somatrem	2-8° C	7 d	ex da	SBWFI	24 h	14 d
Somatropin	2-8° C	72 h	72 h ex da	dil	24 h	14 d

Table 17.4a. Storage, stability and reconstitution of selected biotechnology products[1].
1. all information contained in this table has been obtained from the respective product package insert information on file with the manufacturers as listed in the reference list, and McEvoy 1995.
Table key: d = day; dil = supplied diluent; DNF = do not freeze; D5W = dextrose 5% in water; ex da = see expiration date on package; h = hours; IA = intraarterial; IC = intra coronary; IL = intralesional, IM = intramuscular injection; IO = intraorbital; IP = intraperitoneal; IVB = intravenous bolus; IVIF = intravenous infusion; IVIN = intravenous injection; m = months; mfg = contact manufacturer; NA = not available; NS = normal saline; PP = polypropylene; PVC = polyvinyl chloride; pwd = powder; Ref = refrigerator; RT = room temperature; RTU = ready to use solution; SBWFI = sterile bacteriostatic water for injection; sol = solution; SQ = subcutaneous injection; SQI = subcutaneous infusion; SWFI = sterile water for injection; y = years

For additional information or to check on the most current information on this topic the manufacturer should be contacted.

Storage in IV Solutions

Biotech products may have variable stability when stored in the various available containers or syringes. Some products are only stable in plastic syringes, e.g. somatropin and erythropoietin, while others are stable in glass, polyvinyl chloride and polypropylene, e.g. aldesleukin. See Table 17.4 for a listing of all products and their compatibility with storage equipment. It is important to make sure that the product you wish to provide pre-filled syringes for is stable in the type of syringe you wish to use. This may present a challenge to home health care programs. Batch prefilling of syringes is possible and G-CSF is stable in Becton Dickinson (B-D) disposable plastic syringes for up to 7 days (Amgen, 1992; Amgen, 1995) while erythropoietin is stable for up to 14 days (Amgen, 1993; Amgen, 1995). Aldesleukin by Chiron Therapeutics (Chiron, 1995) is stable when administered in glass, PVC, and polypropylene while GM-CSF and G-CSF can be administered in either PVC or polypropylene (Immunex, 1995). See Table 17.4 for information of the other available products.

Product Name	Compatibility with equipment	Compatibility with solution	Approved admin/route	Non approved admin/route
Aldesleukin	glass, PVC,PP	D5W	IVIF	IV, SQ
Alteplase	glass, PVC	D5W, NS	IVIF	IVB, IC,IA,IO
Antihemophiliac Factor VIII	plastic syringes	NA	IVIN, IVIF	NA
Dornase Alpha	NA	NA	Inhalation	NA
Erythropoetin Alpha	plastic syringes	NA	IVB, SQ	IP
Filgrastim	glass, PVC, plastic syringes	D5W	SQ, SQI, IVIF	IVIF-4h
Interferon Alpha 2a	glass, plastic syringes	mfg	SQ, IM	IVIF, topical, IL, intravaginal
Interferon Alpha 2b	glass, plastic syringes	mfg	SQ, IM, IL	IVIF, topical, IL, intravaginal
Interferon Beta 1b	plastic syringes	NA	SQ	mfg
Interferon Gamma 1b	glass, plastic syringes	D5W, NS	SQ	IVIF, IM
Sargromastim	PVC, PP syringes	D5W, NS	IVIF-2h	IVIF-continuous SQ
Somatrem	PP syringes	NA	SQ, IM	NA
Somatropin	plastic syringes	NA	SQ, IM	MA

Table 17.4b. Compatibility and administration information on selected biotechnology products[1].

1. all information contained in this table has been obtained from the respective product package insert information on file with the manufacturers as listed in the reference list, and McEvoy 1995.

Table key: d = day; dil = supplied diluent; DNF = do not freeze; D5W = dextrose 5% in water; ex da = see expiration date on package; h = hours; IA = intraarterial; IC = intra coronary; IL = intralesional, IM = intramuscular injection; IO = intraorbital; IP = intraperitoneal; IVB = intravenous bolus; IVIF = intravenous infusion; IVIN = intravenous injection; m = months; mfg = contact manufacturer; NA = not available; NS = normal saline; PP = polypropylene; PVC = polyvinyl chloride; pwd = powder; Ref = refrigerator; RT = room temperature; RTU = ready to use solution; SBWFI = sterile bacteriostatic water for injection; sol = solution; SQ = subcutaneous injection; SQI = subcutaneous infusion; SWFI = sterile water for injection; y = years

Light Protection

Some products are sensitive to light. Dornase alpha is packaged in protective foil pouches by the manufacture to protect it from light degradation. The product should be stored in these original light protective containers. For patients who travel, the manufacturer will provide special travel pouches on request (Berlex, 1994). Alteplase in the lyophilized form also needs to be protected from light, but is not light sensitive when in solution (Genentech, 1995).

As new products become available there will undoubtedly be more that will have specific storage requirements with respect to light.

Handling

Mixing and Shaking

Since the biotech products are complex proteins, improper

handling can lead to denaturation. Shaking and severe agitation of most of these products will result in degradation. Therefore special techniques must be observed in preparing biotech products for use. Biotech products should not be shaken when adding any diluent. Shaking may cause the product to break down. Therefore once the diluent is added to the container it should be swirled as has been the case with insulin over the years. Some shaking during transport may be unavoidable and proper inspection should occur to make sure the products have not been harmed. Usually when this happens one can observe physical separation or frothing within the vial of liquid products. For lyophilized products agitation is not harmful until they have been reconstituted. In distributing individual products to patient or ward areas, pneumatic tubes should be avoided.

Travel Requirements

During travel with these products certain precautions should also be observed. They should be stored in insulated, cool containers. This can be accomplished by using ice packs to keep the biotech drug at the proper temperature in warmer climates, whereas the insulated container in colder climates may be all that is required. In fact, when traveling in sub-freezing weather, the products should be protected from freezing. When ice is used, care should be taken to not place the product directly on the ice. Dry ice should be avoided since it has the potential for freezing the product. When traveling by air, biotech products should be taken onto the plane in insulated packages and not placed in a cargo container. Aeroplane cargo containers may be cold enough to cause freezing (Banga, 1994; Koeller *et al.*, 1991).

Preparation

When preparing biotech products, aseptic technique should be adhered to as it is with other parenteral products. The pharmaceutical should be prepared in a clean room designed for this purpose with laminar air flow hoods, etc. Most of the products require reconstitution with sterile water or bacteriostatic water for injection depending on stability data. The compatibility of individual products varies and limited data is available. As mentioned previously when adding diluent to these products, care should be taken not to shake them, but to swirl the container between the palms of your hands. In the case of lyophilized products, the introduction of the diluent should be directed down the side of the vial and not directly on the powder to avoid denaturing the protein. Table 17.4 provides specific compatibility data regarding individual products. It is important to mention here that stability does not mean sterility. Biotech products are not any different in this regard

than any other parenteral product. The same precautions need to be adhered to and are worth mentioning to be complete. Sterility is a particularly important consideration when pre-filling and pre-mixing various doses for administration at home. Once the manufacturer's provided sterile packaging is entered, sterility can no longer be assured nor will the manufacturer be responsible for any subsequent related problems. Individual manufacturers have not addressed the issue of sterility and each institution or organization must determine its own policy on this issue. Approximately half of the currently available biotechnology-produced products are provided as single-dose vials and thus, should not be reused. This does not, however, prevent preparing batches ("batching") of unit-of-use doses in order to be more cost efficient. Most of the patients receiving these agents are likely to have suppressed immune systems and are vulnerable to infection. Therefore, a policy involving the maintenance of sterility of biotech products should be developed by each health care organization, especially home health care programs. For example, policy at the University of Arizona Medical Center is that all parenteral products that are reconstituted are routinely given a 72 hour expiration date in accordance with infection control policy of the hospital. When products are made in a sterile environment under aseptic procedures they should remain sterile until used and thus could be stored for as long as physical compatibility data dictates. However, most institutions have shorter expiration dates, which are generally 72 hours or less, on reconstituted products. These expiration dates have been arbitrarily set due to lack of good sterility data to the contrary. Sterility studies should be performed in order to determine if reconstituted products could be stored for a longer period of time and still maintain sterility. For products reconstituted for home use in the pharmacy sterile products area, however, a 7 day expiration date is used, provided the product is stable and can be stored in the refrigerator. The American Society of Health-System Pharmacists has published a technical assistance bulletin on sterile products which should be consulted for developing policy on storage of reconstituted parenteral products (American Society of Hospital Pharmacy, 1993). Patients need to be informed about specific storage requirement and expiration dates to assure sterility and stability.

Administration

Prior to administering these products, pharmacists will need to observe extra caution in reviewing dosage regimens. This is primarily because the units of measure for the various products may be radically different. Some products are dosed in micrograms/kilogram (mcg/kg), while others in milligrams/kilograms (mg/kg). Also in some cases, units of measure are used which may be unique to the product, e.g. Chiron or Roche units. Dosage calculations need to be carefully checked to avoid any potential errors.

Routes of Administration

Biotech products, with the exception of dornase alpha, are restricted to parenteral administration. Some products may be given by either the intravenous or subcutaneous route while others are restricted to the subcutaneous route only. Table 17.4 lists the approved and non-approved routes of administration for each product. In some cases, new information may be available and the manufacturer should always be consulted in order to obtain supporting evidence for a particular route that is not approved, but may be more convenient for the patient. For example, G-CSF should be administered by the subcutaneous or intravenous route only, while GM-CSF is given by intravenous infusion over a two hour period (McEvoy, 1995). Aldesleukin is approved for intravenous administration only. But, subcutaneous administration, while not approved, has been used by some (Chiron, 1992). Erythropoietin should only be administered by the intravenous or subcutaneous routes (Amgen, 1993), while alteplase is only approved for the intravenous route (Genentech, 1992; McEvoy, 1995). Alteplase has also been administered by the intracoronary, intraarterial, and intraorbital routes as well (McEvoy, 1995).

Filtration

Filtering biotech products is not generally recommended since most of these proteins will adhere to the filter. Some hospitals and home infusion companies routinely use in line filters for all intravenous solutions to minimize the introduction of particulate matter into the patient. In the case of biotech products, they should be infused below the filter to avoid any possible decrease in the amount of drug delivered to the patient (Banga, 1994; Koeller *et al.*, 1991).

Flushing Solutions

Pharmaceutical biotechnology products are usually flushed with either saline or dextrose 5% in water. The product literature should be consulted and care should be taken to assure that the proper solution is used with each agent. In general, these biotech drugs should not be administered with other fluids or drugs since, in most cases, data does not exist about such compatibilities.

Outpatient/Home Care Issues

The management of patients in the outpatient and home settings is a growing aspect of health care delivery. The use of biotech products outside the hospital is no exception to this trend. Home infusion services is one of the fastest growing sectors of the health care market and they have become involved with all forms of parenterally-administered drugs including biotech products. Just as we have been educating insulin-dependent diabetics on the proper administration techniques, storage, and handling of insulin over the last several decades, we must also do this for patients receiving these other protein biotech products. The main difference with most of these newer products is that, unlike insulin, the dose may need to be prepared in the patient's home.

Patient Assessment and Education

Before a patient can be a candidate for home therapy, an assessment of the patient's capabilities must occur. The patient, family member, or care giver will need to be able to inject the medication and comply with all of the storage, handling, and preparation requirements. If the patient is incapable, then a patient care giver, relative, spouse, or friend will need to be solicited. The patient will need to be educated as to all of the storage, handling, preparation, and administering aspects as previously described. The use of aseptic technique is usually new to most patients and in some cases may be frightening. The health care provider must be sure that the patient is competent and willing to follow these procedures. Self-instructional tapes on specific products may be available from the manufacturer, and if so, should be provided to the patient providing they have the proper equipment for tape reviewing.

Proper storage facilities will need to be available in the patient's home as well as a clean area for preparation and administration. Ideally, the patient will be able to prepare each dose immediately prior to the time of administration. If this is not possible, the pharmacy will have to prepare prefilled syringes and provide appropriate storage and handling requirements to the patient. The patient will also need to be educated as to the proper handling, needed supplies and materials such as needles, syringes, alcohol wipes, etc. The proper disposal of these hazardous wastes must also be reviewed. Specific issues related to patient teaching include rotating injection sites, product handling, drug storage also during transporting/traveling, expiration dates, refrigeration, cleansing the injection site with alcohol, disposal of needles and syringes, drug side effects, and expected therapeutic outcome.

Monitoring

Like other injectables used by patients in the home, it is important that close patient monitoring occurs. This will require frequent phone calls to the patient and periodic home visits. Monitoring parameters should include adverse events, progress to expected outcomes, assessment of administration technique, review of storage and handling procedures, and adherence to aseptic technique.

Reimbursement

Reimbursement issues include third party billing information and availability of forms, cost sharing programs which limit the annual cost of therapy, financial assistance programs for patients who would otherwise have difficulty paying for therapy, and reimbursement assurance programs which are designed to remove reimbursement barriers which may exist when reimbursement has been denied. Any detailed discussion of reimbursement issues is beyond the scope of this book and is subject to practice location. This discussion will deal only with the availability of information to pharmacists to appropriately handle reimbursements for products and services in the United States.

Pharmacists need to know current insurer payment policies such as whether insurance companies will disallow claims for uses other than the labeled indications or if the product is to be used in the home rather than administered in a hospital or physician's office. Prior authorization is required for many products, particularly insurers with managed care or prepaid plans. Some manufacturers will contact the carrier to verify coverage, provide sample prior-approval letters, and will follow up on claims to determine the claim's status and continue to follow up until resolution of the case.

Manufacturers can also provide information that may convince the third-party payer to reconsider a denied claim. Some companies will intervene with the third party payer to determine the cause for denial, provide additional clinical documentation or coding information, and will follow the appeal to conclusion. Pharmacists can act as facilitators to get qualified patients enrolled in programs to provide free medication to those who have insufficient insurance coverage or are otherwise unable to purchase the therapy.

Educational Materials

Therapy with biotech drugs is a rapidly growing, ever changing area of therapeutics. Pharmacists need to keep informed of current information about existing agents such as new indications, management of side effects, results of studies describing drug interactions or changes in information regarding product stability and reconstitution. Pharmacists will also be interested in the status of new agents as they move through the FDA approval process. Some good periodical sources of practical information about products of biotechnology are listed in Table 17.5.

■ **Biotechnology Medicines in Development,** Communications Division, Pharmaceutical Manufacturers Association, Washington, D.C., 202-835-3400, *updated approximately every 18 months.*

■ **FDC Reports, "The Pink Sheet,"** Chevy Chase, MD, *published weekly.*

■ **Biotechnology Update,** *a monthly column in* **Journal of the American Pharmaceutical Association.**

■ **BioWorld Today,** Atlanta: Bioworld Publishing Group, *newspaper, 5 issues per week; also available on Netscape; Tel. (404)-262-7436; Fax (404)-814-0759.*

■ **Bio/Technology,** New York: Nature Publishing Co., *a monthly journal dealing with all aspects of biotechnology.*

■ **Genetic Engineering News,** New York: GEN Publishing, *bimonthly publication, Tel. (914)-834-3100; Fax (914)-834-3771.*

■ **Biotechnology News,** New Jersey: CTB International Publishing,

Table 17.5. Information sources for current trends in biotechnology.

Professional Services

Medical information services provided by manufacturers of biotech drugs are similar to the product, medical and patient management services provided by drug companies for traditional drug products. Information provided via this service generally includes appropriate indications, side effects, contraindications to use, results of clinical trials and investigational uses. Upon request, manufacturers can supply a product monograph and selected research articles that provide valuable information about each product.

EDUCATIONAL MATERIALS FOR HEALTH PROFESSIONALS

Examples of pharmacist/patient educational materials provided by manufacturers are listed in Table 17.6. Numerous educational materials have been developed by manufacturers including continuing education programs for

Betaseron® Patient Training Kit including the video, "Learning To Use Betaseron® ", materials for practicing reconstitution and injection procedures and a patient journal which contains information for patients as well as provides a format for documenting compliance

Ceredase® "Living with Gaucher Disease", a guide for patients, parents, relatives and friends; **Horizons**, a quarterly newsletter for people with Gaucher Disease

Epogen® Epoetin alfa Monograph Series: a comprehensive review covering the use of epoetin alfa in the clinical pharmacy setting; each monograph is accredited for continuing education credit through the Academy of Continuing Education Programs; monograph topics include, "Anemia Associated With Chronic Renal Failure," "Iron Balance in Dialysis Patients," "Epoetin Alfa in Clinical Practice," " Suboptimal Response to Epoetin Therapy in Dialysis Patients With Anemia," "Peritoneal Dialysis and Epoetin Therapy," "Epoetin Therapy and Quality of Life."

Humatrope® Series of brochures on "Short Stature due to Growth Hormone Deficiency" dealing with a variety of social issues; booklet containing instructions and advice on administration of human growth hormone; patient reimbursement handbook describing the "Humatrope Hotline" and tips for seeking reimbursement.

Intron A® Ongoing series of educational monographs carrying continuing education credit; a video on self-administration of Intron A®; ICONSM, a computerized information service providing the latest information on interferons; "Taking Control of Your Therapy for Chronic Hepatitis Non-A, Non-B/C", an information brochure for patients

KoGENate® Manufacturer refers patients and health professionals to the National Hemophilia Foundation, 1-800-42-HANDI for educational materials

Neupogen® Guide to Providing Neupogen® in the Community Pharmacy; "Filgrastim (rG-CSF) a Hematopoietic Growth Factor," an educational program including slides; "How to Give Yourself a Subcutaneous Injection" booklet and video; "What I wish I Knew" video for breast cancer patients by breast cancer survivors; "The First Step in Chemotherapy is Overcoming Your Fear" a booklet; "The Most Important Part of Your Treatment is You" a booklet; Neupogen® (Filgrastim) "Part of the Good News about Today's Chemotherapy" a booklet; patient support paks which includes a thermometer and daily calendar for recording injections and temperature

Proleukin® "Interleukin-2 Therapy, What you should know" a booklet for patient and their families, available from the National Kidney Cancer Association, Suite 200, 1234 Sherman Avenue, Evanston IL 60202.

Pulmozyme® Cystic fibrosis medical reference set; Beneath the Surface, Counseling program for CF patients and parents; Cystic fibrosis, Pathogenesis and New Therapies, modular slide library and lecture support program; Pulmozyme® slide library and lecture support program

ReoPro® "New Approaches to PTCA and Concomitant Pharmacotherapy, The Pharmacist's Expanded Role," a videotape and monograph program approved for continuing pharmacy education credit; ReoPro® treatment algorithm; additional educational materials have not yet been released by the FDA as of 9/1/95.

Roferon-A® Self-administration instructional videotape; managing side effects videotape; pocket-sized Roferon-A® dosing card; syringe disposal container, travel cooler, self-administration flip chart, document organizer, relaxation audiotapes, self-injection practice pad; many of these items are contained in a "personal care kit."

Table 17.6. Examples of pharmacist/patient educational materials available from manufacturers.

physicians, pharmacists and nurses; these programs sometimes include slides, videos and brochures. Since most biotechnology products are parenteral products, several manufacturers have produced videotapes which show the proper procedure for giving a subcutaneous injection. These instructional tapes are beneficial not just for patients but also for pharmacists who may not be skilled in injection techniques.

Amgen provides information on one of its products, Epogen®, through a monograph series which comprehensively reviews the use of the drug in the clinical pharmacy setting. Genentech supplies information on Pulmozyme® via a medical reference set, slide libraries and lecture support program. These and other materials are described in greater detail in Table 17.6.

EDUCATIONAL MATERIALS FOR PATIENTS

Examples of pharmacist/patient educational materials provided by manufacturers are listed in Table 17.6. Detailed patient information booklets exist for many of the products. Patient education materials can assist the patient and family members in learning more about his or her disease and how it will be treated. Education allows the patient to participate more actively in the therapy and to feel a greater level of control over the process. By contacting the manufacturer and acquiring patient educational materials, pharmacists can offer support to the patient in learning to use a new product. Many patients are already overwhelmed by dealing with a diagnosis of serious or chronic disease. Learning about a new therapy, especially if it involves the necessity of subcutaneous self-injection, can cause additional stress for the patient and family.

For example, both Genentech and Lilly have several booklets dealing with short stature, human growth hormone (Protropin®; Humatrope®) therapy and the "how to" of preparing and giving injections to children. A chart is included for recording of injections sites to insure that site rotation is maintained.

Berlex provides a patient training kit for multiple sclerosis patients to learn the reconstitution and injection procedures for Betaseron®. A journal is included for the patient to document compliance and record side effects which can be significant with this drug.

Some manufacturers also provide a referral to associations that can provide valuable information and services including a link to local chapters, meetings and support groups. For example, Bayer refers inquiries for patient information about KoGENate®, a recombinant clotting factor product (cf. Chapter 14), to the National Hemophilia Foundation and Chiron Therapeutic, manufacturer of Proleukin®, refers families to the National Kidney Cancer Association.

Toll-Free Access to Manufacturers' Services

Most manufacturers can be reached by toll-free numbers to request any of the types of information discussed above.

Internet Site	Type of Site	Web Address
A Doctor's Guide to the Internet	Biomedical news	www.pslgroup.com:80/DOCGUIDE.HTML
BioOnline	Information library/catalog	www.bio.com
Biotech Brief	On-line journal	www.lsa.org/btb
Bioworld Today	On-line journal	www.bio.com/home/bioworld/new.html
Current Opinion in Biotechnology	On-line journal	BioMedNet.com/cbiology/bio.html
Genetic Engineering News	On-line journal	www.dc.enews.com/magazines/geng_news/
Nature Biotechnology	On-line journal	biotech.nature.com/
Pharmaceutical Research and Manufacturers of America	Homepage	www.phrma.org/
Physicians Guide to the Internet	Biomedical news	www.webcom.com/pgi/contntpg.html
Reuter's Health Information Services, Inc.	Biomedical news	www.reutershealth.com/
The World Wide Web Virtual Library: Biotechnology	Information library/catalog	www.cato.com/interweb/cato/biotech

Table 17.7. Sampling of some biotech-related Internet sites.

Manufacturers of biotech products may have a separate number for reimbursement questions. Table 17.3 lists the manufacturers' toll-free assistance numbers for obtaining product and reimbursement information in North America. Vaccines and insulin products are not included in this table since these products were previously available in a non-recombinant form which was used in a similar manner. Moreover, the recombinant form is not significantly higher in price than the non-recombinant product.

The Internet and Biotech Information

The Internet has become a valuable site rich in up-to-date information concerning all aspects of pharmaceutical biotechnology. Sites including virtual libraries/catalogs, on-line journals (usually requiring a subscription), biomedical newsletters and biotechnology specific homepages abound on the Internet. Since the number of biotech-related sites are constantly increasing, only a small sampling of sites of interest could be provided in Table 17.7.

Concluding Remarks

Basically, the handling of biotechnology products requires similar skills and techniques as required for the preparation of other parenteral drugs, but there are often slightly difference nuances to the handling, preparation and administration of biotechnology-produced pharmaceuticals. The pharmacist can become an educator to others related to the pharmaceutical aspects of biotechnology products and can serve as a valuable resource to other health care professionals. In addition, biotech products give the pharmacist the opportunity to provide pharmaceutical care since patient education and monitoring is required. To play this role successfully, the pharmacist will need to keep abreast of new developments as new literature and products become available. ■

Further Reading

See Tables 17.1, 17.2 and 17.5 and 17.7 for lists of selected readings.

References

- **American Society of Health-System Pharmacists.** (1993). ASHP technical assistance bulletin on quality assurance for pharmacy-prepared sterile products. *Am J Hosp Pharm*, 50, 2386–2398
- **Amgen Inc.** (1993). Epogen® package insert. Thousand Oaks, CA
- **Amgen Inc.** (1992). Neupogen® package insert. Thousand Oaks, CA
- **Amgen Inc.** (1995). Written information on storage, stability, compatibility, and administration. Thousand Oaks, CA
- **Banga AK, Reddy IK.** (1994). Biotechnology drugs: pharmaceutical issues. *Pharmacy Times*, March, 68–76
- **Bayer AG, Co.** (1993). Kogenate® package insert. Elkart, IN
- **Baxter Health Care Corporation.** (1992). Recombinate® package insert. Glendale, CA
- **Berlex Laboratories.** (1994). Betaseron® package insert. Richmond, CA
- **Check WA.** (1984). New drug and drug-delivery systems in the year 2000. *Am J Hosp Pharm*, 41, 1536–15417
- **Chiron Therapeutics.** (1994). Proleukin® package insert. Emeryville, CA
- **Chiron Corporation.** (1995). Proleukin® written information on storage, reconstitution, compatibility, stability, and administration on file. Emeryville, CA
- **Genentech, Inc.** (1990). Actimune® package insert. South San Francisco, CA
- **Genentech, Inc.** (1991). Protropin® package insert. South San Francisco, CA
- **Genentech, Inc.** (1994). Activase® package insert. South San Francisco, CA
- **Genentech, Inc.** (1994b). Pulmozyme® package insert. South San Francisco, CA
- **Genentech, Inc.** (1995). Written information on storage, reconstituion, compatibility, stability, and administratin on file. South San Francisco, CA
- **Immunex Corporation.** (1992). Leukine® package insert. Seattle, WA
- **Immunex Corporation.** (1995). Written information on storage, reconstitution, compatibility, stability, and administration on file. Seattle, WA
- **Koeller J, Fields S.** (1991). The pharmacist's role with biotechnology products. Kalamazoo, MI: The Upjohn Company
- **Lilly, Eli Company.** (1994). Humatrope® package insert. Indianapolis, IN
- **Lilly, Eli Company.** (1995). Written informatin on storage, reconstitution, compatibility, stability, and administration on file. Indianapolis, IN

- **McEvoy GK.** (1995). American Hospital Formulary Service Drug Information, American Society of Health-System Pharmacists. Bethesda, MD
- **Roche Laboratories.** (1992). Roferon® package insert. Nutley, NJ
- **Schering Laboratories.** (1994). Intron® package insert. Kennilworth, NJ
- **Schering Laboratories.** (1995). Written information on storage, reconstitution, compatibility, stability and administration on file. Kennilworth, NJ
- **Stewart CF, Fleming RA.** (1989). Biotechnology products: new opportunities and responsibilities for the pharmacist. *Am J Hosp Pharm*, 46 (suppl 2) S4–S8

Self-Assessment Questions

Question 1: *What are some of the causes of pharmacist reluctance to handling biotech products?*

Question 2: *In what areas of study do pharmacists and pharmacy students need to engage to be best prepared to provide pharmaceutical care services to patients receiving biotechnology therapeutic agents?*

Question 3: *What resources are available to pharmacy practitioners to learn more about biotechnology and the drug products of biotechnology?*

Question 4: *How do the storage requirements of biotech products differ from the majority of products pharmacists normally dispense?*

Question 5: *What is the most common temperature for the storage of biotech pharmaceuticals?*

Question 6: *Why is human serum albumin added to the solution of many biotech drugs?*

Question 7: *Why should biotech products not be shaken when adding any diluent?*

Question 8: *During travel, what precautions should also be observed with biotech products?*

Question 9: *Should biotech products be filtered prior to administration?*

Question 10: *What assessments must be done by the pharmacist before a patient can be considered a candidate for home therapy with a biotech product?*

Question 11: *What types of professional services information are provided by manufacturers of biotech drugs.*

Answers

Answer 1: Lack of understanding of the basics of biotechnology, lack of understanding of the therapeutics of recombinant protein products; unfamiliarity with the side effects and patient counseling information; lack of familiarity with the storage, handling and reconstitution of proteins; and the difficulty of handling reimbursement issues.

Answer 2: Basic biotechnology/immunological methods; protein chemistry; therapeutics of biotechnology agents; storage, handling, reconstitution and administration of biotechnology products

Answer 3: Biotechnology/immunology texts, continuing education programs, manufacturers' information and toll-free assistance, biotechnology-oriented journals, the Internet (as described in Tables 17.1–17.7).

Answer 4: The shelf life of these products is often considerably shorter than has been the case with more traditional compounds. These products need to be kept at refrigerated temperatures. There are, of course, exceptions to this rule.

Answer 5: In general, most biotech products are shipped by the manufacturer in gel ice containers and need to be stored at 2–8°C. Once reconstituted, they should be kept under refrigeration until just prior to use.

Answer 6: Most biotech products may adhere to either plastic or glass containers such as syringes and polyvinyl chloride (PVC) intravenous bags reducing effectiveness of the product. Human serum albumin is usually added to the solutions to prevent adherence.

Answer 7: Shaking may cause the product to break down (aggregation). Usually when this happens one can observe physical separation or frothing within the vial of liquid products.

Answer 8: They should be stored in insulated, cool containers. This can be accomplished by using ice packs to keep the biotech drug at the proper temperature in warmer climates, whereas the insulated container in colder climates may be all that is required. In fact, when traveling in sub-freezing weather, the products should be protected from freezing.

Answer 9: Filtering biotech products is not generally recommended since most of the proteins will adhere to the filter.

Answer 10: Before a patient can be a candidate for home therapy, an assessment of the patient's capabilities must occur. The patient, family member, or care giver will need to be able to inject the medication and comply with all of the storage, handling, and preparation requirements.

Answer 11: Medical information services provided by manufacturers of biotech drugs are similar to the product, medical and patient management services provided by drug companies for traditional drug products. Information provided via this service generally includes appropriate indications, side effects, contraindications to use, results of clinical trials and investigational uses. Upon request, manufacturers can supply a product monograph and selected research articles that provide valuable information about each product.

18 Biotechnology Products in the Pipeline

by: Ronald P. Evens and Robert D. Sindelar

Introduction

The information assembled in this book provides ample evidence to support the statement that biotechnology represents an enormous resource for drug discovery and development. In the coming years it will continue to expand its contributions to modern pharmaceutical care. These contributions include, (1) a greater understanding of the cause and progression of diseases, (2) the development of novel pharmacological screening methods to identify new pharmaceuticals, (3) the production of biopharmaceuticals being tested for the first time against several diseases, (4) the creation of innovative technologies for optimizing drug development and, finally, (5) improvements in the methods used to manufacture protein and peptide-based biopharmaceuticals. Thus, biotechnology and various related techniques will expand its influence in all areas of the drug discovery process and is playing a major role in shaping the pharmaceuticals that will be dispensed in the future.

Drug Development and Biotechnology

Over the past 20 years, from the mid-1970's when the first human gene was cloned to the mid 1990's, molecular biological technologies have assumed an important position along with established disciplines, such as organic chemistry and medicinal chemistry, in the field of drug discovery and development. Biotechnology has been responsible for developing and marketing over 50 products for therapeutic use, comprised of 27 different molecules, in the United States, Europe and Japan from 1982 to 1996 (Table 18.1). Most of the molecules are (glyco)proteins and include biological response modifiers (BRMs), colony stimulating factors (CSFs), enzymes, hormones, monoclonal antibodies (MAbs), and vaccines. About 25 different companies are responsible for these 50 products; however, over 1300 biotechnology companies in US and 400 in Europe are conducting basic research, and over 100 companies have over 250 molecules in human clinical trials in 1995 and early 1996 in the USA alone (Lee Jr. and Burrill, 1995; Evens et al., 1995a; Evens et al., 1995b; Pharmaceutical Research and Manufacturers of America, 1996).

Product *)	Class **)
Abciximab	MAb
Acelluvax	vaccine
Aldesleukin	BRM
Alteplase	enzyme
Antihemophilic Factor VIII (2)	enzyme
DNase	enzyme
Epoetin Alfa (6)	CSF
Filgrastim	CSF
Factor IX	enzyme
Glatiramer	BRM
Hepatitis B Vaccine (2)	vaccine
Imiglucerase	enzyme
Insulin (3)	hormone
Interferon Alfa (5)	BRM
Interferon Beta (2)	BRM
Interferon Gamma	BRM
Lenograstim	CSF
Liposomal Agents (5)	Liposome
Molgramostim	CSF
Muromonab-CD3	MAb
Panorex	MAb
Reteplase	enzyme
Sargramostim	CSF
Seprafilm	Surgical Adjunct
Somatrem	hormone
Somatropin (5)	hormone
Satumomab Pendetide	MAb

Table 18.1. Marketed biotechnology-produced pharmaceuticals. *) The numbers in parentheses indicate the approximate number of products of the same molecule manufactured by different companies. **) MAb = monoclonal antibody; CSF = colony stimulating factor; BRM = biological response modifier.

Time and Cost of Modern Drug Discovery

Modern drug development is still a slow and expensive process. The time from discovery of a drug to market availability for a product is quite lengthy, ranging from 8 years to 20 years, as suggested by the New York Times (New York Times, 1995) (Figure 18.1). Research investment is substantial and risky, about $7.7 billion in 1994 by biotech-

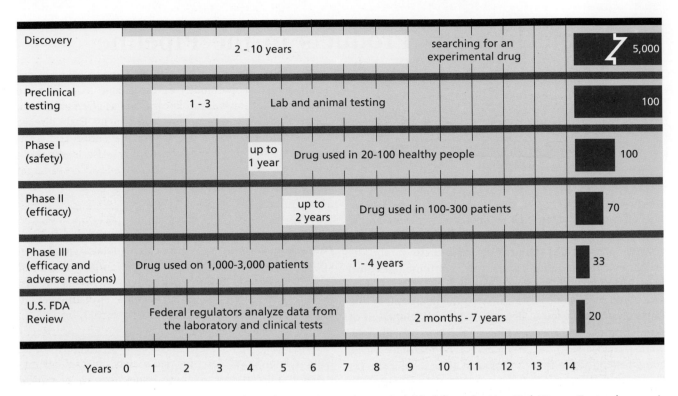

Figure 18.1. The drug development process from discovery to marketing (modified from the New York Times, September 1995).

Techniques of Biotech Drug Discovery

nology companies, along with $14.9 billion by traditional drug manufacturers, of which a significant percentage is devoted to biotechnology as well (Lee Jr. and Burrill, 1995). The cost to bring a conventional, small molecule drug to market was estimated to be about $350 million, according to the US. Congressional Budget Office. A study of drug development by Merck and Co. found only a marketing success rate of 5% for 140 leading drug candidates: all 140 drugs made it through preclinical animal testing, 65 made it through Phase I trials (human safety), 27 made it through Phase II trials (efficacy), 9 made it through Phase III trials (large-scale safety and efficacy), and 7 were approved for marketing (Shapiro, 1995). An approximate time frame for each phase of these trials is Phase I – up to 1 year, II – up to 2 years, and III – 1–4 years with a FDA review time of 2 months–7 years (New York Times, 1995). Biotechnology products experience a similar complex process in success rates and time frames. For 1993 and 1994, clinical research was terminated on over 20 biologicals during Phase III, after successful Phase II trials, while product approvals numbered only four. The time frame for clinical trials with biologicals was calculated to be 3.4 years. In addition, based on a 1993 study, the regular review time in the US takes 1.7 years; in comparison, in Europe the total time was 3 years and in Japan 4.7 years (Bienz-Tadmor, 1993; Struck, 1994).

Drug research (including discovery, preclinical, formulation efforts, etc.) and drug development (including safety studies, proof of efficacy, etc.) in biotechnology are evolving rapidly with many new technologies and types of molecules. During the 1970's and 1980's, organs, tissues, and cells were studied successfully to find proteins responsible for physiological or cellular responses in animals. For example, erythropoietin (Epoetin alpha) is produced by kidney cells, is secreted into the blood, and stimulates bone marrow to produce red blood cells. This conventional technique of drug discovery still accounts for most biologicals in clinical research to date and biotechnology has made major contributions to such discoveries. Innovations in small molecule drug-development technology, however, are providing ways of narrowing down choices and then screening likely candidates. As described in detail in Chapter 6, one of the most powerful tools in the 1990's is combinatorial chemistry (Figure 18.2), a mix-and-match process in which a simple subunit (e.g., a six-membered–heterocycle with an ethylene substituent, a modified peptide, etc.) is joined to one or more other simple subunits (e.g., a four carbon olefin, a modified amino acid, etc.) in every possible combination (Ecker and Crooke, 1995). Assigning the task to automated synthesizing equipment results in the rapid

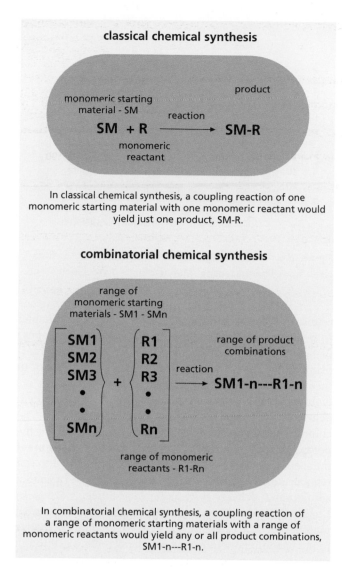

classical chemical synthesis

monomeric starting
material - SM

product

$$SM + R \xrightarrow{\text{reaction}} SM\text{-}R$$

monomeric
reactant

In classical chemical synthesis, a coupling reaction of one
monomeric starting material with one monomeric reactant would
yield just one product, SM-R.

combinatorial chemical synthesis

range of
monomeric starting
materials - SM1 - SMn

$$\begin{Bmatrix} SM1 \\ SM2 \\ SM3 \\ \bullet \\ \bullet \\ SMn \end{Bmatrix} + \begin{Bmatrix} R1 \\ R2 \\ R3 \\ \bullet \\ \bullet \\ Rn \end{Bmatrix} \xrightarrow{\text{reaction}} SM1\text{-}n\text{---}R1\text{-}n$$

range of product
combinations

range of monomeric
reactants - R1-Rn

In combinatorial chemical synthesis, a coupling reaction of
a range of monomeric starting materials with a range of
monomeric reactants would yield any or all product combinations,
SM1-n---R1-n.

Figure 18.2. Representation of the process of combinatorial
chemistry (cf. Chapter 6, Figure 6.22).

creation of large collections or "libraries" of diverse molecules, which quickly can be screened pharmacologically via
high throughput screening (see Chapter 6) to identify the
most active compound for a given therapeutic target. In
most cases today, biotechnology contributes directly to the
understanding, identification and/or the generation of the
drug target being screened (e.g., radioligand binding displacement from a cloned protein receptor). Thousands of
compounds can be generated, screened, and evaluated for
further development in a matter of weeks.

Biotechnology contributes to another major resource for
drug development; the identification and localization of
gene sequence databases generated by the Human Genome
Project and other large-scale genome-sequencing programs.

An international venture, the Human Genome Project is to
construct detailed genetic and physical maps of each of the
23 different human chromosomes. Identifying the exact
location and identity of all the human genes increases
significantly the possibility of being able to predict the
occurrence of thousands of known, and as of yet unknown,
diseases with a strong genetic component. Early disease
detection and increased options for prevention and treatment are likely to be products of these efforts. As mentioned in Chapter 6, critically important and novel target
databases for drug design are resulting from discoveries
generated by the Human Genome Project. Automated
sequencing equipment, sequencing by hybridization, and
"DNA on a chip" methods ensure that these already large
databases will continue to grow rapidly. Major social, ethical and legal concerns, however, can accompany the use of
any new technology. The unprecedented insights into human
genetics and disease resulting from the Human Genome
Project and efforts to realize its full potential raise societal
questions concerning an individual's right to privacy
versus who should have access to this rapidly increasing
bank of knowledge. An informed society must initiate discussion and consider all these issues that are of critical
importance.

Other information, including drug target structural data
generated by X-ray crystallography and nuclear magnetic
resonance techniques, also continue to accrue rapidly. Fast
computers with cheap memory, massive storage, and 3-D
simulation redrawing programs have made possible the
large scale accessing and manipulation of this biological
information for drug development. Large-scale gene-transfer techniques, perfected by Jaenisch and others in the
early 1990s, enabled the creation of transgenic rats and
mice in which human diseases can be mimicked (see Chapter
6 for details). Also important is the use of rodents with one
gene turned off, or "knocked out." These knockout animals
provide insights into the causes of disease and 'how missing proteins function', and make accelerated development
of new drugs possible. Transgenic mouse models now exist
for hyperglyceridemia, Lesch-Nynan syndrome, hypertension, liver cancer, rheumatoid arthritis, cystic fibrosis, brain
cancer, kidney cancer, scrapie/prion disease, and many
others.

Classes of Molecules Being Discovered and Studied through Biotechnology

The types of molecules being discovered and studied through
biotechnology has broadened substantially over the past
decade (Table 18.2). Proteins remain a major emphasis of
research with active classes including additional colony-
stimulating factors (CSFs), biological response modifiers
(BRMs) and other cytokines, enzymes and hormones for

Protein pharmaceuticals

- Colony stimulating factors
- Biological response modifiers and other cytokines
  - Interferons
  - Interleukins
- Enzymes
  - Clotting factors
  - Dismutases
  - Tissue plasminogen activators
- Hormones
- Growth factors
  - Tissue/bone growth factors
  - Neurotropic factors
- Recombinant protein vaccines
- Monoclonal antibodies
  - Diagnostic antibodies
  - Therapeutic antibodies
- Recombinant soluble receptors
- Fusion molecules

Peptides and peptidomimetics

Nucleic acid therapies with

- Genes
- Oncogenes
- Ribozymes
- Antisense molecules
- Telomers and telomerase

Carbohydrate-based pharmaceuticals and other products of glycobiology

Whole cells

Delivery systems for biotechnology drugs

Table 18.2. Types of biotechnology pharmaceuticals, adjunct pharmaceuticals and technologies in development today.

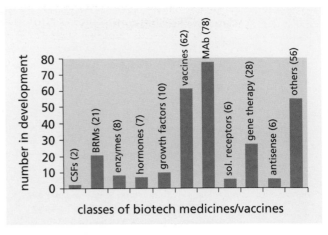

Figure 18.3. Biotech drugs in development in the U.S. Data taken from Pharmaceutical Manufacturers Association, 1996.

ceuticals and other products of glycobiology (see Chapter 6) being examined. Exciting technologies are developing using whole cells such as stem cells in autologous transplant therapy of cancer and in allogenic transplants in utero for blood-borne genetic diseases.

In Chapter 4 attention is paid to the issue of protein delivery by microencapsulated, secretory cells. The first clinical trials are now in progress to further evaluate the potentials and limitations of this exciting concept of microencapsulated protein secreting cells designed to self regulate protein-drug release. The bottom line of Table 18.2 speaks about delivery systems for biotechnology drugs. In Chapters 3 and 4, the problems regarding the delivery of protein drugs are extensively discussed. Finding alternative routes of administration to the parenteral route, e.g. through a safe absorption enhancing system, would be highly desirable as it would make the use of biotech products more patient friendly. A lot of efforts are being made to improve drug efficiency and reduce toxicity through the development of systems for release rate control (e.g. implants), or for site specific delivery (e.g. 'drug targeting' with liposomes).

It is always difficult to predict which new products might be approved by regulatory agencies worldwide in any given year and what their impact on pharmaceutical care will be. For instance, several monoclonal antibodies and a soluble receptor protein have been hailed, in recent years, as major advances in therapy for the treatment of septic shock. The US Food and Drug Administration, however, has denied approval of these products because Phase III pivotal trials failed to demonstrate efficacy.

For the remainder of this section, we present a selection of some potential biotechnology pharmaceuticals that are in the development pipeline. Figure 18.3 and Tables 18.3–18.9 provide a breakdown by class of the biotech drugs in development in the US. The tables are not intended to be definitive or all inclusive and will be somewhat dated due

disease (e.g., clotting factors, tissue plasminogen activators, etc.), vaccines (for cancer, AIDS, rheumatoid arthritis and multiple sclerosis, to list a few), and monoclonal antibodies (Table 18.2). Other novel classes of drug protein molecules are now being discovered including tissue/bone and nerve growth factors, soluble receptors and fusion molecules (see below). Peptide drugs and peptidomimetics (see Chapter 6) are important adjuncts to typical biotechnology strategies. Nucleic acid based therapies, e.g., gene therapies (please see Chapter 7), and therapies using antisense molecules (please see Chapter 6), and ribozymes (see Chapter 6), are being tested. Gene therapy is the fastest growing category of biotechnology products under development (Pharmaceutical Research and Manufacturers of America, 1996). We also have carbohydrate-based pharma-

Colony Stimulating Factors (CSFs)		
Product	Company	Indication
Sargramostim (GM-CSF)	Immunex	prophylaxis and treatment of chemotherapy-induced neutropenia
		reduction of post-operative infections, neonatal sepsis, prevention of infection in very low birth weight infants
Filgrastim (rG-CSF)	Amgen	infectious diseases
Platelet Factors		
Product	Company	Indication
MGDF	Amgen	treatment of chemotherapy-induced thrombocytopenia
TPO	Genentech	platelet donation
Interferons (INFs)		
Product	Company	Indication
Consensus interferon	Amgen	hepatitis C, cancerchemotherapy
Recombinant interferon beta	Serono Laboratories	malignant diseases unresponsive to standard therapies, hepatitis C; relapsing, remitting and secondary progressive multiple sclerosis

Table 18.3a. Some biotechnology-derived protein products in various stages of clinical trials: CSFs and INFs (Source: Pharmaceutical Research and Manufacturers of America, 1996).

to the rapid changes occurring each day in the pharmaceutical and biotech industries. Brief explanatory notes will be provided for some, but not all of the products.

Some Protein Pharmaceuticals in Development

The "early" period of biotechnology (1970s and 1980s) was defined by the development of proteins of known sequence and function. Recombinant insulin, tissue plasminogen activator, factor VIII, granulocyte colony-stimulating factor (G-CSF), and interferons all derive from this style of biotechnology drug development, and the trend continues as many new native proteins with therapeutic value are discovered. Protein products in clinical trials as of 1996 include at least nine categories of proteins and over 200 molecules (Pharmaceutical Research and Manufacturers of America, 1996).

Colony-Stimulating Factors, Interferons and Interleukins

A list of some biotechnology-derived colony-stimulating factors, interferons, and interleukins in various stages of clinical trials (Pharmaceutical Research and Manufacturers of America, 1996) can be found in Table 18.3a,b. Some examples are described below.

COLONY-STIMULATING FACTORS

Many times, clinical trials examine currently approved protein products for additional therapeutic indications. Examples include the use of filgrastim (recombinant granulocyte colony stimulating factor, rG-CSF) in infectious disease and sargramostim (granulocyte macrophage-colony stimulating factor, GM-CSF) for the prophylaxis and treatment of chemotherapy-induced neutropenia, and the prevention of infection in very low birth weight infants.

Interleukins (ILs)		
Product	Company	Indication
Recombinant human interleukin-3 (rhIL-3)	Sandoz Pharmaceuticals	acceleration of engraftment of platelets following bone marrow transplantation or peripheral blood stem cell transplantation in patients receiving myeloablative chemotherapy
Recombinant human interleukin-4	Schering-Plough	non-small-cell lung cancer
Recombinant human interleukin-6 (rhIL-6)	Sandoz Pharmaceuticals	acceleration of engraftment of platelets following myelo-suppressive chemotherapy for various cancers
Interleukin-6 mutein	Imclone Systems	thrombocytopenia secondary to chemotherapy
Recombinant human interleukin-11	Genetics Institute	platelet enhancement
Recombinant human interleukin-12 (rhIL-12)	Genetics Institute and Wyeth-Ayerst Laboratories	HIV infection, cancer
Liposomal IL-2	Biomira USA	renal cell carcinoma
IL-3 fusion GM-CSF	Immunex	hematopoietic reconstituition after myeoablative chemotherapy
IL-2 fusion protein, DAB389 IL-2	Seragen	cutaneous T-cell lymphoma
		psoriasis
		HIV infection, lymphomas, severe rheumatoid arthritis, recent onset type 1 diabetes

Table 18.3b. Some biotechnology-derived protein products in various stages of clinical trials: ILs (Source: Pharmaceutical Research and Manufacturers of America, 1996).

INTERFERONS

Interferons in each sub class (α, β, or γ) are available, and clinical research primarily focuses on new indications with only a few new products, principally of second generation nature, e.g. consensus α interferon.

INTERLEUKINS

Interleukins, as intercellular communication proteins, continue to be targets for drug development. As described earlier in this text, they bind to receptors on the surface of target cells and stimulate cellular activity including proliferation and cytotoxicity. Many different cells display interleukin receptors, including monocytes, megakaryocytes, neutrophils, myeloma cells, and blast cells. Because of their proliferative effect on hematopoietic stem cells, several ILs currently are in clinical trials for treatment of thrombocytopenia or acceleration of platelet engraftment following bone marrow transplantation or peripheral blood progenitor cell transplantation. These include IL-3, IL-6, and IL-11 (cf. Chapter 9.1). With the discovery of thrombopoietin in 1994, however, further development of these less specific molecules for a platelet indication may not be warranted. Several ILs are also under development for cancer indications and for the treatment of HIV infection, e.g. IL-4, IL-10 and IL-12.

LIPOSOMAL IL-2

Liposomal IL-2 is an example of attempts to improve drug delivery of proteins (see Chapter 4 and Table 18.3 of this section). While Proleukin (aldesleukin, IL-2) is already used for the treatment of renal cell carcinoma, satisfactory drug

Enzymes (Clotting factors, Dismutases, Tissue Plasminogen Activators, and Others)		
Product	Company	Indication
Recombinant factor VIIa	Novo Nordisk Pharmaceuticals	treatment of hemophilia A & B with and without antibodies against factors VII/IX
Recombinant human factor IX (rhFIX)	Genetics Institute	hemophilia B
Recombinant factor VII	Pharmacia & Upjohn	hemophilia
Superoxide dismutase	Bio-Technology I Genera	oxygen toxicity in premature infants
nPA	Bristol-Myers Squibb	acute myocardial infarction
Second-generation t-PA	Genentech	heart attacks and related cardiovascular disorders
Carboxypeptidase G-2	National Cancer Institute	methotrexate overdose following intrathecal administration
PEG - glucocerebrosidase	Enzon	Gaucher's disease
Platelet activating factor - acetylhydrolase	ICOS	adult respiratory distress syndrome (ARDS)
		pancreatitis
		asthma
DNase (dornase alpha)	Genentech	lupus nephritis
Urate oxidase (recombinantly-produced enzyme)	Sanofi	prophylaxis for chemotherapy-related hyperuricemia treatment of cancer-related hyperuricemia

Table 18.4. Some biotechnology-derived protein products in various stages of clinical trials: Enzymes (1. Source: Pharmaceutical Research and Manufacturers of America, 1996).

delivery of this protein product is lacking. Now liposomal IL-2 is used to improve therapeutic efficacy in renal cell carcinoma, and also to enhance IL-2 induced adjuvant effects in antitumor vaccines.

FUSION MOLECULES

Using ligation chemistry, researchers have created biologically active molecules that combine the activities of two individual proteins into fusion molecules. Fusion molecules contain portions or the entire amino acid sequences of both parent proteins. One such molecule is Pixykine (interleukin-3 fused with GM-CSF; both hematopoietic growth factors), designed for hematopoietic reconstitution after myeloablative chemotherapy (cf. Chapter 8). Pixykine increases neutrophil and platelet production. Fusion technologies hold promise for developing "custom" molecules expressing a variety of

activities. Another example of a fusion product in clinical trials is IL-2 fusion protein, DAB389 IL-2 being examined for the treatment of cutaneous T-cell lymphoma (Ajinomoto, Seragen, 1994). DAB389 IL-2 (also called IL-2 fusion toxin) is a recombinant protein consisting of the first 389 amino acids of diphtheria toxin "fused" to amino acid residues 2-133 of human IL-2 (the IL-2 residues replace the amino acids of the receptor binding domain of the native diphtheria toxin).

Enzymes

A selection of biotechnology-derived enzymes in clinical development (Pharmaceutical Research and Manufacturers of America, 1996) including clotting factors, dismutases, tissue plasminogen activators and others can be found in Table 18.4. Two examples are described to illustrate the importance of this group.

CLOTTING FACTORS

Blood coagulation, the conversion of fluid blood to a solid gel or clot, requires a complex enzymatic cascade. The ultimate event is the conversion of soluble fibrinogen to insoluble strands of fibrin. The cascade factors are present as inactive precursors of proteolytic enzymes and other enzyme cofactors. The cascade factors themselves require proteolytic activation. Activation of the cascade results in a continually increasing production of the next factor in the clotting sequence. Hemophilia A and B are sex-linked genetic disorders characterized by dysfunction of the blood-clotting mechanism (Sanchez *et al.*, 1993). Hemophilia A is a life-long bleeding disorder resulting from a deficiency of factor VIII (Antihemophiliac factor, AHF). The rarer form of hemophilia, hemophilia B (Christmas disease), results from a deficit of factor IX (Christmas factor). Conventional biotherapy for the treatment of hemophilia has included providing the patient with fresh blood, plasma, or protein concentrate preparations from human plasma collected by transfusion services or commercial organizations. Therefore, these treatments may possibly contain other native human proteins and microorganisms, such as viruses (HIV, hepatitis, etc.), derived from infected blood. Biotechnology provided a major advance in the therapy of hemophilia A when two versions of recombinant factor VIII were approved. Several additional products are in clinical trials including factors VII, VIIa and IX.

SUPEROXIDE DISMUTASE

Superoxide dismutase (SOD) is a ubiquitous copper- and zinc-containing enzyme which destroys oxygen free radicals (see mechanistic scheme below). A familial variant of amyotrophic lateral sclerosis (ALS, Lou Gehrig's disease) has been linked to deficits in human cytosolic SOD (Rosen *et al.*, 1993). Recombinant SOD is in clinical trials for the treatment of oxygen toxicity in premature infants and has the potential to be useful in patients with myocardial infarction, organ transplantation and stroke.

$$O_2\cdot^- + O_2\cdot^- + 2H^+ \text{-----} SOD \text{-----}> O_2 + H_2O_2$$

Hormones, Erythropoietins, and Growth Factors

A list of some biotechnology-derived hormones, erythropoietins, and growth factors in various stages of clinical trials (Pharmaceutical Research and Manufacturers of America, 1996) can be found in Table 18.5a,b. Some examples are described below.

THROMBOPOIETIN

Recombinant human thrombopoietin, a hematopoietic growth factor recently cloned and expressed, is a cytokine

Hormones		
Product	Company	Indication
Human corticotropin-releasing hormone (hCRH)	Neurobiological Technologies	rheumatoid arthritis, brain tumor edema, post-surgical edema
Recombinant human lutinizing hormone	Serono Laboratories	follicular support stimulation of follicular development
Recombinant human parathyroid hormone (rhPTH)	Allelix Biopharmaceuticals	post-menopausal osteoporosis
Recombinant human thyroid stimulating hormone	Genzyme	adjunct in procedures used for detection and treatment of recurrent thyroid cancer
Erythropoietins		
Product	Company	Indication
Epoetin alfa	Ortho Biotech	prevention of anemia associated with surgical blood loss, autologous blood donation adjuvant

Table 18.5a. Some biotechnology-derived protein products in various stages of clinical trials: Hormones and Erythropoietins (Source: Pharmaceutical Research and Manufacturers of America, 1996).

Growth Factors		
Product	Company	Indication
Transforming growth factor-beta	Genzyme	chronic skin ulcers
		multiple sclerosis
Glial-derived neurotrophic factor (GDNF)	Amgen	treatment of Parkinsonism
FIBLAST trafermin	Scios	stroke
Insulin-like growth factor (IGF-1)	Genentech	diabetes
Myotrophin, rhIGF-1	Cephalon	ALS
		peripheral neuropathies
Nerve growth factor	Genentech	peripheral neuropathies
Neurotrophin-3	Amgen-Regeneron Partners	peripheral neuropathies
Recombinant human platelet-derived growth factor-BB (PDGF)	Chiron and R.W. Johnson Pharmaceutical Research Institute	wound healing
Stem cell factor	Amgen	adjunct to chemotherapy

Table 18.5b. Some biotechnology-derived protein products in various stages of clinical trials: Growth Factors (Source: Pharmaceutical Research and Manufacturers of America, 1996).

that selectively stimulates megakaryocyte synthesis and maturation, thus increasing platelet count (Lok *et al.*, 1994; Kaushansky *et al.*, 1994). Administered alone, or in combination with G-CSF, GM-CSF and/or erythropoietin, thrombopoietin is being examined clinically for the treatment of thrombocytopenia related to cancer treatment.

Hematopoietic Pathway to Platelets

---

pluripotent stem cells -----> CFU-GEMM* ----->
CFU-Meg** -----> Megakaryocyte -----> platelets
* CFU = colony-forming unit; GEMM = granulocyte, erythrocyte, monocyte, and megakaryocyte
** Meg = megakaryocyte

NEUROTROPHIC FACTORS

Growth factors (GFs) are cytokines responsible for regulating the production, maturation and function of cells in specific tissues and organs. Each cell type's response will be specific for each particular growth factor and will differ from growth factor to growth factor. Families of GFs and their receptors include many of the CSFs ILs, erythropoietins, and other cytokines already mentioned (See Chapters 8 and 9). Additional classes of GFs are neurotrophic factors and various tissue specific growth factors. Several rDNA-produced growth factors are now undergoing clinical trials.

Neurotrophic factors (NFs or nerve growth factors) have emerged in the 1990s into a significant class of molecules to treat various serious neurologic diseases, such as amyotrophic lateral sclerosis (ALS) and Parkinson's disease; the molecules include brain-derived neurotrophic factor (BDNF), ciliary neurotrophic factor, glial-derived neurotrophic factor (GDNF), nerve growth factor, and neurotrophin-3. Neurotrophic factors exert the ability to regenerate damaged or partially severed nerve cells. With the identification of these nerve growth factors, a long-sought means of repairing neurological trauma appears to be within reach (Hotzman and Mobley, 1994). The dream of repairing nerve damage became a reality in 1991 with a report in the *New England Journal of Medicine* describing the effects of the lipid

"GM-1 ganglioside" (Geisler *et al.*, 1991). This material is present in high concentrations in the outer portion of nerve sheath cells, and it stimulates production of nerve growth factor, which in turn both protects and restores nerve function and growth. The search for protein growth factors that can produce the same effects continues.

Glial-derived neurotrophic factor (GDNF), tiny amounts of which affect survival and differentiation of sensory and motor neurons, is in Phase I trials for treating parkinsonism. A primate animal model of drug-induced parkinsonism showed significant activity in revolving muscle rigidity and other signs of motor disease. Some other neurotrophic

Vaccines		
Product	Company	Indication
Acellular pertussis vaccine	The Biocine Company Chiron	pediatric pertussis (whooping cough)
CMV vaccine	The Biocine Company Chiron	cytomegalovirus
Neutralizing G-17 hormone	Aphton	colorectal cancer
		stomach cancer
		pancreatic cancer
		GERD
		peptic ulcers
		NSAID ulcers
gp 120 vaccine	GenenVax	AIDS
Herpes simplex vaccine (recombinant)	SmithKline Beecham	prevention of herpes simplex infection
		treatment of herpes simplex infection
Herpes vaccine	The Biocine Company Chiron	herpes simplex 2
		genital herpes
HIV vaccine (gp120)	The Biocine Company Chiron	AIDS
Lyme disease vaccine (recombinant)	SmithKline Beecham	prevention of Lyme disease
Recombinant BCG	MedImmune	Lyme disease
Melanoma theraccine	Ribi ImmunoChem	stage IV melanoma with interferon alfa
		stage II melanoma in patients with no evidence of disease to prevent recurrence following surgery to remove primary disease
Neutralizing hCG hormone vaccine	Aphton	female contraception
rCEA Vaccine, recombinant carcinoembryonic antigen	MicroGeneSys	colon and breast cancer

Table 18.6a. Some biotechnology-derived protein products in various stages of clinical trials: Vaccines (Source: Pharmaceutical Research and Manufacturers of America, 1996).

Vaccines (continued)		
Product	Company	Indication
Recombinant canarypox-CEA (human) vaccine	National Cancer Institute	advanced cancers expressing CEA
Recombinant vaccine-CEA (70kD)vaccine	National Cancer Institute	adenocarcinoma of the colon and rectum
RSV subunit vaccine	Wyeth-Ayerst Laboratories	respiratory syncytial virus-mediated lower respiratory disease for at-risk children and elderly
HIV-1 (gp 160)	MicroGeneSys	AIDS

Table 18.6b. Some biotechnology-derived protein products in various stages of clinical trials: Vaccines (Source: Pharmaceutical Research and Manufacturers of America, 1996).

factors in trials include neurotrophin-3 and nerve growth factor (NGF) for peripheral neuropathies.

OTHER GROWTH FACTORS

A non-neurotrophic cytokine with a nerve specific effect is insulin-like growth factor-1 (IGF-1, Myotrophin). First viewed as a candidate for growth disorders and diabetes, it was then discovered that nerve cells also have receptors for this cytokine. Myotrophin exhibited highly positive results in a Phase III clinical study involving 266 ALS patients (Piascik, 1996). A second Phase III study in Europe in 183 patients for ALS, and a Phase II study for other indications including peripheral neuropathies caused by chemotherapy, diabetes and polio are ongoing. Since it causes new nerves to sprout and strengthens interactions between muscle and nerve connections, IGF-1 could possibly be used to repair neurologic damage caused by these conditions.

Tissue growth factors are being discovered and tested for tissue repair. Growth factors regulating bone development have also been identified. They belong to the tissue growth factor β (TGF-β) superfamily of growth-regulating cytokines. They guide bone stem cells through their various differentiation pathways and very specifically regulate skeletal development. Bone growth factor research is of great interest to develop a bone-mending putty for repairing severe fractures, in treating osteoporosis and connective tissue damage, and for dental reconstruction. Other growth factors such as β Kine (transforming growth factor β) and platelet-derived growth factor (PDGF) are in clinical trials to promote healing of wounds and skin ulcers.

Epidermal growth factor and fibroblast growth factor are other tissue growth factors with potential therapeutic use. Epidermal growth factor (EGF) stimulates epidermal cell proliferation. Fibroblast growth factor (FGF) is a member of a family of heparin-binding growth factors. Indications for EGF and FGF being explored include tissue repair in corneal and cataract surgeries, angiogenesis (new capillary formation), and improvement in wound healing including burns and tendon repair.

Another exciting growth factor being studied by the pharmaceutical industry is stem cell factor (SCF; also known as c-kit ligand and steel factor). A protein on the surface of bone marrow stromal cells, SCF stimulates early pluripotent and committed stem cells, acts synergistically with various other cytokines, increases B cell formation and stimulates mast cells and melanocytes (Huang *et al.*, 1990). SCF is being studied as an adjunct to cancer chemotherapy to facilitate hematopoiesis.

Vaccines

Some biotechnology-derived vaccines in clinical development (Pharmaceutical Research and Manufacturers of America, 1996) are listed in Table 18.6. Thanks to molecular techniques, vaccines are undergoing a renaissance (see Chapter 12 and references contained therein). Live attenuated vaccines made non-pathogenic by a gene deletion may elicit a greater immune response. With the availability of entire bacterial genomic sequences such as that of Haemophilus influenzae, this method is likely to be improved by engineering out (or in) specific genes to create non-pathogenic live vaccines. Genetic engineering also makes it possible to express combinations of elements that would never occur in natural selection. Recombinant methods have given us new types of vaccines including the subunit vaccine or DNA vaccines that deliver a code to the host to produce subunits endogenously, such as "naked DNA".

An antihormone vaccine is under development directed against gastrin, a peptide hormone that regulates digestion and is present at elevated levels in cancers of the gut, stomach, pancreas, and other organs. This vaccine may also be useful in gastroesophageal reflux disease (GERD), peptic ulcers and ulcers induced by non-steroidal antiinflammatory drugs (NSAIDs). Another target is gonadotropin-releasing hormone, which regulates testosterone and estrogen levels, and is involved in prostate, breast, and endometrial cancers.

Vaccines for herpes simplex infection, HIV disease (AIDS), and cytomegalovirus disease (CMV) are now in clinical trials. An acellular (i.e., subunit) vaccine for diphtheria-pertussis tetanus successfully completed a large trial. Other vaccines in late-stage trials are for the prevention of Lyme disease, and Melacine, a therapeutic vaccine based on interferon α to treat stage IV melanoma. Another trial of Melacine for stage II melanoma with no evidence of disseminated disease, to prevent recurrence after surgery to remove primary disease is also in late clinical trials.

A new class of vaccine, the fusion vaccine is an extenuation of the idea of mobilizing the immune system against undesirable entities. One example of the fusion vaccine is a contraceptive vaccine that is directed against chorionic gonadotropin, a hormone essential to implantation of the embryo. Chorionic gonadotropin is normally not recognized as a foreign protein, for obvious reasons. A strong antigenic response to the vaccine is elicited by attaching the β chain of the hormone to a bacterial toxoid. The effects of the vaccine are said to be reversible, and the vaccine lacks the burdensome side effects of steroid contraceptives. Eighty percent of the women in early clinical trials produced large amounts of antibody in response to it. The vaccine holds great promise for population control especially in developing countries (Aldous, 1994). The fusion vaccine concept has considerable potential and may be extended to many new indications.

Recombinant Soluble Receptors

Receptors are macromolecules (generally, but not always proteins) which specifically recognize a binding ligand. Receptor-ligand binding initiates a specific biological response directly or causes an intracellular signal transduction resulting in the observed biological effect. Natural protein receptors may be soluble, circulating proteins (such as enzymes and released cell surface proteins), cell surface proteins, proteins found embedded in and spanning a cellular membrane (transmembrane receptors), or entirely intracellular proteins. Many small molecular drugs act at specific receptors. With the advent of DNA cloning and other recombinant DNA techniques, it is possible to produce receptor proteins found on the surface of cells and portions of transmembrane proteins in soluble forms. A recombinant soluble receptor may be the entire cellular receptor amino acid sequence, or a portion of the sequence, i.e., the rDNA-produced extracellular portion of a transmembrane receptor lacking the membrane spanning and intracellular amino acids. A selection of recombinant soluble receptors in clinical develoment (Pharmaceutical Research and Manufacturers of America, 1996) can be found in Table 18.7. Examples of soluble receptor molecules in clinical develop-

Recombinant Soluble Receptors		
Product	Company	Indication
Interleukin-1 receptor (dry powder inhalant)	Immunex and Inhale Therapeutic Systems	asthma
Interleukin-4 receptor	Immunex	asthma
TNF-receptor fusion protein	Hoffmann-La Roche	septic shock, severe sepsis
		rheumatoid arthritis, multiple sclerosis
Soluble complement receptor CR1	T Cell Sciences	adult respiratory distress syndrome (ARDS)
		reperfusion injury following first-time myocardial infarction
Tumor necrosis factor (TNF) receptor	Immunex Wyeth-Ayerst Laboratories	rheumatoid arthritis

Table 18.7. Some recombinant soluble receptors in clinical development (Source: Pharmaceutical Research and Manufacturers of America, 1996).

Monoclonal Antibodies	
Indication	**Indication (continued)**
Acute kidney rejection, graft v. host disease	Inflammatory bowel disease
Acute myeloid leukemia	Leukemia and metastatic melanoma
All EGFR positive malignancies	Multiple sclerosis
All Her2/neu positive malignancies	Neuroblastoma (pediatric)
Allergic diseases, including allergic rhinitis and asthma	Non-Hodgkin's B-cell lymphoma
Asthma	Pancreatic cancer
Atherosclerotic plague imaging agent	Poison ivy, poison oak
Blood clot imaging agent	Prevention of respiratory syncytial virus (RSV) disease
Breast cancer	Prevention of secondary cataract
Cardiac imaging agent	Reduction of restinosis (vascular remodeling) following balloon angioplasty
CMV infections in AIDS patients	Refractory unstable angina
Colorectal cancer	Relapsed AML
Diagnosis of osteomyelitis, infected prosthesis, appendicitis	Renal prophylaxis
Epidermal growth factor receptor positive cancers	Rheumatoid arthritis
Extent of disease staging of breast cancer	Sepsis syndrome
Extent of disease staging of liver and germ cell cancers	Stroke
Extent of disease staging of lung cancer	Targeted radiotherapy for prostrate malignancies
Gram-negative sepsis	T-cell lymphoma
Hemorrhagic shock	Thermal injury
HIV-infection, AIDS	Thromolytic complications of PTCA

Table 18.8. Indications of some therapeutic and diagnostic monoclonal antibodies in development (Source: Pharmaceutical Research and Manufacturers of America, 1996).

ment include tumor necrosis factor receptor, IL-1 receptor, IL-4 receptor, and a human complement cascade receptor. The therapeutic aim of these receptor molecules is to bind to their normal ligands, preventing the ligands from binding to the cellular receptors, thus interrupting the expected specific biological response or signal transduction event.

Monoclonal Antibodies

Indications for some of the therapeutic and diagnostic MAbs that are in development (Pharmaceutical Research and Manufacturers of America, 1996) are listed in Table 18.8. A brief discussion of some areas of current development follows.

THERAPEUTIC MONOCLONAL ANTIBODIES

Therapeutic MAbs as potential products from drug development helped propel the early biotechnology industry, but thus far diagnostic MAbs have proved to be more useful. Some of biotechnology's biggest disappointments have been therapeutic MAb products, such as several high-profile products for septic shock that failed to show efficacy in large-scale trials in 1994: Centoxin®, E-5, T-88, and Bradycor®. A MAb that received FDA marketing approval in 1995 was ReoPro®, a human/murine chimeric antibody aimed at blocking the aggregation of platelets and fibrin in angioplasty patients, in order to prevent cardiovascular complications (see Chapter 13, appendix B).

Technological advances (see Chapter 13) are addressing some of the challenges encountered in developing MAbs and have increased their therapeutic potential (Burton and Barbas, 1994; Owens and Young, 1994). For example, earlier versions of MAbs had "human"-variable (i.e., molecular-recognition) sites but also partially mouse-constant regions, which could lead to possible immune recognition. This murine structure limited them to one time-only therapeutic uses and rendered repeated uses, as in chronic disease states, inappropriate. "Humanized" mice now can be created by transferring the complete segment of the human heavy-chain antibody gene into mouse blastocysts generating completely human MAbs for treating rheumatoid arthritis, transplant rejection, chronic inflammation, and other conditions. Also, MAbs conjugated to toxins or radioisotopes are being developed as therapeutic agents (see Chapter 4).

DIAGNOSTIC MONOCLONAL ANTIBODIES

Diagnostic MAbs are in wide use in the familiar enzyme-linked immunosorbent assay (ELISA) for detecting food contaminants and environmental toxins. In human medicine, they are most typically utilized in the form of conjugates composed of a recognition site that is specific to a tumor antigen or another pathological marker and an imaging moiety like technetium Tc99m or gadolinium that emits a detectable signal when excited by an appropriate impulse during magnetic resonance imaging or other scanning procedures.

Some Nucleic Acid Therapies in Development

Early development of nucleic acid therapy concentrated on the use of gene therapy aimed at genetic deficiency diseases amenable to gene replacement (see Chapter 7). Recently, interest in the use of antisense oligonucleotides (see Chapter 6) which suppress or block selected protein expression by interacting with genes or mRNA has expanded rapidly (Crooke, 1992). The potential use of oligonucleotides in therapy now goes well beyond their ability to interact with nucleic acid receptors (genes or mRNA). Oligonucleotides targeted toward non-nucleic acid receptors such as proteins (i.e., aptamer technology) are also under intense investigation. There is little doubt that the intense investigations of nucleic acid therapy will provide interesting therapeutics for clinical development. Some recent progress in the development of nucleic acid therapies is described.

Gene Therapy

Chapter 7 provides a good overview of the development of gene therapies. By mid-1995, 112 gene therapy trials were open or pending in the US; 87 trials attempt various therapeutic approaches to treating cancer and infectious and genetic diseases. The remaining 25 trials insert a marker gene only in order to test the efficacy of the transfer process (NIH, 1995). The triple major challenge in gene therapy is: 1) identification and reproduction of the required gene,

Gene Therapy Trials
Indication
Asymptomatic HIV-1-infection
Brain cancer
Breast cancer
Chemoprotection of hematopoietic stem cells from toxicity of chemotherapy
Colon cancer
Cystic fibrosis, sinusitis
Disseminated malignant melanoma
Gaucher's disease
HIV infection
Metastatic renal cell carcinoma
Neuroblastoma
Non-small cell lung cancer

Table 18.9. Gene therapy trials (Source: Pharmaceutical Research and Manufacturers of America, 1996).

(2) creation of a vector for carrying the gene into human cells that offers high cell delivery, high expression and persistence, and (3) clinical testing of this gene-vector product for safety and efficacy (Mulligan, 1993; Goldspiel *et al.*, 1993). Table 18.9 provides a list of indications for the gene therapy protocols currently approved (Pharmaceutical Research and Manufacturers of America, 1996).

Antisense Oligonucleotides

Antisense technology is highly sequence-specific, and thus is expected to have few side effects. Also, antisense molecules have the additional advantages of morphologic simplicity and of being easy to synthesize (Nagel *et al.*, 1993). As discussed in Chapter 6, native antisense molecules are subject to rapid degradation by endogenous RNAses, but the half-lives and binding affinity of antisense constructs can be increased by chemically modifying their phosphodiester backbones by substituting moieties such as methylphosphonate or methylphosphorothionate. Thus, future developments will address these issues. While early in clinical trials, antisense molecules are being examined for their use in HIV infection, CMV retinitis in AIDS patients, various cancers and inflammatory diseases (Pharmaceutical Research and Manufacturers of America, 1996).

Development of Adhesion Molecules, Glycoproteins, Carbohydrate-Based Pharmaceuticals and Other Products of Glycobiology

Glycobiology

As described in Chapter 6, glycobiology is an emerging field that has opened up a whole new realm of possibilities for drug development. Carbohydrate recognition and adhesion by molecules, viruses, and cells to cells are mediated by transmembrane proteins called selectins (E-selectin and P-selectin are expressed on endothelium and platelets; L-selectin is expressed on some leukocytes) and other cell surface carbohydrate-binding proteins. The structure of the oligosaccharides present on glycoproteins, glycolipids and these component's presentation on cell surfaces may dramatically alter cell biological function. Because of the immense number of combinations possible in rearranging a small number of carbohydrate subunits, complex specificities are possible. Highly specific drug/target interactions at the cell surface involving carbohydrates of adhe-

sion molecules are thus attractive points for intervention (Cheresh, 1994).

Fibronectin and Fibronectin Receptor Antagonists

Fibronectin is a type of adhesion glycoprotein. It is a component of the extracellular matrix, the fibrous scaffolding that surrounds the exteriors of cells (Nichols *et al.*, 1994). It holds the cells in their proper positions, and also helps them to move from place to place during normal transport and turnover processes such as wound healing. Fibronectin binds integrins, and in a wound cavity provides a temporary scaffolding whereby fibroblasts can more easily commute to the wound site. Other fibronectin receptors (integrins) are located on platelets, which produce fibrinogen, which in turn clogs the area, slows down the migration of fibroblasts, and retards wound healing.

By preventing or reducing the action of platelets, wound healing can be promoted. Non-healing wounds plague persons with diabetes, bedridden patients, and others with circulatory problems. Conversely, blocking the binding of fibronectin to integrins could slow down the clotting process in heart attacks or could retard the build-up of excess scar tissue in the corneal disease known as dry eye (Sjögren's syndrome) or in the glomerular membrane of the kidney, another threat to persons with diabetes. Among the drugs in clinical trials aimed at carbohydrate moieties is Integrelin, for arterial thrombosis. Integrelin prevents platelet binding to the fibronectin receptor, GPIIb-IIIa (also called α_{IIb}/β_3 or CD41/CD61) (Nichols *et al.*, 1994). The fibronectin receptor is a member of the integrin family of adhesion molecules. Integrelin is in Phase III trials for coronary angioplasty and in Phase II trials for acute myocardial infarction and unstable angina.

Concluding Remarks

Pharmaceutical biotechnology and its various related techniques will continue to expand its influence in all areas of the drug discovery process. The development of novel pharmacological screening methods to identify new pharmaceuticals, the production of biopharmaceuticals being tested for the first time against several diseases, and the creation of innovative technologies for optimizing drug development will play a defining role in the genesis of pharmaceuticals that will serve as the foundation of modern pharmaceutical care. With the number of biotechnology-derived products in clinical development increasing each year, the prospects for continued innovation of our therapeutic arsenal look bright. ■

Further Reading

- **Biotechnology Update Column.** In *Journal of the American Pharmaceutical Association*, edited by P Piascik. The column appears each month and frequently contains information about biotech products in development.
- **Pharmaceutical Research and Manufacturers of America.** *Biotechnology Medicines in Development.* Washington, DC. This publication appears approximately once each year.

References

- **Ajinomoto S.** (1994). DAB$_{389}$IL-2. *Ann Drug Data Report*, 16, 313–314
- **Aldous P.** (1994). A booster for contraceptive vaccines. *Science*, 266, 1484
- **Bienz-Tadmor B.** (1993). Biopharmaceuticals go to market; patterns of worldwide development. *Bio/Technology*, 11, 168–172
- **Burton DR, Barbas CF.** (1994). Human monoclonal antibodies: recent achievements. *Hosp Prac*, 15, 111–122
- **Cheresh DA.** (1994). The biological function of b3 integrins and other vitronectin receptors. In *Cellular Adhesion Molecular Definition to Therapeutic Potential*, edited by BW Metcalf, BJ Dalton, G Poste. New York, New York: Plenum Press, pp. 213–237
- **Crooke ST.** (1992). Therapeutic applications of oligonucleotides. *Annu Rev Biochem*, 32, 329–376
- **Ecker DJ, Crooke ST.** (1995). Combinatorial drug discovery: which methods will produce the greatest value? *Bio/Technology*, 13, 351–360
- **Evens RP, Dinarello GA, Browne J, Fenton D.** (1995a). Biotechnology and clinical medicine, Part 1. *Hospital Physician*, 31, (11), 27–36
- **Evens RP, Dinarello GA, Browne J, Fenton D.** (1995b). Biotechnology and clinical medicine, Part 2. *Hospital Physician*, 31 (12), 26–31
- **Geisler FH, Dorsey FC, Coleman WP.** (1991). Recovery of motor function after spinal-cord injury – a randomized, placebo-controlled trial with GM-1 ganglioside. *N Engl J Med*, 324, 1829–1838
- **Goldspiel BR, Breen L, Calis KA.** (1993). Human gene therapy. *Clin Pharm*, 12, 488–505
- **Hotzman DM, Mobley WC.** (1994). Neurotrophic factors and neurologic disease. *West J Med*, 161, 246–254
- **Huang E, Nocka K, Beier DR, Chu TY, Buck J, Lahm HW, Wellner D, Leder P, Besmer P.** (1990). The hematopoietic growth factor K1 is encoded at the S1 locus and it is the ligand of the c-kit receptor, gene product of the W locus. *Cell*, 63, 225–233
- **Kaushansky K, Lok S, Holly RD, Broudy VC, Lin N, Bailey MC, Forstrom JW, Buddle MM, Dort PJ, Hagen FS, Roth GJ, Papayannopoulou T, Foster DC.** (1994). Promotion of megakaryocyte progenitor expansion and differentiation by the c-Mpl ligand thrombopoietin. *Nature*, 369, 568–571

- **Lee Jr KB, Burrill GS.** (1995). Biotech 96: The Industry Annual Report. Ernst and Young LLP
- **Lok S, Kaushansky K, Holly RD, Kuijpen JL, Lofton-Day CE, Oort PJ, Grant FJ, Heipel MD, Burkhead SK, Kramer JM, Ching AFT, Mathewes SL, Bailey MC, Forstrom JW, Buddle MM, Osborn SG, Evans SJ, Sheppard PO, Presnell SR, O'Hara PJ, Hagen FS, Roth GJ, Foster DC.** (1994). Cloning and expression of murine thrombopoietin cDNA and stimulation of platelet production *in vivo*. *Nature*, 369, 565–568
- **Mulligan RC.** (1993). The basic science of gene therapy. *Science*, 260, 926–932
- **Nagel KM, Holstad SG, Isenberg KE.** (1993). Oligonucleotide pharmacotherapy: An antisense strategy. *Pharmacotherapy*, 13, 177–188
- **New York Times.** (1995). September
- **Nichols AJ, Vasko JA, Koster PF, Valocik RE, Samanen JM.** (1994). GPIIb/IIIa Antagonists as Novel Antithrombic Drugs. In *Cellular Adhesion Molecular Definition to Therapeutic Potential*, edited by BW Metcalf, BJ Dalton, G Poste. New York, New York: Plenum Press, pp. 213–237
- **NIH.** (1995). Communication, Office of Recombinant DNA Activities (ORDA), August
- **Owens RJ, Young RJ.** (1994). The genetic engineering of monoclonal antibodies. *J Immunol Methods*, 168, 149–165
- **Pharmaceutical Research and Manufacturers of America.** (1996). *Biotechnology Medicines in Development.* Washington, DC
- **Piascik P.** (1996). New hope for treatment of Lou Gehrig's disease. *Amer Pharm*, NS36 (6), 355–356
- **Rosen DR, Siddique T, Patterson D, Figlewicz DA, Sapp P, Hentati A, Donaldson D, Groto J, O'Regan JP, Deng HX, Zohra R, Krizus A, McKenna-Yasik D, Cayabyab A, Gaston SM, Berger R, Tanzi RE, Haperin JJ, Hertzfeld B, Van den Bergh R, Hung WY, Bird T, Deng G, Mulder DW, Smyth C, Laing NG, Soriano E, Pericak-Vance MA, Haines J, Rouleau GA, Gusella JF, Horvitz HR, Brown RH.** (1993). Mutations in Cu/Zn superoxide dismutase gene are associated with familial amyotrophic lateral sclerosis. *Nature*, 362, 59–62. [Published erratum appears (1993). *Nature*, 364, 362.]
- **Sanchez J, Rodvold KA, Friedenberg WR.** (1993). Coagulation Disorders. In *Pharmacotherapy: A Pathophysiologic Approach, Second Edition*, edited by JT DiPiro, RL Talbert, PE Hayes, GC Yee, GR Matzke, LM Posey. East Norwalk, Connecticut: Appleton & Lange, pp. 1443–1461

- In *Cellular Adhesion Molecular Definition to Therapeutic Potential*, edited by BW Metcalf, BJ Dalton, G Poste. New York, New York: Plenum Press, pp. 213–237
- **Sharpiro B, Merck and Co.** (1995). The impact of biotechnology on drug discovery. *9th International Congress of Immunology*. San Francisco, California
- **Struck MM.** (1994). Biopharmaceutical R&D success rates and development times. *Bio/Technology*, 12, 674–677

Self-Assessment Questions

Question 1: What are some of the contributions of pharmaceutical biotechnology to modern pharmaceutical care?

Question 2: Briefly describe the time and costs of developing a pharmaceutical product.

Question 3: Briefly describe the process of combinatorial chemistry.

Question 4: The types of molecules being discovered and studied through biotechnology have broadened over the past decade. What are these types?

Question 5: Which recombinant interleukin (IL) products are under development for the treatment of cancer and HIV infection?

Question 6: What are recombinant fusion molecules?

Question 7: Briefly explain the importance of superoxide dismutase.

Question 8: What are neurotrophic factors (NFs)? Give some examples of recombinant NFs in development?

Question 9: What are some of the indications for new recombinant vaccines?

Question 10: What are recombinant soluble receptors?

Question 11: What are some of the indications for new monoclonal antibodies?

Question 12: What are nucleic acid therapies?

Question 13: What may be the therapeutic role of blocking the binding of fibronectin to integrins?

Answers

Answer 1: A greater understanding of the cause and progression of diseases, the development of novel pharmacological screening methods to identify new pharmaceuticals, the production of biopharmaceuticals being tested for the first time against several diseases, the creation of innovative technologies for optimizing drug development and, improvements in the methods used to manufacture protein and peptide-based biopharmaceuticals.

Answer 2: Figure 18.1 gives an overview of these issues.

Answer 3: Figure 18.2 provides a schematic overview of the process. Combinatorial chemistry is a mix-and-match process in which a simple subunit is joined to one or more other simple subunits in every possible combination. Assigning the task to automated synthesizing equipment results in the rapid creation of large collections or "libraries" of diverse molecules, which can be quickly pharmacologically screened to identify the most active compound for a given therapeutic target.

Answer 4: Table 18.2 provides a list.

Answer 5: Several ILs are also under development for cancer indications and for the treatment of HIV infection, e.g. IL-4, IL-10 and IL-12.

Answer 6: Using ligation chemistry, fusion molecules combine the activities of individual proteins by containing portions or the entire amino acid sequences of both parent proteins.

Answer 7: Superoxide dismutase (SOD) is a ubiquitous copper- and zinc-containing enzyme which destroys oxygen free radicals. A familial variant of amyotrophic lateral sclerosis (ALS, Lou Gehrig's disease) has been linked to deficits in human cytosolic SOD. Recombinant SOD is in clinical trials for the treatment of oxygen toxicity in premature infants and has the potential to be useful in patients with myocardial infarction, organ transplantation and stroke.

Answer 8: NFs are cytokines responsible for regulating the production, maturation and function of nerve cells. Neurotrophic factors have emerged into a significant class of molecules to treat various serious neurological diseases, such as amyotrophic lateral sclerosis (ALS) and Parkinson's disease; the molecules include brain-derived neurotrophic factor (BDNF), ciliary neurotrophic factor, glial-derived neurotrophic factor, nerve growth factor, and neurotrophin-3.

Answer 9: Table 18.6 provides a list.

Answer 10: A recombinant soluble receptor may be the entire cellular receptor amino acid sequence, or a portion of the sequence, i.e., the rDNA-produced extracellular portion of a transmembrane receptor lacking the membrane spanning and intracellular amino acids. A selection of recombinant soluble receptors in clinical development can be found in Table 18.7.

Answer 11: Table 18.8 provides a list.

Answer 12: Gene therapy (Chapter 7) and therapy with antisense oligonucleotides (Chapter 6).

Answer 13: Slow down the clotting process in heart attacks, retard the buildup of excess scar tissue in the corneal disease known as dry eye (Sjögren's syndrome) or in the glomerular membrane of the kidney, another threat to persons with diabetes.

Index